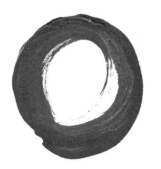

Nurse Coaching
Integrative Approaches for Health and Wellbeing

BARBARA MONTGOMERY DOSSEY

SUSAN LUCK

BONNEY GULINO SCHAUB

D1604515

International Nurse Coach Association
North Miami, Florida
www.inursecoach.com

Library of Congress Cataloging-in-Publication data
Nurse Coaching: Integrative Approaches for Health and Wellbeing/
Barbara Dossey ... [et al.].

Includes bibliographical references and index.

ISBN: 13-978-0615943299   ISBN: 10-0615943292

I. Dossey, Barbara Montgomery II. International Nurse Coach Association (INCA).

1. Nurse Coaching. 2. Theory of Integrative Nurse Coaching. 3. Nurse Coach Role.
4. Integrative Nurse Coach Certificate Program (INCCP).

The International Nurse Coach Association (INCA) is an international nursing organization that recognizes and supports Nurse Coaches, local to global, and that is bringing coaching skills and competencies into all healthcare settings. *Nurse Coaching: Integrative Approaches for Health and Wellbeing* reflects the knowledge of Nurse Coaches on various topics and issues and should be reviewed in conjunction with state boards of nursing policies and practices. *Nurse Coaching: Integrative Approaches for Health and Wellbeing* guides registered nurses in the application of their professional skills and responsibilities.

Published by the International Nurse Coach Association
640 N.E. 124th Street
North Miami, FL 33161
1.888.494.4469
www.inursecoach.com

For information on the Integrative Nurse Coach Certificate Program go to
www.inursecoach.com/programs/

To order: CreateSpace (www.createspace.com/4432832) or
Amazon (www.amazon.com/dp/0615943292)

Copyright © 2015 by the International Nurse Coach Association. All rights reserved. No part of this book may be reproduced or used in any form or any means, electronic, or mechanical, including photocopying and recording, or by any information storage and retrieval system, without permission in writing from the publisher.

ISBN: 13-978-0615943299   ISBN: 10-0615943292
First printing: October 2014

The Flame of Florence Nightingale's Legacy

Today, our world needs healing and to be rekindled with Love.
Once, Florence Nightingale lit her beacon of lamplight
     to comfort the wounded
And her Light has blazed a path of service across a Century to us,
Through her example and through the countless Nurses and Healers
     who have followed in her footsteps.

Today, we celebrate the flame of Florence Nightingale's Legacy.
Let that same Light be rekindled to burn brightly in our hearts.
Let us take up our own Lanterns of Caring, each in our own ways.
To more brightly walk our own paths of service to the World.
To more clearly share our own Noble Purpose with each other.

May Human Caring become the Lantern for the 21st Century.
May we better learn to care for ourselves,
     for each other and for all Creation.
Through our Caring, may we be the Keepers of that Flame.
That Our Spirits may burn brightly
To kindle the hearts of our children and great-grandchildren
As they too follow in these footsteps.

Copyright © 1996 by Deva-Marie Beck, PhD, RN
International Co-Director, Nightingale Initiative for Global Health
Neepawa, Manitoba, Canada, and Washington, DC
www.nightingaledeclaration.net

To Our Colleagues in Nursing

In honor of Florence Nightingale's (1820–1910) legacy and the 21st-century Nightingales—the 19.6 million nurses and midwives worldwide—who advocate for health as a basic human right. Their endeavors are raising consciousness about healthy people living in a healthy world—local to global.

Cover Design

The enso titled "Miracle in Each Moment" by the renowned Japanese calligraphic painter Kazuaki Tanahashi* is a single unbroken brushstroke that expresses the moment when the mind is unhindered and free to be creative.

The enso represents an emergent process of wholeness, bringing together aspects of one's body–mind–spirit–culture–environment at deep levels of inner knowing and healing, each aspect having equal importance and value, leading toward integration and balance.

The Nurse Coach engages in reflective practice that guides inner development and an immersion in the pool of universal truth. Reflective practice permits entry into the flow and dance of wholeness and unity. The Nurse Coach strives always to be in the present moment while coaching the client/patient and others, and in all nurse coaching endeavors.

*Source. Used with permission. Copyright © 2008. Kazuaki Tanahashi. www.brushmind.net

Contents

10

11

12

13

Case Studies: Awareness and Choice 257
Bonney Gulino Schaub

CORE VALUE 3   *Nurse Coach Communication, Coaching Environment*   **281**

14

Integral Perspectives and Change 283
Barbara Montgomery Dossey

CORE VALUE 4   *Nurse Coach Education, Research, Leadership*   **349**

19

20

Contents

Foreword

The growing emphasis on health promotion is essential in an age of healthcare reform. We are spending over $2.7 *trillion* a year on healthcare, without getting the outcomes we need. Why? Because our healthcare system has been built around acute care rather than primary care, health promotion, and wellness. We cannot afford the system we have. While most people know the Affordable Care Act as the law that is reducing the ranks of the uninsured by extending private health insurance and Medicaid to a significant portion of those living in the United States, it also includes steps to reform care delivery through approaches such as transitional care, primary care, and wellness programs.

But the healthcare system itself is only one part of the solution to helping people live healthier lives. We must have clinicians who know how to help their patients develop a plan for healthy living and to support them in making the step-by-step journey to health. Doing so also requires a framework of health and health promotion that embraces the integration of body, mind, and spirit. Indeed, there is a growing body of literature that documents a connection between happiness and health and the use of meditation and energy work to "heal" and "tune up," as well as other integrative approaches to health promotion. While the nursing community often claims to be the profession that can provide such health promotion services, we too often fail to teach integrative approaches in schools of nursing and in healthcare organizations. This must change.

As an educator, I realize that nursing education's emphasis on patient teaching is essential but not sufficient for promoting the health of people. In fact, I continue to be struck by the number of graduate students in my courses who want to teach patients out of their "non-adherence" to treatment regimens or unhealthy lifestyles. When I ask how many of the students in my class are living a healthy life, few hands emerge amidst the chuckles of embarrassment over their own challenges to change—even in the face of knowing what they ought to do.

Patient teaching is important, and I want nurses who are skilled in helping patients to understand the nuances of health and illness. But they must also understand how to promote health and to better manage their chronic illnesses.

Nurse Coaching: Integrative Approaches for Health and Wellbeing is a timely, essential resource for an age of health promotion. It provides the framework for an integrative view of health and the tools and resources for coaching. Every school of nursing should require this book at the undergraduate and graduate levels. Practicing nurses can use the book to develop their knowledge and skill in helping the patient with diabetes or congestive heart failure or obesity to no longer be controlled by their illnesses, but rather be able to live full and vibrant lives.

It is time to recognize that changing health behaviors is difficult and requires a long-term commitment and coaching. Because of our orientation to relationship-centered care, nurses are ideal coaches. I commend the authors of this important book for helping nurses to fulfill this essential role.

Diana J. Mason, PhD, RN, FAAN
Rudin Professor of Nursing
Co-Director, Center for Health, Media & Policy at Hunter College
Professor, Graduate Center, City University of New York
President, American Academy of Nursing

Preface

Nurse Coaching: Integrative Approaches for Health and Wellbeing is the *first* comprehensive textbook for nurse coaching practice, education, research, and healthcare policy. As pioneers on the vast frontier of healthcare—local to global—Nurse Coaches are inspired leaders practicing at the forefront of an integrative healthcare paradigm that understands the interconnected, multidimensional aspects that influence health and wellbeing throughout the life cycle.

The hope and intention of this innovative nurse coaching approach for transforming healthcare is to share this information with nurses and other interprofessional colleagues and concerned citizens around the world (International Nurse Coach Association, n.d.). This will lead to healthy people living in a healthy nation and on a healthy planet by 2020 (Nightingale Initiative for Global Health, n.d.).

The nurse coaching movement recognizes and addresses the resiliency and capacity of individuals and communities to adapt healthier lifestyles with the support, guidance, expertise, and advocacy of Nurse Coaches. As change agents, their mission is to improve the health of the nation and the world, addressing the wellness and "health span" of all people.

Nurse Coaches are focused on "upstream factors," the social and environmental determinants of health. The *social determinants of health* include the family composition, friends, religion, race, gender, socioeconomic status, education, occupation, or profession. The social, economic, and political forces and conditions under which people live determine their state of health, or disease or illness. The *environmental determinants of health* are those external agents (biological, chemical, physical, social, or cultural factors) that can be linked to a change in health status (food, water, air pollution, secondhand smoke, and home and workplace environment).

The roots of nurse coaching began with the legacy of Florence Nightingale (1820–1910), and her words continue to inspire us today; thus, Nightingale quotes appear at the beginning of each book chapter. In the 1880s, Nightingale began to write that it would take 100–150 years before educated and experienced nurses would arrive to change the healthcare system. Nurse Coaches are the generation of 21st-century Nightingales who have arrived to transform healthcare and carry forth her vision of social action and sacred activism to create a healthy world. She is a model for us in accomplishing our own work in today's world (Dossey, 2010).

Nurse Coaches have recognized the importance of the emerging role in this major shift from disease care to disease prevention, and to improved health and enhanced wellbeing (Dossey & Keegan, 2013). In 2010, the Institute of Medicine *Future of Nursing* report (IOM, 2010) published an action-oriented blueprint for the future of nursing with four key messages:

- Nurses should practice to the full extent of their education and training.
- Nurses should achieve higher levels of education and training through an improved education system that promotes seamless academic progression.
- Nurses should be full partners, with physicians and other healthcare professionals, in redesigning healthcare in the United States.
- Effective workforce planning and policy-making require better data collection and information infrastructure.

Two Nurse Coach initiatives towards implementing the IOM recommendations occurred from 2008 through 2012. The *first* endeavor included the efforts of the Professional Nurse Coach Work Group (PNCW) composed of six Nurse Coaches—Darlene Hess,

Barbara Dossey, Mary Elaine Southard, Susan Luck, Bonney Gulino Schaub, and Linda Bark. They worked in collaboration with an Advisory Committee and Review Committee through a peer-reviewed process to establish professional Nurse Coach definitions, scope of practice, and competencies. In 2013, the American Nurses Association (ANA) and 20 other professional nursing organizations endorsed their work that was published by the ANA, *The Art and Science of Nurse Coaching: A Provider's Guide to Coaching Scope and Competencies* (Hess et al., 2013). This document clearly established the Nurse Coach role.

The *second* endeavor began as the PNCW members entered into a conversation with the American Holistic Nurse Credentialing Corporation (AHNCC, n.d.), regarding the paradigm shift toward health and wellness inherent in the Affordable Care Act (The Patient Protection and Affordable Care Act [PPACA] [2010]), and *Healthy People 2020* (U.S. Department of Health and Human Services, n.d.), and the importance of developing a role and certification program for the Professional Nurse Coach. Given that the American Holistic Nurses Association (AHNA, 2012) had achieved holistic nurse specialization in the practice of health and wellness, it was mutually determined that AHNCC was the appropriate venue for a national certification program for Nurse Coaches.

The AHNCC and the Professional Testing Corporation of New York (PTC) collaborated to develop a set of competencies, extrapolated from the literature and in accordance with ANA's *Nursing: Scope and Standards of Practice*, 2nd edition (ANA, 2010). The competencies, reviewed by three expert panels, were revised until approved, and then used for a Role-Delineation Study (RDS). The results from the RDS were used to develop a blueprint and guide the development of the Nurse Coach Certification Examination that began in January 2013. The PNCW collaborated with the AHNCC Board in the early stages of this certification process. Those nurses who successfully completed the AHNCC Nurse Coach examination and who were already holistic nursing-board certified received the designation of Health and Wellness Nurse Coach-Board Certified (HWNC-BC). Those who were not holistic nursing-board-certified received the Nurse Coach-Board Certified (NC-BC).

This textbook is organized by the recognized Nurse Coach five core values that are as follows (Hess et al., 2013):

Core Value 1: Nurse Coach Philosophy, Theories, Ethics
Core Value 2: Nurse Coaching Process
Core Value 3: Nurse Coach Communication, Coaching Environment
Core Value 4: Nurse Coach Education, Research, Leadership
Core Value 5: Nurse Coach Self-Development

Core Value 1 presents the philosophical concepts of nurse coaching and how a deeper understanding of inner knowledge and wisdom and the transpersonal human caring process and healing are essential in nurse coaching. In this section, the roots of nurse coaching are provided, which includes extant nurse coaching review of the literature. Using the integrative nurse coaching lens, the Theory of Integrative Nurse Coaching (TINC), a middle-range nursing theory, is presented and has three intentions as follows: (1) demonstrate the unique Integrative Nurse Coach role and competencies for health and wellbeing; (2) explore the direct application of integrative nurse coaching in all healthcare and community settings, and in interprofessional collaboration; and (3) expand Integrative Nurse Coaches' capacities as 21st-century Nightingales and health diplomats who are coaching for health and wellness—local to global. Nurse coaching and ethics covers an ethics review, relational knowing and embodied knowing, meaning of respect, authentic advocacy, and Earth ethics.

Core Value 2 presents the peer-reviewed nurse coaching competencies, nursing process, and the identified nurse coaching process. This is a *shift* in terminology and meaning to understand and incorporate the client's subjective experience. This section includes story theory, story-health model, positive psychology, and how to develop strengths to support and deepen the Nurse Coach and client therapeutic relationship. The Integrative Health and Wellness Assessment™ (IHWA), a designated tool for the TINC, identifies specific areas that Nurse Coaches assess in working with clients, families, and communities towards healthy behaviors and change. Nutritional health and environmental health, awareness and choice, and awareness practices are addressed as these are major nurse coaching interventions used in coaching towards changing lifestyle behaviors with new actions and how to sustain health and change. This section also presents client/patient stories and coaching sessions that include the clinical setting, client narrative, triggers, antecedents, mediators, and Nurse Coach narratives. These case studies reveal the art and science of nurse coaching and journeying with the client who sources from personal wisdom to discover the answers for improved health. Many examples are given about how to coach and not teach, and to release being the expert who tries to "fix" the client. Nurse Coach and client dialogues show how to conduct a coaching session and to continue with follow-up sessions and Nurse Coach notes.

Core Value 3 provides strategies to enhance Nurse Coach communication and the coaching environment. Topics covered are integral perspectives, change and two perspectives towards achieving goals, motivational interviewing and nonviolent communication, appreciative inquiry, and cultural perspectives and rituals of healing.

Core Value 4 examines nurse coaching and education and offers examples of Nurse Coach course descriptions, objectives, topics, and activities/assignments for a 3 semester credit hour (SCH) graduate course, a 3 SCH undergraduate course, and a 1 SCH undergraduate course. A one-day INCA Introductory Nurse Coach workshop and a one-day workshop for self-care are also presented. The nurse coaching and research section guides the Nurse Coach in how to engage in research at various levels. The Nurse Coach leadership exploration shows steps towards being a change agent for true integrative healthcare and transformational organizational changes.

Core Value 5 presentation is a unique approach to Nurse Coach self-development in four areas—self-reflection, self-assessment, self-evaluation, and self-care. Nurse Coach self-development is foundational for being an authentic Nurse Coach.

The textbook provides a rich *Nurse Coach Resources and Toolkit* section that includes Nurse Coach and client guiding principles and contract, specifics on coaching sessions, Integrative Health and Wellness Assessment (short and long forms), personal health history, and integral perspectives. The integrative lifestyle health and wellbeing resources include Nurse Coach intake, symptoms checklist, food, exercise, environment, personalized lifestyle plan, and awareness practices, including breath awareness, meaning, purpose, inner wisdom, and imagery rehearsal.

Nurse Coaches recognize that our time demands a new paradigm and a new language to once again give attention to the heart of nursing, for "sacred" and "heart" reflect a common meaning, which is generating the vision, courage, and hope for profound healing and to address the challenges in these troubled times—local to global. This is not a matter of philosophy, but of survival.

Barbara Montgomery Dossey
Susan Luck
Bonney Gulino Schaub

INTEGRATIVE NURSE COACH CERTIFICATE PROGRAM (INCCP)

For information on the INCCP see http://www.inursecoach.co/programs/

REFERENCES

American Holistic Nurses Association and American Nurses Association (AHNA/ANA) (2013). *Holistic nursing: Scope and standards of practice* (2nd ed.). Silver Spring, MD: Author.

American Holistic Nurses Credentialing Corporation (AHNCC). *AHNCC nurse coach certification*. Retrieved from http://www.ahncc.org/certification/nursecoachnchwnc .html

American Nurses Association (ANA) (2010). *Nursing: Scope and standards of nursing practice* (2nd ed.). Silver Spring, MD: Nursesbooks.org.

Dossey, B. M. (2010). *Florence Nightingale: Mystic, visionary, healer* (Commemorative ed.) Philadelphia: F. A. Davis.

Dossey, B. M., & Keegan, L. (2013). *Holistic nursing: A handbook for practice* (6th ed.). Burlington, MA: Jones & Bartlett Learning.

Hess, D. R., Dossey, B. M., Southard, M. E., Luck, S., Schaub, B. G., & Bark, L. (2013). *The art and science of nurse coaching: The provider's guide to coaching scope and competencies*. Silver Spring, MD: Nursesbooks.org.

Institute of Medicine (IOM) (2010). The *future of nursing: Leading change, advancing health*. Washington, DC: National Academies Press. Retrieved from http://www.iom.edu/Reports/2010/The-Future-of-Nursing-Leading-Change-Advancing-Health.aspx

International Nurse Coach Association (n.d.). Retrieved from www.inursecoach.com

Nightingale Initiative for a Healthy World (n.d.). Retrieved from http://www.nightingaledeclaration.net/the-declaration

The Patient Protection and Affordable Care Act (PPACA) (2010). Retrieved from http://democrats.senate.gov/pdfs/reform/patient-protection-affordable-care-act-as-passed.pdf

U.S. Department of Health and Human Services, Office of Disease Prevention and Health Promotion (n.d.). *Introducing healthy people 2020*. Retrieved from http://www.healthypeople.gov/2020/about/default.aspx

Lead Authors and Contributors

LEAD AUTHORS

Barbara M. Dossey, PhD, RN, AHN-BC, FAAN, HWNC-BC
Co-Director, International Nurse Coach Association
Core Faculty, Integrative Nurse Coach Certificate Program
North Miami, Florida
International Co-Director, Nightingale Initiative for Global Health Washington, DC, and
    Neepewa, Manitoba, Canada
Director, Holistic Nursing Consultants, Santa Fe, New Mexico

Susan Luck, MA, RN, HNB-BC, CCN, HWNC-BC
Co-Director, International Nurse Coach Association
Core Faculty, Integrative Nurse Coach Certificate Program
North Miami, Florida
Founder, EarthRose Institute
Director, Integrative Nursing Institute
Miami, Florida

Bonney Gulino Schaub, MS, RN, PMHCNS-BC, NC-BC
Co-Director and Core Faculty, Huntington Meditation and Imagery Center
Huntington, New York
Co-Director, New York Psychosynthesis Institute
Huntington, New York
Faculty, Italian Society for Psychosynthesis Psychotherapy
Florence, Italy

CONTRIBUTORS

Deva-Marie Beck, PhD, RN
International Co-Director, Nightingale Initiative for Global Health
Neepawa, Manitoba, Canada, and Washington, DC

Lisa A. Davis, PhD, MPH, RN, NC-BC
Professor, Department of Nursing
Associate Department Head for Graduate Studies, Research, and Grants, West Texas
    A&M University
Certified Holistic Stress Management Instructor
Canyon, Texas

Christine Gilchrist, MSN, MPH, RN, NC-BC
Associate Faculty, International Nurse Coach Association
Clinical Nurse Specialist, Department of Integrative Medicine, Mount Sinai Beth Israel
Associate Director, Student Health and Counseling Services, School of Visual Arts
Adjunct Lecturer, Hunter-Bellevue School of Nursing, City University of New York
New York, New York

Diana J. Mason, PhD, RN, FAAN
Rudin Professor of Nursing
Co-Director, Center for Health, Media & Policy at Hunter College
Professor, Graduate Center, City University of New York
New York, New York
President, American Academy of Nursing

Deborah McElligott, DNP, AHN-BC, ANP-BC, HWNC-BC, CDE
Associate Faculty, International Nurse Coach Association
Assistant Professor, Hofstra-North Shore LIJ School of Medicine
Hempstead, New York
Nurse Practitioner, Women's Heart Health Program, The Katz Institute for Women's
    Health, NSLIJ Health System
Bayshore, New York

Heidi Taylor, PhD, RN, NC-BC
Professor
Department of Nursing, West Texas A&M University
Canyon, Texas

Acknowledgments

A collaborative process inspired this book. We thank all of our many students who have joined us on the Nurse Coach journey and have completed our Integrative Nurse Coach Certificate Program (INCCP). Together, we continue to develop the Nurse Coach role and integrate nurse coaching into many diverse settings in healthcare, communities, corporations, and other areas. We thank our International Nurse Coach Association (INCA) Affiliates who joined us in our Advanced Integrative Nurse Coach Program (AINCP). Many are now serving as Associate Faculty teaching with us across the United States and globally.

We honor our Nurse Coach colleagues, Darlene Hess, Mary Elaine Southard, and Linda Bark, who collaborated with us to bring the Nurse Coach role and competencies to the forefront in the nursing profession. We are grateful to the American Holistic Nurses Credentialing Corporation (AHNCC), and Margaret Erickson, Helen Erickson, Mary Brekke, Kay Sandor, and AHNCC Board Members (past and present) for establishing the Nurse Coach Certification process.

We thank the many clients that we have worked with over the years. We have taken every effort to respectfully protect their confidentiality in the sharing of the Nurse Coach and client caring process and coaching sessions.

Special thanks are due to Jocelyn Rudert, for her attention to editorial details and keeping our writing clear; to Cheryl Allen-Bush, for her book design and layout; and to Keith Groesbeck for his graphic designs.

Most of all, for their understanding, encouragement, and love in seeing us through this book—Barbara to Larry Dossey; Susan to Robert Daigler; and Bonney to Richard Schaub—who share our interconnectedness.

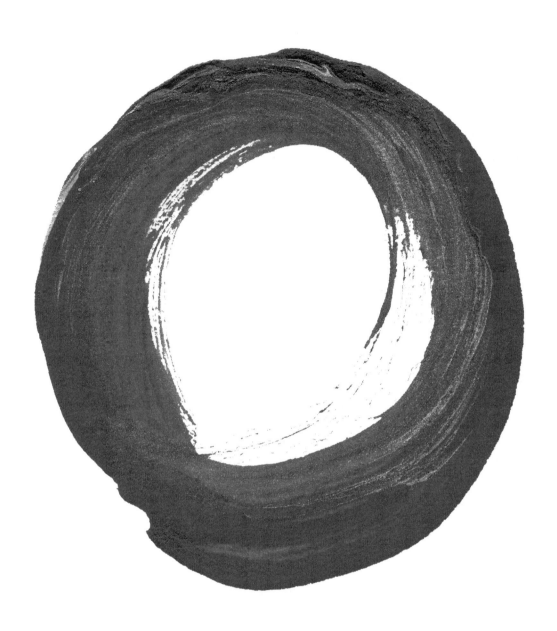

CORE VALUE 1

*Nurse Coach Philosophy,
Theories, Ethics*

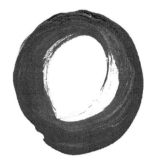

CHAPTER 1

Nurse Coaching

Barbara Montgomery Dossey

In the future, which I shall not see, for I am old, may a better way be opened! May the methods by which every infant, every human being will have the best chance at health — the methods by which every sick person will have the best chance at recovery, be learned and practiced. Hospitals are only an intermediate stage of civilization, never intended, at all events, to take in the whole sick population.

Florence Nightingale, 1893

LOOKING AHEAD...

After reading this chapter, you will be able to:

*   Define Professional Nurse Coach and Professional Nurse Coaching.
*   Explore the concept of collaboratory in nurse coaching.
*   Explore the history of the health and wellness coaching and nurse coaching movements.
*   Examine national and global strategies for healthcare transformation.

DEFINITIONS

Note: The terms "client" and "patient" are interchangeable throughout this book.

Collaboratory: Composite of "collaboration" (collaborate) and "laboratory" (place where experiments take place). In nurse coaching, a Nurse Coach and the client enter into a co-creative process in the most important laboratory of all—an individual's life.

Global health: Worldwide focus on the health of all people with a priority of achieving equity, reducing disparities, and protecting against global threats that disregard national borders—local to global; it is a global commons, a bridge across boundaries, and a path to world peace (NIGH, n.d.)

Health: Process through which individuals reshape basic assumptions and worldviews, which includes aspects of physical, mental, emotional, social, spiritual, cultural, and environmental wellbeing, and not merely the absence of disease; may include living with a disease, illness, or symptoms. It includes death...as a natural process of living.

Professional Nurse Coach: A registered nurse who integrates coaching competencies into any setting or specialty area of practice to facilitate a process of change or development that assists individuals or groups to realize their potential.

Professional nurse coaching: A skilled, purposeful, results-oriented, and structured relationship-centered interaction with clients provided by registered nurses for the purpose of promoting achievement of client goals.

Wellbeing: A general term for the condition of an individual or group and their social, economic, psychological, spiritual, or medical state; based on the idea that the way each person thinks and feels about his or her life is meaningful and important.

PROFESSIONAL NURSE COACH AND PROFESSIONAL NURSE COACHING

The professional Nurse Coach is a registered nurse who integrates coaching competencies into any setting or specialty area of practice to facilitate a process of change or development that assists individuals or groups to realize their potential (Hess et al., 2013). The change process is grounded in an awareness that effective change evolves from within before it can be manifested and maintained externally. The professional Nurse Coach works with the whole person using principles and modalities that integrate the bio-psycho-social-spiritual-cultural-environmental dimensions towards human flourishing.

Professional nurse coaching is a skilled, purposeful, results-oriented, and structured relationship-centered interaction with clients provided by registered nurses for the purpose of promoting achievement of client goals. The Nurse Coach establishes a co-creative partnership with the client where the client is the expert and identifies priorities and areas for change. Goals originate from clarifying and identifying the client's agenda.

Nurse Coaches are 21st-century Nightingales and are advocates for health as a basic human right (Beck, Dossey, & Rushton, 2014; Dossey, Beck, & Rushton, 2011). As part of the 3.1 million nurses in the United States (American Association of Colleges of Nursing [AACN], 2011; American Nurses Association [ANA], 2010a) and the 19.6 million nurses and midwives worldwide (World Health Organization, 2009), their endeavors are uniting nurses in healing and raising consciousness about a healthy world. An example is the Nightingale Declaration for a Healthy World (NIGH, n.d.) as seen in **Figure 1-1**. In the next section the concept of collaboratory is explored as an analogy for our individual and collective Nurse Coach endeavors, which includes technology.

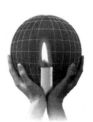

Nightingale Declaration for A Healthy World

"We, the nurses and concerned citizens of the global community, hereby dedicate ourselves to achieve a healthy world by 2020.

We declare our willingness to unite in a program of action, to share information and solutions and to improve health conditions for all humanity—locally, nationally and globally.

We further resolve to adopt personal practices and to implement public policies in our communities and nations—making this goal achievable and inevitable by the year 2020, beginning today in our own lives, in the life of our nations and in the world at large."

www.NightingaleDeclaration.net

Figure 1-1 Nightingale Declaration for a Healthy World by 2020.
Source: Used with permission. Nightingale Initiative for Global Health (n.d.).
www.nightingaledeclaration.net

COLLABORATORY

The term "collaboratory" is a neologism, or a newly coined word, that captures the essence of nurse coaching. Collaboratory is a composite of "collaboration" and "laboratory." Collaborate comes from Latin words meaning "to work together." Laboratory is derived from the Latin word for "labor," and its modern meaning is an area where experiments take place. Wulf (1989) coined collaboratory as a "center without walls" where researchers perform their research without regard to physical location, interacting with colleagues, accessing instrumentation, sharing data and computational resources, [and] accessing information in digital libraries (Wulf, 1989). Bly (1998, p. 31) refined the definition to "a system that combines the interests of the scientific community at large with those of the computer science and engineering community to create integrated, tool-oriented computing and communication systems to support scientific collaboration."

We can expand this definition to include the nurse coaching process. The collaboratory consists of the Nurse Coach and the client, who agree to an experiment of sorts that takes place in the most important laboratory of all—an individual's life. In a true experiment, one is never certain of the outcome; one puts the pieces in place and patiently awaits the results. So it is in nurse coaching. The outcome of a coaching encounter can never be known for certain; it is unpredictable in essence. Both the Nurse Coach and client do their best to structure a favorable result, which cannot be forced, but must be left to unfold and enfold. This process recognizes the source of all sustained energy and action and includes sourcing from personal awareness and wisdom that results in transformation (Sharma, 2006).

Effective nurse coaching interactions involve the ability to develop a coaching partnership, to create a safe space, and to be sensitive to client issues of trust and vulnerability as a basis for further exploration, self-discovery, and action-planning related to desired goals and outcomes. It builds on the client's strengths rather than attempting to "fix" weaknesses. Nurse coaching engages the co-creative process with clients, families, communities, and colleagues in either individual or group sessions or in interprofessional collaboration. The purpose of this co-creating partnering process allows for reflection and addressing challenges, where a heightened degree of awareness and choice, imagination, creativity, and healthy lifestyle behaviors emerge. This process has the potential to enhance health and wellbeing and stop illness, injuries, and the chronic disease epidemic.

Nurse Coaches have many opportunities to work with clients, families, colleagues, and communities, and to enter into various collaboratories through practice, education, research, and healthcare policy—local to global. The current technology—Internet, Skype, iPads, smartphones, face-to-face Internet meetings, e-mail, social media, messaging, apps for all kinds of record keeping and tracking new health behaviors such as food diaries, exercise, and more—expands the Nurse Coach role. As we become comfortable with the new technology and understand how technology can be enhancing our nurse coaching endeavors we also are able to share our nursing endeavors and stories with the media and others (Wilson, 2013). In the next section health and wellbeing are discussed.

HEALTH AND WELLBEING

What is health, and what is wellbeing? Health is how the individual defines her or his state and experiences related to a sense of growth, harmony, and unity. Health is that process through which individuals reshape basic assumptions and worldviews, which includes aspects of physical, mental, emotional, social, spiritual, cultural, and environmental wellbeing, and not merely the absence of disease; it also includes death as a natural part of living. It is that process in which the individual's (nurse, client, family, group, or community) subjective experiences about health, health beliefs, and values are honored. It is a process of opening and deepening personal awareness and expanding our consciousness (Newman, 1994).

Wellbeing is a general term for the condition of an individual or group and their social, economic, psychological, spiritual, or medical state. Wellbeing is based on the idea that how each person thinks and feels about his or her life is meaningful and important.

Nurse Coaches support and empower others to find common ground and engage in the cooperative consensus process to build healthy communities, remembering that the environment is everything that surrounds the person, both the external and the internal (physical, mental, emotional, spiritual, and cultural) environment as well as patterns not yet understood (Dossey, B. M., 2013). They are part of the co-creative partnering process and energy field with clients and other concerned individuals about how to become more aware and make healthy choices towards health and wellbeing—at the individual, community, and global levels. Nurse Coaches also demonstrate *authentic advocacy*, which is described as the actions taken on behalf of others that arise from a deep alignment of one's beliefs, values, and behaviors (term coined by Rushton, in press).

Nurse Coaches and clients examine the internal and external factors that contribute to health and wellbeing. These include the environmental and social determinants of health (Beck et al., 2014). The environmental determinants of health are those external agents (biological, chemical, physical, social, or cultural factors) that can be linked to a change in health status (food, water, air pollution, secondhand smoke, home and workplace environment) (see Chapter 9 for details). The social determinants of health include the family composition, friends, religion, race, gender, socioeconomic status, education, occupation, or profession. The social, economic, and political forces and conditions under which people live determine their state of health, or disease or illness. We are all called into the collaboratory of life, "the one mind", so that we can consider how our individual efforts are part of a greater consciousness and discover why it matters (Dossey, L., 2013). In the next section the evolution of health coaching and nurse coaching is explored.

EVOLUTION OF THE FIELD OF HEALTH COACHING AND PROFESSIONAL NURSE COACHING

Health and Wellness Coaching

Prior to the 1980s, the term "coach" was used to refer to a role in the field of human performance, specifically in the field of athletics. Coaches training athletes for the Olympic Games began introducing relaxation, imagery rehearsal, and somatic awareness practices to enhance athletic performance. Winners of the Olympic Games popularized these practices.

During the 1960s, with the beginning of the human potential movement, coaching moved outside of sports and into organizational settings. An increased demand for greater productivity and enhanced employee performance led to programs and coaching designed to promote employee self-development. Additionally, there was a desire to be able to measure and document the effectiveness of these initiatives in meaningful ways. New challenges emerged with the increase in technology, globalization, and multicultural teams located in different countries. Professional and executive coaching became an important factor in business. Formal coaching programs were still in their infancy.

By the 1990s, formal coaching programs, courses, and certifications emerged outside of the nursing profession. For the last 20 years, many professional disciplines have explored health and wellness coaching.

In 2010 the National Consortium for the Credentialing of Health and Wellness Coaches (NCCHWC) convened to develop consensus around health and wellness coaching (NCCHWC, 2011; Wolever & Eisenberg, 2011). Over 80 individuals and organizations representing coaching, healthcare, and wellness discussed the development of credentialing and professional standards for health and wellness coaching, and the need to integrate coaching skills across the healthcare professions. In the next section the roots of professional nurse coaching and an overview of nurse coaching are explored.

Roots of Professional Nurse Coaching

Florence Nightingale (1820–1910)—the foundational philosopher of modern nursing—established nursing practice that could be measured by evaluating outcomes. Nightingale was the first recognized nurse theorist—a clinical educator, scientist, statistician, environmentalist, policy maker, social activist, facilitator, communicator, and visionary. Her contributions to nursing theory, research, statistics, public health, healthcare reform, and nurse coaching are foundational and inspirational (Beck, 2013; Dossey et al., 2011).

Nightingale established the imperative of evidence-based practice, a nursing standard now widely known to be as important as she had known them to be. She advocated, identified, and focused on factors that promote health and are recognized today as environmental and social determinants of health previously discussed. These are the same factors that Nurse Coaches promote to achieve optimal health and wellbeing (Dossey, B. M., 2013; Dossey, 2010; Dossey et al., 2005; Nightingale, 1859, 1860, 1893). Nightingale emphasized the necessity for nursing to be a profession, and that nurses must be educated, and not "trained."

In the 1950s, nursing theorists Hildegard Peplau and Dorothea Orem introduced several concepts and practices that are now seen as important elements of nurse coaching. Peplau (1952) described the nurse's role as recognizing and mobilizing the person's innate capacity for self-healing and growth. Orem (1971) first wrote of her self-care model of nursing in 1953. Her work emerged from a philosophy of health as a state of wholeness. Patricia Benner (1985), the prominent nurse leader, theorist, and author of the nursing textbook *From Novice to Expert* (Benner, 1984) used the term "Nurse Coach" over 25 years ago to describe the client and nurse partnership and a conceptual framework based on social support theory. See Chapter 2 for the Theory of Integrative Nurse Coaching and other nursing theories used in nurse coaching.

The United States healthcare system is undergoing a transformation from a disease-focused healthcare system to one focused on wellness, health promotion, and disease prevention. Nursing, recognizing the importance of its emerging role, is claiming its rightful position in this major shift from disease care to disease prevention, and improved health and enhanced wellbeing. Nurses constitute the largest group of healthcare providers and are uniquely situated for the Nurse Coach role. They have been taking the lead by engaging clients in self-care and management of healthcare practices and client-centered outcomes. In 2010 the Institute of Medicine (IOM, 2010) published an action-oriented blueprint for the future of nursing with four key messages as follows:

- Nurses should practice to the full extent of their education and training.
- Nurses should achieve higher levels of education and training through an improved education system that promotes seamless academic progression.

- Nurses should be full partners, with physicians and other healthcare professionals, in redesigning healthcare in the United States.
- Effective workforce planning and policy-making require better data collection and information infrastructure.

One endeavor towards implementing the IOM recommendations occurred from 2008 through 2012 with a group of six nurse coaches—Darlene Hess, Barbara Dossey, Mary Elaine Southard, Susan Luck, Bonney Gulino Schaub, and Linda Bark. They worked with an Advisory Committee and Review Committee through a peer-reviewed process to establish professional Nurse Coach definitions, scope of practice, and competencies. In 2013 the American Nurses Association (ANA) and 21 other professional nursing organizations endorsed their work published by the ANA, *The Art and Science of Nurse Coaching: A Provider's Guide to Coaching Scope and Competencies* (Hess et al., 2013). In the next section an overview of the professional Nurse Coach role is discussed.

Professional Nurse Coaching Scope of Practice

Nurse Coaches are addressing the bio–psycho–social–spiritual–cultural–environmental dimensions of health. They are aware of integrating the new paradigm of medicine and health while releasing the old paradigm as seen in **Table 1-1**. They recognize the masculine and feminine archetypes in healing as seen in **Table 1-2**.

Nurse coaching interactions are based on research findings related to Nurse Coach theories (see Chapter 2), Transtheoretical Model of Behavioral Change (Prochaska, Norcross, & DiClemente, 1995), Appreciative Inquiry (Cooperrider & Whitney, 2005), Motivational Interviewing (Miller & Rollnick, 2002), and Positive Psychology (Csikszentmihalyi, 1990; Seligman, 1990).

Effective nurse coaching interactions involve the ability to develop a coaching partnership, to create a safe space, and to be sensitive to client issues of trust and vulnerability as a basis for further exploration. The Nurse Coach must be able to structure a coaching session, explore client readiness for coaching, facilitate achievement of the client's desired goals, and co-create a means of determining and evaluating desired outcomes and goals.

Nurse Coaches use mindfulness, presence, deep listening, and skillful questioning as the foundation of the coaching relationship. They listen for the client's innate inner potential and wisdom. They use referrals to other professionals as part of the coaching action plan when needed. They also receive ongoing training and supervision in enhancing nurse coaching competencies. See International Nurse Coach Association (INCA, n.d.).

Table 1-1 Old and New Paradigms of Medicine and Health: Assumptions.

Old Paradigm	New Paradigm
Treatment of symptoms	Search for patterns and causes
Specialized	Integrated and interconnected; concerned with whole person
Emphasis on efficiency	Emphasis on human values
Professional should be emotionally neutral	Caring and compassion are part of healing process
Pain and disease are negative	Pain and dis-ease are information about disharmony

(continues on next page)

Table 1-1 (*Continued*)

Old Paradigm	New Paradigm
Primary intervention—drugs, surgery	Noninvasive techniques including diet, exercise, stress reduction
Body viewed as a machine in need of repair	Body as a dynamic system and field of energy
Disease or disability as an "entity" or thing	Disease as a process
Emphasis on eliminating symptoms	Emphasis on wellness and healing
Patient as dependent	Patient as empowered
Professional as authority	Professional as therapeutic partner
Mind as secondary factor	Mind as co-equal factor in all illness
Placebo effects show power of suggestion	Placebo shows the mind's role in healing
Primary reliance on quantitative information (charts, data, tests, statistics)	Primary reliance on qualitative information including patient story and profession intuition
Prevention refers to immunization, testing, etc.	Prevention is synonymous with wholeness, lifestyle, and behaviors

Source: Adapted from: Ferguson, M. (1987). *The Aquarian Conspiracy: Personal and Social Transformation in Our Time* (revised ed., pp. 246–248). Los Angeles, CA: J. P. Tarcher.

Table 1-2 Masculine and Feminine Archetypes.

Masculine	Feminine
Curing	Healing
Masculine	Feminine
Knowledge	Understanding
Objective (external)	Subjective (internal)
Linear	Relational (holistic)
Active	Receptive
Doing	Being
Technical	Natural
Mastery	Mystery
Individual	Relationship
How	Why
Form	Process
Sky	Earth
Analytical	Intuitive

Source: Copyright © 2014 by the International Nurse Coach Association. www.inursecoach.com

Nurse Coach Practice Areas

Nurse Coaches are found in all areas of nursing practice and work with individuals and groups. They are staff nurses, ambulatory care nurses, case managers, advanced practice nurses, nursing faculty, nurse researchers, educators, administrators, Nurse Coach consultants, or nurse entrepreneurs. Nurse Coaches may practice in a specialty area such as diabetes education, cardiac rehabilitation, or end-of-life care.

Nurse Coaches may focus on health and wellness coaching, executive coaching, faculty development coaching, managerial coaching, business coaching, or life coaching. The extent to which registered nurses engage in the Nurse Coach role is dependent on coach-specific education, Nurse Coach certification, experience, position, and the population they serve.

With a renewed focus on prevention and wellness promotion, the nursing profession is expanding its visibility in the emerging health and wellness coaching paradigm. As various strategies gain momentum, Nurse Coaches are uniquely positioned to coach and engage individuals in the process of behavior change that can be sustained.

Nurse Coaches are emerging as leaders who are informing governments, regulatory agencies, businesses, and organizations about the important part they play in achieving the goal of improving both the health of our nation and the health of the world. **Table 1-3** (see end of chapter) provides an overview of the role of Nurse Coaches to support the role in health coaching (Dossey & Hess, 2013). Nurse coaching is grounded in the principles and core values of professional nursing as discussed next.

Nurse Coaching Core Values

The Nurse Coach role is based upon the following five core values: (1) Nurse Coach Philosophy, Theories, Ethics; (2) Nurse Coaching Process; (3) Nurse Coach Communication, Coaching Environment; (4) Nurse Coach Education, Research, Leadership; and (5) Nurse Coach Self-Development (Self-Reflection, Self-Assessment, Self-Evaluation, Self-Care). This book is organized by these core values.

Professional Nurse Coaching Practice and Performance Competencies

Nurse Coaches understand that the professional Nurse Coach role, scope of practice, and competencies are linked to each of the ANA six standards of practice and ten standards of professional performance (ANA, 2010a). The professional nurse coaching competencies are authoritative statements of the duties that all Nurse Coaches are expected to perform competently, regardless of setting or specialization. The Nurse Coach competencies are discussed in Chapter 4. (*Note:* The competencies include the International Coach Federation (ICF, n.d.) competencies).

Nurse Coaches understand that professional nurse coaching practice is defined by these core values and competencies. Professional nurse coaching enhances foundational professional nursing knowledge and competencies that are acquired by additional training (International Nurse Coach Association, n.d.).

Professional Nurse Coaching Resources

Nurse Coaches are guided in their thinking and decision-making by three professional resources: *Nursing: Scope and Standards of Practice* (2nd ed.) (ANA, 2010a), *Code of Ethics for Nurses with Interpretive Statements* (ANA, 2001), and *Nursing's Social Policy Statement: The Essence of the Profession* (ANA, 2010b).

Nurse Coaches are also guided by *The Art and Science of Nurse Coaching: The Provider's Guide to Coaching Scope and Competencies* (Hess et. al., 2013) and the American Holistic Nurses Association (AHNA) and the American Nurses Association *Holistic Nursing: Scope and Standards of Practice* (2nd ed.) (AHNA/ANA, 2013). All nursing specialty standards also inform Nurse Coaches. Nurse Coaches practice within the scope of practice within the state where they live. If Nurse Coaches practice in compact states, they adhere to these guidelines (National Council of State Boards of Nursing, n.d.).

Professional Nurse Coach Certification Process

Beginning in 2009 through 2012, establishing the Nurse Coach Certification process was begun by the American Holistic Nurses Credentialing Corporation (AHNCC) (American Holistic Nurses Credentialing Corporation, n.d.) and the Professional Testing Corporation (PTC) of New York City, New York. This collaboration resulted in a Role-Delineation Study (RDS) that was completed in 2012. The results were used to develop a blueprint and guide the development of the Nurse Coach Certification Examination that was a multiple-step process, overseen by PTC, including item-writing to assess specified competencies, item-reviews to assess content validity, and an exam-development process to assess content and construct validity. The prepublication of *The Art and Science of Nurse Coaching: A Provider's Guide to Coaching Scope and Competencies* also informed this process (Hess et al., 2013). The first Professional Nurse Coach Certification Examination was offered in January 2013 with the Nurse Coach Recertification process and criteria.

NATIONAL AND GLOBAL TRANSFORMATION: IMPLICATIONS FOR NURSE COACHING

Currently, the United States is in an economic crisis, and health promotion and cost-effective behavioral change strategies are needed. There is an urgent need to develop initiatives to help shift the focus of healthcare by empowering individuals to take control of their own health and wellbeing. Nurse Coaches are engaged in efforts to assist people towards sustained health as we shift from a disease-focused and reactive healthcare system to one proactively focused on culturally sensitive wellness, health promotion, and disease prevention. The Nurse Coach role will be part of the successful implementation of the following national initiatives.

National Initiatives

Patient Protection and Affordable Care Act

In March 2010, the Patient Protection and Affordable Care Act (PPACA) became law (HR3590) (The Patient Protection and Affordable Care Act, 2010) and PPACA Phase One was implemented in January 2014. In Section 4001 the language references partnerships with a diverse group of licensed health professionals including practitioners of integrative health, preventive medicine, health coaching, public education, and more.

Many provisions in the medical home and accountable care models are based on interprofessional care coordination that is patient-centered. The Agency for Healthcare Research and Quality (AHRQ) has funded and published projects that clearly address the need for a revitalized care system where decisions are based within the context of the patient's values and preferences (Meyers et al., 2010). Asking patients and families what matters most to them is a critical step in engaging them in care. Coordinated patient-centered care that includes actively engaged patients requires a new set of skills for providers, patients, and families (Scholle et al., 2010).

Healthy People Initiative 2020

The Healthy People 2020 initiative continues the work started in 2000 with the Healthy People 2010 initiative for improving the Nation's health. Healthy People 2020 is the result of a multiyear process that reflects input from a diverse group of individuals and organizations (U.S. Department of Health and Human Services, n.d.). The leading health indicators are physical activity, weight and obesity, tobacco use, substance abuse, responsible healthy sexual behavior, mental health, injury and violence, environmental quality, immunization, and access to healthcare. These health indicators were selected on the basis of their ability to motivate action, the availability of data to measure progress, and their importance as public health issues.

The vision, mission, and overarching goals provide structure and guidance for achieving the Healthy People 2020 objectives. While general in nature, they offer specific, important areas of emphasis where action must be taken if the United States is to achieve better health by the year 2020. Developed under the leadership of the Federal Interagency Workgroup (FIW), the Healthy People 2020 framework is the product of an exhaustive collaborative process among the U.S. Department of Health and Human Services (HHS) and other federal agencies, public stakeholders, and the advisory committee.

National Prevention Strategy

In June 2011, the National Prevention, Health Promotion, and Public Health Council announced the release of the National Prevention and Health Promotion Strategy, a comprehensive plan that will help increase the number of Americans who are healthy at every stage of life (National Prevention, Health Promotion, and Public Health Council, 2011). The Strategy addresses the importance of healthy foods, clean air and water, and safe worksites, which are directly related to national and global healthcare transformation discussed next.

Global Transformation

Throughout the world, there are many conversations and initiatives with "health" as the common thread focusing on health promotion, health maintenance, disease prevention, and how to prevent the catastrophic impact of diseases as well as the cost burden. To see global changes in health, Nurse Coaches are aware of what it means to engage with an integrative, integral, and holistic approach and explore the root cause/s of a problem or condition using appropriate technologies (Donner & Wheeler, 2009).

The concept of health of the global commons is yet another aspect of the globalization trend that affects many areas of human endeavor. Where once people thought about and worked within the narrow confines of their communities and regions, now people are interacting within a wide geographic and regional lens of health—the social and environmental determinants of health.

As Monica Sharma, MD, (Sharma, 2006; 2007) has noted, "today, the most urgent and sustainable response to the world's problems is to expand solutions for problems—that are driven solely by technology—[to those solutions] generated from personally-aware leadership." This type of leadership, which Sharma calls "global architecture for personal to planetary transformation," can arise from applying Nightingale's broader and deeper legacy. This can inspire and instill world-centric leadership values and capacities. It is also a transformative approach to develop nurses and global citizens—beyond the tasks of coping with the problems of today—local to global—to become agents of transformation creating new solutions.

SUMMARY

- The Nurse Coach and the client enter into a co-creative process in the most important laboratory of all—an individual's life.
- Health is a process through which individuals reshape basic assumptions and world-views, which includes aspects of physical, mental, emotional, social, spiritual, cultural, and environmental wellbeing. It is not merely the absence of disease; it includes death as a natural process of living.
- Wellbeing is a general term for the condition of an individual or group and their social, economic, psychological, spiritual, or medical state. Wellbeing is based on the idea that the way each person thinks and feels about his or her life is meaningful and important.
- The roots of professional nurse coaching began with Florence Nightingale (1820–1910), the foundational philosopher of modern nursing.
- The professional Nurse Coach is a registered nurse who integrates coaching competencies into any setting or specialty area of practice to facilitate a process of change or development that assists individuals or groups to realize their potential.
- Professional nurse coaching is a skilled, purposeful, results-oriented, and structured relationship-centered interaction with clients provided by registered nurses for the purpose of promoting achievement of client goals.
- Global health is a worldwide focus on the health of all people with a priority of achieving equity, reducing disparities, and protecting against global threats that disregard national borders—local to global. It is a global commons, a bridge across boundaries, and a path to world peace (Beck et al., 2014).

NURSE COACH REFLECTIONS

After reading this chapter, the Nurse Coach will be able to bring awareness and personal insight to the following questions:

- What new insights do I have about my role as a Nurse Coach?
- What is my vision for nurse coaching—local to global?
- What are my beliefs, values, and assumptions about my contributions to the field of nurse coaching?
- When I reflect on my Nurse Coach role as an agent for transformation, what do I experience?

Table 1-3 Overview of Extant Nurse Coach and Nurse Coaching Literature Review.

Allison, M. J., & Keller, C. (2004). Self-efficacy intervention effect on physical activity in older adults. *Western Journal of Nursing Research, 26*(1), 31–46.	Nurse Coaches used verbal persuasion and monitored achievements and awareness of physiological arousal to help increase physical activity self-efficacy of older adults (n = 83). It appears that participants received telephone coaching every 2 weeks for 12 weeks.
Ammentorp, J., & Kofoed, P. E. (2010). Coach training can improve the self-efficacy of neonatal nurses: A pilot study. *Patient Education and Counseling, 79*(2), 258–261.	Neonatal nurses were offered a 3-day coaching training to assess their ability to meet the needs of mothers and fathers. Coach training improved nurses' self-efficacy scores by 14.8% in relation to meeting the needs of mothers and fathers.

Beliveau, L. (2004). Comfort coaching. *Canadian Association Nephrology Nurses and Technologists Journal, 14*(2), 35–36.	Coaching was used to encourage, counsel, educate, and support patients. This article is a self-reflective narrative of the (nurse) author's experience serving as coach to two women receiving dialysis while also dealing with cancer.
Berg, J., Tichacek, M. J., & Theodorakis, R. (2004). Evaluation of an educational program for adolescents with asthma. *The Journal of School Nursing, 20*(1), 29–35.	Three weeks of individual nurse coaching took place after participating in a Power Breathing program, a 3-week educational program about asthma. Each student met with a Nurse Coach 3 times each week for 15 minutes to help tailor the education program to his/her needs. Coaching was seen as a separate intervention from the educational program.
Bennett, J. A., Perrin, N. A., Hanson, G., Bennett, D., Gaynor, W., Flaherty-Robb, M., Joseph, C., Butterworth, S., & Potempa, K. (2005). Healthy aging demonstration project: Nurse coaching for behavior change in older adults. *Research in Nursing & Health, 28*(3), 187–197.	Two registered nurses provided coaching after receiving 24 hours of motivational interviewing training that consisted of didactic instruction and role-playing. Motivational interviewing consisted of: a) expressing empathy; b) supporting self-efficacy; c) working with resistance; and d) acknowledging and working with discrepancy between behavior and goals.
Bloom, S. L., Casey, B. M., Schaffer, J. I., McIntire, D. D., & Leveno, K. J. (2006). A randomized trial of coached versus uncoached maternal pushing during the second stage of labor. *American Journal of Obstetrics and Gynecology, 194*, 10–13.	Coaches were certified nurse midwives who attended training sessions to ensure compliance with the training protocol. The coaching protocol consisted of positioning the head of the bed, positioning the patient, coaching the patient to pull back on both knees and tuck-in the chin while the partner supports the legs, and coaching the patient on breathing techniques during contractions.
Bos, A., Remmen, J. J., Aengevaeren, W. R. M., Verheugt, F. W. A., Hoefnagels, W. H. L., & Jansen, R. W. M. M. (2002). Recruitment and coaching of healthy elderly subjects for invasive cardiovascular research with right-sided catheterisation. *The European Journal of Cardiovascular Nursing, 1*(4), 289–298.	A research nurse with extensive experience in geriatric nursing provided the coaching. Coaching consisted of providing the participants with extensive information about the procedure. There was no set protocol for coaching, and the research nurse did not receive any training.
Bridges, R. A., Holden-Huchton, P., & Armstrong, M. L. (2013). Accelerated second degree baccalaureate student transition to nursing practice using clinical coaches. *Journal of Continuing Education in Nursing, 44*(5), 225–229.	The clinical coach model involves placing a student nurse with an experienced, baccalaureate-prepared staff nurse for 12 months of clinical experience during a second-degree accelerated baccalaureate program. The student works the same schedule as the coach, rather than with a series of preceptors on different units. Coaches attend training conducted by school of nursing faculty, using high-fidelity simulation with clinical scenarios. Coaches and students are supported through weekly visits by clinical faculty.

Brinkert, R. (2011). Conflict coaching training for nurse managers: A case study of a two-hospital health system. *Journal of Nursing Management, 19*(1), 80–91.	Twenty nurse managers were trained over an 8-month period as conflict coaches, and each coached a supervisee. Conflict coaching was a practical and effective means of developing conflict communication competencies of nurse managers and supervisees. This type of program works best when supported by a positive conflict culture and integrated with other conflict intervention processes.
Broscious, S. K., & Saunders, D. J. (2001). Peer coaching. *Nurse Educator, 26*(5), 212–214.	Coaching took place for two days during the first four hours of junior nursing students' clinical shift to support and assist junior students during clinical rounds to reduce stress. Five senior students were responsible for coaching three junior students. Coach training consisted of watching a video entitled "The Helping Hand" produced in 1990.
Butterworth, S., Linden, A., & McClay, W. (2007). Health coaching as an intervention in health management programs. *Disease Management & Health Outcomes, 15*(5), 299–307.	Article provides evidence-based support for the potential role of nurse coaches in tobacco cessation programs. Motivational interviewing methods were used as part of the coaching technique. Coaching was identified as a cost-effective strategy compared to counseling.
Carrieri-Kohlman, V., Gormley, J. M., Douglas, M. K., Paul, S. M., & Stulbarg, M. S. (1996). Exercise training decreases dyspnea and the distress and anxiety associated with it: Monitoring alone may be as effective as coaching. *CHEST, 110*(6), 1526–1535.	A master's-prepared nurse coach provided the coaching. At the beginning of each coaching session, the Nurse Coach helped participants (*n* = 51) set goals related to their clinical status. Coaching was based on guided mastery techniques that included vicarious experiences, verbal persuasion, and physiological feedback.
Carrieri-Kohlman, V., Gormley, J. M., Douglas, M. K., Paul, S. M., & Stulbarg, M. S. (2001). Dyspnea and the affective response during exercise training in obstructive pulmonary disease. *Nursing Research, 50*(3), 136–146.	A master's-prepared Nurse Coach provided the coaching. At the beginning of each coaching session, the Nurse Coach helped participants (*n* = 45) set goals related to their clinical status. Coaching was based on guided mastery techniques that included vicarious experiences, verbal persuasion, and physiological feedback.
Cohen, L. L., Blount, R. L., & Panopoulos, G. (1997). Nurse coaching and cartoon distraction: An effective and practical intervention to reduce child, parent, and nurse distress during immunizations. *Journal of Pediatric Psychology, 22*(3), 355–370.	Two nurses provided coaching to 92 children ages 4–6 and their parents. Both nurses received approximately 15 minutes of intervention training prior to the study. Coaching consisted of making sure children watched a movie while being immunized, and attending to the child's distress.
DeCampli, P., Kirby, K. K., & Baldwin, C. (2010). Beyond the classroom to coaching: Preparing new nurse managers. *Critical Care Nursing Quarterly, 33*(2), 132–137.	A suburban Philadelphia Magnet-designated hospital engaged an experienced nurse executive to coach new nurse managers for four months on site. Face-to-face coaching was agreed as the most important component of the program. Having a seasoned coach also helped increase confidence in the new role.

Dodd, M. J., & Miaskowski, C. (2000). The PRO-SELF program: A self-care intervention program for patients receiving cancer treatment. *Seminars in Oncology Nursing*, *16*(4), 300–308.

An intervention nurse provided the coaching. No formal training was discussed. Coaching consisted of: instructing patients how to use the PRO-SELF program; providing support and encouragement to expand self-care abilities; and positively reinforcing behavior change. No other coaching details were provided.

Donner, G., & Wheeler, M. M. (2009). Coaching in nursing: An introduction. Geneva, Switzerland: International Council of Nursing and Indianapolis, IN: *The Honor Society of Nursing, Sigma Theta Tau International.*

This document provides an overview of nurse coaching. Nurse coaching is based upon ICF core competencies.

Dossey, B. M., Luck, S., Schaub, B. G., & Hess, D. R. (2013). Nurse coaching. In B. M. Dossey & L. Keegan, *Holistic nursing: A handbook for practice* (6th ed., pp. 189–204). Burlington, MA: Jones & Bartlett Learning.

The evolution of health coaching and nurse coaching introduces the topic of nurse coaching. The professional nurse coach scope of practice and competencies is described, including nurse coaching core values. Application of the Theory of Integral Nursing and the Integrative Nurse Coach Method and Process is applied to a discussion of nurse coaching and change. The nurse coaching process is compared to the nursing process.

Dossey, B. M., & Hess, D. R. (2013). Professional nurse coaching: Advances in national and global transformation. *Global Advances in Health and Medicine, 2*(4), 10–16.

The goals of this review were as follows: (1) to identify how the health and wellness coach role was embedded in nursing practice; (2) to identify areas where nurse coaching skills were used and integrated; (3) to determine how nurse coaches defined their roles, practices, and competencies; (4) to explore emerging trends within professional nurse coaching practice; and (5) to identify areas of future research in nurse coaching.

Dowd, T., Kolcaba, K., & Steiner, R. (2003). The addition of coaching to cognitive strategies: Interventions for persons with compromised urinary bladder syndrome. *Journal of Wound, Ostomy, & Continence Nursing*, *30*(2), 90–99.

Coaching was used to provide support to patients. Participants (*n* = 35) received weekly coaching calls for 12 weeks. Coaching enhanced selected outcomes. Information regarding the length of the coaching and the training received was not provided. A nursing role (as coaching) to augment other interventions (education) is supported.

Driscoll, J., & Cooper, R. (2005). Coaching for clinicians. *Nursing Management*, *12*(1), 18–22.

Coaching is a holistic term for the support of continuing personal and professional development. The clients' experiences and needs determine the degree to which coaching is directive or non-directive and may involve skills coaching, performance coaching, or development coaching. The ICF core competencies underpin the work of professional coaches. Professional coaching is an eclectic discipline based on knowledge from counseling, social sciences, neurolinguistics, management and business consulting, philosophy, and motivational psychology. It adopts an appreciative approach with clients. Key differences between coaching and clinical supervision are presented.

Fahey, K. F., Rao, S. M., Douglas, M. K., Thomas, M. L., Elliott, J. E., & Miaskowski, C. (2008). Nurse coaching to explore and modify patient attitudinal barriers interfering with effective cancer pain management. *Oncology Nursing Forum, 35*(2), 233–240.

Nurse coaching was used with patients with cancer pain to explore beliefs and attitudinal barriers interfering with pain management that included communication about pain management and the use of analgesics and non-pharmacologic interventions. Nurse coaching reduced ineffective behaviors and improved pain treatment.

Fielden, S. L., Davidson, M. J., & Sutherland, V. J. (2009). Innovations in coaching and mentoring: Implications for nurse leadership development. *Health Services Management Research, 22*(2), 92–99. doi:10.1258/hsmr.2008.008021

Coaching and mentoring are compared. Transformational coaching is a coaching process that involves development of rapport, relationship building, information gathering through assessment and review, negotiation of carefully defined goals, development of an action plan, and implementation of problem solving. Coaching is not telling people what to do or how to do it. There are differences and similarities in coaching and mentoring. While mentoring was perceived to be "support" and coaching was described as "action," the actual process and content were quite similar. Mentoring may include aspects of coaching more than coaching incorporates aspects of mentoring.

Gortner, S. R., Gilliss, C. L., Shinn, J. A., Sparacino, P. A., Rankin, S., Leavitt, M., Price, M., & Hudes, M. (1988). Improving recovery following cardiac surgery: a randomized clinical trial. *Journal of Advanced Nursing, 13,* 649–661.

Nurses who provided a telephone monitoring intervention on post-hospital cardiac surgery recovery and rehabilitation at home taught and coached on a variety of emotional and physical issues and assisted with problem solving. Master's- and doctoral-level nurses provided coaching. No set coaching protocol or training was discussed. No operational definition of coaching was provided.

Hayes, E., & Kalmakis, K. (2007). From the sidelines: Coaching as a nurse practitioner strategy for improving health outcomes. *Journal of the American Academy of Nurse Practitioners, 19*(11), 555–562. doi:10.1111/j.1745-7599.2007.00264.x

The coaching process for nurse practitioners is described as a method of developing "interpersonal communication skills" that promote the client's engagement in the health and wellness process. The client's needs, life experiences, and goals are the center of the relationship. The NP must be a good listener and assist the client in decision-making. Client characteristics are the driving force of the coaching interaction. Concepts can be applied to nurses in a variety of roles other than NP. This approach also supports the transtheoretical stages of change model and motivational interviewing techniques.

Heath, J., Kelley, F. J., Andrews, J., Crowell, N., et al. (2007). Evaluation of a tobacco cessation curricular intervention among acute care nurse practitioner faculty members. *American Journal of Critical Care, 16*(3), 284–289.

Nurse coaching is expanding, and NPs need to have tools that can assist tobacco users in deciding to stop. There is an opportunity to add nurse coaching to educational nursing programs.

Heckerson, E. W. (2006, February). Nurse leader as coach. *Nurse Leader,* 29–31. doi:10.1016/j.mnl.2005.11.006	Nurses are natural coaches, and coaching is an inherent responsibility of nurse leaders. High-performing leaders focus on coaching. Essential attributes of a coach are passion, integrity, energy, creativity, and excellent communication. Coaching strategies include asking questions; listening carefully without judgment; considering all options; offering specific constructive, direct, and supportive feedback; and building on strengths. Open dialogue and a relationship of mutual trust are essential. Nurse coaching is an exciting new role for the 21st century.
Hennessey, B., & Suter, P. (2011). The community-based transitions model: One agency's experience. *Home Healthcare Nurse,* 29(4), 218–230. doi:10.1097/NHH.0b013e318211986d	Transitional care is a central part of the Patient Protection and Affordable Care Act of 2010. CMS is working with states to design, implement, and evaluate care transition improvement programs. One model involves the use of a health coach—one who abandons the traditional role of "doing" for the patient in favor of role modeling self-care. Another model utilizes advanced practice nurses as transition coaches. Common characteristics necessary for health coaches are presented. "Health coach" is a term that is not uniformly defined, but may include home health nurses as coaches—a role that is compatible with professional nursing practice and requires minimal retooling.
Hess, D. (2011, Winter). Defining holistic nurse coaching. *Beginnings,* 16–19.	This article is excerpted from a white paper presented at the 2010 Summit on Standards and Credentialing of Professional Coaches in Healthcare and Wellness. Nurse coaching is grounded on the foundation of the Scope and Standards of Holistic Nursing Practice. Coaching as it relates to holistic nursing is defined. An overview of holistic nurse coaching is presented, and the evolution of holistic nurse coaching is described. Four behavioral change models for nurse coaching interventions are briefly described: transtheoretical stages of the change model, health belief model, motivational interviewing, and unitary appreciative inquiry.
Huffman, M. (2007). Health coaching: A new and exciting technique to enhance patient self-management and improve outcomes. *Home Healthcare News,* 25(4), 271–274. doi:10.1097/01.NHH.0000267287.84952.8f	Health coaching is described as a partnering with clients to enhance self-management. A Medicare pilot testing this approach for patients with CHF and DM is described.
Johnson, V. D. (2007). Promoting behavior change: Making healthy choices in wellness and healing choices in illness—use of self-determination theory in nursing practice. *Nursing Clinics of North America,* 42(2), 229–241.	Holistic nurses can use Self-Determination Theory (SDT) to promote healthy behavior change. As nurses act in ways to support clients' innate needs for autonomy, competence, and relatedness, clients may be more successful at internalizing self-regulation and more inclined to adopt and maintain lifelong behavioral changes.

Jones, D., Dufy, M. E., & Flanagan, J. (2011). Randomized clinical trial testing efficacy of a nurse-coached intervention in arthroscopy patients. *Nursing Research, 60*(2), 92–99.	The nurse-coached intervention "focused on giving information, interpreting the experience, and validating and clarifying responses and actions related to the surgical experience directed toward making a difference in recovery outcomes" (p. 93). Nurse Coaches received three 2-hour classes related to the study. The coaching intervention was delivered by telephone. Nurse Coaches were provided with clinical guidelines and a set of questions to guide the discussion with the patient.
Kelly, M., & Starr, T. (2008). From hospital to home: An innovative program eases discharged patients back into the community. *Advance for Nurses, 5*(18), 12.	Senior-level BSN students provided coaching based on the Coleman Transition Intervention, a method designed to promote client empowerment and self-advocacy skills through a coaching intervention model. "As today's healthcare paradigm shifts patients toward shared decision-making with their providers, the next generation of nurses will need specific competencies that facilitate their clients' empowerment of their personal healthcare management" (p. 1).
Kelly, J., Crowe, P., & Shearer, M. (2005). The Good Life Project: Telephone coaching for chronic disease self management. *Australian Family Physician, 34*(1/2), 31–34.	Coaching was provided monthly over 12 months by student nurses to promote client empowerment and self-advocacy skills through the use of a coaching intervention model. Coaches received 2 days of motivational interviewing training that also included identifying depression, anxiety, and levels of social support in participants. Patients were specifically encouraged to adhere to recommended treatment.
Leveille, S. G., Huang, A., Tsai, S. B., Allen, M., Weingart, S. N., & Lezzoni, L. I. (2009). Health coaching via an Internet portal for primary care patients with chronic conditions: A randomized control trial. *Medical Care, 47*(1), 41–47.	This randomized study tested the effectiveness of an Internet portal-based nurse coaching intervention to enhance patient-primary care physician visits to discuss three chronic conditions (depression, chronic pain, mobility difficulty). Internet portal-based coaching produced some possible benefits in care for chronic conditions but without significantly changing patient outcomes.
Manne, S. L., Bakeman, R., Jacobsen, P. B., Gorfinkle, K., & Redd, W. H. (1994). An analysis of a behavioural intervention for children undergoing venipuncture. *Health Psychology, 13*(6), 556–566.	Nurse Coaches received one hour of training on how to properly coach parents while their child (ages 36–107 months) experienced venipuncture. The nurse coached parents to encourage the child to use a party blower and to verbally help them through the procedure.
Medland, J., & Stern, M. (2009). Coaching as a successful strategy for advancing new manager competency and performance. *Journal of Nurses Staff Development, 25*(3), 141–147.	Employing the expertise of a dedicated coach is a unique approach to advance competency of new nurse managers in the formative stage of development. This article describes how coaching is emerging as an essential tool for new manager development.

Miakowski, C., Dodd, M., West, C., Schumacher, K., Paul, S. M., Tripathy, D., & Koo, P. (2004). Randomized clinical trial of the effectiveness of a self-care intervention to improve cancer pain management. *Journal of Clinical Oncology*, *22*(9), 1713–1720.

A specially trained oncology nurse provided the coaching. The nurse coached patients in the following areas: improving pain relief by altering the times and frequency of analgesic intake; how to assess pain and the need for analgesics; strategies to prevent side-effects; and how to speak to their healthcare provider about the need for a change in their analgesic prescription. The coaching method utilized was not specified.

Miller, C. (2011). An integrated approach to worker self-management and health outcomes: Chronic conditions, evidence-based practice, and health coaching. *American Association of Occupational Health Nurses*, *59*(11), 491–501.

Occupational health nursing practice will be impacted by the new trends in health coaching, evidence-based practice, and standards of care. Occupational health nurses possess scientific knowledge related to acute and chronic disease and symptoms, stress-management, and relationships. By incorporating new health coaching skills, they can assist employees to learn self-discovery and self-management that have the potential to produce optimal health outcomes.

Mitchell, G. J., Cross, N., Wilson, M., Biernacki, W. W., Adib, B., & Rush, D. (2013). Complexity and health coaching: Synergies in nursing. *Nursing Research & Practice*. Article ID238620. http://dx.doi.org/10.1155/2013/238620

Human beings are complex and are living in complex systems and evolving in nonlinear ways and are influenced by the systems in which they live. Informed by complexity science, the RN Health Coach (RNHC) role is a creative innovation in community settings to care for people with acute and chronic illnesses. This article explores complexity science and its implication for the RNHC role.

Moore, J. O., Marshall, M. A., Judge, D. C., Crocker, B. J., & Zusman, R. M. (2014). Technology-supported apprenticeship in the management of hypertension. *Journal of Clinical Outcome Management*, *21*(3), 110–122.

This study investigates the effectiveness of the remote (home-base) use of a software platform for collaborative hypertension management coupled with nurse coaching in controlling hypertension. The primary outcomes evaluated were: the achievement of blood pressure to goal, patient experience, and cost effectiveness. Forty-two of the 44 subjects completed the study. Intervention subjects achieved a greater decrease in SBP at 12 weeks than control subjects (26.3 mmHG vs 16.0 mmHg, p = 0.009). A greater percentage of patients in the intervention group achieved a goal SBP < 130 mmHg (80.0% vs 45.5%, p = 0.03), and rated a higher scale of satisfaction with their care (8.9 vs 7.6 out of 10, p = 0.12). Intervention patients required more nurse coaching time than controls (0.85 hours vs 0.57 hours, p = 0.15), but this corresponded to less than 1/5 of the clinician cost of standard care ($42.50 vs $248) for optimal outcomes (100% < 140/90 at 3 months). Technology-supported nurse coaching may serve as a new, cost-effective paradigm in the management of hypertension. The success of this trial warrants its study of scalability (across larger populations) as well as its use across a broader spectrum of chronic disease management.

Mott, M. (1992). Cognitive coaching for nurse educators. *The Journal of Nursing Education*, *31*(4), 188–190.	Coaching model is described as peer cognitive coaching to enhance faculty development and thus student achievement. Coaching involves positive feedback to enhance and reinforce desired behavior. The model allows for personal and professional growth through trust, openness, and curiosity. Discussion and critique of others' views are promoted.
Naylor, M., & Keating, S. A. (2008). Transitional care. *Journal of Social Work Education*, Supplement, *44*(3), 65–73.	Nurse-led multidisciplinary care transition models that engage the patient and caregivers in discharge planning have consistently improved quality and cost-savings. One intervention model described as care transition coaching encourages older patients and family caregivers to assume more active roles during care transitions. An advanced practice nurse serves as a "transitions coach" to engage, teach, and promote cross-site continuity of care. Coaching begins in hospital and for 30 days after discharge. Available studies indicate that a focus on patient and caregiver needs, preferences, and goals is one of four key elements of improving care transition.
Old, N. (2012). Positive health coaching: the way forward in nursing. *Australian Nursing Journal, 20*(2), 32.	Nursing is moving into a new phase of health delivery that involves assisting clients to increase healthy behaviors. A Nurse Coach model of care is described. A Nurse Coach supports people to develop the skills of self-awareness to achieve their health goals. Self-empowerment is encouraged. Nurse Coaches focus on client perspectives, expectations, and specific concerns. The Transtheoretical Model, positive psychology, and a focus on client motivation and on what is working rather than what is not, provide frameworks for successful nurse coaching.
Ponte, P. R., Gross, A. H., Galante, A., & Glazer, G. (2006). Using an executive coach to increase leadership effectiveness. *Journal of Nursing Administration, 36*(6), 319–324.	Engaging a leadership coach is a trend and being used as innovative nursing leadership self-development programs and practices. Reporting on four coaches and four nurse leaders, this article reports on the effectiveness of coaching as a leadership development tool and makes recommendations for leaders interested in engaging a coach.
Potempa, K. M., Butterworth, S. W., Flaherty-Robb, M. K., & Gaynor, W. L. (2010). The Healthy Ageing Model: Health behaviour change for older adults. *Collegian*: Royal College of Nursing, Australia, *17*(2), 51–55.	The Healthy Ageing Model focuses on aging adults and has four elements—client-centered, goal-driven approach, individualized coaching strategy of behavioral change, and personal health system. Care is delivered by a nurse practitioner or a primary care physician via in-person clinic visits or home visits, telephone, or e-mail. Behavioral coaching is the core strategy with the ongoing shift to a client-centered relationship of health promotion with the coach as the client's support partner.

Rivers, R., Pesata, V., Beasley, M., & Dietrich, M. (2011, October). Transformational leadership: Creating a prosperity-planning coaching model for RN retention. *Nurse Leader*. doi:10.1016/j.mnl/2011.01.013	To assist nurses to develop resilience to the effects of compassion stress, 30 nurse managers and staff nurses enrolled in a 20-week program with a life coach. All who completed the program viewed it as a positive experience and indicated that the most helpful aspect was having a consistent, nonjudgmental person to provide feedback and suggestions. An overall theme of self-awareness was noted by participants. Improved resilience and retention indicators were evident.
Samarel, N., Fawcett, J., & Tulman, L. (1997). Effect of support groups with coaching on adaptation to early state breast cancer. *Research in Nursing & Health*, 20, 15–26.	A nurse/social worker team referred to as "expert clinicians" led coaching support groups. The coaches were significant others of participants. No formal definition of coaching was provided. Clinician team training consisted of a 4-hour training session with a manual for them to follow.
Schaub, B. G., Luck, S., & Dossey, B. (2012). Integrative nurse coaching for health and wellness. *Alternative and Complementary Therapies*, 18(1), 14–20. doi:10.1089/act.2012.18110	The Samueli Institute in its Wellness Initiative for the Nation recommended the education of health and wellness coaches to improve the nation's healthcare system by changing to a wellness model. This recommendation was written into the PPACA law. This article addresses the implementation of this transition through the development of the Nurse Coach role. Professional nurse coaches are in every healthcare setting and are ideally positioned to take leading roles in implementing new models of care that emphasize health and wellness. Integrative nursing principles and the Integrative Nurse Coach Model are described. The Theory of Integral Nursing is presented as a framework for integrative nurse coaching.
Schenak, S. (2002). Nurse coaching: Healthcare resource for this millennium. *Nursing Forum*, 37(3), 16–20.	Nurse coaching is described as a new role for nurses. It is client-directed as opposed to illness-directed. The nurse coach can provide a structure and an approach with the patient/client to custom fit towards attainable behavioral change. Specific aspects of the nurse coach role include integration of self-efficacy, promoting lifestyle changes, readiness for change, and motivation.
Schumacher, K. L., Koresawa, S., West, C., Hawkins, C., Johnson, C., Wais, E., Dodd, M., Paul, S. M., Tripathy, D., Koo, P., & Miaskowski, C. (2002). Putting cancer pain management regimens into practice at home. *Journal of Pain and Symptom Management*, 23(5), 369–382.	A specially trained oncology nurse provided the coaching. The nurse coached patients in the following areas: improving pain relief by altering the times and frequency of analgesic intake; how to assess pain and the need for analgesics; strategies to prevent side-effects; and how to speak to their healthcare provider about the need for a change in their analgesic prescription. No other coaching details were provided.
Sethares, K. A. (2003). Supporting the self-care behaviors of women with heart failure through an individualized nursing intervention (Doctoral dissertation) Boston College, Boston, MA). Available from *Dissertation Abstracts Online* (363).	Coaching was provided by an advance practice nurse and followed the Individualized Nursing Care Model of Self-care for Women with heart failure. Coaching was used to educate and support. The Nurse Coach visited each participant (*n* = 7) for one hour once per week for 4 weeks. Each session was audio-taped.

Southard, M. E., Hess, D. R., & Bark, L. (2013). Facilitating change: Motivational interviewing and appreciative inquiry. In B. M. Dossey & L. Keegan, *Holistic nursing: A handbook for practice* (6th ed.) (pp. 205–219). Burlington, MA: Jones & Bartlett Learning.	This book chapter focuses on two strategies used by nurse coaches—motivational interviewing (MI) and appreciative inquiry (AI). MI is a skillful interaction for eliciting motivation for change. The guiding principles of MI—partnering with clients and communication skills needed for successfully negotiating behavior change—are discussed. AI originated from organizational systems development. It is a way of asking questions that is based on the basic goodness of people, situations, and organizations. The main precept of AI is that it is a method of co-creating a future that inspires new possibilities. Foundational assumptions of AI, the 4-D cycle of AI are presented. Several case studies that illustrate the application of MI and AI to professional nursing practice are provided.
Stefancyk, A., Hancock, B., & Meadows, M. T. (2013). The nurse manager: Change agent, change coach? *Nursing Administration Quarterly*, *37*(1), 13–17. doi:10.1097/ NAQ.0b013e31827514f4	A change coach, building upon the nurse manager's foundations skill of coaching, uses coaching skills to inspire others towards change. Being a change coach reflects the art of change, which includes mobilizing the resources toward innovation and improvement. Three categories of coaching behavior are discussed: guidance, facilitation, and inspiration. Change coaching is viewed as a leadership imperative and a skill needed by successful nurse managers. A greater emphasis on coaching to influence change requires further development to expand the skills and behaviors of all nurse leaders.
Stulbarg, M. S., Carrieri-Kohlman, V., Gormley, J. M., Tsang, A., & Paul, S. (1999). Accuracy of recall of dyspnea after exercise training sessions. *Journal of Cardiopulmonary Rehabilitation*, *19*(4), 242–248.	A master's-prepared Nurse Coach provided the coaching. At the beginning of each coaching session, the nurse coach helped participants (*n* = 44) set goals related to their clinical status. Coaching was based on guided mastery techniques that included vicarious experiences, verbal persuasion, and physiological feedback.
Sutters, K. A., Miaskowski, C., Holdridge-Zeuner, D., Waite, S., Paul, S. M., Savedra, M., & Lanier, B. (2004). A randomized clinical trial of the effectiveness of a scheduled oral analgesic dosing regimen for the management of postoperative pain in children following tonsillectomy. *Pain*, *110*(1–2), 49–55.	A research nurse provided nurse coaching via telephone calls to parents on days 1 and 2 post-surgery that consisted of an evaluation of the child's condition, review of pain intensity, verification that the child was taking the medication, re-education of the rationale for the dosing, review of strategies to give the medication to the child, and repeat education concerning potential side-effects of the medication. One nurse coach delivered the same information during all the coaching calls to maintain consistency.

Sutters, K. A., Miaskowski, C., Holdridge-Zeuner, D., Waite, S., Paul, S. M., Savedra, M., & Lanier, B. (2005). Time-contingent dosing of an opioid analgesic after tonsillectomy does not increase moderate-to-severe side effects in children. *Pain Management Nursing, 6*(2), 49–57.	A research nurse provided nurse coaching via telephone calls to parents on days 1 and 2 post-surgery that consisted of a discussion of postoperative pain experiences, an explanation of the administration of a non-opioid with an opioid analgesic, a review of the ordered dosing regimen, strategies for improving adherence, teaching regarding possible side-effects, and an explanation about myths about psychological addiction. The nurse also evaluated the child's condition, reviewed pain levels, and verified the child was taking the medication. One Nurse Coach delivered the same information during all the coaching calls to maintain consistency.
Tidwell, L., Holland, S., Greenberg, J., Malone, J., Mullan, J., & Newcomer, R. (2004). Community-based nurse health coaching and its effect on fitness participation. *Lippincott's Case Management, 9*(6), 267–279.	Coaching was part of a program provided by a nurse coach, a social worker, and a geriatrician that included using a client-developed health action plan, patient education instruction and classes, and a fitness program to increase physical activity. A focus was to improve chronic disease self-management, and improve self-confidence in communicating with a primary care provider. Nurse coaching was used to empower participants (504 members of the California Public Employees Retirement system) through encouragement to make healthy choices towards a healthier way of living as outlined by the Case Management Society of America. The Nurse Coach provided health education, counseling, and medication management coaching. The article did not report how each participant was coached.
Tripp, S. B., Templeton, P., Romney, S., & Blood-Siegfried, J. (2011). Providers as weight coaches: Using practice guides and motivational interview to treat obesity in the pediatric office. *Journal of Pediatric Nursing, 26,* 474–479. doi:10.1016/j.pedn.2011.07.009	Motivational interviewing (MI) techniques (following, directing, guiding) a perceived efficacy scale, and lab results were used by healthcare providers (95% of care was provided by FNP) to develop a self-directed provider-assisted plan to remove barriers and move forward to achieve weight loss. Clients were assessed for depression and a three-generation family history was obtained. Support systems were identified by the patient. Clients were seen monthly for 6 months. With consistent use of MI and diet and exercise counseling, a trend toward decreased BMI and waist measurement was noted.
Vale, M., Jelinek, M., Grigg, L., & Newman, R. (2003). Coaching patients on achieving cardiovascular health (COACH). *Archives of Internal Medicine, 163,* 2775–2783.	The coaches for this program were four nurses and two dieticians that were hospital-based. The coaches used telephone calls and mailings to coach patients. Coaches underwent two weeks of part-time coaching training using the COACH model developed by the authors.
Vincent, A. E., & Sanchez Birkhead, A. C. (2013). Evaluation of the effectiveness of nurse coaching in improving health outcomes in chronic conditions. *Holistic Nursing Practice, 27*(3), 148–161.	Nurse coaching was explored as a legitimate, holistic enhancement to Western medicine. Thirteen research studies were reviewed and outcomes discussed that were related to nurse coaching interventions in patients with various chronic conditions. All but two of these studies reported at least some statistically significant positive health outcomes.

Vojta, D., De Sa, J., Prospect, T., & Stevens, S. (2012). Effective interventions for stemming the growing crisis of diabetes and prediabetes: A national payer's perspective. *Health Affairs, 31*(1), 20–26. doi:10.1377/hlthaff.2011.0327	New evidence-based consumer care models that support and encourage lifestyle changes for those with diabetic conditions include partnerships with pharmacists, nurses, and health coaches. Health plans are participating in projects designed to dramatically impact diabetes risk through carefully tailored lifestyle interventions led by lifestyle coaches.
Whittemore, R. (2000). A coaching intervention to integrate lifestyle change in adults with non-insulin dependent diabetes mellitus (Doctoral dissertation, Boston College, 2000). *Dissertation Abstracts Online*, 285.	Participants (*n* = 9) received eight weeks of nurse coaching aimed at facilitating diabetes self-care patients' existing lifestyle. Four coaching sessions were completed throughout the eight-week period and each session was in-person for approximately 60 minutes. Coaching was used to educate, support, and provide guidance to participants. How the coaching was implemented was not described.
Whittemore, R., Chase, S. K., Mandle, C. L., & Roy, C. (2002). Lifestyle change in type 2 diabetes. *Nursing Research, 51*(1), 18–25.	The nurse coaching model used for this study was a modified version of the Adaptation of Chronic Illness Model. Nurse coaching consisted of: providing diabetes information; identifying barriers and facilitators to lifestyle change; providing motivational support; giving feedback and positive encouragement; and goal setting. Nurse coaching was delivered by an advanced practice nurse and consisted of individual four 45-minute sessions every two weeks.
Whittemore, R., D'Eramo Melkus, G., Sullivan, A., & Grey, M. (2004). A nurse-coaching intervention for women with type 2 diabetes. *The Diabetes Educator, 30*(5), 795–804.	A Nurse Coach provided coaching to educate, assist, and provide support to increase maintenance of patient self-management. Participants (*n* = 49) received six personal coaching sessions, using a coaching model developed by the primary author (and others), over a 6-month period. It was not clear how the coaching was done.
Wilkie, D. J., Williams, A. R., Grevstad, & P. Mekwa, J. (1995). Coaching persons with lung cancer to report sensory pain: Literature review and pilot study findings. *Cancer Nursing, 18*(1), 7–15.	Coaching was defined as a method for patients to become more educated and active in their own pain management. Coaching was an interactive process that assumed patients are active processors of information; can elicit beliefs and attitudes to promote change; can learn more adoptive ways of thinking, feeling, and behaving; and be active in their own behavior change. Patients in the coached group were instructed how to self-monitor pain, how to qualify the pattern and intensity of their pain, and how to best report the pain to a clinician. This information was reinforced one week later during a telephone call.

Source: Used with permission. Dossey, B. M., & Hess, D. R. (2013). Professional nurse coaching: Advances in national and global transformation. *Global Advances in Health and Medicine 2*(4), 10–16.

REFERENCES

American Association of Colleges of Nursing (AACN) (2011). *Fact sheet*. Retrieved from http://www.aacn.nche.edu/Media/FactSheets/nursfact.htm

American Holistic Nurses Association and American Nurses Association (AHNA/ANA) (2013). *Holistic nursing: Scope and standards of practice* (2nd ed.). Silver Spring, MD: Author.

American Holistic Nurses Credentialing Corporation (AHNCC) (n.d.). *AHNCC nurse coach certification*. Retrieved from http://www.ahncc.org/certification/nursecoachnch-wnc.html

American Nurses Association (ANA) (2001). *Code of ethics for nurses with interpretive statements*. Washington, DC: Author.

American Nurses Association (ANA) (2010a). *Nursing: Scope and standards of nursing practice* (2nd ed.). Silver Spring, MD: Author.

American Nurses Association (ANA) (2010b). *Nursing's social policy statement: The essence of the profession*. Silver Spring, MD: Author

Beck, D. M. (2013). Empowering women and girls—Empowering nurses: Discovering Florence Nightingale's global citizenship legacy. In S. G. Mijares, A. Rafea, & N. Angha (Eds.), *A force such as the world has never known: Women creating change*. Toronto, ON: Innana Publications.

Beck, D. M., Dossey, B. M., & Rushton, C. H. (2014). Global activism, advocacy and transformation: Florence Nightingale's legacy for the 21st-century. In M. J. Kreitzer & M. Koithan (Eds.), *Integrative nursing*. New York, NY: Oxford University Press.

Benner P. (1984). *Novice to expert: Excellence and power in clinical nursing practice*. Menlo Park, CA: Addison-Wesley.

Benner P. (1985). The oncology clinical specialist: An expert coach. *Oncology Nursing Forum, 12*, 40–44.

Bly, S. (1998). Special section on collaboratories. *Interactions, 5*(3), 31, New York, NY: ACM Press. Retrieved from http://en.wikipedia.org/wiki/Collaboratory

Cooperrider, D. L., & Whitney, D. (2005). *Appreciative inquiry: A positive revolution in change*. San Francisco, CA: Berrett-Koehler.

Csikszentmihalyi, M. (1990). *Flow: The psychology of optimal experience*. New York, NY: Harper and Row.

Donner, G., & Wheeler, M. (2009). *Coaching in nursing: An introduction*. Indianapolis, IN: International Council of Nursing & Sigma Theta Tau. Retrieved from http://www.icn.ch/images/stories/documents/pillars/sew/coaching/Coaching_in_Nursing.pdf

Dossey, B. M. (2010). *Florence Nightingale: Mystic, visionary, healer* (Commemorative ed.). Philadelphia, PA: F. A. Davis.

Dossey, B. M. (2013). Nursing: Integral, integrative, and holistic—local to global. In B. M. Dossey & L. Keegan (Eds.), *Holistic nursing: A handbook for practice* (6th ed., pp. 1–57). Burlington, MA: Jones & Bartlett Learning.

Dossey, B. M., Beck, D. M, & Rushton, C. H. (2011). Integral nursing and the Nightingale Initiative for Global Health: Florence Nightingale's legacy for the 21st century. *Journal of Integral Theory and Practice, 6*(4), 71–92.

Dossey, B. M., & Hess, D. R. (2013). Professional nurse coaching: Advances in national and global healthcare transformation. *Global Advances in Health and Medicine, 2*(4/July), 10–16.

Dossey, B. M., Selanders, L. C., Beck, D. M., & Attewell, A. (2005). *Florence Nightingale today: Healing, leadership, global action*. Silver Spring, MD: Nursesbooks.org.

Dossey, L. (2013). *One mind: How our individual mind is part of a greater mind and why it matters* (pp. xxviii–xxix). Carlsbad, CA: Hay House.

Hess, D. R., Dossey, B. M., Southard, M. E., Luck, S., Schaub, B. G., & Bark, L. (2013). *The art and science of nurse coaching: The provider's guide to coaching scope and competencies*. Silver Spring, MD: Nursesbooks.org.

Institute of Medicine (IOM) (2010). *Future of nursing: Leading change, advancing health*. Washington, DC: The National Academies Press. Retrieved from http://www.iom.edu/Reports/2010/The-Future-of-Nursing-Leading-Change-Advancing-Health.aspx

International Coach Federation (ICF) (n.d.). ICF core competencies. Retrieved from http://www.coachfederation.org/icfcredentials/core-competencies

International Nurse Coach Association (INCA) (n.d.). Retrieved from http://www.inurse coach.com

Meyers, D., Peikes, D., Genevro, J., Peterson, G., Taylor, E. F., Lake, T., & Grumbach, K. (2010). The roles of patient-centered medical homes and accountable care organizations in coordinating patient care. AHRQ Publication No. 11-M005-EF. Rockville, MD: Agency for Healthcare Research and Quality. Retrieved from http://www.ahrq.gov/

Miller, W. R., & Rollnick, S. (2002). *Motivational interviewing: Preparing people for change*. New York, NY: Guilford Press.

National Consortium for the Credentialing of Health and Wellness Coaches (NCCHWC). Progress Report—July, 2011 (2011). Retrieved from http://www.wellcoaches.com/images/pdf/progressreport-nationalteam-jul-2011.pdf

National Council of State Boards of Nursing (n.d.). Nurse License Compact. Retrieved from https://www.ncsbn.org/nlc.htm

National Prevention, Health Promotion, and Public Health Council (2011). National prevention strategy: American's plan for better health and wellness Retrieved from http://www.surgeongeneral.gov/initiatives/prevention/index.html

Newman, M. A. (1994). *Health as expanding consciousness* (2nd ed.). St. Louis, MO: C.V. Mosby.

Nightingale, F. (1859). *Notes on hospitals*. London, UK: John W. Parker.

Nightingale, F. (1860). *Notes on nursing: What it is and what it is not*. London, UK: Harrison.

Nightingale, F. (1893). Sick-nursing and health-nursing. In B. M. Dossey, D. M. Beck, L. C. Selanders, & A. Attewell (2005). *Florence Nightingale today: Healing, leadership, global action* (pp. 296–297). Silver Spring, MD: Nursesbooks.org.

Nightingale Initiative for Global Health (NIGH) (2013). Retrieved from http:www.nightingaledeclaration.net

Orem, D. E. (1971). *Nursing concepts of practice.* New York, NY: McGraw Hill.

Patient Protection and Affordable Care Act (PPACA) (2010). Retrieved from http://democrats.senate.gov/pdfs/reform/patient-protection-affordable-care-act-as-passed.pdf

Peplau, H. E. (1952). *Interpersonal relations in nursing.* New York, NY: G.P. Putnam.

Prochaska, J. O., Norcross, J. C., & DiClemente, C. C. (1995). *Changing for good: A revolutionary six-stage program for overcoming bad habits and moving your life positively forward.* New York, NY: Harper Collins.

Rushton, C. H. (in press). *One heart: The art of compassion based ethics in healthcare.*

Scholle, S. H., Torda, P., Peikes, D., Han, E., & Genevro, J. (2010). *Engaging patients and families in the medical home.* AHRQ Publication No. 10-0083-EF. Rockville, MD: Agency for Healthcare Research and Quality. Retrieved from http://www.ahrq.gov/

Seligman, M. E. P. (1990). *Learned optimism: How to change your mind and your life.* New York, NY: Free Press.

Sharma, M. (2006). Conscious leadership at the crossroads of change. *Shift, 12*(September–October), 17–21.

Sharma, M. (2007). World wisdom in action: Personal to planetary transformation. *Kosmos,* (Fall/Winter): 31–35.

U.S. Department of Health and Human Services, Office of Disease Prevention and Health Promotion (n.d.). *Introducing healthy people 2020.* Retrieved from http://www.healthypeople.gov/2020/about/default.aspx

Wilson, B. (2013). *The nerdy nurse's guide to technology.* Indianapolis, IN: Sigma Theta Tau, International.

Wolever, R. Q., & Eisenberg, D. M. (2011). What is health coaching anyway? Standards needed to enable rigorous research. *Archives of Internal Medicine, 171*(22), 2017–2018. Epub 2011 Oct 10. Retrieved from doi:10.1001/archinternmed.2011.508

World Health Organization. *World Health Organization Statistics Report 2009.* Retrieved from http://www.who.int/hrh/resources/gpw/en/

Wulf, W. (1989). Retrieved from http://en.wikipedia.org/wiki/Collaboratory

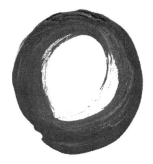

Theory of Integrative Nurse Coaching

Barbara Montgomery Dossey

> If we can transform by a few years of quiet, persistent effort, the habits of centuries, our progress will have been slow, but amazingly rapid.
>
> *Florence Nightingale, 1894*

LOOKING AHEAD...

After reading this chapter, you will be able to:

- Describe the Theory of Integrative Nurse Coaching© (TINC) five components, philosophical assumptions, content, context, and process.
- Examine the metaparadigm in nursing theory and the patterns of knowing in nursing.
- Define a middle-range nursing theory and its implications for Nurse Coaches.
- Use the TINC to guide Nurse Coach practice, education, research, and healthcare policy.

DEFINITIONS

Note: The terms "client" and "patient" and "Integrative Nurse Coach" and "Nurse Coach" are interchangeable throughout this chapter.

Integrative Nurse Coach: A registered nurse who views clients/patients as integrated whole beings; honors and emphasizes each person's unique history, culture, beliefs, and story; and recognizes each person's health and wellbeing as influenced by her/his internal and external environments.

Integrative nurse coaching: The emergence of a distinct nursing role that places clients/patients at the center and assists them in establishing health goals, creating change in lifestyle behaviors for health promotion and disease management, and implementing integrative modalities as appropriate.

Integrative Nurse Coaching Five Components: (1) Integrative Nurse Coach Self-Development (Self-Reflection, Self-Assessment, Self-Evaluation, Self-Care); (2) Integral Perspectives and Change; (3) Integrative Lifestyle Health and Wellbeing; (4) Awareness and Choice; and (5) Listening with HEART (**H**ealing, **E**nergy, **A**wareness, **R**esiliency, **T**ransformation).

Metaparadigm in nursing theory: Four recognized components (nurse, person, health, and environment [society]) in nursing theory.

Middle-range nursing theory: Focused on a specific nursing phenomena; offers a bridge between grand nursing theories that encompass the fullest range or the most global phenomena in the nursing discipline; broad enough to be useful in complex situations;

and leads to implications for instrument development, theory testing through research, and nursing practice strategies.

Patterns of knowing in nursing: Six recognized patterns of knowing in nursing (personal, empirical, aesthetic, ethical, not knowing, and sociopolitical) that are a way to organize nursing knowledge and impact nursing practice, education, research, and healthcare policy.

Theory of Integrative Nurse Coaching (TINC): A middle-range nursing theory that contains healing, the metaparadigm in nursing theory, patterns of knowing, five components [(1) Integrative Nurse Coach Self-Development (Self-Reflection, Self-Assessment, Self-Evaluation, Self-Care); (2) Integral Perspectives and Change; (3) Integrative Lifestyle Health and Wellbeing; (4) Awareness and Choice; and (5) Listening with HEART (Healing, **E**nergy, **A**wareness, **R**esiliency, **T**ransformation)], and energy fields and internal and external healing environments.

THEORY OF INTEGRATIVE NURSE COACHING (TINC)*: OVERVIEW

Health and wellness coaching is a multidimensional concept across the healthcare professions, and it acquires multiple meanings depending on the discipline from which it is viewed. This chapter provides an overview of the Theory of Integrative Nurse Coaching (TINC) that contains healing, the metaparadigm in nursing theory, patterns of knowing in nursing, and the five components of integrative nurse coaching, referred to as theoretical niches that acquire the TINC meaning and context within the component in which it resides. The TINC coauthors—Barbara Dossey, Susan Luck, and Bonney Gulino Schaub—believe that the TINC is essential to the continued evolution of the Nurse Coach role. They also believe that Nurse Coaches, with their leadership capacities, interactions with clients/patients, and other interprofessional collaborations, are leaders in the evolution of healthy people living in a healthy world. See Chapter 21 for the Integrative Nurse Coach Leadership Model (INCLM). See specific book chapters for each of the TINC five components to clearly explicate each component.

TINC: A Middle-Range Nursing Theory

The TINC is a middle-range nursing theory to guide nurse coaching practice, education, research, and healthcare policy. A middle-range nursing theory is focused in scope on a specific nursing phenomenon. It offers a bridge between grand nursing theories that encompass the fullest range or the most global phenomena in the nursing discipline. It is broad enough to be useful in complex situations and leads to implications for instrument development, theory testing through research, and nursing practice strategies (Smith & Parker, 2014).

TINC Definitions

An Integrative Nurse Coach views clients/patients as integrated whole beings, honoring and emphasizing each person's unique history, culture, beliefs, and story. The Integrative

---

*Note: The TINC is the organizational framework for the International Nurse Coach Association's (INCA) (International Nurse Coach Association, n.d.) Integrative Nurse Coach Certificate Program (INCCP) (Integrative Nurse Coach Certificate Program, n.d.), a 3 semester credit hour (SCH) undergraduate Nurse Coach course, a 3 SCH graduate-level Nurse Coach course, a 1 SCH undergraduate Nurse Coach course, and a 1-day Introduction to Integrative Nurse Coaching workshop (6.5 contact hours). See Chapter 19 and Tables 19-5, 19-6, 19-7, and 19-8. For information on INCCP programs, see www.inursecoach.com/programs

Nurse Coach recognizes each person's health and wellbeing as influenced by her/his internal and external environments. Through a self-discovery process Nurse Coaches implement integrative modalities with self and clients/patients.

Integrative nurse coaching is the emergence of a distinct nursing role for assisting clients/patients in establishing health goals, creating change in lifestyle behaviors for health promotion, and in disease management. This role can be integrated into all healthcare settings. Integrative nurse coaching arises out of the tradition of Florence Nightingale who left a legacy to guide nurses for improving the health and wellbeing of humanity (Dossey, 2010; Dossey, Selanders, Beck, & Attewell, 2005; Nightingale Declaration, n.d.).

TINC Intentions

The intention (purpose) in a nursing theory is the aim of the theory. Using the integrative nurse coaching lens, the TINC has three intentions as follows:

1. Demonstrate the unique Integrative Nurse Coach role and competencies for health and wellness.
2. Explore the direct application of integrative nurse coaching in all healthcare and community settings and in interprofessional collaboration.
3. Expand Integrative Nurse Coaches' capacities as 21st-century Nightingales and health diplomats who are coaching for health and wellness—local to global. (See Chapter 1 for more on the roots of professional nurse coaching and Florence Nightingale's legacy.)

TINC Developmental Process

Early in the TINC developmental process the TINC coauthors asked the following three questions to move forward with a nursing lens focused on the TINC development process:

Question 1: What are the implications and relevance of integrative nurse coaching to healing, the metaparadigm in nursing theory, patterns of knowing in nursing, Nurse Coach self-development, integral perspectives for change, integrative lifestyle health and wellbeing, awareness and choice, energy, resilience, and transformation?

Question 2: Which of the existing nursing paradigms and worldviews most closely explains integrative nurse coaching?

Question 3: What are the substantive domains of health and wellness coaching knowledge, qualities, and competencies through a Nurse Coach lens?

The *first* question was answered by reviewing Barbara Dossey's Theory of Integral Nursing (TIN) (Dossey, 2013) and other specific concepts: healing (Achterberg, Dossey, & Kolkmeier, 1994; Dossey, 2013); the metaparadigm in nursing theory (nurse, person, health, environment [society]) (Fawcett & DeSanto-Madeya, 2000); the recognized patterns of knowing in nursing (personal, empirical, aesthetic, ethical, not knowing, sociopolitical) (Carper, 1978; Munhall, 1993; White, 1995); self-development and integral perspectives (Dossey, 2013; Wilber, 2013); integrative lifestyle health (Luck, 2013; Luck & Keegan, 2013); mindfulness, awareness, and choice (Schaub & Burt, 2013); energy (Slater, 2013); resiliency (Maddi & Khoshaba, 2005; McCraty & Childres, 2010; Seaward, 2015); and transformation (Schaub & Schaub, 2013).

Healing, the metaparadigm in nursing theory, patterns of knowing, self-development, integral perspective for changes, and awareness and choice were determined as being relevant for Integrative Nurse Coaches to bring themselves into the full expression of being present in the moment with self and clients/patients, and in all of their knowing, doing, and being in nurse coaching. Healing is seen in **Figure 2-1a** and described in **Table 2-1**. The metaparadigm in nursing theory is seen in **Figure 2-1b** and described in **Table 2-2**. The patterns of knowing in nursing are seen in **Figure 2-1c** and described in **Table 2-3**. These patterns continue to be refined and reframed with new applications and interpretations (Chinn & Kramer, 2010). The TINC five components are developed later and are seen in **Figure 2-1d**.

Figure 2-1a Healing.
Source: Copyright © 2014 by the International Nurse Coach Association. www.inursecoach.com

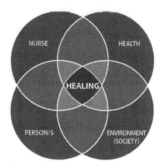

Figure 2-1b Healing and Metaparadigm in Nurse Theory.
Source: Copyright © 2014 by the International Nurse Coach Association. www.inursecoach.com

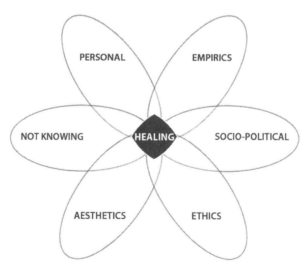

Figure 2-1c Healing and Patterns of Knowing in Nursing.
Source: Copyright © 2014 by the International Nurse Coach Association. www.inursecoach.com

Table 2-1 Healing Concepts.

- A lifelong journey of seeking harmony and balance in one's own life and in family, community, and global relations.
- An emergent process of the whole system bringing together aspects of one's self and the body-mind-spirit-culture-environment at deeper levels of inner knowing, leading toward integration and balance, with each aspect having equal importance and value.
- Includes evolving one's state of consciousness to higher levels of personal and collective understanding that acknowledges the individual's interior and exterior experiences and the shared collective interior and exterior experiences with others where authentic power is recognized within each person.
- Disease and illness at the physical level may manifest for many reasons and variables. It is important *not* to equate physical health, mental health, and spiritual health, as they are not the same thing. They are facets of the whole jewel of health.
- Involves recovery, repair, renewal, and transformation that increase wholeness and often (though not invariably) order and coherence.
- Leads to more complex levels of personal understanding and meaning, and may be synchronous but not synonymous with curing.
- Healing with self or another can happen until the moment of death.

Source: Copyright © 2008 by Barbara Dossey.

Table 2-2 Metaparadigm in Nursing Theory.

Nurse	A registered nurse who is a 21st-century Nightingale engaged in social action and sacred activism. The nurse is an instrument in the healing process where she/he brings one's whole self into relationship to the whole self of another or a group of significant others that reinforces the meaning and experience of oneness and unity.
Person	An individual (client/patient, family member, significant other) who engages with a nurse in a manner that is respectful of a person's subjective experiences about health, health beliefs, values, sexual orientation, and personal preferences. It also includes an individual nurse who interacts with a nursing colleague, other healthcare team members, or a group of community members, other groups, or concerned citizens around health issues.
Health	A state or process defined by an individual in which one's experiences a sense of growth, wellbeing, harmony, and unity. Each individual reshapes basic assumptions and worldviews about wellbeing and see death as a natural process of living. Health places the client/patient at the center of care and addresses the bio-psycho-social-spiritual-cultural-environmental aspects that influence health.
Environment (Society)	Includes both interior and exterior aspects. The interior environment includes the individual's feelings, meaning, and mental, emotional, and spiritual dimensions; it also includes a person's physiology, which is an internal (inside) aspect of the exterior self. The exterior environment includes objects that can be seen and measured and that are related to the physical and social in some form in any of the gross, subtle, and infinite levels.

Source: Copyright ©2014 by the International Nurse Coach Association. www.inursecoach.com

Table 2-3 Patterns of Knowing in Nursing.

Personal Knowing	The nurse's dynamic process and awareness of wholeness that focuses on the synthesis of perceptions and being with self. It may be developed through art, meditation, dance, music, stories, and other expressions of the authentic and genuine self in daily life and nursing practice. This may be related to living and nonliving people and things, such as a deceased relative, animal, or a lost precious object through flashes of memories stimulated by a current situation (a touch may bring forth past memories of abuse or suffering). Insights gained through dreams and other reflective practices that reveal symbols, images, and other connections also influence one's interior environment.
Empirical Knowing	The science of nursing that focuses on formal expression, replication, and validation of scientific competence in nursing education and practice. It is expressed in models and theories and can be integrated into evidence-based practice. Empirical indicators are accessed through the known senses that are subject to direct observation, measurement, and verification.
Aesthetic Knowing	The art of nursing that focuses on how to explore experiences and meaning in life with self or another that includes authentic presence, the nurse as a facilitator of healing, and the artfulness of a healing environment. It is the combination of knowledge, experience, instinct, and intuition that connects the nurse with a patient or client in order to explore the meaning of a situation about the human experiences of life, health, illness, and death. It calls forth resources and inner strengths from the nurse to be a facilitator in the healing process. It is the integration and expression of all the other patterns of knowing in nursing praxis.
Ethical Knowing	The moral knowledge in nursing that focuses on behaviors, expressions, and dimensions of both morality and ethics. It includes valuing and clarifying situations to create formal moral and ethical behaviors intersecting with legally prescribed duties. It emphasizes respect for the person, the family, and the community, which encourages connectedness and relationships that enhance attentiveness, responsiveness, communication, and moral action.
Not Knowing	The capacity to use healing presence, to be open spontaneously to the moment with no preconceived answers or goals to be obtained. It engages authenticity, mindfulness, openness, receptivity, surprise, mystery, and discovery with self and others in the subjective space and the intersubjective space that allows for new solutions, possibilities, and insights to emerge. It acknowledges the patterns that may not be understood and that may manifest related to various situations or relationships.
Sociopolitical Knowing	Addresses the important contextual variables of social, economic, geographic, cultural, political, historical, and other key factors in theoretical, evidence-based practice and research. This pattern includes informed critique and social justice for the voices of the underserved in all areas of society along with protocols to reduce health disparities.

Source: Copyright © 2014 by Barbara M. Dossey. Adapted from Carper, 1978; Munhall, 1993; White, 1995.

The *second* question was answered by reviewing the recognized nursing paradigms, the integrative–interactive paradigm, the unitary–transformative paradigm, the caring theories paradigm, and different grand nursing theories and middle-range theories relevant in each paradigm. Although nursing is in a phase where multiple paradigms can coexist, the TINC coauthors believed that the paradigm that most informed and best suited their theory was the interactive–integrative paradigm, which is described as follows (Beck, Dossey, & Rushton, 2014; Smith & Liehr, 2013; Smith & Parker, 2014).

Interactive–integrative Paradigm

- Individuals (person/s, families, groups, communities) are seen as integrated wholes or integrated systems interacting with the larger environmental system.
- The individual (person/s, families, groups, communities) dimensions of each person are integrated and are influenced by environmental factors leading to some change that enhances health and wellbeing.
- The individual's subjective experiences and interpretation and the multidimensional nature of any outcome are significant.
- Individuals are seen as reciprocal interactive entities, and change is probalistic. This implies that there may be more than one way to change that is related to many factors, and an individual follows the one that seems best. Knowledge is grounded in the perspective of the social sciences.
- Individuals change in a reciprocal interactive process where they exercise influence over what they do and decide how to behave.
- Concepts at the theoretical level include self-efficiency expectations and self-efficacy outcomes. Examples include learning about proper nutrition and eating real food, exploring movement and exercise options, addressing stress and unpleasant sensations, cueing in to stress and choosing to integrate stress management skills, and examining home and work environments for toxicity, which leads to awareness and choice for healthier behaviors and how to sustain these behaviors.

The *third* question concerning the substantive domains of health and wellness coaching knowledge, qualities, and competencies was determined by the TINC coauthors' extensive work from 2009 to 2012, as Professional Nurse Coach Workgroup (PNCW) members with Nurse Coach colleagues Darlene Hess, Mary Elaine Southard, and Linda Bark. Together as coauthors on *The Art and Science of Nurse Coaching: A Provider's Guide to Coaching Scope of Practice and Competencies* (Hess et al., 2013), this document brought the Nurse Coach role in healthcare reform to the forefront. (See Chapter 1, Table 1-3, and Chapter 4.) *The Art and Science of Nurse Coaching* determined these five goals: (1) identify how the health and wellness coach role was embedded in nursing practice; (2) identify areas where nurse coaching skills were used and integrated; (3) determine how Nurse Coaches defined their roles, practices, and competencies; (4) explore emerging trends within professional nurse coaching practice; and (5) identify areas for research in nurse coaching.

The Art and Science of Nurse Coaching (Hess et al., 2013) demonstrates nursing's proactive stance in healthcare transformation and clarifies nursing perspectives concerning the role of the Nurse Coach in four key ways: (1) it specifies the philosophy, beliefs, and values of the Nurse Coach and the Nurse Coach's scope of practice; (2) it articulates the relationship between *The Art and Science of Nurse Coaching* and the American Nurses Association's *Nursing: Scope and Standards of Practice* (2nd ed.) (ANA, 2010a), the ANA *Code of Ethics for Nurses with Interpretive Statements* (ANA, 2001), the ANA's *Nursing's Social Policy Statement* (ANA, 2010b), and the *AHNA and ANA Holistic Nursing: Scope and Standards* (2nd ed.) (AHNA & ANA, 2013); (3) it provides the basis for continued interdisciplinary conversations related to professional health and wellness coaches and lay health and wellness coaches (NCCHWC, 2011); and (4) it provides the foundation for a national and an international certification process in professional nurse coaching. See details of the American Holistic Nurses Credentialing Corporation (AHNCC) Nurse Coach Certification Process (AHNCC, n.d.).

The TINC coauthors reviewed *Holistic Nursing: A Handbook for Practice* (Dossey & Keegan, 2013) book chapters, other holistic and integrative healthcare textbooks, and integrative interprofessional journals. Other topics included reflective practice (Freshwater, Taylor, & Sherwood, 2008; Johns, 2013) and select nursing theorists (see Hess et al., 2013, Appendix D). Social science theories reviewed were change theories with specific topics that included Transtheoretical Model of Behavioral Change (Moore & Tschannen-Moran, 2010; Prochaska, Norcross, & DiClemente, 1995); motivational interviewing (Dart, 2011; Rollnick, Miller, & Butler, 2008); appreciative inquiry (Cooperrider & Whitney, 2005); functional medicine (Institute for Functional Medicine, n.d.); personalized lifestyle medicine (Personalized Lifestyle Medicine Institute, n.d.), vulnerability (Brown, 2012; Schaub & Schaub, 2013), positive psychology (Csikszentmihalyi, 1990; Seligman, 1990); flow theory (Csikszentmihalyi, 1990), resilience and heart math (McCraty & Childres, 2010); sense-of-coherence theory (Antonovsky, 1996); and complexity science (Davidson, Ray, & Turkel, 2011). (See specific book chapters for additional topics and resources.) In the next section, the TINC content, context, and process are discussed.

TINC CONTENT, CONTEXT, AND PROCESS

To present the TINC, Barbara Barnum's (2005) framework to critique a nursing theory includes content, context, and process, and highlights what is most critical to understand a theory. This framework provides an organizing framework that avoids duplication of explanations within the theory. The TINC philosophical assumptions are listed in **Table 2-4**.

Table 2-4 Theory of Integrative Nurse Coaching Philosophical Assumptions.

1. An integrative understanding recognizes the wholeness of humanity and humans and the world as energy that is open, dynamic, interdependent, fluid, and continuously interacting with changing variables that can lead to greater complexity and order.

2. Nurse coaching is a developmental process of personal growth and expanding states of consciousness to deeper levels of personal and collective understanding of one's physical, mental, emotional, social, spiritual, cultural, and environmental dimensions.

3. Health is how the individual defines her/his state or process in which one experiences a sense of growth, wellbeing, harmony, and unity.

4. Health is a process through which individuals reshape basic assumptions and worldviews that includes aspects of physical, mental, emotional, social, spiritual, cultural, and environmental wellbeing, and not merely the absence of disease; it includes death as a natural process of living.

5. Wellness is a multidimensional state of existence experienced as wellbeing and integration and has a congruent functional quality aiming towards one's highest potentials.

6. The Integrative Nurse Coach is an instrument in the healing process and facilitates healing through her/his presence and knowing, doing, and being.

7. Integrative nurse coaching is a reflective practice that integrates all ways of knowing (personal, empirics, aesthetics, ethics, not knowing, and sociopolitical).

8. The Nurse Coach uses an integral perspective in coaching sessions that is a comprehensive way to organize multiple phenomenon of human experience from four perspectives of reality: 1) individual interior (subjective, personal); 2) individual exterior (objective, behavioral); 3) collective interior (interobjective, cultural); and 4) collective exterior (interobjective, systems/structures).

9. Integrative nurse coaching is applicable in practice, education, research, and healthcare policy.

Source: © 2014 by the International Nurse Coach Association. www.inursecoach.com

Content

The *content* of a nursing theory includes the subject matter and building blocks that give a theory its form. It comprises the stable elements that are acted on or that do the acting. After the TINC coauthors established the theoretical linkage to the interactive–integrative paradigm, and that healing, the metaparadigm in nursing theory, and patterns of knowing in nursing were important to integrative nurse coaching, the specific five nurse coaching components were explicated as follows: (1) Nurse Coach Self-Development (Self-Reflection, Self-Assessment, Self-Evaluation, Self-Care); (2) Integral Perspectives and Change; (3) Integrative Lifestyle Health and Wellbeing; (4) Awareness and Choice; and (5) Listening with HEART (Healing, Energy, Awareness, Resiliency, Transformation). All five components are *fully integrated* and have equal value as seen in **Figure 2-1d** and **Table 2-5**. An overview of each component follows, and these details are expanded in specific chapters in this book as indicated for each component. See Chapter 21 on the Integrative Nurse Coach Leadership Model© (INCLM) as it contains the same components that are integrated to expand Nurse Coach leadership qualities and capacities.

Table 2-5 Theory of Integrative Nurse Coaching (TINC) Five Components.

THEORY OF INTEGRATIVE NURSE COACHING (TINC)© FIVE COMPONENTS	
Component 1:	Nurse Coach Self-Development (Self-Reflection, Self-Assessment, Self-Evaluation, Self-Care)
Component 2:	Integral Perspectives and Change
Component 3:	Integrative Lifestyle Health and Wellbeing (ILHWB)
Component 4:	Awareness and Choice
Component 5:	Listening with HEART (Healing, Energy, Awareness, Resilience, Transformation)

Source: © 2014 by the International Nurse Coach Association. www.inursecoach.com

TINC Component 1: Nurse Coach Self-Development

Nurse Coach Self-Development includes the following four areas: self-reflection, self-assessment, self-evaluation, and self-care. See Chapter 22 for details. The Nurse Coach understands the importance of deepening personal self-exploration to identify one's personal goals, action plans, and readiness, priority, and commitment to change. Through this process the Nurse Coach identifies and strengthens her/his Nurse Coach qualities and leadership capacities as seen in Chapter 21, Tables 21-4 through 21-8.

Self-reflection. Self-reflection is being in a present state of mindfulness with the inner awareness of our thoughts, feelings, judgments, beliefs, and perceptions that brings us into the present moment. See Chapter 12 and Appendix F. As Nurse Coaches increase their understanding and experience of mindfulness practice and healing through self-reflection, they declare their deep intention for presence in their nurse coaching endeavors. Presence is the essential state or core in healing, and in approaching an individual in a way that respects and honors her/his essence. It is relating in a way that reflects a quality of *being with* and *in collaboration with* rather than *doing to*.

Nurse Coaches enter into a shared experience (or field of consciousness) with the client that promotes healing potential and an experience of wellbeing. Consciousness is the capacity to react to, attend to, and be aware of self and other. Consciousness subsumes all categories of experience, including perception, cognition, intuition, instinct, will, and emotion, at all levels, including those commonly termed "conscious," "subconscious," "superconscious," or "unconscious," "intention," and "attention," without presumption of

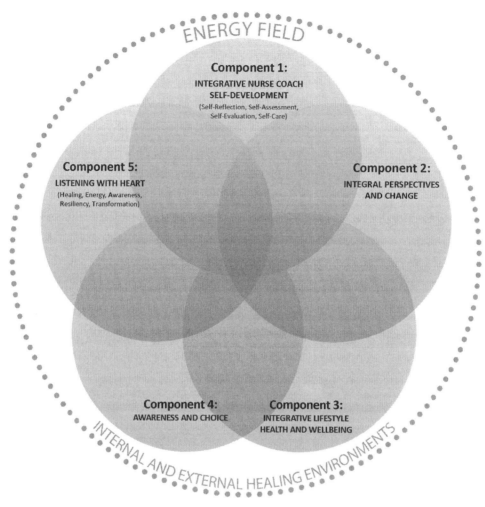

Figure 2-1d Integrative Nurse Coaching Five Components (1) Nurse Coach Self-Development (Self-Reflection, Self-Assessment, Self-Evaluation, Self-Care); (2) Integral Perspectives and Change; (3) Integrative Lifestyle Health and Wellbeing; (4) Awareness and Choice; and (5) Listening with HEART (Healing, Energy, Awareness, Resiliency, Transformation).
Source: Copyright © 2014 by the International Nurse Coach Association. www.inursecoach.com

specific psychological or physiological mechanisms. Neither consciousness nor its environment exists in isolation; they can be represented only in interaction and exchange of information (Dossey, L., 2013; Jahn & Dunne, 1987).

Self-reflection is about valuing who we are and recognizing that we must be willing to experience and face our fears, worries, and self-deceptions. This also includes exploring our own dying as well as old habitual patterns each day and releasing relationships or projects that no longer work in our life. Self-reflection leads to deeper understanding of impermanence and surrendering to our capacity for healing.

Self-assessment. Nurse Coaches use self-assessment in an informal or formal manner to deepen the experience of understanding our present way of life, feelings, and personal habits. See Chapter 6 for details. There are many ways of engaging in self-assessment that may be done in an informal or formal manner, such as the IHWA (Appendix C-1, short form and Appendix C-2, long form) and other appendices. These are some of the ways Nurse Coaches deepen their experiences of understanding their own present patterns, feelings, health behaviors, and personal strengths to assist them in establishing goals and a personal plan of care to enhance health and wellness.

Through identifying personal goals related to health and wellness, Nurse Coaches deepen their capacities around life balance and satisfaction, relationships, spiritual, mental, emotional, physical (nutrition, exercise, weight), and health responsibility processes of recovery, repair, renewal, and transformation that increase wholeness and often (though not invariably) order and coherence.

Self-evaluation. Self-evaluation invites exploration around many areas that may assist in letting go of fixed ideas about self or others. Learning to bear witness to personal joy as well as personal suffering is essential for coaching others. How might we welcome everything that occurs? What allows us to embrace all experiences directly? We learn to use all the ingredients of life. Self-evaluation requires that we explore our understanding and experience of deep attention, intention, compassion, presence, empathy, humility, resilience, and healing.

Self-care. Self-care assists Nurse Coaches with creating more balance and harmony in daily life. These are activities that are initiated and performed to maintain wellbeing. It includes the ability to increase awareness and choice, leading to behaviors and activities and integration of body, mind, and spirit. Self-care is valuing and recognizing how to care for self in order to be able to serve others. It is a willingness to experience and face personal fears, worries, and self-deceptions. Self-care also means Nurse Coaches will be able to bring more of themselves to all aspects of their work and life (Clark & Paraska, 2014; Richards, Sheen, & Mazzer, 2014).

TINC Component 2: Integral Perspectives and Change

The Nurse Coach explores integral perspectives in daily life and in coaching sessions. See Chapter 14 and Figure 14-1, Figure 14-2, and Table 14-1 for details. This is a comprehensive way to organize multiple phenomenon of human experience from four perspectives (four quadrants) of reality (Dossey, 2013; Wilber, 2000):

1. Individual interior "I" (subjective, personal)
2. Individual exterior "It" (objective, behavioral)
3. Collective interior "We" (interobjective, cultural)
4. Collective exterior "Its" (interobjective, systems/structures)

An integral process assists Nurse Coaches to help clients become more aware of their wholeness and power in knowing, which leads to freedom to choose new health patterns and behaviors, to identify their desired goals and make changes, and then to learn how to sustain these changes (Barrett, 2003). An integral perspective provides the Nurse Coach with a powerful framework for coaching clients to become more aware of their personal, current way of being and envisioning a transforming self. This process includes a creative process of both embracing self and opening to a capacity to transcend and go beyond old patterns. Leaving any one quadrant out will compromise the coaching process.

Integral perspectives assist the Nurse Coach in appreciating patterns that are expressed as the coming to know the uniqueness of the other. It can be described as "connecting the dots" of one's storyline. Meaning in these patterns is often revealed as the wholeness of the person where creative insight and the unfolding and enfolding of self-discovery emerge, along with revealing obstacles and where one is stuck in a life pattern. This occurs very frequently when the Nurse Coach uses the nurse coaching process and resists labeling, diagnosis, and naming specific concrete goals to be achieved. See Chapter 4. This allows for attuning to "dancing in the moment" with the dynamic flow of the client's story where both the Nurse Coach and client can feel an inner shift as their energy fields come together. See Chapter 5 Nurse Coach 5-Step Process and Figure 5-3.

TINC Component 3: Integrative Lifestyle Health and Wellbeing (ILHWB)

Nurse Coaches recognized Integrative Lifestyle Health and Wellbeing (ILHWB) as a personalized approach that deals with primary prevention and underlying causality through a whole person perspective rather than traditional labels and codes for symptoms and diagnoses of disease. See Chapter 7, Figure 7-1, Chapters 8–9, and Appendix E for details. The ILHWB holds the worldview that human health is the microcosm of the macrocosm in the web of life (Luck, 2013; Luck & Keegan, 2013). This is a science-based approach to health that is grounded in the following principles:

- **Energy field principles and dynamics:** Thoughts, stress, toxic environments, social and cultural isolation, and nutrient imbalances can disrupt our human energy field.
- **Interconnectedness:** All communication is an orchestrated network of interconnected messenger pathways and signaling systems and not autonomous or in isolation.
- **Promotion of optimizing our internal and external healing environments:** All-encompassing worldview that human health is the microcosm and reflects the macrocosm in the web of life.
- **Patient-centered:** Honors and emphasizes each person's unique history, culture, beliefs, and story rather than a medical diagnosis and disease labels.
- **Biochemical individuality:** Recognizes the importance of variations in metabolic function that derive from genetics, epigenetics, strengths, and vulnerabilities unique to each individual.
- **Health on a wellness continuum:** Views health as a dynamic balance on multiple levels and trusts that our human capacity seeks to identify, restore, and support our innate resilience and reserve to enhance wellbeing and healing throughout the life cycle.

TINC Component 4: Awareness and Choice

Nurse Coaches cultivate awareness and choice through knowledge and self-regulation skills of mindfulness; it is a volitional act of love. Mindfulness is the practice of giving attention to what is happening in the present moment such as thoughts, feelings, emotions, and sensation. Through awareness practices of mindfulness, four qualities are cultivated—lovingkindness, calmness, concentration, and insight. Learning awareness practices increases one's capacities towards more helpful choices. See Chapters 11–13 and Appendix F for details.

The Nurse Coach assists the client to increase her/his awareness and choice/s, which are both essential for achieving inner balance and harmony and determining specific health goals and desired behavioral changes. With increased capacities of awareness and choice, the individual may more easily access her/his vulnerability, which is a universal human awareness that our physical lives are transitory; vulnerability can serve as a bridge among all people (Schaub & Burt, 2013; Schaub & Schaub, 2013). This speaks to the essential truth that everyone, without exception, is subject to change and loss at any moment. It is the human condition. When we become aware of how we react to vulnerability, we become *response-able* to make new healthier life-affirming choices. People respond to vulnerability in different ways that are described below (Chapter 11 and Figures 11-1, 11-2, and 11-3):

- **Willful:** This is the behavior of instinctive, fight–flight patterns of protective and fight-activated behaviors.
- **Will-lessness:** This is the behavior of flight-activated responses that are manifestations of the bio–psycho–social–spiritual–cultural–environmental aspects of the person's behavior. [*Note*: Willfulness (fight) and will-lessness (flight) are reactions at the most instinctual, physiological level.]
- **Willingness:** This is the behavior of becoming aware of how to develop awareness and choice so that the individual recognizes different patterns of fight–flight behaviors and learns that there is the possibility of choosing the best response.

TINC Component 5: Listening with HEART

Listening with HEART© (**H**ealing, **E**nergy, **A**wareness, **R**esiliency, **T**ransformation) captures the dynamic elements within all TINC components as seen below. These elements are threaded throughout this book.

Healing: Healing is the emergent process of the whole system bringing together one's self and the bio–psycho–social–spiritual–cultural–environmental aspects at deeper levels of inner knowing, leading towards integration and balance, with each aspect having equal importance and value. See Table 2-1.

Energy: Energy is a state and a process of an individual's unfolding and enfolding and becoming aware of her/his energy field with the internal and external healing environments. It includes finding balance and increasing awareness and choice/s in life's journey. The Nurse Coach enters into this dynamic energy flow with presence, intention, and a state of consciousness of human wholeness with nothing "to fix," and to participate knowingly to uncover the many levels and patterns within the client's story. See Chapter 5.

This relationship allows a flow of energy in each person that may manifest as new meaning, insight, and creativity, or suffering, anxiety, fear, and frustration. The Nurse Coach holds the space for what the client wants or needs to express. In the coaching relationship there may be various shifts in consciousness, intrapersonal dynamics, interpersonal relationships, and expressions of the lived experiences of disconnection or of connection, unity, and oneness with the larger environment, cosmos, or spirit, however defined.

Awareness: Awareness is mindfulness in the present moment to increases one's capacities towards more helpful choices for achieving inner balance and harmony, and determining specific health goals and desired behavioral changes. See TINC Component 4 above for more details.

Resiliency: Resiliency is generally considered to be a positive trait involving the capacity to cope with stress and adversity (McCraty & Childres, 2010). *Physical resilience* is reflected in physical flexibility, endurance, and strength. *Mental resilience* is reflected in one's attention span, mental flexibility, optimistic worldview, and ability to integrate multiple points of view. *Emotional resilience* is related to one's ability to self-regulate the expression of one's emotions. *Spiritual resilience* is related to one's commitment to personal core values, the ability to trust one's intuition, and tolerance of others' values and beliefs.

Transformation: Transformation is the process of the continual changing and evolution of one's self, which includes reflecting on meaning, beliefs, values, and purpose in living. It may lead to developing the transpersonal self that transcends personal, individual identity and opens to connecting to unitive experiences and universal principles that occur with a person's life maturity whereby a sense of self expands.

Listening with HEART reflective questions in **Table 2-6** may potentiate and lead to the client's greater understanding, meaning, and insight around lifestyle behaviors, awareness, and choice/s. This enhances creative emergence towards desired goals and behaviors, sustained change, and human flourishing. As a Nurse Coach, listening from your HEART mode, reflect on the questions that you might ask a client or perhaps just ask yourself. These are not formulaic questions. They are for you to consider within the context of the person you are working with. The key is to not make any assumptions about what this person needs or wants. Allow time to be curious and "not know" rather than thinking about what the next question should be. Trust in the therapeutic effect of what happens when one is being deeply listened to and her/his story unfolds. Remember to take a breath and know the value of being fully present in the energy field that you are sharing with the client.

Table 2-6 Listening with HEART©.

H—HEALING
- What are you hoping for?
- What would a healing outcome be?
- What do you believe is the meaning of this challenge?
- What do you imagine success will feel like?

E—ENERGY
- What are your feelings about moving forward with this challenge?
- What has given you the energy or will to succeed at other times?
- What would be a step in the right direction for now?
- What do you need to take that step?

A—AWARENESS
- What do you understand about the challenge you are facing?
- What support do you have or need in following through with choices you have made?
- How have you taken care of yourself in the past?
- Where do you feel most comfortable or comforted?

R—RESILIENCY
- What has worked for you in other challenging times?
- What do you trust the most about yourself?
- Tell me about a time when you had success in dealing with a challenge?
- What have you learned from that success?

T—TRANSFORMATION
- In facing challenges, what brings you experiences of joy?
- What brings out your creativity when you are facing challenges?
- In facing these challenges, what has brought you deep feelings of love?
- When, during this challenging time, have you felt a deep sense of peacefulness?

Source: © 2014 by the International Nurse Coach Association. www.inursecoach.com

Context

Context in a nursing theory is the environment in which nursing acts occur and the nature of the world of nursing. In an integrative nurse coaching environment, the Nurse Coach and the client enter into a unique relationship of trust and mutual respect and engage in a manner that allows for a shift in consciousness and exploration of the client's life's journey, health and wellness goals, healing, and transformation. See Chapter 4 and Nurse Coach competencies.

The Nurse Coach is an instrument in the healing process and a major part of the external healing environment of a client/patient, family, or another person. Nurse Coaches assist and facilitate the individual person/s (client/patient, family, community, etc.) to access their own healing process and potentials; Nurse Coaches do not do the actual healing. The Nurse Coach recognizes her- or himself as a healing environment interacting with a person, family, or colleague in *being with* rather than an always *doing to* or *doing for* another person, and enters into a shared experience (or field of consciousness) that promotes healing potentials and an experience of wellbeing.

A key concept in an integrative healing environment, both interior and exterior, is *meaning*, which addresses that which is indicated, referred to, or signified. See Chapter 5 for details. Relationship-centered care is valued and integrated as it provides the map and highlights the most direct routes to achieve the highest levels of integrative nurse coaching. Context also provides for the creating of a theory structure as discussed next.

Structure

The structure of the Theory of Integrative Nurse Coaching (TINC) is seen in **Figure 2-1e**. All content components are seen as an overlay together. The Nurse Coach and the client enter into a unique relationship of trust and mutual respect and engage in a manner that allows for a shift in consciousness and exploration of the client's life's journey, health and wellness goals, healing, and transformation.

Healing is placed at the center, then the metaparadigm in nursing theory (nurse, person, health, environment [society]), and the patterns of knowing in nursing (personal, empirics, aesthetics, ethics, not knowing, sociopolitical). The TINC five components are represented as a five-circle Venn diagram: (1) Nurse Coach Self-Development, (2) Integral Perspectives and Change, (3) Integrative Lifestyle Health and Wellbeing, (4) Awareness and Choice, and (5) Listening with HEART. The outside dotted circle denotes the exchanging movement of the energy field with the internal and external healing environments that impact all aspects of health and wellbeing, which is described next under the process of a nursing theory.

Process

Process in a nursing theory is the method by which the theory works. Nurse Coaches assist others to discover their own healing path by incorporating integrative modalities in coaching sessions as seen in **Table 2-7**. An integrative *healing process* contains both Nurse Coach processes and client/patient/family and healthcare team and community processes (individual interior and individual exterior), and collective healing processes of individuals and of systems/structures (interior and exterior). This is the understanding of the whole person at the center of care, interacting in mutual process with the environment.

TINC Designated Tool: Integrative Health and Wellness Assessment (IHWA)

The TINC has a designated tool that supports research in the field of nurse coaching—the Integrative Health and Wellness Assessment (IHWA), which is described in Chapter 6 and seen in IHWA (Appendix C-1, short form and Appendix C-2, long form). See Chapter 20 for a discussion of specific research using the IHWA tool and other empirical indicators that can guide clinical practice and nursing education, and generate research questions or develop other paths for healthcare policy.

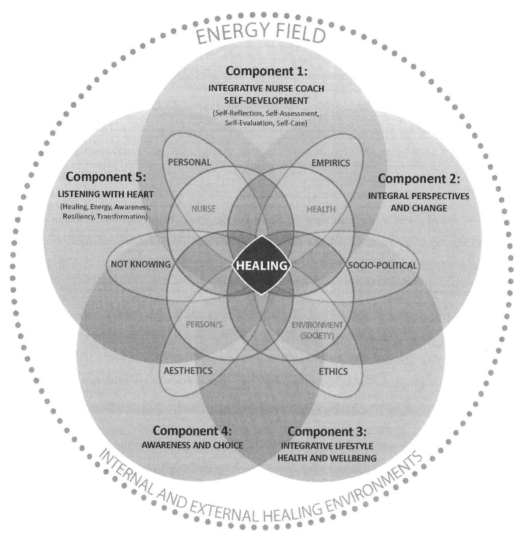

Figure 2-1e Theory of Integrative Nurse Coaching.
Legend. The TINC is an overlay of Healing, Metaparadigm in a Nursing Theory, Patterns of Knowing in Nursing, TINC Five Components, and Energy Field and Internal and External Healing Environments.
Source: Copyright © 2014 by the International Nurse Coach Association. www.inursecoach.com

Table 2-7 Interventions Most Frequently Used in Integrative Nurse Coaching.

Affirmations	Humor and laughter	Presence
Appreciative inquiry	Intention	Probing questions
Aromatherapy	Journaling	Reflection
Art and drawing	Meditation	Relaxation modalities
Celebration	Mindfulness practice	Ritual
Client assessments	Motivational interviewing	Rulers
Cognitive reframing	Movement	Self-assessments
Contracts	Music and sound	Self-care interventions
Deep listening	Nature walks	Self-reflection
Energy practices	Observation	Silence
Exercise	Play	Somatic awareness
Goal setting	Open-ended questions	Stories
Guided imagery	Prayer	Visioning

Source: © 2014 by the International Nurse Coach Association. www.inursecoach.com

SUMMARY

- The Theory of Integrative Nurse Coaching (TINC) is a middle-range theory and is composed of healing, the metaparadigm in nursing theory, patterns of knowing in nursing, five Nurse Coach components [(1) Nurse Coach Self-Development (Self-Reflection, Self-Assessment, Self-Evaluation, and Self-Care; (2) Integral Perspectives and Change; (3) Integrative Lifestyle Health and Wellbeing; (4) Awareness and Choice; and (5) Listening with HEART (**H**ealing, **E**nergy, **A**wareness, **R**esiliency, **T**ransformation)], and energy field and internal and external healing environments. All five Nurse Coach components are *fully integrated* and have equal value.
- The TINC is a middle-range nursing theory to guide nurse coaching practice that is broad enough to be useful in complex situations and leads to implications for education, instrument development, theory testing through research, and nursing practice strategies, and for healthcare policy and reform.
- A middle-range nursing theory is focused in scope on a specific nursing phenomenon that offers a bridge between grand nursing theories that encompass the fullest range or the most global phenomena in the nursing discipline.
- The TINC has a designated tool, the Integrative Health and Wellness Assessment (IHWA), which supports research in the field of nurse coaching.

NURSE COACH REFLECTIONS

After reading this chapter, the Nurse Coach will be able to bring awareness and personal insight to the following questions:

- How am I guided by the Theory of Integrative Nurse Coaching (TINC) in my personal and professional endeavors?
- How do I describe the role of an Integrative Nurse Coach and integrative nurse coaching to colleagues and others?

REFERENCES

Achterberg, J., Dossey, B. M., & Kolkmeier, L. (1994). *Rituals of healing: Using imagery for health and wellness*. New York, NY: Bantam Books.

American Holistic Nurses Association & American Nurses Association (AHNA/ANA) (2013). *Holistic nursing: Scope and standards of practice* (2nd ed.). Silver Spring, MD: Author.

American Holistic Nurses Credentialing Corporation (AHNCC) (n.d.). *AHNCC Nurse Coach Certification*. Retrieved from http://www.ahncc.org/certification/nursecoachnch-wnc.html

American Nurses Association (ANA) (2001). *Code of ethics for nurses with interpretive statements*. Washington, DC: Nursesbooks.org.

American Nurses Association (ANA) (2010a). *Nursing: Scope and standards of nursing practice* (2nd ed.). Silver Spring, MD: Nursesbooks.org.

American Nurses Association (ANA) (2010b). *Nursing's social policy statement: The essence of the profession*. Silver Spring, MD: Nursesbooks.org.

Antonovsky, A. (1996). The salutogenic model as a theory to guide health promotion. *Health Promotion International, 11*(1), 11–18.

Barnum, B. S. (2005). *Nursing theory: Analysis, application, evaluation* (6th ed.). Philadelphia, PA: Lippincott Williams & Wilkins.

Barrett, E. A. M. (2003). Update on a measure of power as knowing participation in change. In O. L. Strickland & C. DiIorio (Eds.), *Measurement of nursing outcomes: Focus on patient/client outcomes* (Vol. 4, pp. 21–39). New York, NY: Springer.

Brown, B. (2012). *Daring greatly. How the courage to be vulnerable transforms the way we live, love, parent, and lead*. New York, NY: Gotham Books.

Carper, B. A. (1978). Fundamental patterns of knowing in nursing. *Advances in Nursing Science 1*(1), 13–23.

Chinn, P. L., & Kramer, M. K. (2010*). Integrated theory and knowledge in nursing* (8th ed.). St. Louis, MO: C. V. Mosby.

Clark, C. C., & Paraska, K. K. (2014). *Health promotion for nurses: A practical guide*. Burlington, MA: Jones & Bartlett Learning.

Cooperrider, D. L., & Whitney, D. (2005). *Appreciative inquiry: A positive revolution in change*. San Francisco, CA: Berrett-Koehler.

Csikszentmihalyi, M. (1990). *Flow: The psychology of optimal experience*. New York, NY: Harper and Row.

Dart, M. A. (2011). *Motivational interviewing in nursing practice*. Sudbury, MA: Jones & Bartlett Learning.

Davidson, A. W., Ray, M. A., & Turkel, M. C. (2011). *Nursing, caring, and complexity science: For human-environment well-being*. New York, NY: Springer.

Dossey, B. M. (2010). *Florence Nightingale: Mystic, visionary, healer* (Commemorative ed.). Philadelphia, PA: F. A. Davis.

Dossey, B. M. (2013). Nursing: Integral, integrative, and holistic—local to global. In B. M. Dossey & L. Keegan (Eds.), *Holistic nursing: A handbook for practice* (6th ed., pp. 1–57). Burlington, MA: Jones & Bartlett Learning.

Dossey, B. M., & Hess, D. R. (2013). Professional nurse coaching: Advances in national and global transformation. *Global Advances in Health and Medicine 2*(4), 10–16.

Dossey, B. M., & Keegan, L. (2013). *Holistic nursing: A handbook for practice* (6th ed., pp. 1–57). Burlington, MA: Jones & Bartlett Learning.

Dossey, B. M., Selanders, L. C., Beck, D. M., & Attewell, A. (2005). *Florence Nightingale today: Healing, leadership, global action*. Silver Spring, MD: Nursesbooks.org.

Dossey, L. (2013). *One mind: How our individual mind is part of a greater consciousness and why it matters*. Carlsbad, CA: Hay House.

Fawcett, J., & DeSanto-Madeya, S. (2000). *Contemporary nursing knowledge: Analysis and evaluation of nursing models and theories* (3rd ed). Philadelphia, PA: F. A. Davis.

Freshwater, D., Taylor, B. J., & Sherwood, G. C. (Eds.) (2008). *The international textbook of reflective practice in nursing*. Chichester, UK: Wiley-Blackwell.

Hess, D. R., Dossey, B. M., Southard, M. E., Luck, S., Schaub, B. G., & Bark, L. (2013). *The art and science of nurse coaching: A provider's guide to scope of practice and competencies*. Silver Spring, MD: Nursesbooks.org.

Institute of Lifestyle Medicine (n.d.). Retrieved from http://www.institutelifestyle medicine.org

Institute of Medicine Future of Nursing Report (2010). Retrieved from http://www.iom.edu/Reports/2010/The-Future-of-Nursing-Leading-Change-Advancing-Health.aspx

Institute for Functional Medicine (n.d.). Retrieved from http://www.ifunctionalmedicine.org

Integrative Nurse Coach Certificate Program (n.d.). Retrieved from http://www.inursecoach.com/programs

International Coach Federation (2011). Individual credentialing core competencies. Retrieved from http://www.coachfederation.org/icfcredentials/core-competencies

International Nurse Coach Association (INCA) (n.d.). Retrieved from http://www.inursecoach.com

Jahn, R. G., & Dunne, B. J. (1987). *Margins of reality: The role of consciousness in the physical world*. New York, NY: Harcourt Brace Jovanovich.

Johns, C. (2013). *Becoming a reflective practitioner* (4th ed.). Hoboken, NJ: Wiley-Blackwell.

Luck, S. (2013). Nutrition. In B. M. Dossey & L. Keegan (Eds.), *Holistic nursing: A handbook for practice* (6th ed., pp. 261–292). Burlington, MA: Jones & Bartlett Learning.

Luck, S., & Keegan, L. (2013). Environmental health. In B. M. Dossey & L. Keegan (Eds.), *Holistic nursing: A handbook for practice* (6th ed., pp. 633–676). Burlington, MA: Jones & Bartlett Learning.

Maddi, S. R., & Khoshaba, D. (2005). *Resilience and work: How to succeed, no matter what life throws at you*. New York, NY: AMACOM.

McCraty, R., & Childres, D. (2010). Coherence: Bridging personal, social, and global health. *Alternative Therapies in Health and Medicine, 16*(4), 10–24.

Miller, W. R., & Rollnick, S. (2002). *Motivational interviewing: Preparing people for change* (2nd ed.). New York, NY: Guilford Press.

Moore, M., & Tschannen-Moran, B. (2010). *Coaching psychology manual*. Philadelphia, PA: Lippincott Williams & Wilkins.

Munhall, P. L. (1993). Unknowing: Toward another pattern of knowing in nursing. *Nursing Outlook 41*(3), 125–128.

National Consortium for the Credentialing of Health and Wellness Coaches (NCCHWC) (2011). *National Consortium for the Credentialing of Health and Wellness Coaches Progress Report—July, 2011*. Retrieved from http://www.wellcoaches.com/images/pdf/progressreport-nationalteam-jul-2011.pdf

Nightingale, F. (1894). Health teaching in towns and villages. In Seymer, L. R. (Ed.). *Selected works of Florence Nightingale* (p. 377). New York, NY: MacMillan.

Nightingale Declaration for a Healthy World (n.d.). Retrieved from http://www.nightingaledeclaration.net/the-declaration

Personalized Lifestyle Medicine Institute (n.d.). Retrieved from http://www.plminstitute.org

Prochaska, J. O., Norcross, J. C., & DiClemente, C. C. (1995). *Changing for good: A revolutionary six-stage program for overcoming bad habits and moving your life positively forward*. New York, NY: Harper Collins.

Richards, K., Sheen, E., & Mazzer, M. C. (2014). *Self-care and you: Caring for the caregiver*. Silver Spring, MD: Nursesbooks.org.

Rollnick, S., Miller, W. R., & Butler, C. C. (2008). *Motivational interviewing in healthcare: Helping patients change behavior*. New York, NY: Guilford Press.

Schaub, B. G., & Burt, M. (2013). Addictions and recovery counseling. In B. M. Dossey & L. Keegan (Eds.), *Holistic nursing: A handbook for practice* (6th ed., pp. 539–562). Burlington, MA: Jones & Bartlett Learning.

Schaub, R., & Schaub, B. G. (2013). *Transpersonal development: Cultivating the human resources of peace, wisdom, purpose and oneness*. Huntington, NY: Florence Press.

Seaward, B. L. (2015). *Managing stress: Principles and strategies for health and well-being*. Burlington, MA: Jones & Bartlett Learning.

Seligman, M. E. P. (1990). *Learned optimism: How to change your mind and your life*. New York, NY: Free Press.

Slater, V. (2013). Energy healing. In B. M. Dossey & L. Keegan (Eds.), *Holistic nursing: A handbook for practice* (6th ed., pp. 751–773). Burlington, MA: Jones & Bartlett Learning.

Smith, M. C., & Parker, M. E. (2014). *Nursing theories and nursing practice* (4th ed.). Philadelphia, PA: F. A. Davis.

Smith, M. J., & Liehr, P. R. (2013). *Middle range theory in nursing* (3rd ed.). New York, NY: Springer.

White, J. (1995). Patterns of knowing: Review, critique, and update. *Advances in Nursing Science 17*(2), 73–86.

Wilber, K. (2000). *Integral psychology: Consciousness, spirit, psychology, therapy*. Boston, MA: Shambhala.

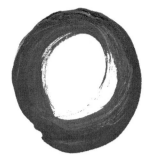

CHAPTER 3

Nurse Coaching and Ethics

Barbara Montgomery Dossey

And how can a Certificate or public register show this? Rather, she ought to have a moral 'Clinical' Thermometer in herself... Nursing work must be quiet work—An individual work—Anything else is contrary to the whole realness of the work. Where am I, the individual, in my utmost soul? What am I, the inner woman, called 'I'?—That is the question.

Florence Nightingale, 1888

LOOKING AHEAD...

After reading this chapter, you will be able to:

- Identify how nurse coaching embodies the ethics of caring and compassion.
- Examine ethics principles, traditional ethical theories, and a typology of moral concerns that influence life, work, and society.
- Analyze ethical principles presented in three different nursing codes of ethics that are applicable in nurse coaching.
- Examine how respect is central to a Nurse Coach ethical framework.
- Explore how relational knowing and embodied knowing are a starting point for ethical inquiry in nurse coaching.
- Discuss advocacy as part of nursing's moral foundation.
- Define decent care.

DEFINITIONS

Authentic advocacy: Refers to actions—taken on behalf of others—that arise from a deep alignment of one's beliefs, values, and behaviors; the ability to be present for all levels of suffering, to acknowledge the suffering of others, to transform this suffering, and to engage in helping those who suffer (Rushton, in press).

Earth ethics: A code of behavior that incorporates the understanding that the Earth community has core value in and of itself and includes ethical treatment of the nonhuman world and the Earth as a whole. This code influences the way that we individually and collectively interact with the environment and all beings of the Earth (Burkhardt & Keegan, 2013).

Embodied knowing: Recognition of every person as living in her/his body in-the-world, which is a way of coming to know the relationship of self-to-self and self-to-others.

Engagement: A capacity to connect and be with another in an intersubjective, mutual, and authentic manner while honoring complexity and ambiguity.

Ethics: Offers a critical, rational, defensible, systematic, and intellectual approach to determining what the right way to behave is. Concerned with our behavior, the choices we make, our intentions, and our character.

Ethical deliberation: Informs ethical reflection and involves a process of discernment, analysis, and articulation of ethically defensible solutions. The goal is not absolute certainty but reliability in our behavior, choices, and character.

Ethical reasoning: Involves disciplined and critical reflection on ambiguity. There may be uncertainty about what is the "right" or proper thing to do or end to pursue or value conflicts about what ought to be done or what ends we seek.

Holistic ethics: The basic underlying concept of the study of unity and integral wholeness of all people and of all nature, which is identified and pursued by finding unity and wholeness within one's self and within humanity. In this framework, acts are not performed for the sake of law, precedent, or social norms, but rather from a desire to do good freely and to witness, identify, and contribute to unity (Burkhardt & Keegan, 2013).

Morals: Standards of right and wrong that are learned through socialization.

Nursing ethics: A discipline-specific code of values and behaviors that influence the way nurses work with clients/patients in their care, with one another, and with society.

Personal ethics: A person's code of beliefs and values that guides her/his actions.

Relational knowing: Coming to know the client and her/his autonomy and respecting the wishes as a person who has decision-making capacity and ability to choose.

Respect: The act of feeling esteem for or honoring another; an act that demands we have a sense of authenticity, integrity, and self-knowledge to appreciate the uniqueness and essence of another; exhibited through words, deeds, and behaviors; the recipient experiences reverence, worthiness, a sense of being seen, heard, and honored (Rushton, in press).

Values: The capacity for choosing and caring about what is moral and ethical in personal behavior/s and action/s.

Values clarification: A process of becoming more aware of how life values are established and how these values influence one's life.

NURSE COACHING, CARING, AND COMPASSION

Nurse coaching is indeed an ethics of caring and compassion. Nurses Coaches strive to maximize the good (autonomy, comfort, dignity, quality of life) and minimize the bad (pain, suffering). It is listening with intention and from a heart space to the client's stories/narratives, history, experiences, and perceptions. The Nurse Coach conveys the ethics of caring and compassion by asking curious questions that are interspersed with authentic statements such as, "What do you want to discuss today?" "I see you," "I hear you," "I am walking with you," "What do you want me to know most about you?" "I am learning and understanding how you relate to the world and others," "In our session today where do you want to be by the end of the session?" "What was one 'pearl of insight' for you in today's coaching session?"

From an integral perspective, these Nurse Coach curious questions and authentic statements reflect the subjective "I" that explores the many dimensions of being in the world, while assisting the client to reflect and respond in her/his own time to what is manifesting and emergent in the moment and in the coaching relationship. It is also the "We" of the shared intersubjective presence and the interactions between the Nurse Coach and client. See Chapter 14.

Nurse Coach actions are performed for a desire to do good freely and to witness, identify, and contribute to unity; they are not performed for the sake of law, precedent, or social norms. Nurse Coaches fully engage with clients, which implies a capacity to connect to and be with another in an intersubjective, mutual, and authentic manner while honoring complexity and ambiguity. Nurse Coaches view clients, others, and society from a unity and integral wholeness that reflect the fundamental values of a client-centered, integrative, integral, and holistic relationship (Dossey, 2013).

The purpose of this chapter is to first present a review of ethical principles, traditional ethical theories and systems, and a typology of ethical concerns. Three professional nursing organizations' codes of ethics that Nurse Coaches adhere to in nurse coaching will be presented. Next, the topics of respect, relational knowing and embodied knowing, authentic advocacy, and Earth ethics are discussed with their relevance to nurse coaching. For a full discussion on nursing ethics and ethical theories, see Burkhardt & Keegan (2013) and Burkhardt and Nathanial (2013), and other books and articles on nursing, medical, and interprofessional ethics. In the next section, an ethics overview is presented.

ETHICS OVERVIEW

Ethics is the study or discipline concerned with our behavior, the choices we make, our intentions, and our character. This includes judgments of right and wrong, approval and disapproval, good and bad, virtue and vice, and desirability and wisdom of actions, as well as dispositions, ends, objectives, states of affairs, and the disciplined reflections on the moral choices that people make (Burkhardt & Keegan, 2013). Nurse Coaches recognize nursing ethics as a discipline-specific code of values and behaviors that influence the way they work with clients/patients in their care, with one another, and with society. Values are the capacity for choosing and caring about what is moral and ethical in personal behavior/s and action/s. Values clarification is a process of becoming more aware of how life values are established and how these values influence one's life.

Nurse Coaches follow ethical guidelines set by the nursing profession as they coach clients/patients and families/significant others on topics and concerns related to healthier lifestyles, life balance, healthcare decisions, treatments, and/or ending treatments, and how to build healthy communities and more. Nurse Coaches explore ethical principles and theories to fully participate in ethical decision-making. Holding an integrative, integral, and holistic worldview, Nurse Coaches incorporate the bio–psycho–social–spiritual–cultural–environmental aspects in coaching around ethical issues. Ethical principles listed in **Table 3-1** suggest direction and proposed behaviors and moral actions for resolving conflicts or competing claims. They are neither rules (means) nor values (ends). These principles are universal in nature and not absolute, and are unchangeable and discovered by individuals rather than invented. **Table 3-2** provides an overview of the traditional ethical theories and styles. **Table 3-3** presents a typology of ethical concerns.

When ethical concerns arise, Nurse Coaches seek the consultation of nurse ethicists and nurse colleagues and others with experience in dealing with the ethical deliberation and ethical reasoning within the complexity of ethical dilemmas and circumstances (Rushton, 2007). Ethical deliberation informs ethical reflection and involves a process of discernment, analysis, and articulation of ethically defensible solutions. The goal is not absolute certainty but reliability in our behavior, choices, and character. Ethical reasoning involves disciplined and critical reflection on ambiguity. There may be uncertainty about what is the "right" or proper thing to do or end to pursue or value conflicts about what ought to be done or what ends we seek. To apply this information in everyday practice, three different nursing codes of ethics are discussed in the next section.

Table 3-1 Ethics Principles.

Beneficence:	To engage in actions that benefits others.
Nonmaleficence:	To do no harm to others.
Veracity:	To be truthful and to disclose information.
Justice:	To distribute benefits and harms fairly.
Fidelity:	To keep promises and contracts.
Reparation:	To make up for a wrong.
Gratitude:	To make up for a good.
Autonomy:	To respect the wishes of a person who is required to have decision-making capacity in order to choose.
Informed consent:	Four elements as follows: (1) The person must possess decision-making capacity; (2) Pertinent information is disclosed; (3) Comprehension or understanding of the information is assured; (4) Consent is given voluntarily without coercion.
Confidentiality:	To respect privacy and protect confidential information.
Utility:	The greatest good or least harm for the greatest number.
Universality:	The same principle must hold for everyone regardless of time, place, or persons involved.

Source: Adapted by Barbara M. Dossey. With permission from Burkhardt, M. A., & Keegan, L. (2013). Holistic ethics. In B. M. Dossey & L. Keegan (Eds.), *Holistic nursing: A handbook for practice* (6th ed., pp. 129–141). Burlington, MA: Jones & Bartlett Learning.

Table 3-2 Traditional Ethical Theories and Styles.

Aristotelian Theory. Aristotle (384–322 BCE) believed that an individual who practices the virtues of courage, temperance, integrity, justice, honesty, and truthfulness will know almost intuitively what to do in a particular situation or conflict.

Kantian Theory. Emmanuel Kant (1724–1804) formulated the categorical imperative that acts on all people, regardless of their interests or desires; it is the historical Christian idea known as the Golden Rule, "So act in such a way as your act becomes a universal for all mankind." Kant was concerned with the "personhood" of human beings and "persons" as moral agents.

Utilitarianism Theory. Jeremy Bentham (1748–1832) and John Stuart Mill (1806–1873) held that the proper course of action is the one that maximizes total benefit and reduces suffering or the negatives. It helps in the art of decision-making. The consequences of man's actions are the primary concern, "it is the greatest happiness of the greatest number that is the measure of right and wrong."

Natural Rights Theory. John Locke (1632–1714) declared that individuals have fundamental inalienable rights of life, liberty, and property that can never be taken away. Most fundamental human law was preservation of humankind, and they are free to make choices about how to conduct their lives. Property not only included land and goods, but ownership of one's self and a right to personal wellbeing.

Social Contract Theory or Contractarian Theory. Thomas Hobbes (1588–1679) declared that humans by their very nature have a self-interest, thus he contended that all morality involves a social contract indicating what individuals can and cannot do.

(continues on next page)

Table 3-2 (*Continued*).

Deontologic System and Teleologic System. (Two traditional forms)

> **Deontologic System.** (Greek root meaning "knowledge of that which is binding and proper"). Focuses upon adherence to independent moral rules or duties. By understanding our moral duties and the correct rules that exist to regulate those duties, we can make correct moral choices. By following our duty, we are behaving morally. When we fail to follow our duty, we are behaving immorally.

> **Teleologic System** (Greek root meaning "knowledge of the ends"). Assigns duty or obligation based on the consequences of the act. Action is morally defensible on the basis of its extrinsic value or outcome.

Source: Adapted by Barbara M. Dossey. With permission from Burkhardt, M. A., & Keegan, L. (2013). Holistic ethics. In B. M. Dossey & L. Keegan (Eds.), *Holistic nursing: A handbook for practice* (6th ed., pp. 129–141). Burlington, MA: Jones & Bartlett Learning.

Table 3-3 Typology of Ethical Concerns.

Moral uncertainty:	Occurs when one is unable to define the moral problem or is unsure what moral principles apply.
Moral conflict:	Occurs when a tension exists between moral values or principles, or there is disagreement about which moral values or principles apply or about the proper course of action to pursue in a situation. Conflicts are often amenable to clarification, dialogue, and negotiation.
Moral dilemmas:	Occur when there are two or more clear moral principles applied but they support mutually inconsistent courses of action. Pursuing either course of action violates important principles. There is an irreconcilable conflict that no amount of clarification and application can erase. Moral dilemmas are reserved for refractory moral conflicts. They often involve unyielding elements, grave harms, moral crisis, and tragic choices. Resolution of a dilemma requires fundamental changes in attitudes and/or actions.
Moral distress:	Occurs when one knows the "right" thing to do but is unable to act upon it. The inability to act threatens one's integrity.

Source: Used with permission from Jameton, A. (1984). *Nursing practice: The ethical issues.* Englewood Cliffs, NJ: Prentice-Hall.

NURSING CODES OF ETHICS

Nurse Coaches adhere to the professional code of ethics set forth by the American Nurses Association and the specific nursing specialty organization codes of ethics. For the purpose of this chapter, three codes of ethics are presented: (1) the American Nurses Association (ANA) Code of Ethics with Interpretative Statements (ANA, 2001), **Table 3-4**; (2) the American Holistic Nurses Association (AHNA) Code of Ethics (AHNA, 2012), **Table 3-5**; and (3) the International Council of Nurses (ICN) Code of Ethics (ICN, 2012), **Table 3-6**. See the end of the chapter for Tables 3-4, 3-5, 3-6. The Nurse Coach description below following the ANA Standard 7: Ethics (Hess et al., 2013) (see Chapter 4):

The Nurse Coach:

1. Uses the *Code of Ethics for Nurses with Interpretive Statements* (ANA, 2001) to guide practice and communicate the foundation of the professional nurse coaching practice.
2. Clearly communicates to the client and others the distinctions among coaching, consulting, counseling, and teaching.

3. Provides coaching in a manner that recognizes and respects the client's autonomy, dignity, rights, values, and beliefs.
4. Maintains an effective coaching relationship that is congruent with the coaching agreement and within the boundaries of professional nursing practice.
5. Values all life experiences as opportunities to find personal meaning and cultivate self-awareness, self-reflection, and growth.
6. Maintains client confidentiality within legal and regulatory parameters.

The ANA, AHNA, and ICN codes of ethics contain content of the International Coach Federation (ICF) Code of Ethics (ICF, 2011). To further the understanding of ethics concepts, the meaning of respect is discussed next.

MEANING OF RESPECT

Nurse Coaches understand that respect is foundational to understanding professional roles, relationships, and responsibilities. Respect is the act of feeling esteem for or honoring another; it is an act that demands we have a sense of authenticity, integrity, self-knowledge, and appreciation of the uniqueness of another, as well as for ourselves (Rushton, in press). It is rooted in our internal beliefs about how we value another human being. Respect is central to a Nurse Coach ethical framework and for appreciation of the dimensions of multiculturalism, understandings of culture, and the rich understanding of self and others (Rushton, 2007; 2009). See Chapter 18.

Understanding of these ethical imperatives highlights the many opportunities for expanding our notion of what respect requires of us in our everyday interactions. Nurse Coaches engage with the client and others with respect that allows for the deep trusting relationship that honors the wholeness and the essence of the other. As Nurse Coaches demonstrate respect through words, behaviors, and actions, the client or others experience a sense of being heard, seen, and honored. The client feels honored and open to discovery about different choices. This includes respecting their boundaries for privacy by telling the truth, keeping promises, and being trustworthy (Dossey, 2013).

Nurse Coaches are aware that in our interprofessional endeavors, respect should not become confused or trivial. Respect is not about liking someone, condoning the decisions or behaviors of others, or avoiding conflict. Respecting clients, colleagues, or others because they are human beings is different from respecting them for what they know or for their title or position (Rushton, in press). Demonstrating respect becomes very challenging when we find ourselves in situations where our values conflict, or we do not agree with the decisions of others, or we find the personality of the person offensive. This is extremely important in nurse coaching when a client makes decisions that Nurse Coaches do not endorse. This requires deep listening to what clients are saying and to be careful not to engage in behaviors aimed at convincing them of our way of thinking, rather than accepting their informed choices.

RELATIONAL KNOWING AND EMBODIED KNOWING

Nurse Coaches enter into a coaching relationship that is both relational knowing and embodied knowing and a starting point for ethical inquiry (Wright & Brajtman, 2011). Relational knowing is coming to know the client through narratives that start with her/his autonomy and respecting the wishes of a person who has decision-making capacity and ability to choose. Autonomy, as a lived experience, is a relational experience that involves both independence and interdependence.

Embodied knowing is the recognition of every person as living in her/his body in-the-world, which is a way of coming to know self-to-self and self-to-others. Being a nurse implies an intimacy that is part of nursing practice and education. At some point in the everyday of nursing practice, nurses come to know people in the most intimate ways, particularly when a person is very ill and her/his bodily functions are beyond control. Every nurse knows this intimacy as a past experience or a present lived experience that resides in the deep understanding of another and in the nursing role. This has been called the "ethic of intimates" and is consistent with nursing's history of orienting our moral compass towards issues of everyday practice (Wright & Brajtman, 2011). Thus, this embedded consciousness and intimacy lives within the soul of each Nurse Coach and is part of "being with" another.

Within the coaching relationship the Nurse Coach recognizes the client's uniqueness and individuality that is always emerging. It is through the discovery process and rediscovery that hunches, intuition, and new insights are allowed to emerge. Nurse Coaching is listening to the client and to the meaning that is constructed in the moment. This is the meaning-making that is placed within the context and situation/s that are arising in the client's life. From this emerges the client's potential to become more aware and to make choices that reflect personal values and beliefs towards her/his health, which is embodied in the coaching process.

As the Nurse Coach and client relationship evolves, it becomes a co-created lived story with a new sense of meaning through insights that lead to healthy life choices, new possibilities and experiences, ways to form healthier relationships, and much more. Wright & Brajtman (2011), quoting Gadow (1996), state that the existential meaning of an ethical dilemma is "the lack of a livable story describing the good." Gadow further suggests that for a story to be habitable, it must be coauthored by both nurse and patient in contextual relation. See Chapter 5 on Story Theory and Story-Health Model.

A central question of a relational ethic becomes "Can we (authors of the ethical story) live with this?" Nurse Coaches must reflect on their own desires and motivations, remembering that the client is the author of the story. In a relational approach to ethical decision-making, the boundaries of traditional decision-making models (describing the problem, elucidating conflicts, identifying principles, implementing solutions, etc.) require that more basic questions about moral experience are asked, such as "What are you going through right now?" "What is the best thing to do in this situation?" "How might I understand your experience?" The following vignette illustrates the relational knowing and embodied knowing that occur within a Nurse Coach and client coaching relationship.

Vignette: Mary

Mary is a 74-year-old, vibrant community educator and national leader, who has recently been diagnosed with breast cancer. Her oncologist wanted her to have a mastectomy, radiation, and chemotherapy within a week of diagnosis. However, Mary felt overwhelmed and wanted time to make sense of her diagnosis and to decide what she needed with the support of her family and a few close friends. Mary was referred to a Nurse Coach, who listened deeply to her story and also shared some breath awareness practices and imagery during this challenging time. A month later Mary made the decision to have a mastectomy, radiation, and chemotherapy while also receiving acupuncture, massage, and a new vitamin regimen to boost her immune system. Below is a note that Mary wrote to her Nurse Coach three months after her surgery, radiation, and chemotherapy.

> I tend to live so much in my head and thinking self that I find it quite challenging to let go of this and simply be...and allow next steps to unfold. When I first began work with Dr. R, he made a statement which I immediately knew was toxic and one I did

not want to internalize. He said innocently and honestly that cancer can be seemingly eliminated and then unexpectedly for unknown reasons "come roaring back" and that was so scary and alarming. The power of hearing this from a highly respected oncologist, I knew could have a potentially negative power (reverse placebo effect) that I did not want to internalize. I knew the power of strongly believing in my body's capacity to heal itself. Yet try as I may I could not erase this powerful visual thought from my mind. It was like trying to NOT think of pink elephants. They rebelliously dance in front of my eyes and through my mind endlessly. The harder I try to NOT think of them, the more they take center stage.

Thanks for your support and helping me to know that I didn't have to race to have surgery, radiation, and chemo the next week, but to take the time to sort out my options. I think you will enjoy this discovery about my immune system. As I was listening to your relaxation and imagery tape, I realized I could instead use the phrase, "now shine the powerful light on a long bone, perhaps a leg bone and see the millions, billions of white blood cells being born every minute and see them moving through your body, searching out anything that does not contribute to your health and destroying it..." Now I smile warmly anytime the thought comes to me that I choose not to own regarding cancer cells and simply "shine the light on a long bone and visualize and feel the power of my amazing immune system guarding, protecting and preserving the magical balance of wellness by searching out and destroying any unwelcomed invaders."

Thanks for standing with me during those dark times of trying to decide on surgery, radiation, and chemo, while you gave me some ways to find my center again. I find myself in a very different space now with a very different awareness. I am learning to release the sense of control that I have for so long focused to achieve in every area of my life. Something new is emerging that I can't express in words but that I feel blessed by. I have a greater sense of simply showing up to serve, learn, participate and appreciate.

I am so happy that seeing a Nurse Coach was offered to me. You did an incredibly thorough job of studying my personal health history and advising me. I made an appointment with the functional medicine doctor you recommended before my surgery and treatment. You have validated the message from all the healers I am working with. I was very impressed that you were so familiar with all the modalities and even the individuals I was working with. You helped me hear my own intuition even more clearly and feel very, very encouraged by where I am already.

I am confident that I will heal completely and will be eager to help women around me learn from my journey...and am amazed at how my body-mind-spirit is responding. Each time I open myself to new learning, something amazing happens. I get confused as my logic tries to sort everything out as in, "Which way is the right way? Just show me that one right way and don't confuse me." Then I realize that surrendering into new modes of learning might be part of the journey.

One of many gifts from my journey through cancer and back to perfect health is the much deeper sense of transformation thanks to new daily practices such as deep breathing, meditation, long walks...in addition to other long enjoyed practices. And when I say, "perfect health" I mean to include the ambiguity that will always be part of this. How can we know we are in perfect health? Yet, daring to believe that our body-mind-spirit knows how to bring this powerful balance.

My role is to make daily choices that nurture unconditional love and bring healing energy not just to me but also to the community around us. Surrendering into not knowing yet daring to believe is for me part of the journey of faith. I find that I am very much in my head and this can limit my ability to listen to and trust my body and the many nonlogical ways of being in the world.

I find it very encouraging that there seems to be an awakening that is growing around health and wellness and our personal responsibility for our choices and ways of being. This is to do the best we can and then surrender to what is without judging.

In Mary's story we see how the Nurse Coach entered into full engagement, to connect and be with Mary in an intersubjective, mutual, and authentic manner while honoring complexity and ambiguity. The Nurse Coach interaction reveals the genuine engagement and ethics of caring and compassion and an integrative approach using the Integrative Health and Wellness Assessment (Appendix C-2). The Nurse Coach listened to and supported Mary so that she could drop into her suffering and despair, tap into her inner wisdom and find her own answers without feeling rushed, and come to terms with her situation. She chose surgery, chemotherapy, and radiation and chose her own integrative practitioners and integrative approaches that were powerful for her fast healing. See Chapter 5 on suffering and the Nurse Coach Five-Step Process. To further this discussion of relational knowing and embodied knowing in ethics, authentic advocacy is discussed next.

AUTHENTIC ADVOCACY

Nursing organizations have codes of ethics recognizing advocacy as nursing's moral foundation as seen in the ANA (Table 3-4), AHNA (Table 3-5), and ICN codes of ethics (Table 3-6). The word "advocacy" is derived from the Latin *advocatus,* "counselor," and *advocare,* "to summon or to aid." Coined by Rushton (Rushton, in press), "authentic advocacy" refers to actions—taken on behalf of others—that arise from a deep alignment of one's beliefs, values, and behaviors, which is in her model of "compassion-based ethics"—the ability to be present for all levels of suffering, to acknowledge the suffering of others, to transform this suffering, and to engage in helping those who suffer.

Nurse Coaches strive for authenticity in action as a foundational element of integrity, as well as a foundation that allows for meaning, service, and fulfillment to arise. Similarly, in this context, authenticity also refers to alignment with the beliefs, values, and desired actions of those who are in need of advocacy. This connotes an "egoless" engagement with the other—or others—for the purpose of both benefitting them and serving from one's own highest purpose.

When applied to nurse coaching, authentic advocacy and compassion-based ethics are the intrinsic moral foundation of Nurse Coaches. We are each morally required to demonstrate—in all interactions—*respect* for the inherent human dignity of individuals, including the "self" of each nurse, as well as for patients and continuity of care. An authentic advocate understands the foundational principle of respect—the act of esteeming one another and attending to the whole person perspectives marked by cultural humility. As authentic advocates, Nurse Coaches demonstrate self-awareness with clearly defined values and the knowledge and skills of ethical discernment, analysis, and action. These authentic advocacy concepts are directly linked to decent care, which is discussed next.

DECENT CARE

Nurse Coaches extend their nurse coaching into communities to reach the underserved and to recognize concepts within decent care. Decent care is about health for all, which leads to flourishing (NIGH, n.d.). Human flourishing begins with building healthy people, neighborhoods, communities, and nations (Beck, Dossey, & Rushton, 2014).

Decent care is a comprehensive, care continuum approach that is integral, integrative, and holistic (Ferguson, Karpf, Weait, & Swift, 2010). It is inclusive where individuals are afforded dignity and a destigmatized space to take control of their own destinies. It considers the care and health-related services (physical, preventative, therapeutic, economic, emotional, and spiritual aspects, etc.), and the person's (includes family, significant others) needs, expectations, and desires. Decent care has six key values that parallel an integral perspective (see Chapter 14) as follows:

1. Agency and 2. Dignity—*individual level.*
3. Interdependence and 4. Solidarity—*social level.*
5. Subsidiarity and 6. Sustainability—*systemic level.*

Agency comes from the Latin verb *agere*, which means to drive, lead, act, or do. Agency is the heart of decent care. Without providing the space for, acknowledging, and responding to and respecting the agency of the individual, care is not decent. This is crucial to anyone in a position of vulnerability to own her/his individual response/s. This means that every person has the capacity to direct her or his own care. *Dignity* represents the humanity of decent care. Without honoring the unique individuality and worth of the "life world" the individual has constructed—her/his needs, desires, relationships, and values—care is not decent (Ferguson et al., 2010).

Interdependence represents the reciprocity of decent care. Without actively participating in our own caring process and the caring process of others, care is not decent. *Solidarity* represents the communal spirit of decent care. Without being actively responsible for each other's wellbeing and advocating for each other's needs, care is not decent (Ferguson et al., 2010).

Subsidiarity instructs that people closest to where the care is being offered should allocate resources responsibly. *Sustainability* is the future and legacy of decent care. Without careful stewardship of resources and short- and long-term planning to ensure the ongoing regeneration and evolution of care processes, care is not decent (Karpf, Ferguson, Swift, & Lazarus, 2008).

Nurse Coaches are aware of the challenges of a changing world of individuals' unmet healthcare needs. Three basic questions shape the Nurse Coach approach, the course, and the purpose of decent care in their nurse coaching endeavors (Ferguson et al., 2010):

*   What do (I/you/we) need now?
*   How do (I/you/we) live in the face of life/death/wellness/disease?
*   How might (I/you/we) flourish?

With an awareness of the decent care model, nurse coaching can further advance the health framework—local to global. The main reason is that Nurse Coaches have an approach to "be with" and do not tell clients/patients and others what to do. There is a balance of power between the Nurse Coach and the client—between those who are receiving care and those providing care. To further understand decent care, Nurse Coaches also address Earth ethics, which is explored next.

EARTH ETHICS

Nurse Coaches believe that Earth ethics are essential for healthy people living on a healthy planet. This is a code of behavior that incorporates the understanding that the Earth community has core value in and of itself and includes ethical treatment of the nonhuman world and the Earth as a whole which influences the way that we individually and collectively interact with the environment and all beings of the Earth (Burkhardt & Keegan, 2013).

To further this commitment to Earth ethics, the Earth Charter is a declaration of fundamental principles for building a just, sustainable, and peaceful global society in the

21st century (Earth Charter, n.d.). It seeks to inspire in all peoples a new sense of global interdependence and shared responsibility for the wellbeing of the human family and the larger living world. It is an expression of hope and a call to help create a global partnership at a critical juncture in history. The Charter for Compassion (Charter for Compassion, 2008) urges the peoples and religions of the world to embrace the core value of compassion. The Nightingale Initiative for Global Health (NIGH, n.d.) and its *Nightingale Declaration for a Healthy World* (Nightingale Declaration, n.d.) are also a way to increase global public awareness about the priority of human health and an Earth ethic. See Chapter 1, Figure 1-1.

Nurse Coaches understand that Earth ethics requires a shift in consciousness and in our beliefs, attitudes, and worldviews about the interdependence of all of life. An Earth ethic declares that we are all "one mind" and that our individual minds are part of a greater consciousness, and this matters in how we see our role with all humanity and a healthy world—local to global (Dossey, L. 2013).

SUMMARY

- Ethics is the study or discipline concerned with our behavior, the choices we make, our intentions, and our character.
- Nurses Coaches strive to maximize the good (autonomy, comfort, dignity, quality of life) and minimize the bad (pain, suffering), which is the ethics of caring and compassion.
- Nurse Coaches adhere to the professional code of ethics set forth by the American Nurses Association and other specific nursing specialty organization codes of ethics.
- Nurse Coaches enter into a coaching relationship that is both relational knowing and embodied knowing and a starting point for ethical inquiry.
- Nursing organizations have codes of ethics recognizing advocacy as nursing's moral foundation.
- Decent care is a comprehensive, care continuum approach that is integral, integrative, and holistic.

NURSE COACH REFLECTIONS

After reading this chapter, the Nurse Coach will be able to bring awareness and personal insight to the following questions:

- What ethical principles can I identify in each of the ANA, AHNA, and ICN codes of ethics?
- What do each of these ANA, AHNA, and ICN codes of ethics statements mean to me as related to my coaching clients/patients and others?
- What new insights do I have about nurse coaching and ethics and my personal values that influence my life, work, and society.
- In what ways do I understand the concept of respect in coaching clients and others?
- What new insights do I have about relational knowing and embodied knowing in nurse coaching?
- How do I advocate for myself and my needs at home and work?
- What new insights do I have about Earth ethics?

Table 3-4 American Nurses Association (ANA) Code of Ethics for Nurses with Interpretative Statements.

1. The nurse, in all professional relationships, practices with compassion and respect for the inherent dignity, worth, and uniqueness of every individual, unrestricted by considerations of social or economic status, personal attributes, or the nature of health problems.
2. The nurse's primary commitment is to the patient, whether an individual, family, group, or community.
3. The nurse promotes, advocates for, and strives to protect the health, safety, and rights of the patient.
4. The nurse is responsible and accountable for individual nursing practice and determines the appropriate delegation of tasks consistent with the nurse's obligation to provide optimum patient care.
5. The nurse owes the same duties to self as to others, including the responsibility to preserve integrity and safety, to maintain competence, and to continue personal and professional growth.
6. The nurse participates in establishing, maintaining, and improving healthcare environments and conditions of employment conducive to the provision of quality healthcare and consistent with the values of the profession through individual and collective action.
7. The nurse participates in the advancement of the profession through contributions to practice, education, administration, and knowledge development.
8. The nurse collaborates with other health professionals and the public in promoting community, national, and international efforts to meet health needs.
9. The profession of nursing, as represented by associations and their members, is responsible for articulating nursing values, for maintaining the integrity of the profession and its practice, and for shaping social policy.

Source: Used with permission. Copyright © 2001 by the American Nurses Association, Silver Spring, MD: Nursesbooks.org. http://www.nursingworld.org

Table 3-5 American Holistic Nurses Association (AHNA) Code of Ethics for Holistic Nurses.

We believe that the fundamental responsibilities of the nurse are to promote health, facilitate healing and alleviate suffering. The need for nursing is universal. Inherent in nursing is the respect for life, dignity and right of all persons. Nursing care is given a context mindful of the holistic nature of humans, understanding the body–mind–emotion–spirit. Nursing care is unrestricted by considerations of nationality, race, creed, color, age, sex, sexual preferences, politics or social status. Given that nurses practice in culturally diverse settings, professional nurses must have an understanding of the cultural background of clients in order to provide culturally appropriate interventions. Nurses render services to clients who can be individuals, families, groups or communities. The client is an active participant in health care and should be included in all nursing care planning decisions. To provide services to others, each nurse has a responsibility towards the client, co-workers, nursing practice, the profession of nursing, society and the environment.

Nurses and Self
The nurse has a responsibility to model health care behaviors. Holistic nurses strive to achieve harmony in their own lives and assist others striving to do the same.

Nurses and the Client
The nurse's primary responsibility is to the client needing nursing care. The nurse strives to see the client as a whole and provides care that is professionally appropriate and culturally consonant. The nurse holds in confidence all information obtained in professional practice and uses professional judgment in disclosing such information. The nurse enters into a relationship with the client that is guided by mutual respect and a desire for growth and development.

(continues on next page)

Table 3-5 (*Continued*).

Nurses and Co-Workers

The nurse maintains cooperative relationships with co-workers in nursing and other fields. Nurses have a responsibility to nurture each other and to assist nurses to work as a team in the interest of client care. If a client's care is endangered by a co-worker, the nurse must take appropriate action on behalf of the client.

Nurses and Nursing Practice

The nurse carries personal responsibility for practice and for maintaining continued competence. Nurses have the right to use all appropriate nursing interventions, and have the obligation to determine the efficacy and safety of all nursing actions. Wherever applicable, nurses use research findings in directing practice.

Nurses and the Profession

The nurse plays a role in determining and implementing desirable standards of nursing practice and education and research. Holistic nurses may assume a leadership position to guide the profession towards a holistic philosophy of practices. Nurses support nursing research and the development of holistically oriented nursing theories. The nurse participates in establishing and maintaining equitable social and economic working conditions in nursing.

Nurses and Society

The nurse, along with other citizens, has the responsibility for initiating and supporting actions to meet the health and social needs of all society.

Nurses and the Environment

Nurses strive to create a client environment to be one of peace, harmony, and nurturance so that healing may take place. The nurse considers the health of the ecosystem in relation to the need for health, safety and peace of all persons.

Source: Used with permission. Copyright © 2012 by the American Holistic Nurses Association. http://www.ahna.org

Table 3-6 International Council of Nurses (ICN) Elements of the Code of Ethics.

An international code of ethics for nurses was first adopted by the International Council of Nurses (ICN) in 1953. It has been revised and reaffirmed at various times since, most recently with this review and revision completed in 2012.

Nurses have four fundamental responsibilities: to promote health, to prevent illness, to restore health and to alleviate suffering. The need for nursing is universal.

Inherent in nursing is a respect for human rights, including cultural rights, the right to life and choice, to dignity and to be treated with respect. Nursing care is respectful of and unrestricted by considerations of age, colour, creed, culture, disability or illness, gender, sexual orientation, nationality, politics, race or social status.

Nurses render health services to the individual, the family and the community and coordinate their services with those of related groups.

The ICN Code of Ethics for Nurses has four principal elements that outline the standards of ethical conduct.

1. Nurses and people

- The nurse's primary professional responsibility is to people requiring nursing care. In providing care, the nurse promotes an environment in which the human rights, values, customs and spiritual beliefs of the individual, family and community are respected.
- The nurse ensures that the individual receives sufficient information on which to base consent for care and related treatment.

(continues on next page)

Table 3-6 (*Continued*).

- The nurse holds in confidence personal information and uses judgment in sharing this information.
- The nurse shares with society the responsibility for initiating and supporting action to meet the health and social needs of the public, in particular those of vulnerable populations.
- The nurse also shares responsibility to sustain and protect the natural environment from depletion, pollution, degradation and destruction.

2. Nurses and practice
- The nurse carries personal responsibility and accountability for nursing practice, and for maintaining competence by continual learning.
- The nurse maintains a standard of personal health such that the ability to provide care is not compromised.
- The nurse uses judgment regarding individual competence when accepting and delegating responsibility.
- The nurse at all times maintains standards of personal conduct which reflect well on the profession and enhance public confidence.
- The nurse, in providing care, ensures that use of technology and scientific advances are compatible with the safety, dignity and rights of people.

3. Nurses and the profession
- The nurse assumes the major role in determining and implementing acceptable standards of clinical nursing practice, management, research and education.
- The nurse is active in developing a core of research-based professional knowledge.
- The nurse, acting through the professional organisation, participates in creating and maintaining equitable social and economic working conditions in nursing.

4. Nurses and co-workers
- The nurse sustains a co-operative relationship with co-workers in nursing and other fields.
- The nurse takes appropriate action to safeguard individuals when their care is endangered by a co-worker or any other person.

SUGGESTIONS FOR USE of the ICN Code of Ethics for Nurses

The ICN Code of Ethics for Nurses is a guide for action based on social values and needs. It will have meaning only as a living document if applied to the realities of nursing and health care in a changing society. To achieve its purpose the Code must be understood, internalised and used by nurses in all aspects of their work. It must be available to students and nurses throughout their study and work lives.

Source: Used with permission. Copyright © 2012 by the International Council of Nurses, Geneva, Switzerland. http://www.icn.ch

REFERENCES

American Holistic Nurses Association (AHNA) (2012). *AHNA position statement on holistic nursing ethics.* Topeka, KS: Author.

American Nurses Association (ANA) (2001). *Code of ethics with interpretative statements.* Washington, DC: Nursesbooks.org.

Beck, D. M., Dossey, B. M., & Rushton, C. H. (2014). Global activism, advocacy, and transformation: Florence Nightingale's legacy for the twenty-first-century. In M. J. Kreitzer & M. Koithan (Eds.), *Integrative nursing* (pp. 526–537). New York, NY: Oxford University Press.

Burkhardt, M. A., & Keegan, L. (2013). Holistic ethics. In B. M. Dossey & L. Keegan (Eds.), *Holistic nursing: A handbook for practice* (6th ed., pp. 129–141). Burlington, MA: Jones & Bartlett Learning.

Burkhardt, M. A., & Nathanial, A. K. (2013). *Ethics and issues in contemporary nursing* (4th ed.). Boston, MA: Cengage Learning.

Charter for Compassion (2008). Retrieved from http://charterforcompassion.org

Dossey, B. M. (2010). *Florence Nightingale: Mystic, visionary, healer* (Commemorative ed.). Philadelphia, PA: F. A. Davis.

Dossey, B. M. (2013). Nursing: Integral, integrative, and holistic—Local to global. In B. M. Dossey & L. Keegan (Eds.), *Holistic nursing: A handbook for practice* (6th ed., pp. 3–57). Burlington, MA: Jones & Bartlett Learning.

Dossey, B. M., Beck, D. M., & Rushton, C. H. (2011). Integral nursing and the Nightingale initiative for global health: Florence Nightingale's legacy for the 21st century. *Journal of Integral Theory and Practice* 6(4), 71–92.

Dossey, L. (2013). *One mind: How our individual mind is part of a greater consciousness and why it matters*. Carlsbad, CA: Hay House.

Earth Charter (n.d.). Retrieved from http://www.earthcharterinaction.org

Ferguson, J. T., Karpf, T., Weait, M., & Swift, R. Y. (2010). *Decent care: Living values, health justice and human flourishing*. WHO Summative Report to the Ford Foundation. Geneva, Switzerland: World Health Organization.

Gadow, S. (1996). Ethical narratives in practice. *Nursing Science Quarterly* 9(1), 8–9.

Hess, D. R., Dossey, B. M., Southard, M. E., Luck, S., Schaub, B. G., & Bark, L. (2013). *The art and science of nurse coaching: A provider's guide to coaching scope and competencies*. Silver Spring, MD: Nursesbooks.org.

International Coach Federation (ICF) (n.d.). *ICF code of ethics*. Retrieved from http://www.coachfederation.org/icfcredentials/ethics/

International Council of Nurses (ICN) (2012). *The ICN code of ethics for nurses*. Geneva, Switzerland: Author. Retrieved from http://www.icn.ch/about-icn/code-of-ethics-for-nurses

Jameton, A. (1984). *Nursing practice: The ethical issues*. Englewood Cliffs, NJ: Prentice-Hall.

Karpf, T., Ferguson, T., Swift, R., & Lazarus, J. (2008). *Restoring hope: Decent care in the midst of HIV/AIDS*. London, UK: Palgrave Macmillan.

Nightingale, F. (1888). *To the probationer-nurses in the Nightingale Fund School at St. Thomas' Hospital from Florence Nightingale 16th May 1888* (pp. 3–4). (Privately printed).

Nightingale Declaration for a Healthy World (n.d.). Retrieved from http://www.nightingaledeclaration.net/the-declaration

Nightingale Initiative for Global Health (NIGH) (n.d.). Retrieved from http://www.nightingaledeclaration.net

Rushton, C. H. (2007). Ethical issues at the end-of-life. In J. Halifax, B. M. Dossey, & C. H. Rushton (Eds.), *Being with dying: Compassionate end-of-life care training guide* (pp. 117–129). Santa Fe, NM: Prajna Mountain Publishers.

Rushton, C. H. (2009). Caregiver suffering: Finding meaning when integrity is threatened. In W. Ellenchild-Pinch & A. M. Haddad (Eds.), *Nursing and health care ethics: A legacy and a vision* (pp. 293–306). Silver Spring, MD: Nursesbooks.org.

Rushton, C. H. (in press). *One heart: The art of compassion based ethics in health care.*

Wright, D., & Brajtman, S. (2011). Relational and embodied knowing: Nursing ethics within the interprofessional team. *Nursing Ethics 18*, 20–30. doi:10.1177/0969733010386165

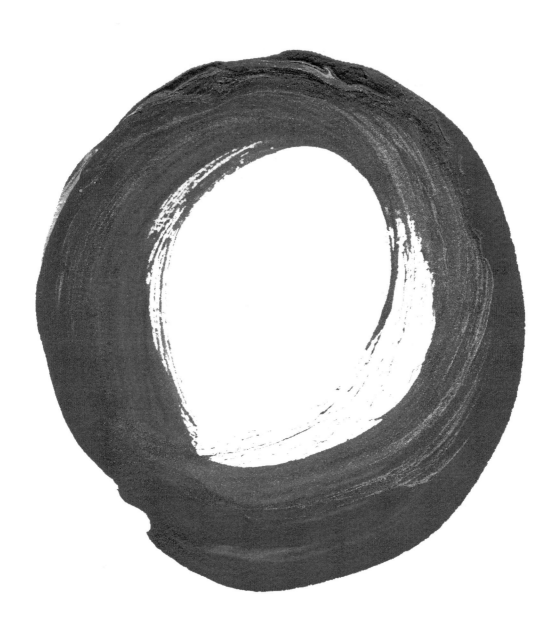

CORE VALUE 2
Nurse Coaching Process

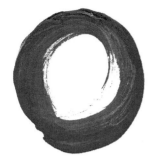

CHAPTER 4

Nurse Coaching Process and Nurse Coach Practice Competencies*

Barbara Montgomery Dossey

No set form of words is of any use. And patients are so quick to see whether a Nurse is consistent always in herself—whether she is what she says to them. And if she is not, it is no use. If she is, of how much use may the simplest word of soothing, of comfort, or even of reproof—especially in the quiet night... But if she wishes to do this, she must keep up a sort of divine calm, and high sense of duty in her own mind.

Florence Nightingale, 1873

LOOKING AHEAD...

After reading this chapter, you will be able to:

- Define the terms "nursing process" and the "nurse coaching process".
- Identify Nurse Coach Practice Competencies.
- Analyze the Nurse Coach Practice Competencies and how they are linked to the American Nurses Association Standards of Practice (six) and Standards of Professional Performance (ten).

DEFINITIONS

Nurse Coach competency: An expected level of performance that integrates knowledge, skills, abilities, and judgment.

Nurse coaching process: A six-step process that is a shift in terminology from the nursing process (see above) as follows: (1) Establishing Relationship and Identifying Readiness for Change (Assessment); (2) Identifying Opportunities, Issues, and Concerns (Diagnosis); (3) Establishing Client-Centered Goals (Outcomes Identification); (4) Creating the Structure of the Coaching Interaction (Planning); (5) Empowering and Motivating Client to Reach Goals (Implementation); and (6) Assisting Client to Determine the Extent to which Goals were achieved (Evaluation).

---

*Note: The chapter is adapted and includes definitions and Nurse Coach Practice Competencies that are published with permission from the American Nurses Association and Nursesbooks.org, and appear in Hess, D. R., Dossey, B. M., Southard, M. E., Luck, S., Schaub, B. G., & Bark, L. (2013). *The art and science of nurse coaching: A provider's guide to coaching scope and competencies*. Silver Spring, MD: Nursesbooks.org.

Nursing process: The original model describing the "work" of nursing as six steps used to fulfill the purposes of nursing: (1) Assessment, (2) Diagnosis, (3) Outcomes Identification*, (4) Plans, (5) Implementation, and (6) Evaluation.

Standards of practice: Describes a competent level of nursing care as demonstrated by the critical thinking model known as the nursing process and the nurse coaching process.

Standards of professional performance: Describes a competent level of behavior in the professional role, including activities related to ethics, education, evidence-based practice and research, quality of practice, communication, leadership, collaboration, professional practice evaluation, resource utilization, and environmental health.

NURSING PROCESS AND THE NURSE COACHING PROCESS

Nursing Process

The nurse coaching process recognizes the essence and transpersonal dimension of the caring/healing relationship between the Nurse Coach and client. The Nurse Coach understands that growth and improved health, wholeness, and wellbeing are the result of an ongoing journey that is ever-expanding and transformative. The *nursing process* is the original model describing the "work" of nursing, defined as the steps used to fulfill the purposes of nursing (Potter & Frisch, 2013). The nursing process involves six focal areas: assessment, diagnosis, outcomes identification, planning, implementation, and evaluation. These six areas are conceptualized as bidirectional feedback loops from each component (ANA, 2010a).

Nurse Coaching Process

The Nurse Coach uses the nursing process as a framework for the nurse coaching process. This is a *shift* in terminology and meaning to understand and incorporate the client's subjective experience as follows: from *assessment* to establishing a relationship and identifying readiness for change and the resources available to the client for change; from *nursing diagnosis* to identifying opportunities and issues; from *outcomes* to having the client set the agenda for achievement of the client's goals; from *planning* to creating the structure of the coaching interaction; from *intervention* to empowering the client to reach goals; and from *evaluating* to assisting the client to determine the extent to which goals were achieved (Hess et al., 2013). This is a circular process; these six steps may occur simultaneously and are now described:

1. Establishing Relationship and Identifying Readiness for Change (Assessment): The Nurse Coach begins by becoming fully present with self and client before initiating the coaching interaction. Cultivating and establishing a relationship with the client is a priority for effective coaching. Nurse coaching is a relationship-centered caring process. Assessment involves identifying the client's strengths and what the client wants to change, and assisting the client to determine her or his readiness for change. Assessment is dynamic and ongoing.

2. Identifying Opportunities, Issues, and Concerns (Diagnosis): The Nurse Coach, in partnership with the client, identifies opportunities and issues related to growth, overall health, wholeness, and wellbeing. Opportunities for celebrating wellbeing are explored. The Nurse Coach understands that acknowledgment promotes and reinforces previous successes and serves to enhance further achievements. *Note:* There is no attempt or need to assign labels or to establish a diagnosis when coaching. Instead, the Nurse Coach is open to multiple interpretations of an unfolding interaction.

3. Establishing Client-Centered Goals (Outcomes Identification): The Nurse Coach employs an overall approach to each coaching interaction that is designed to facilitate achievement of client goals and desired results.

4. Creating the Structure of the Coaching Interaction (Planning): The Nurse Coach may structure the coaching interaction with a coaching agreement that identifies specific parameters of the coaching relationship, including coach and client responsibilities and action plans.

5. Empowering and Motivating Client to Reach Goals (Implementation): The Nurse Coach employs effective communication skills such as deep listening, powerful questioning, and directed dialogue as key components of the coaching interaction. In partnership with the client, the Nurse Coach facilitates learning and results by co-creating awareness, designing actions, setting goals, planning, and addressing progress and accountability. The Nurse Coach skillfully chooses interventions based on the client's statements and actions, and interacts with intention and curiosity in a manner that assists the client toward achievement of the client's goals. The Nurse Coach effectively uses her/his nursing knowledge and a variety of skills acquired with additional coach training.

6. Assisting Client to Determine the Extent to which Goals were Achieved (Evaluation): The Nurse Coach is aware that evaluation of coaching (the nursing intervention) is done primarily by the client and is based on the client's perception of success and achievement of client-centered goals. The nurse partners with the client to evaluate progress toward goals.

COMPETENCY AND NURSE COACH PRACTICE

Competence is dynamic and situational, and is recognized as an ongoing process resulting in appropriate outcome/s. Competence is evaluated using qualitative and quantitative measurement tools related to the nurse coaching basic knowledge and performance. Nurse coaching competence can be taught, defined, measured, and evaluated. The context of a coaching relationship/coaching interaction determines what competencies are necessary. Assurance of competence is the shared responsibility of each Nurse Coach, professional nursing organizations, credentialing and certification entities, and other key stakeholders. Challenges, barriers, and factors that either enhance or detract from the ability to conduct coaching interactions are assessed and evaluated.

Mitchell et al. (2013) describe Nurse Coach competencies in terms of relationships with clients, communities, and other health professionals. For clients, Nurse Coach competencies include: using inquiry to promote health through pattern recognition and change; using complexity science and established tools to assist clients assess readiness for change, identifying individual and environmental patterns, and changing obsolete views; and enabling self-knowledge and self-care activities considering social justice and accessibility. The Nurse Coach also needs to work with and provide leadership for families and communities to identify assets and barriers for self-care and wellbeing, becoming a partner to enable health-promoting activities. Mitchell et al. (2013) also identifies additional needed competencies of the Nurse Coach as mentoring students and other professionals in health coaching competencies, advocating for needed structural changes to enhance health promotion and participating in and disseminating the needed research in the nurse health coach arena.

Nurse Coaches continually assess and reassess their competencies and identify areas where new knowledge; integrative, integral, and holistic learning experiences; and self-development can enhance personal and professional endeavors. The ability to perform at the expected level requires lifelong learning and self-development (self-reflection, self-assessment, self-evaluation, and self-care). See Chapter 22. **Table 4-1** provides a list of competency concepts related to nurse coaching. In the next section the professional Nurse Coach competencies are presented.

Table 4-1 Nurse Coach Competency Concepts.

- A Nurse Coach competency is an expected level of performance that integrates knowledge, skills, abilities, and judgment.
- A Nurse Coach who demonstrates "competence" is performing at an expected level.
- A Nurse Coach integrates knowledge, skills, abilities, and judgment in formal, informal, and reflective learning experiences.
- A Nurse Coach has integrity.
- A Nurse Coach is aware of her/his own strengths and weaknesses, has positive self-regard, and is open to feedback.
- A Nurse Coach values and uses intuitive knowing.
- Nurse coaching involves emotional, moral, and spiritual intelligence.
- Nurse coaching demonstrates an understanding of science and humanities, professional standards of practice, coaching competencies, insights gained from experiences, personal strengths, resources, capabilities, and leadership performance.
- Nurse coaching includes psychomotor, communication, interpersonal, and environmental skills.
- Nurse coaching judgment includes critical thinking, problem-solving, ethical reasoning, decision-making, and clinical leadership.
- Nurse Coach learning may occur in academic settings, professional practice environments, structured certificate programs, and online educational offerings.
- Nurse Coach reflective learning is recurrent thoughtful self-assessment, analysis, and synthesis of strengths and opportunities for improvement.

Source: Used with permission. American Nurses Association. Adapted from Hess, D. R., et al. (2013). *The art and science of nurse coaching: The provider's guide to coaching scope and competencies* (pp. 9–10). Silver Spring, MD: Nursesbooks.org.

NURSE COACH PRACTICE AND PERFORMANCE COMPETENCIES RESOURCES

Nurse Coaches are guided in their thinking and decision-making by four professional resources. The American Nurses Association's *Nursing: Scope and Standards of Practice,* 2nd edition (ANA, 2010a) outlines the expectations of the professional role of registered nurses and the scope of practice and standards of professional nurse practice and their accompanying competencies. *Code of Ethics for Nurses with Interpretive Statements* (ANA, 2001) lists the nine provisions that establish the ethical framework for registered nurses across all roles, levels, and settings. *Nursing's Social Policy Statement: The Essence of the Profession* (ANA, 2010b) conceptualizes nursing practice, describes the social context of nursing, and provides the definition of nursing. *Holistic Nursing: Scope and Standards of Practice* (AHNA & ANA, 2013) provides the philosophical underpinnings of a holistic nurse coaching practice.

ANA STANDARDS AS ORGANIZING FRAMEWORK FOR PROFESSIONAL NURSE COACHING PRACTICE COMPETENCIES

Nursing: Scope and Standards of Practice, 2nd edition (ANA, 2010a) is the organizing framework for the professional Nurse Coach competencies. This includes six standards of practice and ten standards of professional performance as seen in **Table 4-2**. A description of the professional Nurse Coach role pertaining to each standard is provided followed by the specific Nurse Coach competencies related to that standard. *Note*: These Professional

Nurse Coach Practice Competencies were established through a peer-review process and endorsed by 21 nursing organizations (Hess et al., 2013, vii–ix, pp. 27–47). These competencies include the International Coach Federation (ICF) competencies (ICF, n.d.).

Table 4-2 ANA Standards of Practice (6) and Standards of Performance (10).

Standards of Practice	Standards of Professional Performance
The Standards of Practice describe a competent level of nursing care as demonstrated by the critical thinking model known as the nursing process. The nursing process includes the components of assessment, diagnosis, outcomes identification, planning, implementation, and evaluation. Accordingly, the nursing process encompasses significant actions taken by registered nurses and forms the foundation of the nurse's decision-making.	The Standards of Professional Performance describe a competent level of behavior in the professional role, including activities related to ethics, education, evidence-based practice and research, quality of practice, communication, leadership, collaboration, professional practice evaluation, resource utilization, and environmental health. All registered nurses are expected to engage in professional role activities, including leadership, appropriate to their education and position. Registered nurses are accountable for their professional actions to themselves, their healthcare consumers, their peers, and ultimately to society.
Standard 1. Assessment The registered nurse collects comprehensive data pertinent to the healthcare consumer's health and/or the situation.	**Standard 7. Ethics** The registered nurse practices ethically.
Standard 2. Diagnosis The registered nurse analyzes the assessment data to determine the diagnoses or the issues.	**Standard 8. Education** The registered nurse attains knowledge and competence that reflects current nursing practice.
Standard 3. Outcomes Identification The registered nurse identifies expected outcomes for a plan individualized to the healthcare consumer or the situation.	**Standard 9. Evidence-Based Practice and Research** The registered nurse integrates evidence and research findings into practice.
Standard 4. Planning The registered nurse develops a plan that prescribes strategies and alternatives to attain expected outcomes.	**Standard 10. Quality of Practice** The registered nurse contributes to quality nursing practice.
Standard 5. Implementation The registered nurse implements the identified plan.	**Standard 11. Communication** The registered nurse communicates effectively in a variety of formats in all areas of practice.
Standard 6. Evaluation The registered nurse evaluates progress toward attainment of outcomes.	**Standard 12. Leadership** The registered nurse demonstrates leadership in the professional practice setting and the profession.

(continues on next page)

Table 4-2 (*Continued*).

Standards of Practice	Standards of Professional Performance
	Standard 13. Collaboration The registered nurse collaborates with healthcare consumer, family, and others in the conduct of nursing practice.
	Standard 14. Professional Practice Evaluation The registered nurse evaluates her or his own nursing practice in relation to professional practice standards and guidelines, relevant statutes, and regulations.
	Standard 15. Resource Utilization The registered nurse utilizes appropriate resources to plan and provide nursing services that are safe, effective, and financially responsible.
	Standard 16. Environmental Health The registered nurse practices in an environmentally safe and healthy manner.

Source: Copyright © 2010 by the American Nurses Association. Used with permission. American Nurses Association: *Nursing: Scope and standards of nursing practice,* (2nd ed., pp. 8–9). Silver Spring, MD: Nursesbooks.org.

PROFESSIONAL NURSE COACH PRACTICE COMPETENCIES

ANA Standard 1. Assessment

The registered nurse collects comprehensive data pertinent to the healthcare consumer's health and/or the situation.

Professional Nurse Coach Role

Setting the foundation for coaching begins during the assessment phase of the coaching interaction. Assessment begins by becoming fully present with self and client before initiating the coaching interaction. Assessment proceeds to establishing a relationship with the client and access to the client's subjective experience/story and internal frame of reference through the cultivation and establishment of a relationship. The Nurse Coach determines if the client's concerns are appropriate for the coaching role. The Nurse Coach helps the client assess readiness and available resources for change. Assessment is dynamic and ongoing.

Professional Nurse Coach Competencies

The Nurse Coach:

1. Becomes fully present to self and client prior to collecting data pertinent to the coaching interaction.
2. Co-creates a relationship between the Nurse Coach and the client that promotes trust and intimacy.

3. Recognizes and respects the client as the authority on her or his own health and well-being.
4. Explores with the client why coaching is being considered at this time and what the client wants to address during the coaching interaction.
5. Ensures the client sets the agenda for the coaching session and holds the client's agenda throughout the session.
6. Helps the client assess stage of readiness for change (pre-contemplation, contemplation, preparation, action, maintenance).
7. Incorporates various types of knowing, including intuition, and validates this intuitive knowledge with the client when appropriate.
8. Explores, through powerful questions and feedback, multiple sources of information to assist the client to become aware of areas for coaching.
9. Uses appropriate evidence-informed whole person assessment techniques and instruments, with the client's permission, and with appropriate training.
10. Determines the need for and refers client to other professionals and services as appropriate.
11. Assesses if there is an effective working match between the coach and the prospective client.
12. Understands and effectively discusses with the client the ethical guidelines and specific parameters of the nurse coaching relationship (e.g., logistics, fees, scheduling).
13. Co-creates with the client an agreement that identifies the role of the Nurse Coach and the role of the client.

ANA Standard 2. Diagnosis

The registered nurse analyzes the assessment data to determine the diagnoses or the issues.

Professional Nurse Coach Process and Role: Identifying Opportunities, Issues, and Concerns (Diagnosis)

The Nurse Coach and the client together explore assessment data to determine areas for change.

Professional Nurse Coach Competencies

The Nurse Coach:

1. Clarifies the client's issues and concerns and/or opportunities for change based on the whole person assessment data.
2. Confirms the client's issues and concerns and/or opportunities with the client.
3. Tracks the client's issues and concerns and/or opportunities in a manner that leads to identification of the client's goals that will be the focus of the coaching process.

ANA Standard 3. Outcomes Identification

The registered nurse identifies expected outcomes for a plan individualized to the healthcare consumer or the situation.

Professional Nurse Coach Process and Role: Establishing Client-Centered Goals (Outcomes)

The Nurse Coach assists the client to identify goals that will lead to the desired change. The Nurse Coach values the evolution and the process of change as it unfolds.

Professional Nurse Coach Competencies

The Nurse Coach:

1. Involves the client in formulating goals that are specific, measurable, action-oriented, realistic, and time-lined.
2. Facilitates the client's process of self-discovery related to establishment of the client's goals.
3. Facilitates the client's exploration of alternative ideas and options relevant to goal-setting.
4. Supports the client's inner wisdom, intuition, and innate ability for knowing what is best for self.
5. Realizes that new goals will emerge as the client changes and evolves.

ANA Standard 4. Planning

The registered nurse develops a plan that prescribes strategies and alternatives to attain expected outcomes.

Professional Nurse Coach Process and Role: Creating the Structure of the Coaching Interaction (Plan)

The Nurse Coach and the client develop a coaching plan that identifies strategies to attain goals.

Professional Nurse Coach Competencies

The Nurse Coach:

1. Assists the client to identify strategies to attain goals.
2. Creates with the client an action plan with clearly defined steps and anticipated results.
3. Explores with client potential obstacles to goal attainment and possible responses to these challenges.
4. Adjusts plan as desired by the client.

ANA Standard 5. Implementation

The registered nurse implements the identified plan.

Professional Nurse Coach Process and Role: Empowering and Motivating Clients to Reach Goals (Implementation)

The Nurse Coach supports the client's coaching plan while simultaneously remaining open to emerging goals based on new insights, learning, and achievements. The Nurse Coach supports the client in reaching for new and expanded goals. The Nurse Coach utilizes a variety of specific coaching and communication skills to facilitate learning and growth.

Professional Nurse Coach Competencies

The Nurse Coach:

Before the coaching interaction:

1. Becomes fully present, centered, and grounded.
2. Reviews client status and/or progress from previously obtained data.
3. Minimizes distractions for self and encourages client to do the same.

At the beginning of the coaching interaction:

4. Explores, with the client, an outcome for the coaching session that is achievable in the time allotted.
5. Briefly explores progress since last coaching session, with particular attention to accomplishments, challenges, or barriers relevant to current session.

Throughout the coaching interaction:

6. Remains fully present, centered, and grounded.
    a. Supports the client in directing the agenda/focus of the coaching session.
    b. Acknowledges client and identifies strengths for change.
    c. Maintains an interested, open, and reflective approach to the client.
    d. Is comfortable with silence or pausing to assist the client with reflection and finding new understanding or next steps.
    e. Accesses and trusts her/his own intuition and perceptions of the client.
    f. Draws upon the precepts of the human energy field/system to assist client in achievement of goals.
7. Creates a safe, supportive environment that fosters intimacy and trust.
8. Continuously exhibits authenticity (honesty, sincerity, personal integrity).
9. Demonstrates respect for client's subjective experiences/story, perceptions, learning style, and culture (e.g., beliefs, values, and customs).
10. Provides ongoing support for new ideas, behaviors, and actions that may involve risk-taking and fear of failure and/or fear of success.
11. Obtains client's consent to coach client in areas of vulnerability.
12. Chooses what is most effective in the moment from a variety of coaching strategies and implements as appropriate.
13. Focuses on what the client is saying and is not saying to understand the meaning in the context of the client's desires and to support the client's self-expression by employing such skills as deep listening, relevant use of language, powerful questioning, and direct communication.
    a. Deep Listening
        i.   Accepts, explores, reinforces, and encourages the client's expression of perceptions, concerns, beliefs, suggestions, etc.
        ii. Recognizes incongruities between body language, words used, and the tone of voice.
        iii. Paraphrases, reiterates, and summarizes what client has said to ensure understanding and clarity.
        iv. Focuses on the essence of the client's communication when client becomes involved in long explanatory descriptions.
        v.   Allows the client to express strong feelings without judgment in order to facilitate movement towards achievement of goals.
        vi. Acknowledges client's ambivalence to change and helps identify barriers.
    b. Relevant Use of Language
        i.   Uses language, including metaphors and analogies, which assist the client to explore perspectives, uncertainties, or opportunities for change.
        ii. Uses language that is nonjudgmental, appropriate, and respectful.
        iii. Uses language that reflects the client's worldview, beliefs, and values.
    c. Powerful Questioning
        i.   Asks open-ended questions that create greater insight, clarity, and/or new possibilities and learning.

        ii. Asks questions that move the client towards desired goals.

        iii. Asks questions that evoke discovery, insight, commitment, or action (e.g., those that challenge the client's assumptions).

        iv. Uses inquiry for greater awareness, clarity, and understanding.

    d. Direct Communication

        i. Provides feedback in a clear and direct manner.

        ii. Shares insights with client in ways that are practical and meaningful.

        iii. Explores the client's assumptions and perspectives to evoke new ideas and discover new possibilities for action.

        iv. Challenges the client to stretch and be challenged, while maintaining a comfortable pace with the client.

14. Employs integrated, holistic communication skills including deep listening, relevant use of language, powerful questions, and direct communication, allowing a client to fully explore and articulate what she or he hopes to achieve through the coaching relationship.

    a. Supports the client's inner wisdom, intuition, and innate ability for learning.

    b. Identifies with the client additional areas for learning and development.

    c. Assists the client in uncovering underlying ambivalence, concerns, typical and fixed ways of perceiving self and the world, interpretations of experiences, and differences between thoughts, feelings, and actions.

    d. Helps the client identify barriers to change.

    e. Helps the client identify strengths and opportunities for learning and growth.

    f. Acknowledges client resistance as an opportunity for self-awareness and growth.

    g. Shares information with client that inspires broader perspectives.

    h. Encourages and supports the client to experiment and to apply what has been learned from the coaching interaction.

    i. Assists the client to determine actions that will enable the client to demonstrate, practice, and deepen new learning.

    j. Facilitates the client in taking action that will most effectively lead to achievement of desired goals and prevent relapse.

At the end of the coaching interaction:

15. Inquires of the client if coaching session outcomes have been achieved.
16. Identifies the connection between where the client is and where she/he wishes to go.
17. Identifies with the client the next specific action steps and a timeline that will lead to achievement of desired goals.
18. Assists the client to manage progress by holding the client accountable for stated actions, results, and related time frames, while maintaining a positive and trusting relationship with the client.
19. Determines with the client when the next coaching interaction will occur.
20. Periodically, if relevant, prepares, organizes, and reviews information, including past and current actions, with the client that promotes achievement of client goals.
21. Periodically, as indicated, reviews and revises the coaching plan with the client.
22. Ends the coaching interaction in an energetic, positive, and supportive manner.

ANA Standard 6. Evaluation

The registered nurse evaluates progress toward attainment of outcomes.

Professional Nurse Coach Process and Role: Assisting Client to Determine the Extent to which Goals were Achieved (Evaluation)

The Nurse Coach partners with the client to evaluate progress toward attainment of goals.

Professional Nurse Coach Competencies

The Nurse Coach:

1. Assists the client to evaluate effectiveness of strategies in relation to the client's responses and the attainment of the expected and unfolding goals.
2. Supports client autonomy by recognizing the client is the determinant of progress and success.
3. Documents evaluation of progress and attainment of coaching goals.

ANA Standard 7. Ethics

The registered nurse practices ethically.

Professional Nurse Coach Role

The Nurse Coach integrates ethical provisions in all coaching interactions.

Professional Nurse Coach Competencies

The Nurse Coach:

1. Uses the *Code of Ethics for Nurses with Interpretive Statements* (ANA, 2001) to guide practice and communicate the foundation of the professional nurse coaching practice.
2. Clearly communicates to the client and others the distinctions among coaching, consulting, counseling, and teaching.
3. Provides coaching in a manner that recognizes and respects the client's autonomy, dignity, rights, values, and beliefs.
4. Maintains an effective coaching relationship that is congruent with the coaching agreement and within the boundaries of professional nursing practice.
5. Values all life experiences as opportunities to find personal meaning and cultivate self-awareness, self-reflection, and growth.
6. Maintains client confidentiality within legal and regulatory parameters.

ANA Standard 8. Education

The registered nurse attains knowledge and competence that reflects current nursing practice.

Professional Nurse Coach Role

The Nurse Coach attains knowledge and competency that reflects current nurse coaching practice.

Professional Nurse Coach Competencies

The Nurse Coach:

1. Participates in ongoing educational activities to enhance the nurse coaching role.
2. Documents and maintains evidence of nurse coaching competency.

3. Develops and uses a broad knowledge base related to holistic/integral nursing, integrative health, health systems, professional coaching competencies, counseling, health education, health promotion, and nursing practice issues.

ANA Standard 9. Evidence-Based Practice and Research

The registered nurse integrates evidence and research findings into practice.

Professional Nurse Coach Role

The Nurse Coach integrates evidence and research into nurse coaching practice.

Professional Nurse Coach Competencies

The Nurse Coach:

1. Uses the best available evidence, including theories and research findings, to guide and enhance professional nurse coaching practice.
2. Participates with others to establish research priorities and to identify research questions or areas for inquiry related to professional nurse coaching practice.
3. Participates in research activities related to professional nurse coaching practice.

ANA Standard 10. Quality of Practice

The registered nurse contributes to quality nursing practice.

Professional Nurse Coach Role

The Nurse Coach systematically enhances the quality and effectiveness of nurse coaching practice.

Professional Nurse Coach Competencies

The Nurse Coach:

1. Participates in quality improvement to enhance the professional nurse coaching practice.
2. Contributes to the education of others concerning professional nurse coaching practice.
3. Documents nurse coaching interactions in a responsible, accountable, and ethical manner to facilitate quality review and promotion of effective nurse coaching practice.
4. Uses creativity and innovation in nurse coaching practice to improve client outcomes.
5. Analyzes organizational systems for barriers to effective implementation of the professional nurse coaching practice.
6. Advocates use of *The Art and Science of Nurse Coaching: A Provider's Guide to Scope and Competencies* (Hess et al., 2013) to evaluate and enhance the quality of practice.

ANA Standard 11. Communication

The registered nurse communicates effectively in a variety of formats in all areas of practice.

Professional Nurse Coach Role

The Nurse Coach employs skillful communication in all aspects of the coaching interaction.

Professional Nurse Coach Competencies

The Nurse Coach:

1. Understands that skillful communication is a fundamental component of professional nurse coaching practice.
2. Communicates, when requested by client, with family, significant others, caregivers, healthcare providers, and others to assist and enhance the client's achievement of coaching goals.

ANA Standard 12. Leadership

The registered nurse demonstrates leadership in the professional practice setting and the profession.

Professional Nurse Coach Role

The Nurse Coach demonstrates leadership in the promotion of effective nurse coaching for clients.

Professional Nurse Coach Competencies

The Nurse Coach:

1. Advances the role of the Nurse Coach among health professional and coaching colleagues and in professional organizations.
2. Develops cognitive, emotional, moral, and spiritual intelligence to enhance leadership skills.
3. Promotes the success of others by using effective nurse coaching interventions.
4. Demonstrates energy, excitement, and a passion for quality nurse coaching.
5. Willingly accepts that mistakes will be made by self and others when taking risks to achieve goals.
6. Displays the ability to define a clear vision, associated goals, and a plan to implement and measure progress toward goals.

ANA Standard 13. Collaboration

The registered nurse collaborates with healthcare consumer, family, and others in the conduct of nursing practice.

Professional Nurse Coach Role

The Nurse Coach collaborates with others to assist clients in achieving goals.

Professional Nurse Coach Competencies

The Nurse Coach:

1. Uses effective communication and change skills with individuals and groups to collaboratively identify and achieve individual, group, and organizational goals.
2. Works collaboratively with other health and wellness coaches in interprofessional development initiatives.
3. Collaborates with others to promote nurse coaching as a way to enhance client outcomes.

ANA Standard 14. Professional Practice Evaluation

The registered nurse evaluates her or his own nursing practice in relation to professional practice standards and guidelines, relevant statutes, and regulations.

Professional Nurse Coach Role

The Nurse Coach evaluates her or his own nurse coaching practice in relation to professional practice standards and guidelines, relevant statutes, rules, and regulations. The Nurse Coach is engaged in ongoing personal and professional self-development.

Professional Nurse Coach Competencies

The Nurse Coach:

1. Utilizes *The Art and Science of Nurse Coaching: A Provider's Guide to Scope and Competencies* (Hess et al., 2013) to evaluate and enhance quality of practice.
2. Considers the effect of one's personal values, culture, spiritual beliefs, experiences, biases, and education on the provision of nurse coaching services to individuals, groups, and organizations.
3. Provides nurse coaching services in a manner that is appropriate and sensitive to culture and ethnicity.
4. Engages in self-evaluation of nurse coaching practice on a regular basis, identifying areas of strength as well as areas in which additional development would be beneficial.
5. Obtains evaluative feedback regarding one's own coaching from clients, peers, and professional colleagues and takes appropriate action based upon the feedback.
6. Pursues Nurse Coach certification as a way to demonstrate competency and to promote the nurse coaching role to employers, clients, and the public.
7. Recognizes that the professional nurse coaching practice is enhanced by ongoing self-development to promote physical, mental, emotional, social, moral, and spiritual wellbeing.
8. Receives personal and professional coaching to enhance quality of nurse coaching practice.
9. Integrates knowledge from research on coaching into practice.

ANA Standard 15. Resource Utilization

The registered nurse utilizes appropriate resources to plan and provide nursing services that are safe, effective, and financially responsible.

Professional Nurse Coach Role

The Nurse Coach considers factors related to safety, effectiveness, cost, and impact on practice in the planning and delivery of nurse coaching services.

Professional Nurse Coach Competencies

The Nurse Coach:

1. Evaluates factors such as safety, effectiveness, availability, cost and benefits, efficiencies, and impact on nurse coaching practice when suggesting options for the client that would result in the same expected outcome.
2. Assists the client, as appropriate, in identifying and securing appropriate and available services to facilitate achievement of client goals.

ANA Standard 16. Environmental Health

The registered nurse practices in an environmentally safe and healthy manner.

Professional Nurse Coach Role

The Nurse Coach considers the impact of the internal and external environment of self and client when providing nurse coaching services.

Professional Nurse Coach Competencies

The Nurse Coach:

1. Understands that healthy environments encompass both internal and external environments.
2. Recognizes that individual (physical, psychological, emotional, spiritual) and cultural, social, and historical factors influence internal and external environments.
3. Considers the internal and external healing environments of self and client regarding contribution to client goal achievement.

SUMMARY

- The Nurse Coach recognizes the nursing process as the original model describing the "work" of nursing as the steps used to fulfill the purposes of nursing.
- The nursing process involves six focal areas: (1) assessment, (2) diagnosis, (3) outcomes identification, (4) planning, (5) implementation, and (6) evaluation.
- The nurse coaching process is a six-step process that is a shift in terminology from the nursing process (see above) as follows: (1) Establishing Relationship and Identifying Readiness for Change (Assessment); (2) Identifying Opportunities, Issues, and Concerns (Diagnosis); (3) Establishing Client-Centered Goals (Outcomes Identification); (4) Creating the Structure of the Coaching Interaction (Planning); (5) Empowering and Motivating Client to Reach Goals (Implementation); and (6) Assisting Client to Determine the Extent to which Goals were Achieved (Evaluation).
- The Nurse Coach competencies are linked to the American Nurses Association six Standards of Practice and the ten Standards of Professional Performance (ANA).

NURSE COACH REFLECTIONS

After reading this chapter, the Nurse Coach will be able to bring awareness and personal insight to the following questions:

- How am I guided in my nurse coaching by the nurse coaching process?
- Do I systematically apply the nurse coaching process to help me in coaching clients?
- What is my reaction when clients state they are not ready to change to healthier behaviors?
- How can I cultivate my intuitive knowing for moving deeper into a coaching session?

REFERENCES

American Holistic Nurses Association and American Nurses Association (AHNA/ANA) (2013). *Holistic nursing: Scope and standards of practice* (2nd ed.). Silver Spring, MD: Author.

American Nurses Association (ANA) (2001). *Code of ethics for nurses with interpretive statements*. Washington, DC: Author.

American Nurses Association (ANA) (2010a). *Nursing: Scope and standards of practice* (2nd ed). Silver Spring, MD: Author.

American Nurses Association (ANA) (2010b). *Nursing's social policy statement: The essence of the profession.* Silver Spring, MD: Author.

Hess, D. R., Dossey, B. M., Southard, M. E., Luck, S., Schaub, B. G., & Bark, L. (2013). *The art and science of nurse coaching: A provider's guide to coaching scope and competencies*. Silver Spring, MD: Nursesbooks.org.

International Coach Federation (ICF) (n.d.). ICF core competencies. Retrieved from http://www.coachfederation.org/icfcredentials/core-competencies

Mitchell, G., Cross, N., Wilson, Biernacki, S., Wong, W., Adib, B., & Rush, D. (2013). Complexity and health coaching: Synergies in nursing. *Nursing Research and Practice*, Article ID 238620. http://dx.doi.org/10.1155/2013/238620

Nightingale, F. (1873). *Letter from Miss Nightingale to the probationer-nurses in the 'Nightingale Fund' at St. Thomas's Hospital, and the nurses who were formerly trained there* (p. 2). London, UK: Spottiswoode.

Potter, P. J., & Frisch, N. C. (2013). The nursing process. In B. M. Dossey & L. Keegan (Eds.), *Holistic nursing: A handbook for practice* (6th ed., pp. 145–160). Burlington, MA: Jones & Bartlett Learning.

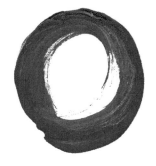

CHAPTER 5

Stories, Strengths, and the Nurse Coach 5-Step Process

Barbara Montgomery Dossey

Nursing is an art; and if it is to be made an art, it requires as exclusive a devotion, as hard a preparation, as any painter's or sculptor's work; for what is the having to do with dead canvas or cold marble, compared with having to do with the living spirit—the temple of God's spirit? It is one of the Fine Arts; I had almost said, the finest of the Fine Arts.

Florence Nightingale, 1868

LOOKING AHEAD...

After reading this chapter, you will be able to:

- Explore presence and meaning in nurse coaching.
- Identify ways to increase strengths.
- Examine Story Theory.
- Analyze the Story-Health Model.
- Identify the Nurse Coach 5-step process for coaching clients.

DEFINITIONS

Bearing witness: Being present for things as they are, which involves developing the qualities of stillness in order to be present for self, clients/patients, and others.

Compassion: Ability to be present for all levels of suffering with no need to "fix" the suffering; It is the tenderness of the heart in response to suffering.

Deep listening: Presence in the moment to understand what another person is expressing or not expressing; communication between two or more individuals in which the conventional division of self and ego is transcended by a sense of indivisible unity between all involved.

Equanimity: A spacious stillness that accepts things as they are; the invitation to see the present moment as the truth of our human condition and to be present to our experience.

Healing: The emergent process of the whole system bringing together aspects of one's self and the body-mind-spirit-culture-environment at deeper levels of inner knowing, leading to integration and balance, with each aspect having equal importance and value.

Healing intention: The conscious awareness of being in the present moment to help facilitate the healing process; a volitional act of unconditional love.

Meaning: That which is signified, indicated, referred to, or understood. More specifically: *philosophical meaning*—meaning that depends on the symbolic connections that are grasped by reason; *psychological meaning*—meaning that depends on connections that are experienced through intuition or insight; *spiritual meaning*—meaning around the ultimate issues, questions, and concerns such as "Who am I?" "What is my soul's purpose?" "How am I part of the interconnected web of life?"

Not knowing: Willingness to be free of fixed ideas.

Presence: The condition of being consciously and compassionately in the present moment with another, believing in her/his inherent wholeness, whatever the current situation; the essence of nurse coaching; the gift of self.

Reflective practice: A process of learning to be in the moment that guides inner development and permits entry into the flow and dance of wholeness and unity.

Story: A dynamic process where the storyteller embraces the telling of a happening or connected series of happenings; narrative meaning usually combines human actions or events that affect the storyteller, thus impacting the whole person.

Strengths: Preexisting patterns of thought, feeling, and behavior that are authentic, energizing, and lead to best potentials and possibilities.

Suffering: An individual's experience of struggle based on a reinforced story around anxiety, distress, or pain. It can manifest as behavioral, emotional, mental, moral, physical, social, and/or spiritual signs of distress; it is anguish experienced—internal and external—as a threat to one's composure, integrity, sense of self, or the fulfillment of expectations.

NURSE COACHING AND REFLECTIVE PRACTICE

Nurse coaching is a reflective practice where the Nurse Coach engages in self-reflection and a process of learning to be in the moment. Reflection includes "thinking about practice," with critical reflection requiring that practitioners "think about how they are thinking about their practice" (Freshwater, Taylor, & Sherwood, 2008). Reflection is viewed as having two dimensions: reflecting on an experience after an event occurs, and reflecting in action—in real time—during an event. In this latter situation, if a usual pattern of action is frustrated, then the situation may be reframed to decide how best to respond (Johns, 2013).

Reflective practice allows for the entry into the flow and dance of wholeness and unity. It is from this place that the Nurse Coach engages in bearing witness to the client/patient story. Bearing witness is being present for things as they are, which involves developing qualities of deep listening to understand what another person is expressing or not expressing. It is an experience in which the conventional division of self and ego is transcended by a sense of indivisible unity between all involved. This process also includes the capacity to be with not knowing, a willingness to be free of fixed ideas (Freshwater et al., 2008; Johns, 2013). To further understand reflective practice, presence and meaning are explored in the next section.

PRESENCE AND MEANING

Presence

Nurse Coaches are aware that presence and caring compassion are essential for genuine empathy. Entering into the present moment with each client/patient, the Nurse Coach believes in each person's inherent wholeness, whatever the current situation. Presence involves approaching an individual or a situation with respect, and relating in a way that reflects a quality of being with and in collaboration with (Quinn, 2013). The Nurse Coach enters into a shared experience, a field of consciousness that promotes growth, healing, and an experience of wellbeing. When this is done without judgment, the moment allows for a shift in consciousness to one of connection (Dossey, 2013).

Presence is a combination of attributes that include intentionality, mutuality, attention, and client-centered (Koerner, 2007). Presence transforms experiences and adds a deeper and more powerful dimension and atmosphere where growth and healing are promoted for self and others (Newman, 2008). These attributes facilitate exploring dimensions of meaning with another as discussed next.

Meaning

Nurse Coaches explore life meaning and purpose to increase their capacities in nurse coaching. As a Nurse Coach, what do you tell yourself about your state of health? Is your health excellent, good, fair, or poor? This question is a way of asking what our health means to us and what it represents or symbolizes in our thoughts and imagination. What does it mean to be human? What is meaning? Why should you seek out meaning? What do you do with it? How do you keep it? This attention to meaning allows us to be more effective with others as we coach them in searching the meaning in their lives.

Meanings are individual and personal. They have relevance to the person's experiences, events, expectations, belief systems, and core values. Within each person's story are meanings about the past and present life story as well as what one believes about future events that can be explored in one's healing journey. Within the story, one notices patterns, insights, and broad relationships to find or seek out the meanings. Only when meaning is found can an experience become a paradigm experience. Meaningless experiences are seldom retained to form a foundation for future reference.

In nurse coaching, meaning is seen as differences, contrasts, novelty, and heterogeneity—and is necessary for the healthy function of human beings. We seek out meaning because our lives are fuller and richer when it means something positive for us. Take away the important meaning of our lives and it is not worth living. In contrast, a new sense of meaning has been identified as an outcome of the healing process. The more we understand about meaning in life, the more we are able to empower ourselves to recognize more effective ways to cope with life and to learn more effective methods of working on life issues. In doing this, we create richer meaning in our daily lives.

Nurse Coaches skillfully coach clients to seek meaning related to health and wellness, as well as when they coach clients with acute and chronic diseases or illnesses. The Integrative Health and Wellness Assessment (see Chapter 6; Appendices C-1 and C-2) may be used to explore the meanings which a person attaches to seeking lifestyle and behavioral change. This is also important when coaching a client/patient around symptoms or illness because meaning is one of the most important factors that influence the journey with life challenges or when going through a crisis. When a person believes meaning is absent, bodies become bored; bored bodies become the spawning ground for depression, disease, and death. Failure of meaning has become a cliché. Professions, personal lives, and even entire cultures are said to suffer from a breakdown of meaning. Although at times it seems that meaning may be absent from our lives and our universe, in fact, such a thing is not possible, even in principle.

Nurse Coaches recognize that our existence is awash with meaning, and it is only a matter of which meaning we shall choose. And the choices are crucial as we coach clients/patients about life balance and harmony, health and wellness, living with an illness or disease, or during the dying process. It is clear from the wealth of scientific data that it is impossible to separate the biological parts from the psychological, sociological, spiritual, cultural, and environmental parts of our being. The importance of meaning can no longer be ignored for it is directly linked with our consciousness and all body systems that influence strengths, states of happiness, hardiness, resilience, or disease and illness. Meanings and emotions go hand in hand, and these connections are intimate and connected with our strengths, as discussed next.

IDENTIFYING STRENGTHS

Nurse Coaches assist clients to identify strengths and build self-esteem, which leads to a solid foundation for coaching. This is based on positive psychology, a recent branch of psychology that places emphasis on ways to make normal life more fulfilling with increased human flourishing (Seligman, 1990). Research shows that there are increased levels of optimism, happiness, gratitude, joy, confidence, self-esteem, energy, vitality, and resilience. Identifying strengths also helps people to be more likely to achieve goals, improve their work performance, and achieve higher levels of social support and lower rates of depression (Linley, Willars, & Biswas-Diener, 2010; Seligman, 2002). Strengths research also focuses on values, virtues, states of flow, and talents, and how these areas can be enhanced in social systems, organizations, and institutions (Csikszentmihalyi, 1990; Peterson & Seligman, 2004; Seligman, 1990). This field does not replace traditional psychology.

Strengths are preexisting patterns of thought, feeling, and behavior that are authentic and energizing, leading to our best potentials and possibilities (Biswas-Diener, 2010). Authentic means that the strength is descriptive of the true individual. Strengths are not something that we aspire to; rather, they are what come naturally. For example, a nurse may thrive in the high-pressure critical care and emergency room environment, where another nurse is called to work with hospice patients. If they shift their roles and work environments, they probably will find it stressful and unsatisfying, and will be unable to reach their highest potentials and sense of calling in the profession.

Energy is a key feature of strengths and a marker that someone is describing strength. The easiest way to pick up on a strength is to be on the lookout for shifts as a person is talking—changes in voice inflection, facial expressions (genuine smile, laugh, and alive eyes), body postures, and hand gestures, and increased depth of a story being shared with increased use of metaphors and symbols. **Table 5-1** lists 10 recommended strength-spotting tips.

Table 5-1 Strength-Spotting Tips.

1. **Childhood memories:** What do you remember doing as a child that you still do now—but most likely better now? Strengths often have deep roots from our early lives.
2. **Energy:** What activities give you an energetic buzz when you are doing them? These activities are very likely calling on your strengths.
3. **Authenticity:** When do you feel most like the "real you"? The chances are that you will be using your strengths in some way.
4. **Ease:** See what activities come naturally to you and at which you excel—sometimes, it seems, without even trying. These will likely be your strengths.
5. **Attention:** See where you naturally pay attention. You are more likely to focus on things that are playing to your strengths.
6. **Rapid learning:** What are the things that you have picked up quickly, learning them almost effortlessly? Rapid learning often indicates an underlying strength.
7. **Motivation:** What motivates you? When you find activities that you do simply for the love of doing them, they are likely to be working from your strengths.

(continues on next page)

Table 5-1 (*Continued*).

8.   **Voice:** Monitor your tone of voice. When you notice a shift in passion, energy, and engagement, you are probably talking about strength.
9.   **Words and phrases:** Listen to the words you use. When you are saying "I love to..." or "It is just great when..." the chances are that it is a strength to which you are referring.
10. **"To do" lists:** Notice the things that never make it onto your "to do" list. These things that always seem to get done reveal an underlying strength that means we never need to ask twice.

Source: Used with permission. Linley, A., Willars, J., & Biswas-Diener, R. (2010). *The strengths book: Be confident, be successful, and enjoy better relationships by realising the best of you* (pp. 60–61). Coventry, UK: CAPP Press.

Strengths Introduction to Clients

Our society is habituated to modesty and not talking about one's accomplishments, which is seen as bragging or being self-centered. Early in coaching a new client, the Nurse Coach can begin with a strengths introduction that her/his coaching style focuses on strengths and positivity and has a scientific basis as described in the previous section.

A natural way to focus on strengths is to ask the client simple questions about the past, present, and future while integrating the strength-spotting tips listed in Table 5-1: "What are some of the things from your *past* that you are most proud of?" "What energizes you in the *present*?" "What are you looking forward to in the near future?"

The key is to move the client to short-story mode where she/he becomes completely absorbed in the telling of the story that reveals the raw material and capacities (Biswas-Diener, 2010). At this point, the Nurse Coach might follow any of the questions above with "Can you tell me more about that?" This short interchange can often result in five or more strengths. To help the client build her/his strength vocabulary, suggest that the client notice things throughout the day that she/he does that are satisfying and labeling them can lead to increasing strengths.

It is also important to address weaknesses for two different reasons (Linley et al., 2010). First, a weakness is exactly that, a weakness, so naming it allows a person to ask for help to decrease the stress around it. Secondly, a weakness can become an area of development to improve. The negative impact of a weakness needs to be minimized so that it does not undermine performance.

For example, a client tells you that he is about to lose his job, as he has been late to work three times in a week. He sets his alarm to wake up, but then he turns it off and goes back to sleep. Rather than giving the client solutions, the Nurse Coach might ask the client some possibilities about how he can change this scenario. Finally, he declares he will buy a second alarm clock to place away from his bed, and will rehearse waking up and getting out of bed. At this point, engaging the client in an imagery practice of going through these steps and rehearsing exactly what he wants to see happen can be empowering. This practice redirects attention towards success rather than further self-criticism. Working with clients to label, spot, and develop strengths is a way to promote energy, effectiveness, productivity, and a sense of meaning.

There may be situations where clients needs to "dial down" a strength. For example, a person's perfectionism and the desire to make something "perfect" may be exhausting. An example might be the person who always raises her hand to take on a project at work and then regrets that she said yes. In hearing the client's story, areas of anxiety and the fear of losing her job surface. This is a good coaching moment to explore other possibilities for increasing self-esteem and self-efficacy.

In summary, the "golden mean" of strengths is critical—the right strength, to the right amount, in the right way, and at the right time. The following four strategies can assist a person to use her/his strengths for higher strength performance (Linley et al., 2010):

1. Marshall realized strengths for optimal performance.
2. Maximize unrealized strengths for growth and development.
3. Moderate learned behaviors for sustainable performance.
4. Minimize weaknesses to make them irrelevant.

Integral Perspective and Strengths

From an integral perspective (see Chapter 14) and at the *subjective level,* the focus is on the positive subjective experience, which includes wellbeing and satisfaction (past), and flow, joy, the sensual pleasures, and happiness (present), and constructive cognitions (future)—optimism, hope, and faith. At the *individual level*, the focus is on positive individual traits—the capacity for love and vocation, courage, interpersonal skill, aesthetic sensibility, perseverance, forgiveness, originality, future-mindedness, high talent, and wisdom. At the *group level*, the focus is on civic virtues and the institutions that move individuals towards better citizenship—responsibility, nurturance, altruism, civility, moderation, tolerance, and work ethic, which are discussed using the VIA classification.

VIA CLASSIFICATION OF CHARACTER STRENGTHS

The VIA Classification of Character Strengths (VIA, n.d.) is the product of a multi-year research project with the goal of identifying what is best about human beings, and how we use those characteristics to build the best lives for ourselves and others. The VIA Classification of Character Strengths is the "backbone" of the science of positive psychology (Csikszentmihalyi, 1990; Seligman, 1990; VIA, n.d.). The resulting classification of 6 virtues and 24 character strengths is seen in **Table 5-2** and forms a language of common ground, which identifies traits of character that are consistent with traits people universally express across all areas of their lives—home, family, social life, and work.

The VIA (VIA, n.d.) views character strengths as capacities humans have for thinking, feeling, and behaving, which are psychological ingredients for displaying virtues or human goodness. The VIA views each person as having a capacity for expressing any of these 24 universal character strengths. Some strengths are easier and more natural for the individual to express (their signature strengths), other strengths arise in particular situations where they are needed (phasic strengths), and other strengths are expressed to a lesser degree or frequency (lesser strengths) (VIA, n.d.). Over a person's lifespan, character strengths are viewed as stable, however, they can change over time. They are also seen as interacting with and influencing each other and are often shaped by the context a person is in.

Seligman (2002) offers a chronology to assist clients to reflect on positive aspects of the past, present, and future. *Positive Past—Elevating Memories* engages the client with practices of past around gratitude, appreciation, forgiveness, and satisfaction. For example, this may include a gratitude imagery practice to explore 5-10 things for which one is grateful (self, family, colleagues, job, etc.) This may also include letter writings, gratitude letters, and journals. *Positive Present—Elevating Emotions* engages the client with practices around mindfulness, slowing down to savor the moment, being in a flow states and noticing life challenges and what can be managed without stress and anxiety. *Positive Future—Elevating Trajectories* engages the client with practices around visioning the future, anticipating the future and reviewing a journal or imagery practice on a regular basis, and confronting any negative reports. See Chapters 16 and 17. In the next section, Story Theory is discussed as a way to further explore clients' strengths.

Table 5-2 The VIA® Classification of Character Strengths.

- **Wisdom and Knowledge:** Cognitive strengths that entail the acquisition and use of knowledge.
  Creativity (originality, ingenuity): Thinking of novel and productive ways to conceptualize and do things; includes artistic achievement but is not limited to it.
  Curiosity (interest, novelty-seeking, openness to experience): Taking an interest in ongoing experience for its own sake; finding subjects and topics fascinating; exploring and discovering.
  Judgment (critical thinking): Thinking things through and examining them from all sides; not jumping to conclusions; being able to change one's mind in light of evidence; weighing all evidence fairly.
  Love of Learning: Mastering new skills, topics, and bodies of knowledge, whether on one's own or formally; obviously related to the strength of curiosity but goes beyond it to describe the tendency to add systematically to what one knows.
  Perspective (wisdom): Being able to provide wise counsel to others; having ways of looking at the world that make sense to one's self and to other people.

- **Courage:** Emotional strengths that involve the exercise of will to accomplish goals in the face of opposition, external or internal.
  Bravery (valor): Not shrinking from threat, challenge, difficulty, or pain; speaking up for what is right even if there is opposition; acting on convictions even if unpopular; includes physical bravery but is not limited to it.
  Perseverance (persistence, industriousness): Finishing what one starts; persisting in a course of action in spite of obstacles; "getting it out the door;" taking pleasure in completing tasks.
  Honesty (authenticity, integrity): Speaking the truth but more broadly presenting one's self in a genuine way and acting in a sincere way; being without pretense; taking responsibility for one's feelings and actions.
  Zest (vitality, enthusiasm, vigor, energy): Approaching life with excitement and energy; not doing things halfway or halfheartedly; living life as an adventure; feeling alive and activated.

- **Humanity:** Interpersonal strengths that involve tending and befriending others.
  Love: Valuing close relations with others, in particular those in which sharing and caring are reciprocated; being close to people.
  Kindness (generosity, nurturance, care, compassion, altruistic love, "niceness"): Doing favors and good deeds for others; helping them; taking care of them.
  Social Intelligence (emotional intelligence, personal intelligence): Being aware of the motives and feelings of other people and one's self; knowing what to do to fit into different social situations; knowing what makes other people tick.

- **Justice:** Civic strengths that underlie healthy community life.
  Teamwork (citizenship, social responsibility, loyalty): Working well as a member of a group or team; being loyal to the group; doing one's share.
  Fairness: Treating all people the same according to notions of fairness and justice; not letting personal feelings bias decisions about others; giving everyone a fair chance.
  Leadership: Encouraging a group of which one is a member to get things done, and at the same time maintaining good relations within the group; organizing group activities and seeing that they happen.

(continues on next page)

Table 5-2 (*Continued*).

- **Temperance**: Strengths that protect against excess.
  Forgiveness: Forgiving those who have done wrong; accepting the shortcomings of others; giving people a second chance; not being vengeful.
  Humility: Letting one's accomplishments speak for themselves; not regarding one's self as more special than one is.
  Prudence: Being careful about one's choices; not taking undue risks; not saying or doing things that might later be regretted.
  Self-Regulation (self-control): Regulating what one feels and does; being disciplined; controlling one's appetites and emotions.

- **Transcendence**: Strengths that forge connections to the larger universe and provide meaning.
  Appreciation of Beauty and Excellence (awe, wonder, elevation): Noticing and appreciating beauty, excellence, and/or skilled performance in various domains of life, from nature to art to mathematics to science to everyday experience.
  Gratitude: Being aware of and thankful for the good things that happen; taking time to express thanks.
  Hope (optimism, future-mindedness, future orientation): Expecting the best in the future and working to achieve it; believing that a good future is something that can be brought about.
  Humor (playfulness): Liking to laugh and tease; bringing smiles to other people; seeing the light side; making (not necessarily telling) jokes.
  Spirituality (faith, purpose): Having coherent beliefs about the higher purpose and meaning of the universe; knowing where one fits within the larger scheme; having beliefs about the meaning of life that shape conduct and provide comfort.

Legend: The VIA Classification of Strengths is the "backbone" of the science of positive psychology (VIA, n.d.). The resulting classification of 6 virtues (Wisdon and Knowledge, Courage, Humanity, Justice, Temperance, Transcendence) and the 24 character strengths within them form a language of common ground and identifies traits of character that are consistent traits people universally express across all areas of their life—home, family, social life, work. The VIA Survey can be accessed at http://www.viacharacter.org/www/The-Survey
Source: Used with permission. Copyright © 2004–2012 by the VIA® Institute on Character. http://www.viacharacter.org/viainstitute/classification.aspx

STORY THEORY

Stories are an integral part of nurse coaching for accessing the client's strengths, wisdom, self-knowledge, and self-understanding of what is true, right, or lasting, and to discover the ambivalence, resistence, and obstacles in a current situation. Stories are based on the client's personal experience in the world. Story is a dynamic process where a person, the storyteller, embraces the telling of a happening or a connected series of happenings (Smith & Liehr, 2010, 2014). It is the storyteller who gives personal meaning to the narrative that usually combines human actions or events, thus impacting the person telling the story and the person listening to the story.

Stories explore healing and meaning and how to be with what is in the moment, which may transform any part of life at different levels. Thus, stories told one way can also change over time when told and retold. As previously discussed, humans are meaning seekers and meaning makers, and we create symbolic stories and use metaphors that have a universal quality. Story is a personal and aesthetic way of knowing (Baldwin, 2005; Carper, 1978; Chinn & Kramer, 2008). (See Chapter 2 and patterns of knowing.) Mary Jane Smith and Patricia Liehr's Story Theory (Smith & Liehr, 2010, 2014), is a middle-range theory that describes story as a narrative happening wherein a person connects with self-in-relation through nurse-person intentional dialogue to create ease. Nurse coaching practice decisions are also informed by the client's stories that infuse bodily responses (both client and Nurse Coach) with unique meaning.

Story Theory has three assumptions that portray the human story as a health story (Smith & Liehr, 2010, 2014). *First*, people change as they interrelate with their world in a vast array of flowing connected dimensions. *Second*, people live in an expanded present moment where past and future events are transformed into the here and now. *Third*, people experience meaning as a resonating awareness in the creative unfolding of human potential. Story Theory has seven phases of inquiry as seen in **Table 5-3**.

Table 5-3 Story Theory Inquiry and Seven Phases.

Phase 1: Gather a story about what matters most about a complication health challenge (or current situation).

Phase 2: Compose a reconstructed story.

Phase 3: Connect existing literature to the health challenge.

Phase 4: Refine the name of the complicating challenge.

Phase 5: Describe the developing story plot with high points, low points, and turning points.

Phase 6: Identify movement towards resolving.

Phase 7: Collect additional stories about the health challenge.

Source: Smith, J. L., & Liehr, P. (2010). Story Theory. In M. E. Parker & M. C. Smith (Eds.), *Nursing theories and nursing practice* (3rd ed., pp. 439–449). Philadelphia, PA: F. A. Davis.

The Nurse Coach can use these seven phases to further assist the client with strategies for dealing with her/his current situation and to further develop evidence-based practice and knowledge:

Phase 1: Gather a story about what matters most about a complicating health challenge (or current situation). As the Nurse Coach gathers the client's story(ies) of what is the most important part of a complicating health challenge or current situation, this is the coming to know the client's unique story, meaning, and strengths.

Phase 2: Compose a reconstructed story. The Nurse Coach with the client will compose a reconstructed story that is a narrative creation with a beginning, middle, and end. This weaves together the client's and the Nurse Coach's perspective on the current topic, situation, or what is most important about the health challenge or current situation.

Phase 3: Connect existing literature to the health challenge. The Nurse Coach will explore the existing literature on themes and symptoms through literature searches. An example might be how a client/patient has found hope and/or exercise strategies while living with severe cardiac conditions.

Phase 4: Refine the name of the complicating challenge. The Nurse Coach skillfully listens to how the client expresses her/his current situation, noticing expressions of obstacles, frustration, or hopelessness. It is in this step that the Nurse Coach assists the client to explore strengths and new possibilities for dealing with the current health challenges.

Phase 5: Describe the developing story plot with high points, low points, and turning points. To help a client make sense of a complicated story, the strategy of developing the story plot through identification of the high points, low points, and turning points is very useful. The Nurse Coach is aware a client often gets stuck in her/his thinking, and by exploring the story plot new meaning and possibilities often emerge.

Phase 6: Identify movement towards resolving. In this phase, the Nurse Coach identifies how the client is considering new strategies for moving forward to find some life satisfaction and balance.

Phase 7: Collect additional stories about the health challenge. This phase takes the Nurse Coach back into the practice area to substantiate what emerged while completing the first six phases.

Next, Henry's complex journey of living with cardiomyopathy, congestive heart failure, and a pacemaker is shared, followed by a Primary Care Physician (PCP) referral to a Nurse Coach who integrates Story Theory and the seven phases and a story-path, and various resource tools.

Vignette: Henry's Story

Henry is a robust and active 65-year-old, anticipating retirement in a few months and completing work as an assistant dean for fundraising at a leading East Coast graduate school. He shares that this is "my last career stretch," and "I want to find home. This is exciting and scary at the same time as I have always had the next project to start." He is an ordained clergy person who has worked virtually half of his life outside of the ecclesiastical institution. A single gay man, he is the father of two adult children (daughter is 32 and son is 29) to whom he is very close.

While still somewhat sexually active, he is being treated with beta-blockers and diuretics, negatively affecting erectile function, which grows worse with each year. This has been a matter of ongoing concern since receiving his cardiomyopathy diagnosis and first pacemaker in 2006. Henry is intolerant to statin medications and continues to have high LDL, even with diet modification and exercise. He has recently gained 18 pounds from fluid retention and has sought medical attention.

Following his second pacemaker in 2013, and his move to New Mexico in early 2014, Henry met with his new cardiologist for a thorough pacemaker evaluation. Henry was started on Lasix (furosemide) 40 mg twice daily and potassium chloride ER daily.

After two weeks with no substantive effect, Henry again met with his cardiologist who questioned how he was taking his medication and what his fluid intake had been. Henry responded that in reading the drug indications and contraindications there was a strict warning about dehydration. Thus, he concluded that he must drink more water than usual to compensate for the loss. The cardiologist reeducated Henry about the value and risks of diuretic treatment and recommended drastic reduction in fluid intake. Henry's dose of diuretic was increased weekly to 200 mg twice daily (the maximum dose) until an optimum of 201 pounds was reached and a 39-inch girth was maintained. He also sent an e-mail report every four days.

After two weeks, the cardiologist referred Henry back to his PCP to manage all his medications, as he was still 10–12 pounds too heavy. The PCP stopped the Lasix and started Henry on Demadex (torsemide) 81 mg daily (loop diuretic). If he was still gaining weight while monitoring his strict sodium and fluid intake, Henry was to take Metolazone 5 mg (thiazide-like diuretic) one hour before torsemide. Henry's sleep apnea was evaluated with a sleep study. He was started on a VPAP (variable positive airway pressure) device with bi-level setting for inhalation and exhalation.

Henry felt that death might be imminent, and the PCP referred him to the Nurse Coach in his office. She listened deeply to Henry's multiple dynamic and complex stories within stories. Over the first three sessions, the Nurse Coach and Henry together explored the meaning of his cardiac challenges and his turning points, high points, and low points (**Table 5-4**) and his story path (**Figure 5-1**). At the first session Henry completed the Integrative Health and Wellness Assessment (Appendix C-2). Henry also declared that he wanted to make changes in the following areas, and he was given specific resource sheets: to learn how to breath from his belly (Appendix F-3); readiness to change eating habits (Appendix E-3); to eat with awareness (Appendices E-4 and E-7); and to keep a food journal (Appendix E-5).

Session 4 (four weeks later).

NC: Henry, it is so good to see you smiling and lighter in spirit today! What major changes have occurred?

Henry: I'm finally on the right combination of medications and losing weight and have no signs of swelling in my lower extremities. The VPAP helps me sleep 5–7 hours. I have some improvement in my sexual function and energy to either swim a mile or walk a mile every other day. I have learned a lot about breathing easier and new behaviors to eat slowly and with awareness.

NC: Can you share with me some of what you are doing that is new?

Henry: Well, a big thing was when you asked me to define health and I keep thinking about this each day. You gave me some suggestions to spot my strengths [Table 5-1]. I am also waking up and doing strength spotting and naming my strengths each morning. Exploring my heart challenges and the turning, high, and low points [Table 5-4] and doing my story path [Figure 5-1] shows me how much progress I have made. Focusing on celebrating what is going right each day also helps.

NC: Henry, how do you define health for you right now?

Henry: Health for me right now is weighing between 201 and 207 as I was making myself crazy trying to weigh 201 every day.

NC: What new skills do you use to stay healthy?

Henry: Keeping a food journal has become a new practice, particularly around sodium levels in food and how to monitor my fluid intake. I can see how to stabilize my big weight fluctuations. I am using the belly breathing to reduce my frequent worrying and my "poor me" conversation. When that happens I concentrate on the breath in and out. I think of exercise as energizing and something to anticipate with joy.

The following illustrates how the Nurse Coach moved Henry to short-story mode to hear the raw material of his experiences and the meaning for his life at the present time around adjusting to the VPAP.

NC: Can you share some of your strengths that helped you accept using the VPAP?

Henry: I would say that learning to place my attention and intention in the present moment has helped me shift my thoughts to feeling motivated to do new things. I am listening to my self-talk and focusing it on what feels right.

I have been claustrophobic my whole life and really afraid of suffocation. When I finally allowed that I would have to accept the VPAP for my oxygen starvation and ongoing congestive heart failure, I was in shock and resisted it for a very long time. After a month of careful desensitization of having a face mask for sleep and accepting the nose pillow device, I yielded. After a month of use, waking one morning, breathing slowly and deeply with the VPAP, I simply followed my breath...in and out, in and out, slowly...deeply. I found myself awash in tears of gratitude and breathing like a newborn.

Your teaching me about relaxation and deep belly breathing as daily practices have been amazing "ah ha" experiences. Deep from within I felt my belly rising and falling, upper chest still, as the VPAP positive and negative pressure forced air in and allowed exhalation to come...naturally. The tears of gratitude and remembrances poured like a morning rain, gently but full. I now see my VPAP as my new friend and my pacemaker as my old friend.

I remembered stories of my infancy and childhood...of being a colicky baby. Never quite breathing fully, hurting in the belly, gasping for air, even after I had an emergency tonsillectomy and adenoidectomy at ages 2 and 3. Still having trouble breathing 60 years later, I am finally breathing deeply and "normally" like a baby. I have suffered for most of my life from lack of breath and capacity to breathe deeply enough to rest... (long pause).

NC: *Have any other experiences come forth?*

Henry: I'm so glad you introduced me to imagery and healing rituals [see Chapters 12 and 18]. The other night I arose from the bed, and I disconnected myself from the VPAP but left the nose pillow straps around my head with the plastic accordion oxygen tube hanging from the front of my face. I could breathe through my mouth. I looked like a man elephant with my trunk swaying (laughing). As I went into the kitchen to get a glass of water, I gazed out into the dawn light, and there was the large bronze garden statue of Ganesh with his elephant trunk...(long pause).

NC: *Say more about Ganesh and what this means right now?*

Henry: He is the patron of arts and sciences and of intellect and wisdom. As the Hindu god of beginnings, he is honored at the start of rituals and ceremonies. Ganesh is also invoked as the patron of letters and learning during writing sessions—looking back at me in the breaking dawn light...(long pause). Seeing my faint reflection in the window in these waning moments of darkness, there was the image of my face and the affixed swaying plastic trunk was superimposed over this image of Ganesh. We became one— elephant and man, baby and boy, father and son, beginning and ending. The past and present and the future strangely merged as one. For the first time in 60 years, I could breathe as humans were designed, and my heart could take some relief that strength would come.

NC: *What rich imagery and powerful meaning for you! In the middle of your sharing your Ganesh experience you had a very long pause. I have a hunch that something came up for you?*

Henry: (Laughing)...You nailed it! I heard my voice say the words, "I am a good writer... begin, my man!" I am being called to write my life story and ready to begin! But where do I start as I have 40 years of diaries, lectures, sermons, global projects, and more? Since the beginning of our sessions, you have heard me say that I am struggling to find home, and I like worthy projects.

To add to the elements of Story Theory, the next section examines the Story-Health Model to further illustrate how story as a narrative happening allows a client/patient to connect with self-in-relation through Nurse Coach–client/patient intentional dialogue to create ease.

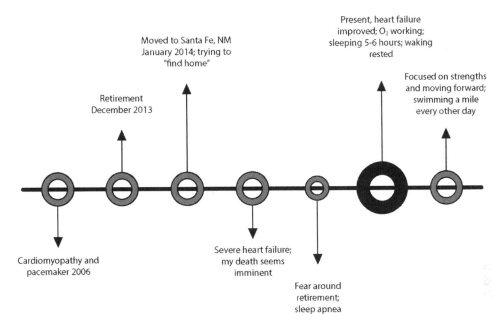

Figure 5-1 Henry's Story Path.
Source: Copyright © 2014 by the International Nurse Coach Association. www.inursecoach.com

Table 5-4 Henry: Turning Points (TP), High Points (HP), Low Points (LP).

Story Event	TP	HP	LP
Cardiomyopathy and pacemaker 2006			X
Retirement December 2013	X		
Moved to Santa Fe, NM, January 2014	X		
Trying to "find home"			X
Heart failure January 2014			X
New cardiologist; extensive pacemaker evaluation		X	
Weight gain of 12 lbs; Lasix 40 mg 2x day; then increased Lasix 200 mg 2x daily	X		
Ace-inhibitors and beta-blockers; impotence			X
New primary care physician; sleep apnea treated with O_2 at night; 5–7 hours sleep; waking rested	X		
Demadex 81 mg and Metolazone 5 mg	X		
Some return of sexual function; walking or swimming a mile every other day		X	
Retirement is freeing work-related stress		X	
Feeling of imminent death has passed for now	X		
Focusing on strengths daily; celebrate living now		X	

Source: Copyright © 2014 by the International Nurse Coach Association. www.inursecoach.com

STORY-HEALTH MODEL

Jennifer L. Reich (2011) developed the Story-Health Model (**Figure 5-2**) as a research model representing the conceptual structure of Story Theory (Smith & Liehr, 2010, 2014). As dis-

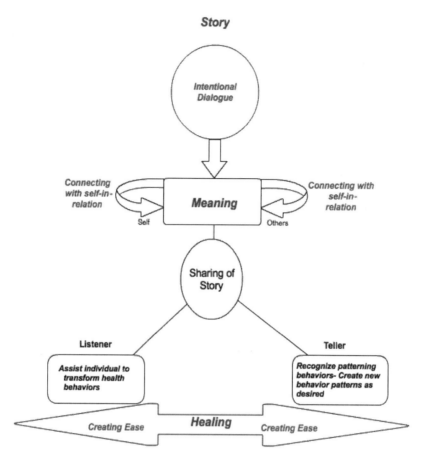

Figure 5-2 Story-Health Model.
Legend: Reich (2010) created the Story-Health Model based on Story Theory (Smith & Liehr, 2010, 2014). The person connects with *self-in-relation* through nurse–person *intentional dialogue* to *create ease*. The *head* represents the whole person from a unitary-transformative perspective. *Intentional dialogue* begins in the head. The Nurse Coach respects the client, the storyteller, as expert. The *heart* level represents meaning, with an expanded awareness of self and others in the developing story plot, represented by the concept of *connecting with self-in-relation*. The client's *gut* represents a deep place inside where there is a power to release stories that do not promote our mental, physical, emotional, and/or spiritual health. This demonstrates client and Nurse Coach connecting with self-in-relation. The *feet* represent the storyteller and the listener, and the concept of *creating ease* in the bottom arrow symbolizes the "flow in the midst of anchoring."
Source: Used with permission from Reich, J. L. (2011). *The anatomy of story.* (Doctoral dissertation, University of Arizona).

cussed under reflective practice, this model can guide the Nurse Coach in new ways to reflect on an experience after an event occurs, and to reflect in action—in real time—during the hearing of a client's story or in other situations.

The *head* of the Story-Health Model is story from a whole person, unitary-transformative perspective. *Intentional dialogue* begins in the head and requires that the Nurse Coach respect the client, the storyteller, as expert. This allows the Nurse Coach to abandon preexisting assumptions and to use the power of the pause before asking the client questions to clarify meaning. The *heart* level represents meaning. As the client shares her/his story, there is the expanded awareness of self and others in the developing story plot as represented by the concept of *connecting with self-in-relation*.

Next, continuing into the client's *gut*, this is a deep place inside where she/he has the power to release stories that do not promote mental, physical, emotional, and/or spiritual health. As the Nurse Coach listens to the client's story, this demonstrates connecting with self-in-relation. The *feet* represent the storyteller and the listener. As the client as storyteller hears her/his story and reflects on what is shared, often there is new awareness, choice, and energy to create new patterns and behaviors. The Nurse Coach's presence as listener may also assist the client to transform health-negating behaviors by offering new strategies that promote health. The concept of *creating ease* is shown in the bottom arrow of Figure 5-2, which is a symbol of "flow in the midst of anchoring" (Smith & Liehr, 2010). This represents when the story moments come together with a feeling of connectedness that is often described as healing where conflicts, fears, or doubts may be resolved and new possibilities emerge (Reich, 2011). In the next section, recurring themes that emerge in client stories are explored.

ADDRESSING SUFFERING, FEAR, AND SPIRITUALITY

Suffering

As Nurse Coaches, we frequently encounter clients' suffering, moral suffering, moral distress, and soul pain, and are often called upon to "be with" these difficult human experiences and to use our nursing presence (**Table 5-5**). Suffering is an individual's experience of struggle based on a reinforced story around anxiety, distress, or pain. It can manifest as behavioral, emotional, mental, moral, physical, social, and/or spiritual signs of distress; it is anguish—internal and external—experienced as a threat to one's composure, integrity, sense of self, or the fulfillment of expectations. See client/patient case studies in Chapters 10 and 13, which include these areas and other health and life challenge topics.

Nurse Coaches cultivate the balance between compassion and equanimity. Compassion is the ability to be present for all levels of suffering with no need to "fix" the suffering. It is the tenderness of the heart in response to suffering. Equanimity is a spacious stillness that accepts things as they are. The balance of compassion and equanimity allows Nurse Coaches to care without becoming overwhelmed. Nurse Coaches are invited to see this balance as the truth of our human condition and to be present to our experience of it in the following ways (Halifax, Dossey, & Rushton, 2007):

1. Acknowledge the suffering.
2. Give voice to the suffering.
3. Bear witness to the suffering.
4. Create and implement a self-care plan.
5. Develop a supportive work environment.

As suffering comes forth, the client is given an opportunity to face the tender parts of her/his personal story that have or are currently causing pain and suffering. It may be due to being hurt by a person, situation (home or workplace abuse, violence, social exclusion), natural hazard, or one's personal perception of an event. It may serve as an awareness bridge to healing, and adhering to positive new steps toward health and wellbeing. Choosing to acknowledge our emotions and feelings with a willingness to engage with this state determines our courage and clarity of purpose.

Our sense of "we" supports us in recognizing the phases of suffering (Table 5-5)—"mute" suffering, "expressive" suffering, and "new identity" in suffering (Reich, 1989). For example, when a person feels alone she/he experiences *mute suffering*, which is an inability to articulate and communicate with others one's own suffering. In coaching sessions, the Nurse Coach skillfully assists clients to enter into the phase of *expressive suffering* wherein sufferers seek language to express their frustrations, feelings, and challenges.

Outcomes of this experience often move toward *new identity* in suffering through new meaning-making where one makes new sense of the past, interprets new meaning in suffering, and can envision a new future. A shift in one's consciousness allows for a shift in one's capacity to be able to transform her/his suffering from causing distress to finding some new truth and meaning of it. Coaching provides time for sharing and giving voice to concerns and vulnerability, and new levels of healing may happen that assist with examining frustrations or fear, which is explored next.

Table 5-5 Suffering, Moral Suffering, Moral Distress, and Soul Pain.

Suffering:	An individual's story around pain where the signs of suffering may be physical, mental, emotional, social, behavioral, and/or spiritual; it is an anguish experienced —internal and external—as a threat to one's composure, integrity, and the fulfillment of intentions.
Moral suffering:	Occurs when an individual experiences tensions or conflicts about what is the right thing to do in a particular situation; it often involves the struggle of finding a balance between competing interests or values.
Moral distress:	Occurs when an individual is unable to translate moral choices into moral actions and when prevented by obstacles, either internal or external, from acting upon it; acting in a manner contrary to personal and professional values undermines the individual's integrity and autheticity.
Soul pain:	The experience of an individual who has become disconnected and alienated from the deepest and most fundamental aspects of one's self.

Sources: Used with permission from Halifax, J., Dossey, B. M., & Rushton, C. H. (2007). *Being with dying: Compassionate end-of-life training guide*. Santa Fe, NM: Prajna Mountain Press. Adapted from Jameton, A. (1984). *Nursing practice: The ethical issues*. Englewood Cliffs, NJ: Prentice Hall; and Kearney, M. (1996). *Mortally wounded*; New York, NY: Scribner.

Fear

Nurse Coaches explore clients' fears. A fear is a worry that can surface at any time and often manifests with contemplating changes in lifestyle patterns. For example, a person who wishes to stop smoking may have many different fears, such as fear of not being able to stop smoking; fear of gaining weight; fear of nicotine withdrawal; fear of offending other people by asking them not to smoke; or fear of not being able to sustain smoking cessation, etc.

Fear only comes in relationship to something else. Then what is fear in relationship to? Is it in relationship to the unknown? If fear is unknown, how can you fear it? Is it possible that the origin of the fear is loss of the known? The known is when we acknowledge that we do not know enough about a situation, such as changing to a healthier lifestyle, not knowing the right thing to say, or not knowing when a family member, friends, or you will die. If this is so, how can a person gain freedom from the fear? This is the healing journey—learning more about one's relationship with all things. See Chapter 15 and Knowing Participation in Change Theory.

Fear somehow can get hold of a person's spirit, lodging somewhere within the physical body. Fear may create separation and aloneness, and it can also become a path that will lead deeper into the present moment. It does not have to be a barrier to the moment. Fear states usually create more of what is feared. However, every time fear surfaces, it can become a moment to learn more about another level of life's journey and courage (Brown, 2012). Fear is useful in that it alerts a person to areas of resistance and not being ready to move through a certain event. Releasing the fear always returns a person to the unconditional core of love. When a person approaches an event with the notion that there is a correct or certain way to be, this may create further distance from one's core of being present in the moment. Fear may also surface around topics of religion, spirituality, and transpersonal experiences, which are discussed next.

Reflections on Religion, Spirituality, and Transpersonal Dimensions

Nurse Coaches often hear stories related to religion and spirituality. Religion is the codified and ritualized beliefs and behaviors of those involved in spirituality, usually taking place within a community of like-minded individuals. The word "spirit" is derived from *spiritus*, which means breath, courage, the soul, life; *spiritus* is the Latin counterpart of the Greek *pneuma*, meaning breath or air. Spirituality is the feelings, thoughts, experiences, and behaviors that arise from a search for that which is generally considered sacred or holy. Spirituality gives meaning to life, and is usually, though not universally, considered to involve a sense of connection with an absolute, imminent, or transcendent spiritual force, however named, as well as the conviction that meaning, value, direction, and purpose are valid aspects of the universe (Dossey, 2003).

The transpersonal can be defined as a person's understanding that is based on personal experiences of temporarily transcending or moving beyond one's usual identification with the limited biological, historical, cultural, and personal self at the deeper and most profound levels of experience possible (Achterberg, Dossey, & Kolkmeier, 1994; Dossey, 2013). It is that which transcends the limits and boundaries of individual ego identities and possibilities to include acknowledgement and appreciation of something greater. From this perspective, the ordinary, biological, historical, cultural, and personal self is seen as important, but only a partial manifestation or expression of this much greater something that is one's deeper origin and destination. In the next section, the Nurse Coach 5-step process in a client coaching session brings together the previous discussion on presence, meaning, strengths, stories, and emerging themes.

NURSE COACH 5-STEP PROCESS IN A CLIENT COACHING SESSION

The Nurse Coach 5-step process as seen in **Figure 5-3** is grounded in clinical knowledge and practice in the full spirit of the coaching movement as a human service. General coaching questions may be used (see Chapter 6, Table 6-1) and also integrated with the Listening with HEART (**H**ealing, **E**nergy, **A**wareness, **R**esilience, **T**ransformation) questions depending on what is occurring in the coaching session (see Chapter 2 Theory of Nurse Coaching Component 5 and Listening with HEART, Table 2-6). The Nurse Coach 5-step process is as follows:

Step 1: Connecting to the story (current self, CS)
Step 2: Deep listening and skillful questioning
Step 3: Inviting opportunities, potentials, and change
Step 4: Integrating, practicing, and embodying change
Step 5: Guiding and supporting the transforming self (TS)

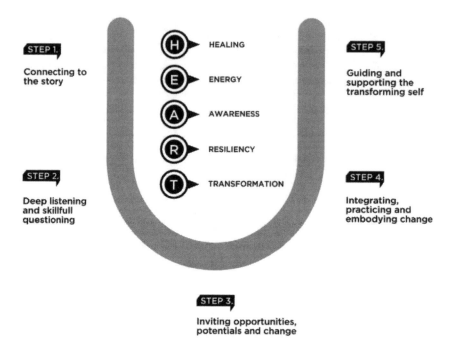

Figure 5-3 Nurse Coach 5-Step Process and Listening With HEART.
Source: Copyright © 2014 by the International Nurse Coach Association. www.inursecoach.com

Step 1: Connecting to the Story (current self, CS)

The Nurse Coach becomes fully present, centered, and grounded. This allows for full attention to the client's chosen topic/s and the elements in the story that are shared. This includes noticing both the affective and energetic state of the client, as well as the content of what is being presented in the session and within any story.

Explore the reason (topic) for the client visit. Walk with the client in self-discovery and let her or him choose the path. At the appropriate time early in a coaching session, review the Nurse Coach and Client Guiding Principles (Appendix A-1) and Agreement (Appendix A-2). (*Note*: Adapt the client contract as needed for whether coaching is done in a private practice or a clinical setting.)

These two forms may also be discussed when a client calls to make an appointment and may be sent before a session via an e-mail attachment or by mail. Allowing the client to be in control of the session will increase self-efficacy and self-confidence. Remember, the client is the expert on her/his life and what works and what does not work. Recognizing where the client is in her/his process of change is very important. Some clients will come to a session highly motivated, and by the end of a session be able to declare clear goals. Other clients may be so overwhelmed with life that setting goals and priorities early on in coaching is impossible. It may be several sessions before even one goal is established. At the beginning of a session it is very useful to ask the client earlier in the session such questions as "What topic do you want to discuss today?" "In our _____minutes together today, where do you want to be by the end of the session?" "Since we met last, what might you want me to know?"

The Nurse Coach aligns her/his intention with the client's goals and attends to the subjective experiences and internal frame of reference. This builds trust and respect. Belief in the client's capacity to connect with inner resources, wisdom, and potentials towards desired changes and goals is essential. Being present with the client's process of discovery assists the Nurse Coach to step back from the nurse expert role, remembering the wisdom of "less is more" in the coaching conversation.

Step 2: Deep Listening and Skillful Questioning

As a starting point, the client may bring a topic or specific intention or goal to the coaching session. If the client cannot identify clearly a topic or goal for the session, the Nurse Coach, through skillful questioning and/or introducing awareness practices (Chapter 12), can assist the client to identify what she or he is hoping for. Topics for exploration may also be generated by the client's responses and reactions to open-ended questions, or from the Integrative Health and Wellness Assessment™ (see Appendices C-1 and C-2) or other tools.

The Nurse Coach conveys curiosity about what the client brings to the coaching session, and is attentive and open to what is presented. The client provides the subject and direction of the coaching conversation. The Nurse Coach lets go of trying "to fix" a client or a situation. Deep listening is achieved by the ability and skill to quiet one's inner dialogue. It has an enormous quality of *nowness*. Nowness is the ability to throw away intellectualizations when the client goes off in an unexpected direction, and to see where the thread of the story might lead.

As previous discussed, a client may be intent on telling a part of her/his story, and deep listening is required to enter into the flow of the story. This frequently leads to the client's gaining some new insight about turning points, high points, and low points as seen in Table 5-4. Nurse Coaches strive to not be intent on a personal viewpoint of what we think should be happening as this starts our own inner dialogue of analysis and intellectualization. As we increase this process of nowness, there is a shift in consciousness that encourages the client to move to a state of nowness to connect with her/his inner wisdom. Questioning and listening that does not structure the answers, except minimally, is a great art.

Any communication process has three components: a sender of the message, a receiver of the message, and the content of the material. In order for us to understand clients, we must move to the present moment. Being quiet while someone else is talking is not equivalent to deep listening. The key to deep listening is *intention* when we focus with someone in order to move with purpose in our responses. This can lead others or us toward effective action steps or forward in personal growth and behavioral change. Deep listening occurs when we have the intention to understand someone, enjoy joy someone, learn something, co-mutually engage with another in the change process as discussed in the Story-Health Model.

Often, clients get impatient and want answers quickly. Reflecting on Rilke's words, "*Live* the questions now. Perhaps you will then gradually, without noticing it, live along some distant day into the answer" (Rilke, 1962). Deep listening facilitates the client's greater acceptance of thoughts and emotions. Thus, the client may be in a better situation to choose the most effective behaviors that lead towards health and wholeness. If and when the client moves into vulnerable moments, bearing witness to the client's narrative is essential. Being curious and open is attending to the present moment, allowing whatever emerges to come forth. By bringing awareness to her/his inner wisdom, wealth of experience and intuition, the Nurse Coach draws from inner resources and intuitions to guide the direction of the questioning.

Cultivating a connection with the client that communicates safety and respect may create more opportunity for the client to explore vulnerability, doubts, and challenges. Skillful questions move the client towards goals by identifying strengths, attitudes, behaviors, and beliefs that have led to past successes and accomplishments. This will also lead to identifying blocks and obstacles, both internal and external, that have created limitations. It supports the client in identifying habits of thought and feeling that are self-defeating. Bringing awareness to these patterns provides the possibility for making different choices.

When the Nurse Coach deals with issues that are outside the scope of her/his expertise, referrals are made. It is essential that the Nurse Coach be knowledgeable about and has information and a team of trusted professional colleagues for referral resources and a full spectrum of community resources (crisis prevention centers, etc.).

Step 3: Inviting Opportunities, Potentials, and Change

The Nurse Coach recognizes and respects the client's subjective experiences, perceptions, learning style, and culture (e.g., beliefs, values, and customs). Additionally, the Nurse Coach continuously exhibits authenticity through honesty, sincerity, personal integrity, and maintaining professional ethics. See Chapter 3. The coaching conversation is a co-creative process with the client in planning and negotiating clear actions and agreements. Following up on agreements and reevaluating their effectiveness or appropriateness is part of the process.

In the returning coaching sessions, an exploration with the client about what goals and plans have been kept and how to reexamine the plans that have not been realized is important. Periodically reviewing the client's action plan stimulates engagement and helps to identify barriers to change. By holding the person accountable for planned actions, SMART goals (see Chapter 15), time frames, and desired outcomes, progress continues as a result of the dynamics within the coaching relationship.

A client's new ideas, behaviors, and actions may feel uncomfortable or even risky as old patterns and habits are challenged. Fear of failure is often an issue. Ongoing support is offered. When unrealistic or unmanageable goals are established, the Nurse Coach often suggests that the client apply the 50% rule—cutting a goal in half to maximize the potential for an initial success.

Step 4: Integrating, Practicing, and Embodying Change

Encouraging and supporting the client to experiment and apply what has been learned from the coaching interaction most often leads to new behaviors and sustained change. Often, if the client works on two goals together such as eating healthier and walking two to three times a week, commitment and confidence may increase. This interaction demonstrates that the Nurse Coach is an ally and supporter in the change process. Being mindful of the power inherent in the coaching relationship, encouragement and feedback that is nonjudgmental, respectful, and appropriate are offered.

Coaching allows the client to express strong feelings without judgment, which facilitates movement towards achievement of goals. The Nurse Coach continues to observe the client's breathing patterns, facial expressions, body language, vocal quality, and energy. Recognizing that change is hard assists the client to identify her/his resistance and/or ambivalence to change. Helping a client to understand patterns of resistance can become an opportunity for self-awareness and growth. See Chapter 16.

Employing deep listening and powerful questioning, the Nurse Coach will focus more completely on what the client is communicating. Changing behavior means integrating and practicing, and embodying change. This implies that the client makes changes that are tangible and bring this awareness into day-to-day activities such as planning for a meal with fresh vegetables and fruit, or identifying when and where a brisk 15-minute walk can be done. This awareness opens up the opportunity for the client to choose to take new actions and create new ways of thinking and being, and planning ahead, rather than engaging in mindless, habituated behavior. Embodied change brings the possibility of being liberated from self-defeating patterns and thoughts.

Step 5: Guiding and Supporting the Transforming Self (TS)

Skillfully, the Nurse Coach assists clients to explore and navigate through the narrative of their story and the turning points, high points, and low points. Profound changes may occur in the coaching journey when clients are also introduced to reflective awareness practices, mindfulness, and imagery awareness practices (Chapter 12 and Appendix F). Integrating motivational interviewing (Chapter 16) and appreciative inquiry (Chapter 17) assists clients to identify stress management skills, as well as metaphors, symbols, images, or words that resonate with their story.

A client's story often brings forth intimate, dynamic, personally meaningful, and quality-of-life experiences that may be aligned with her/his envisioned hopes and intentions. They are not static and become useful resources throughout coaching sessions. These experiences become part of a transformative process where a client may release or reconcile with parts of her/his story that no longer serve. This coaching discovery process inspires the client to be open to broader perspectives and new ways of being.

As shown in **Figure 5-4,** the client's current self (CS) includes one's current reality. As changes are made, the old story remains, but it also opens into another way of being and transcends into the changing and the transforming self (TS). The Nurse Coach recognizes the client's new way of being and acknowledges the changed behaviors and new commitments. Exploring the six lines of development (Chapter 14)—cognitive, emotional, somatic, interpersonal, spiritual, and moral—is also a dynamic way to view the change process, which often leads to sustained change.

Clarity in what is working provides the client with a strong foundation to build on in the future when other challenges occur. This recognition also provides more insights and elicits opportunities for new commitments or actions. The client's old worldview and assumptions have been challenged. The transforming self is becoming integrated into the broadened sense of self, leading to increased self-efficacy, self-esteem, and confidence.

From an integral perspective, every individual is always negotiating her/his experience at many levels. People observe their present interaction at the same time they are affected by, and shaped by, past experiences, some remembered and some forgotten. Both challenges and opportunities can present themselves in any of these aspects of being. This is a dynamic dance and flow of transformation that manifests as creativity between being and becoming in the ever-present change process.

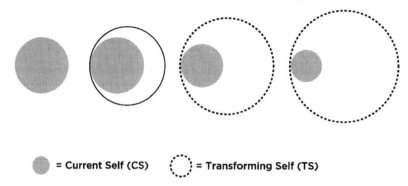

= Current Self (CS)   = Transforming Self (TS)

Figure 5-4 Client Changes Through Coaching.
Legend: Clients bring to coaching their current self (CS) and story (past, present, future). Through coaching, the client's current self opens to new opportunities, potentials, and change. The CS (large gray circle) begins to shift (large gray circle now surrounded by solid black outer circle), to smaller gray circle (with dotted circle of opening and releasing old behaviors/patterns and parts of story that no longer serve), to an even smaller gray circle as the transforming self (TS) emerges where changes can be realized and sustained.
Source: Copyright © 2014 by the International Nurse Coach Association. www.inursecoach.com

SUMMARY

- Stories connect us to our strengths, meaning, resilience, and healing potential.
- Story is an approach for addressing strengths, suffering, fears, spirituality, and human flourishing.
- Story Theory and the Story-Health Model increase capacities for reflective practice and enhance theory-guided and evidence-based nurse coaching practice.
- The Nurse Coach uses the Nurse Coach 5-step process to connect to the client's story: Step 1: Connecting to the story (current self, CS); Step 2: Deep listening and skillful questioning; Step 3: Inviting opportunities, potentials, and change; Step 4: Integrating, practicing and embodying change; and Step 5: Guiding and supporting the transforming self (TS).

NURSE COACH REFLECTIONS

After reading this chapter, the Nurse Coach will be able to bring awareness and personal insight to the following questions:

- How do I use story in my life and nurse coaching practice?
- When I create my story path around being a Nurse Coach and nurse coaching, what do I experience?
- What are my reflective practices that assist me to be present to the client's story?
- How does hearing the client's story assist in promoting health and healing?
- What do I experience when I enter into the flow of the client's story?

REFERENCES

Achterberg, J., Dossey, B. M., & Kolkmeier, L. (1994). *Rituals of healing: Using imagery for health and wellness.* New York, NY: Bantam.

Baldwin, C. (2005). *Storycatcher: Making sense of our lives through the power and practice of story.* Novoto, CA: New World Library.

Biswas-Diener, R. (2010). *Practicing positive psychology coaching: Assessment, activities, and strategies for success* (pp. 19–38). Hoboken, NJ: John Wiley.

Brown, B. (2012). *Daring greatly: How the courage to be vulnerable transforms the way we live, love, parent, and lead.* New York, NY: Gotham Books.

Carper, B. A. (1978). Fundamental patterns of knowing in nursing. *Advances in Nursing Science, 1*(1), 13–23.

Chinn, P., & Kramer, M. (2008). *Theory and nursing: Integrated knowledge development* (7th ed.). St. Louis, MO: C. V. Mosby.

Csikszentmihalyi, M. (1990). *Flow: The psychology of optimal experience.* New York, NY: Harper and Row.

Dossey, B. M. (2013). Nursing: Integral, integrative, and holistic—local to global. In B. M. Dossey & L. Keegan (Eds.), *Holistic nursing: A handbook for practice* (6th ed., pp. 1–57). Burlington, MA: Jones & Bartlett Learning.

Dossey, L. (2003). Samueli conference on definitions and standards in healing research: Working definitions and terms. *Alternative Therapies in Health and Medicine 9*(3), A11.

Freshwater, D., Taylor, B. J., & Sherwood, G. C. (Eds.) (2008). *The international textbook of reflective practice in nursing.* Chichester, UK: Wiley-Blackwell.

Halifax, J., Dossey, B. M., & Rushton, C. H. (2007). *Being with dying: Compassionate end-of-life training guide.* Santa Fe, NM: Prajna Mountain Press.

Johns, C. (2013). *Becoming a reflective practitioner* (4th ed.). Hoboken, NJ: Wiley-Blackwell.

Koerner, J. G. (2007). *Healing presence: The essence of nursing practice.* New York, NY: Springer.

Linley, A., Willars, J., & Biswas-Diener, R. (2010). *The strengths book: Be confident, be successful, and enjoy better relationships by realising the best of you* (pp. 60–61). Coventry, UK: CAPP Press.

Newman, M. (2008). *Transforming presence: The difference that nursing makes.* Philadelphia, PA: F. A. Davis.

Nightingale, F. (1868/June). Una and the lion. *Good words* (p. 362). In B. M. Dossey (2000). *Florence Nightingale: Mystic, visionary, healer* (p. 294). Philadelphia, PA: Lippincott Williams & Wilkins.

Peterson, C., & Seligman, M. E. P. (2004). *Character strengths and virtues: A handbook and classification.* New York, NY: Oxford University Press and Washington, DC: American Psychological Association.

Quinn, J. F. (2013). Transpersonal human caring and healing. In B. M. Dossey & L. Keegan (Eds.), *Holistic nursing: A handbook for practice* (6th ed., pp. 107–114). Burlington, MA: Jones & Bartlett Learning.

Reich, J. L. (2011). *The anatomy of story.* (Doctoral dissertation, University of Arizona).

Reich, W. T. (1989). Speaking of suffering: A moral account. *Soundings 72*, 83–108.

Rilke, R. M. (1962). *Letters to a young poet* (M. D. Herter, trans.) (Revised ed., p. 35). New York, NY: W. W. Norton.

Seligman, M. E. P. (1990). *Learned optimism: How to change your mind and your life.* New York, NY: Free Press.

Seligman, M. E. P. (2002). *Authentic happiness: Using the new positive psychology to realize your potential for lasting fulfillment.* New York, NY: Free Press.

Smith, M. J., & Liehr, P. (2010). Story theory. In M. E. Parker & M. C. Smith (Eds.). *Nursing theories and nursing practice* (3rd ed., pp. 439–449). Philadelphia, PA: F. A. Davis.

Smith, M. J., & Liehr, P. R. (2014). Story theory. In M. J. Smith & P. R. Liehr (Eds.), *Middle range theory for nursing* (3rd ed.). New York, NY: Springer.

VIA Classifications (n.d.). Retrieved from http://www.viacharacter.org/viainstitute/classification.aspx

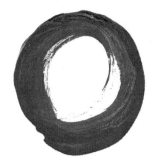

CHAPTER 6

Integrative Health and Wellness Assessment*,†

Barbara Montgomery Dossey

> What is health? Health is not only to be well, but to use well every power we have.
>
> *Florence Nightingale,* 1896

LOOKING AHEAD...

After reading this chapter, you will be able to:

- Examine the Integrative Health and Wellness Assessment™ (IHWA) and the eight components.
- Complete the IHWA to become aware of your current patterns and any areas you wish to change.
- Identify your readiness to change, priority for making a change, and confidence in ability to make the change.
- Coach clients using the IHWA on new health behaviors, goals, and action plans.

DEFINITIONS

Note: The terms "client" and "patient" are interchangeable throughout this chapter.

Healing: A process of understanding and integrating the many aspects of self, leading to a deep connection with inner wisdom and an experience of balance and wholeness.

Healing awareness: A person's conscious recognition of and focused attention on intuitions, subtle feelings, conditions, and circumstances relating to the needs of self or clients.

Healing process: The continual changing and evolution of one's self through life that includes reflecting on meaning and purpose in living.

Health: Process through which individuals reshape basic assumptions and worldviews, which includes aspects of physical, mental, emotional, social, spiritual, cultural, and environmental wellbeing, and not merely the absence of disease; may include living with a disease, illness, or symptoms. It includes death as a natural process of living.

Self-confidence: A person's belief in her/his capacity to make a behavioral change.

***Note:** Contact the International Nurse Coach Association for use of the Integrative Health and Wellness Assessment (IHWA) and survey software at http://www.inursecoach.com/contact-us/

†The chapter is adapted from Dossey, B. M., Luck, S., Schaub, B. G., & Keegan, L. (2013). Self-assessments. In B. M. Dossey & L. Keegan (Eds.), *Holistic nursing: A handbook for practice* (6th ed., pp. 161–187). Burlington, MA: Jones & Bartlett Learning.

Self-efficacy: The belief that one has the capability of initiating and sustaining desired behaviors; includes feeling a sense of empowerment and ability to make healthful choices leading to sustained change.

Self-esteem: The belief that one has personal self-worth.

Wellbeing: A general term for the condition of an individual or group and their social, economic, psychological, spiritual, or medical state; based on the idea that the way each person thinks and feels about her/his life is meaningful and important.

HEALING AND WHOLENESS

Healing is a process of understanding and integrating the many aspects of self, leading to a deep connection with inner wisdom and an experience of balance and wholeness (Dossey, 2013). Healing is more likely to occur on many levels when individuals attend to different aspects of their lives. Daily stress and crisis may emerge, and often we focus only on all the things that are wrong and that can block self-healing. Life is a journey, and our willingness to be present for all that this life journey brings, and cultivating the ability to be fully in the moment with "what is," may lead to a transformative healing process (Luck, 2010). Individuals are complex feedback loops. As we learn about these feedback loops, we are able to understand more about our body–mind–spirit–cultural–environmental connections. Each individual's body is in a constant state of change. Most of these internal energetic, hormonal, biochemical checks and balances are occurring outside of any conscious awareness of what is taking place in the body (Dossey, 2013). However, increasing our awareness and choices about these areas increases our capacity towards balance and harmony and our innate healing potential (Clark & Paraska, 2014; Prochaska, J. O., Norcross, J. C., & DiClemente, C. C., 1995; Robinson, Gould, & Strosahl, 2010; Rollnick, Miller, & Butler, 2008; Weinstein, 2014). Barrett (2010) states that humans can participate knowingly in change. Power as knowing participation in change is being aware of what one is choosing to do, feeling free to do it, and doing it intentionally.

At an even more expansive, organic level, life is a *biodance* (Dossey, L., 1982). We are participating in an endless exchange with all living things, with planet Earth in which all living organisms participate, and at the energetic and cosmic level as well. This energetic dance exists not only as we live, but also as we die. We do not wait until death to make an exchange with planet Earth, for we are constantly returning to the universe while alive.

In every living moment, a portion of the atoms in our body returns to the world outside. This is another idea of wholeness, which explains why the notion of "boundary" begins to seem an arbitrary idea rather than a physical reality. Each of us has the requisite capacity for achieving balanced integration of our human potentials: life balance and satisfaction, relationships, spiritual, mental, emotional, physical, environmental, and health responsibility. We are challenged to learn more about how to gain access to inner wisdom and intuition and apply it in our daily lives. As we take responsibility for making effective choices and changes in our lives, we place ourselves in a better position to be aware of our healthy patterns, purposes, and processes.

As Nurse Coaches, we are challenged each day to actualize our human potentials in order to enhance our self-development (self-reflection, self-assessment, self-evaluation, self-care) (Dossey, Luck, Schaub, & Keegan, 2013). Actualizing human potentials means first recognizing and then accepting all the potentials of our being, even those areas we wish to change. Developing our potentials requires a willingness to assess where we are in our life, to develop an action plan for change, and then to evaluate where we are with this lifelong process. See Chapter 22. Effective change arises and evolves from within before it can be manifested and maintained externally (Dart, 2010; DiClemente, Salazar, & Crosby, 2013; Norcross, 2012).

Nurse Coaches also use the IHWA to deepen their own personal exploration of self, to identify strengths (see Chapter 5, Table 5-1), examine their vulnerabilities, and explore their integrative lifestyle health and wellbeing. This further deepens their exploration with clients around various strategies for changing and choosing new behaviors and how to sustain them. In the next section, the IHWA will be explored for use with clients and our own self-development.

INTEGRATIVE HEALTH AND WELLNESS ASSESSMENT (IHWA)*

The circle is an ancient symbol of wholeness. The IHWA Wheel as seen in **Figure 6-1** has eight components: (1) Life Balance and Satisfaction, (2) Relationships, (3) Spiritual, (4) Mental, (5) Emotional, (6) Physical (Nutrition, Exercise, Weight Management), (7) Environmental, and (8) Health Responsibility (INCA, 2014). All are important components of the self that are interwoven and constantly interacting.

The IHWA (Appendix C-1, short form and Appendix C-2, long form) is based on over 30 years of integrative, integral, and holistic nursing clinical practice, education, and research. This includes coaching clients and patients in self-development, steps in changing lifestyle behaviors, health promotion, health maintenance, disease prevention, and with new self-management knowledge and skills when living with an acute or chronic illness and/or symptoms. The IHWA long form is expanded from Self-Care Assessments (Keegan & Dossey, 1987). Chapter 20 provides a discussion on the construct validity of the IHWA short and long forms.

Following an intake interview with a client (in person, phone, Skype, or Google, or other technologies), the Nurse Coach will determine if the IHWA short form (Appendix C-1) or long form (Appendix C-2) is used. The IHWA short form is most effectively used in an introductory coaching session or in group coaching sessions. The IHWA long form may be used between or throughout coaching sessions over time.

Life Balance and Satisfaction

Assessing our life balance and satisfaction strengthens our capacities and human potentials. See the IHWA Life Balance and Satisfaction section in Appendix C-1 (IHWA short form) and Appendix C-2 (IHWA long form). Recognizing and celebrating the joys and positive things in life adds to experiencing life balance and satisfaction. It attunes us to our healing awareness, which is the innate quality with which all people are born. Healing is recognizing our feelings, attitudes, and emotions, which are not isolated, but are literally translated into body changes. Images cause internal events through mind modulation that simultaneously affect the autonomic, endocrine, immune, and neuropeptide systems.

When assessing our life balance and satisfaction we become more aware of conscious choices we can make each day. Conscious choices involve awareness and skills such as self-reflection, self-care, discipline, persistence, goal setting, priority setting, action steps, discerning best options, and acknowledging and trusting perceptions and intuitions.

*Disclaimer: The Integrative Health and Wellness Assessment (IHWA) is intended for informational purposes only. It is not a substitute for professional medical advice, diagnosis, or treatment. Never ignore professional medical advice in seeking treatment. If you think you may have a medical emergency, immediately call your doctor or dial 911.

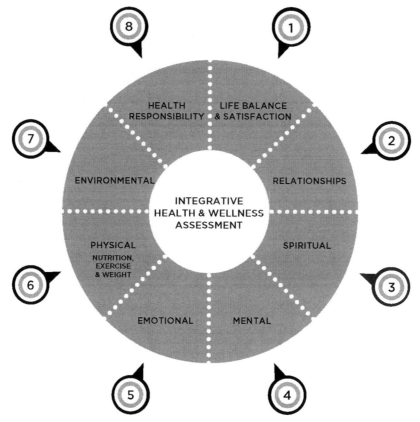

Figure 6-1 Integrative Health and Wellness Assessment™ Wheel.
Source: Copyright © 2014 by the International Nurse Coach Association. www.inursecoach.com

We can be active participants in daily living, not passive observers who hope that life will be good to us.

The unconscious also plays a major role in our choices. Jung (1980) conceived of the unconscious as a series of layers. The layers closest to our awareness may become known; those farthest away are, in principle, inaccessible to our awareness and operate autonomously. Jung saw the unconscious as the home of timeless psychic forces that he called *archetypes*, which generally are invariant throughout all cultures and eras. He felt that every psychic force has its opposite in the unconsciousness—the force of light is always counterposed with that of darkness—good with evil, love with hate, and so on. Jung believed that any psychic energy could become unbalanced. Therefore, one of life's greatest challenges is to achieve a dynamic balance of the innate opposites and make this balancing process as conscious as possible.

Relationships

Healthy people live in intricate networks of relationships and are always in search of new, unifying concepts of the universe and social order. See the IHWA Relationships section in Appendix C-1 (IHWA short form) and Appendix C-2 (IHWA long form). Learning how to understand and nurture our relationships assists us in creating and sustaining meaningful relationships. A healthy person cannot live in isolation. In a given day, we interact with many people: immediate family, extended family, friends, colleagues at work, neighbors in the community, numerous people in organizations, and the ever expanding web of electronic connection with friends, colleagues, and others around the world.

It is essential that we identify relationships that are cohesive and those that are disharmonious. We must be aware of the impact that we have on clients, family, and friends. Something always happens when people meet and spend time together, for life is never a neutral event. Our attitudes, healing awareness, and concern for self and others have a direct effect on the outcome of all our encounters. We also must extend our networks to include our immediate environment and consider that what we do locally has an impact on our larger community—the nation and planet Earth. Each of us must take up the challenge and active role in developing local networks of relationships that can have a ripple effect on global health concerns.

Relationships have different levels of meaning, from the superficial to the deeply connected. The challenges in relationships are multifaceted. First, we need to recognize what we personally are hoping for, and what we are bringing to the variety of relationships in which we are engaged. What do we notice when we are willing to exchange feelings of honesty, trust, intimacy, compassion, openness, and harmony? Many people spend at least half of their waking hours at work with colleagues. Within the context of a work environment, we need to support and nourish these relationships as well.

Sharing life processes requires truthful and caring self-reflection and communication with others. This also includes meaningful dialogues around the dying process and end-of-life care. These conversations require deep, personal contemplation about what is desired and hoped for. The dialogue may begin with the family and/or friends most intimately involved and may need to extend beyond to colleagues, clients, and the community at large.

Spiritual

Spirit comes from our roots—it is a universal need to understand the human experience. It is a vital element and driving force in how we live our lives. Assessing aspects of our spiritual nature can be a profound learning opportunity. See the IHWA Spiritual section in Appendix C-1 (IHWA short form) and Appendix C-2 (IHWA long form).

Usually, though not universally, spirituality is considered to involve a sense of connection with an absolute, imminent, or transcendent spiritual force, however named. It includes the conviction that our values and life's meaning and purpose are considered valid aspects of the individual and universe. It is the essence of being and relatedness that permeates all of life and is manifested in one's knowing, doing, and being. This interconnectedness with self, others, nature, and God/Life Force/Absolute/Transcendent is not necessarily synonymous with religion. Religion is the codified and ritualized beliefs and behaviors of those involved in spirituality, usually taking place within a community of like-minded individuals.

Spirit involves the development of our higher self, also referred to as the transpersonal self that allows for a transpersonal experience. A transpersonal experience (i.e., transcendence) is described as a feeling of oneness, inner peace, harmony, wholeness, and connection with the universe. The meaning and joy that flow from developing this aspect of our human potential allow us to have a transpersonal view. Some of the ways we may come to know this transcendence are through self-reflective practices such as prayer, meditation, philosophy, poetry, stories, music, inspired friends, group work, nature walks, or, for some, being a member of an organized religion.

Our spiritual potential does not develop without some attention and focus. Each day we can acknowledge that our spiritual potential is essential to the development of a healthy value system. We shape our perception of the world through our value system, and our perceptions will influence whether we have positive or negative experiences. Even through the pain of a negative experience (which may be physical, mental, emotional, relational, spiritual, cultural, or environmental), we have the ability to learn. Pain can be a great teacher. On the other side of the experience we may find new wisdom, self-discovery, and the opportunity to make new choices based on awareness and freshly acquired knowledge.

Mental

Assessing our mental capacity helps us examine our belief systems. In our early life we had role models who influenced our beliefs, thoughts, behaviors, and values. See the IHWA Mental section in Appendix C-1 (IHWA short form) and Appendix C-2 (IHWA long form). With maturity and as a result of life experiences, we recognize shifts that occur in regard to these same beliefs, thoughts, behaviors, and values. When we do not take the time to examine our changing perspectives, beliefs, and values, conflicts will often arise.

Our challenge is to use our cognitive capacities to perceive the world with greater clarity. This includes recognizing, to the best of our ability, the variety of perspectives we are presented with both personally and in the world in general. Through both logical and nonlogical mental processes, we become aware of a broad range of subjects that have the potential to enhance our full appreciation of the many great pleasures in life. We can also build our capacity to notice, process, and integrate both logical and intuitive thought.

With reflective practices such as breath awareness, relaxation, imagery, and journaling, we learn to be present in the moment. It is during these moments that we can notice and release the incessant, self-judging, critical inner voice that is constantly engaging part of one's self-dialogue. These are the moments when we expand our mental knowing. We become more capable of focusing our attention away from fear-based, negative thought patterns, and become more open and receptive to life-affirming information and patterns of thought. In this way mental growth can occur. Every aspect of our life is a learning experience and becomes part of a lesson for potential change and healthier repatterning.

Emotional

Assessing our emotional potential assists us in our willingness to acknowledge the presence of feelings, and we value them as important information to notice, and then to express them. See the IHWA Emotional section in Appendix C-1 (IHWA short form) and Appendix C-2 (IHWA long form). Emotional health implies that we have the choice and freedom to process and/or express the full spectrum of emotions, including love, joy, compassion, loving kindness, guilt, forgiveness, fear, and anger. The expression of these emotions can give us immediate feedback about our inner state that may be crying out for a new way of being.

Emotions are responses to the events in our lives. We are living systems that are constantly exchanging with others and our environment. All life events affect our emotions and general wellbeing. When we are willing to confront our emotions, we have the potential to lessen varying degrees of chronic anxiety, depression, worry, fear, guilt, anger, denial, failure, or repression, and experience true healing.

As we start to live in a more balanced way, we allow our humanness to develop. We reach out and seek meaningful dialogue. Increasing emotional potential allows openness, creativity, and spontaneity to be experienced. This contributes to the emergence of a positive, healthy zest for living. We value taking responsibility and allowing our spirit and intuition to blossom to its full potential within us.

Emotions are gifts. Frequently, a first step towards releasing a burden in a relationship is to share deeper feelings with another. There is no such thing as a good or bad emotion; each is part of the human condition. Emotions exist as the light and shadow of the self; thus, we must acknowledge all of them. The only reason that we can identify the light is that we know its opposite, the shadow. When we recognize the value in both types of emotions, we are in a position of new insight and understanding, and we can make more effective choices. As we increase our attention to body–mind–spirit interrelationships, we can focus on the emotions that move us towards wholeness and inner understanding.

Physical

Assessing our physical potential increases our awareness of nutrition, exercise, and weight. See the IHWA Physical sections in Appendix C-1 (IHWA short form) and Appendix C-2 (IHWA long form). See Chapter 8 for nutritional health details. Many people have become obsessed with the physical potential, but have failed to recognize that they are not separate from—or more important than—the other potentials.

All humans share the common biologic experiences of birth, gender, growth, aging, and death. Once each person's basic biologic needs for food, shelter, and clothing have been met, there are many ways to seek wholeness of our physical potential. Health is also more than the absence of pain and symptoms; it is present when there is a balance. As we assess physical needs, we also must take into consideration our perceptions of these areas. Many illnesses have been documented as stress-related because our consciousness plays a major role in health and physical potential.

Our body is a gift to nurture and respect. As we nurture ourselves, we increase our uniqueness in energy, sexuality, vitality, and capacity for language and connection with our other potentials. This nurturance strengthens our self-image, which in turn causes several things to happen: First, our body–mind–spirit responds in a positive and integrated fashion. Second, we embody a positive physical potential and become a role model with a positive influence on others. Finally, we actually enhance our general feeling of wellbeing.

Environmental

Assessing our environment increases our awareness of its impact on our health and wellbeing. See Chapter 9 for environmental details. See the IHWA Environmental section in Appendix C-1 (IHWA short form) and Appendix C-2 (IHWA long form).

The environment is the context or habitat within which all living systems participate and interact. This includes the physical body and its physical habitat, and cultural, psychological, social, and historical influences. It also includes both the external physical space and a person's internal space (physical, mental, emotional, social, and spiritual experiences). A healing environment includes everything that surrounds the Nurse Coach, the client/patient, family, significant others, community, and all healthcare practitioners, as well as patterns not yet understood.

Health Responsibility

Health responsibility occurs when an individual takes an active role in making lifestyle choices to protect and improve her/his health. See the IHWA Health Responsibility section in Appendix C-1 (IHWA short form) and Appendix C-2 (IHWA long form). Health responsibility includes having an annual physical examination and eye examination as recommended for one's age and health status by qualified healthcare practitioners. The Personal

Health Record* (Appendix C-3) is a tool for all baseline personal physiological parameters, personal history, family history, and any current symptoms. The body mass index (BMI) tables (Appendix C-4) are useful for a measure of body fat and are based on an individual's weight and height. In addition, all medications and supplements that are being taken should be noted and evaluated in terms of harmful or potential interactions with prescribed pharmaceuticals, or in combination with supplements. Allergies, hospitalizations, surgeries, and other specific medical factors are also important. In the next section, the IHWA guidelines are offered.

INTEGRATIVE HEALTH AND WELLNESS ASSESSMENT GUIDELINES

The IHWA (Appendix C-1, short form, and Appendix C-2, long form) is used as a personal assessment and as a coaching tool with clients. The Nurse Coach will decide the best way to use the IHWA before, during, or in follow-up coaching sessions. During or immediately following an acute medical crisis, coaching around self-management needs is usually not the best time. However, small steps towards changing unhealthy lifestyle behaviors can be considered. The IHWA is integrated within the Nurse Coach Five-Step Process (Chapter 5). See Chapters 10 and 13 for case studies related to exploration of integrative lifestyle health and wellbeing using the IHWA.

As previously discussed, the IHWA (Appendix C-1, short form) is often used with a client to begin the coaching process around the IHWA eight categories. It is also used in group classes for the purpose of self-reflection, self-assessment, self-evaluation, and self-care. The informal use of the IHWA short form in group classes, workshops, and support groups offers a new perspective on health assessment for many individuals, and a new opportunity for reflection and discussion. The IHWA short form scoring section may assist the participant in prioritizing areas of focus when they need coaching around where to start in addressing self-care. The IHWA short form scoring system may also generate group participation and peer support when a number of individuals identify the same goal. Peer support for self-care can be especially powerful in work situations.

The term "noncompliant" may surface from the client, the family, or another healthcare team member. This author believes that noncompliance is an overused and inaccurate term. There are many reasons that a client does not follow medical guidelines or medications or perceive healthy behaviors such as exercise, good nutrition, stress management, and so forth. The reasons include the client's many stressors, perceived lack of time, too much medical information given at one time, lack of knowledge, fears, denial, financial restraints, religious beliefs, disabilities, lack of family support, and much more. If the client is under medical care, there is almost always a limited amount of time for effective education in a clinic, during an office visit with a physician, or at hospital discharge following an acute illness or a new medical diagnosis (heart, lung, or cancer, etc.).

Depending on the initial phone interview or coaching session, the Nurse Coach will explore why the client seeks coaching around lifestyle changes. The IHWA engages clients in assessing where they are in each of the categories. This tool can be sent electronically via the Internet to a client before a session or given out at the end of a session to complete before the next session. At the appropriate time, the Nurse Coach will enter into a coaching agreement with the client. See Appendices A-1 and A-2. The client agreement can be sent before a session via mail, an e-mail attachment, or after a first coaching session. This facilitates the conversation to prepare for entering a coaching agreement and

*Disclaimer: This Personal Health Record does not provide medical advice. It is intended for individual informational purposes only.

for coaching sessions around the client goals, number and frequency of sessions, action plans, and more.

The following guidelines are offered:

- **Conducting the coaching session.** Review the Nurse Coach 5-Step Process (Chapter 5) and the Nurse Coaching Competencies and the sections marked *Before the coaching interaction*, *Throughout the coaching interaction*, and *At the end of the coaching interaction* (Chapter 4).

- **Opening the session.** Explore the reason (topic) for the client visit. Walk with the client in self-discovery and let her or him choose the path. Discuss the session length. Allowing the client to be in control of the session will increase self-efficacy and self-confidence.

- **Inviting the client to choose the topic for the coaching session.** Each client is the expert on her/his life and what currently works and what does not work. Allow the client to set the pace for the session, and if possible identify at least one goal for the session. Some clients will come to a session with clear goals and may be highly motivated. Other clients will be so overwhelmed with life that they need help with setting priorities.

- **Allowing the client to determine the direction of the coaching conversation.** Let the client direct the conversation around her/his areas of interest. There are many teachable moments that may be offered in a curious question. This also increases the client's motivation, which may invite a possible change. Ask the client's permission before offering unsolicited information.

- **Hearing the client's story.** Listen to the client's story around why she/he seeks coaching and desired goals towards becoming healthier at this time. Explore a typical day related to the chosen topic/s as well as any perceived barriers or stressors. (See Chapter 5 on Story Theory and the Story-Health Model.)

- **Integrative Health and Wellness Assessment (IHWA) statements.** The eight IHWA components engage clients with statements about the present way of life, health behaviors, feelings, and personal habits. Let the client discover patterns and habits related to health and wellness. This leads to new discoveries, options, and action steps that often follow. Explore why the client seeks coaching around lifestyle changes. Remember, the IHWA can be explored over one or many coaching sessions since most clients have most often never taken such an in-depth self-assessment. As the client achieves one goal, the IHWA can elicit further questions and possibilities for changing lifestyle in another area. **Table 6-1** explores various questions that assist with not telling a person what to do. See Chapter 2 on the Theory of Integrative Nurse Coaching Component 5: Listening with HEART questions that are also very helpful.

  Allow time for the client to not feel rushed in answering a question such as, "What areas under Life Balance and Satisfaction sparked some interest, and why are they interesting right now?" "If you can choose one topic for coaching around changing lifestyle behaviors, what might that be?" "What questions are the most interesting to you and why?" Invite the client to "live with a question over time and see what emerges." Coming up with an answer is not always necessary.

- **Listening for client's "shoulds" or "coulds".** A should often connotes a judgment. Something happens when the client shifts the "should" in thoughts and actions to "I could, and I have a choice," and this may be a good place to start. For example, "I should eat healthier but I don't take the time" or "I should exercise but I just don't know how to fit it in my busy day." Through coaching, the client becomes aware that when the "should" moves to "I could eat healthier and I can do some exercise, and I have a choice." Making effective choices is a skill of awareness and declaring self-worth. This requires not being judgmental and releases fears and guilt. See Chapter 14 on Integral Perspectives and Change and the section on Coaching and the Four Quadrants.

- **Exploring stages of change.** Listen closely to determine which of the five stages of change the client is in. These five stages are (1) Precontemplation (not ready for change—"I won't" or "I can't"; (2) Contemplation (thinking about change—"I may"; (3) Preparation (preparing for action)—"I will"; (4) Action (taking action)—"I am"; and, (5) Maintenance ("I still am" maintaining a new behavior). See Chapter 15 for exploring the pros and cons of change, intrinsic and extrinsic motivators, ambivalence and resistance, action plans, and goals. See Chapter 16 for use of rulers.

- **Helping client find strong motivators to change behavior.** Remember to look for the client's *intrinsic* (internal motivators such as more life balance, less stress, better relationships with family and others, hypertension management, or reducing risk factors) and *extrinsic* (family member wants client to change, peer pressure) motivators that can additional information for why clients seek ways to increase healthy lifestyle behaviors.

- **Closing the session.** At the end of the session, review any significant IHWA section specifics. Take time to explore readiness to change, priority for making the change, and confidence in ability to make a positive change. Show appreciation for the client's engagement, and commit to changing lifestyle behaviors. Usually, advice is given only if the client requests it. (*Note:* The exception is if the Nurse Coach is professionally bound to give advice such as around domestic violence, safety issues, etc.)

    Offer confidence statements such as "I am confident that if you decide to exercise two days a week for 20 minutes, you will develop a plan that works and can move forward to meet your goal of 40 minutes." A request for the client to check in via e-mail or phone message is often very helpful. Arrange for the next session and give practice sheets and resources as needed. (See Appendices.)

Table 6-1 Coaching Questions.

BEGINNING QUESTIONS
- What would be important for me to know about you?
- Is there anything else that I have forgotten to ask you before we begin?

WHAT
- What is working best in your life right now?
- What does being healthy mean to you?
- What are three qualities (strengths) that you like about yourself?
- What is motivating you to make this change? Or to go in this direction?
- What small accomplishment/s are you most proud of?
- What is a first step you are willing to take in moving towards (desired change)?
- What difference would this change make in your life?
- What new action are you willing to take?
- What number are you on a scale of 1–10 around this desired change?
- What would a (family member, friend, co-worker) say if you made this change?

(*continues on next page*)

Table 6-1 (*Continued*).

WHO
- Who is there to support you with change?
- Who will be the first to notice that you want to make a change in your life?
- Who is someone that you have learned from in life?
- Who are you becoming as you make this decision to change?
- Who, besides you, needs to be involved in this decision?

WHEN
- When did you first become aware of wanting to make a change with...?
- When will be a good time for you to take a first step towards this change?
- When will you begin to act on creating the changes you want in your life?
- When you make this change/s, who will be the first to notice?
- When will your (family member, co-worker, friend) see your changes or successes?

WHERE
- Where on a scale of 1–10 will you be when you make this change?
- Where do you most typically experience frustration (conflict, confusion)?
- Where in your body will you feel this change/s?
- Where will you recognize the differences about this change?
- Where on a scale of 1–10 do you want to be in (two weeks, a month, three months)?

HOW
- How much do you want to make this change on a scale of 1–10?
- How does what you value apply here?
- How would you evaluate your progress?
- How would you like to move this change forward?
- How have you gotten through challenges before?
- How have you made changes in your life?
- How will you know that this is the right thing to do?
- How will you know when you can let go of this (worry, fear, trouble)?
- How will you recognize when you are on the right path/track?

Source: Copyright © 2014 by the International Nurse Coach Association. www.inursecoach.com

SUMMARY

- The IHWA can engage both clients and Integrative Nurse Coaches in self-development and new awareness related to healthy lifestyle behaviors.
- The IHWA assists individuals to explore perceptions and beliefs about health and wholeness and how to create healthy lifestyle behaviors.
- All IHWA categories are interrelated and create a sense of wholeness.
- Exploration of the IHWA leads to new awareness and choice, insights, action plans, and achieving goals that can be sustained.
- The IHWA assists individuals to integrate strengths, action plans, and affirmations in a creative journey of healing.

NURSE COACH REFLECTIONS

After reading this chapter, the Nurse Coach will be able to answer or begin a process of answering the following questions:

- When I complete the IHWA and its eight components, what new awareness do I have about my life?

- Am I consciously aware of the daily opportunity to increase my health and wellbeing?
- What are my challenges in using the IHWA with myself or with my clients?
- What do clients share as they experience their healing potentials?

REFERENCES

Barrett, E. A. M. (2010). Power as knowing participation in change: What's new and what's next. *Nursing Science Quarterly, 23*(1), 47–54.

Clark, C. C., & Paraska, K. K. (2014). *Health promotion for nurses: A practical guide.* Burlington, MA: Jones & Bartlett Learning.

Dart, M. A. (2010). *Motivational interviewing in nursing practice.* Sudbury, MA: Jones & Bartlett Learning.

DiClemente, R., Salazar, L., & Crosby, R. (2013). *Health behavior theory for public health: Principles, foundations, and applications.* Burlington, MA: Jones & Bartlett Learning.

Dossey, B. M. (2013). Nursing: Integral, integrative, and holistic—local to global. In B. M. Dossey & L. Keegan (Eds.), *Holistic nursing: A handbook for practice* (6th ed., pp. 1–57). Burlington, MA: Jones & Bartlett Learning.

Dossey, B. M., Luck, S., Schaub, B. G., & Keegan, L. (2013). Self-assessments. In B. M. Dossey & L. Keegan (Eds.), *Holistic nursing: A handbook for practice* (6th ed., pp. 161–187). Burlington, MA: Jones & Bartlett Learning.

Dossey, L. (1982). *Space, Time and Medicine* (pp. 72–81). Boston, MA: Shambhala.

International Nurse Coach Association (2014). Integrative Health and Wellness Assessment™. North Miami, FL: Author.

Jung, C. G. (1980). (Translator, R. F. C. Hull). The archetypes and the collective unconscious. In *The collected works of C.G. Jung* (Vol. 9, Part 1). Princeton, NJ: Princeton University Press.

Keegan, L., & Dossey, B. M. (1987). *Self-care: A program to improve your life.* Port Angeles, WA: Holistic Nursing Consultants.

Luck, S. (2010). Changing the health of our nation: The role of nurse coaches. *Alternative Therapies in Health and Medicine, 16*(5), 78–80.

Nightingale, F. (1896). Sick-nursing and health-nursing. In B. M. Dossey, D. M. Beck, L. C. Selanders, & A. Attewell (2005). *Florence Nightingale today: Healing, leadership, global action* (pp. 289; 288–303). Silver Spring, MD: Nursebooks.org.

Norcross, J. (2012). *Changeology: 5 steps to realizing your goals and resolutions.* New York, NY: Simon & Schuster.

Prochaska, J. O., Norcross, J. C., & DiClemente, C. C. (1995). *Changing for good. A revolutionary six-stage program for overcoming bad habits and moving your life positively forward.* New York, NY: Harper Collins.

Robinson, P. J., Gould, D. A., & Strosahl, K. D. (2010). *Real behavior change in primary care: Improving patient outcomes and increasing job satisfaction.* Oakland, CA: New Harbinger.

Rollnick, S. W., Miller, W. R., & Butler, C. C. (2008). *Motivational interviewing in healthcare: Helping patients change behavior*. New York, NY: Guilford Press.

Weinstein, S. (2014). *B is for balance: A nurse's guide for enjoying life at work and at home* (2nd ed.). Indianapolis, IN: Sigma Theta Tau International.

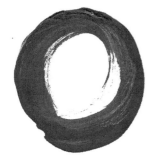

CHAPTER 7

Integrative Lifestyle Health and Wellbeing (ILHWB)

Susan Luck

Shall we begin by taking it as a general principle—that all disease, at some point or other of its course, is more or less a reparative process, not necessarily accompanied with suffering; an effort of nature to remedy a process of poisoning or decay, which has taken place weeks, months, sometimes years beforehand, unnoticed, the termination of the disease being then, while the antecedent process was going on, determined?

Florence Nightingale, 1860

LOOKING AHEAD...

After reading this chapter, you will be able to:

- Describe the Integrative Lifestyle Health and WellBeing (ILHWB) model and its unique contribution to nursing and nurse coaching.
- Explore wellbeing from a nonmedical paradigm that is multidimensional and interconnected.
- Deepen the understanding of the bio–psycho–social–spiritual–cultural–environmental model of health.
- Examine energy and balance in an Integrative Lifestyle Health (ILH) model.

DEFINITIONS

Note: The term "integrative" is used in this chapter to describe both the integration of lifestyle approaches and the philosophy of nurse coaching, both using an expanded model of caring for the whole person.

Health promotion: The process of helping people to take control over and improve their own health. Changing people's expectations of health is the core of heath promotion.
Lifestyle: A manner of living that reflects the person's values and attitudes.
Quality of life: A broad concept that incorporates all aspects of life and has been used in a variety of disciplines such as: geography, philosophy, medical sciences, social sciences, health promotion.
Telomere: The segment of DNA that occurs at the ends of chromosomes.
Wellbeing: A general term for the condition of an individual or group and their social, economic, psychological, spiritual, or medical state; based on the idea that the way each person thinks and feels about her or his life is meaningful and important.

LIFESTYLE INFLUENCES ON HEALTH AND WELLBEING

Nurse Coaches offer the greatest potential for reversing the escalating patterns of illness that we are witnessing today, local to global. The evidence is clear that the root cause of most chronic health conditions today lies within our lifestyle habits and the multitude of daily stressors that challenge our immune, digestive, endocrine, cardiovascular, and neurological systems. Health and wellbeing is affected by the foods we consume, how we manage our stress, the quality of our sleep, physical activity, and the social, environmental, genetic, and epigenetic influences that are part of our internal and external world.

In this chapter, we examine how our lifestyle behaviors are having a profound impact on health and the quality of our lives. Our "evolution" as humans in this modern age has taken an extreme toll, not only on our personal health but on the health of our communities as reflected in the mounting global health crisis of obesity and diabetes. Creating supportive environments and building sustainable communities are fundamental in shaping a healthy future for all.

Lifestyle habits and patterns are deeply embedded in one's culture and worldview and connected with family, community, social group, economic status, and traditions. For example, Yasmine begins her morning with a prayer; Jim begins with exercise at the gym; and Gary jumpstarts his day with four cups of coffee and a donut. Listening to each story and one's daily habits and patterns opens the conversation to share and discover how our choices influence health and wellbeing throughout the life cycle.

In the current medical paradigm, disease is recognized and treated and health and wellbeing is viewed as the diminishing of pain or symptoms. This model is incomplete as it often does not include the whole person within the context of family, community, culture, and environment nor does it strive to empower the client/patient in health-promoting strategies that create lasting behavioral change. Shifting the conversation from the provider directing the expected outcome to the patient guiding her or his process provides an opportunity to increase awareness and explore one's willingness and readiness for change. These steps are critical for attaining and sustaining positive health outcomes. Nurse Coaches support patients/clients along their health continuum.

INTEGRATIVE LIFESTYLE HEALTH AND WELLBEING (ILHWB): A NURSE COACH MODEL

An ILHWB model assesses and addresses core imbalances that underlie various conditions. Imbalances can arise from multiple sources including: inadequate nutrients; poor-quality air and water; lack of exercise and movement; disturbances in our internal and external environment; stress, thoughts, emotions, and trauma; loss of culture and community; lack of social support and relationships; and a longing for connection to others or something greater than oneself.

Lifestyle health and wellbeing is a multidimensional energy matrix that moves along a wellness continuum that centers on restoring balance at multiple levels. Central to wellbeing is the integration of a bio–psycho–social–spiritual–cultural–environmental approach for improving resiliency, function, and capacity for healing. This approach views primary prevention and underlying causality through a whole person perspective rather than through medical labels for symptoms and diagnoses of disease. This model encompasses a personalized approach addressing modern lifestyle influences including food and nutrition, environment exposures, the impact of stress, and the genetic and epigenetic influences on health.

Through assessing all dimensions of wellbeing, and deepening the connection to one's innate capacity for healing, the heart of the art and science in an integrative Nurse Coach model is grounded in the following ILHWB principles:

- **Energy field principles and dynamics:** Thoughts, stress, toxic environments, social and cultural isolation, and nutrient imbalances can disrupt human energy field patterns.
- **Interconnectedness:** All communication is an orchestrated network of interconnected messenger pathways and signaling systems and not autonomous or in isolation.
- **Promotion of optimizing our internal and external healing environments:** All-encompassing worldview that health is the microcosm and reflects the macrocosm in the web of life.
- **Patient-centered:** Honors and emphasizes each person's unique history, culture, beliefs, and story rather than medical diagnosis and disease labels.
- **Biochemical individuality:** Recognizes the importance of variations in metabolic function that derives from genetics, epigenetics, strengths, and vulnerabilities unique to each individual.

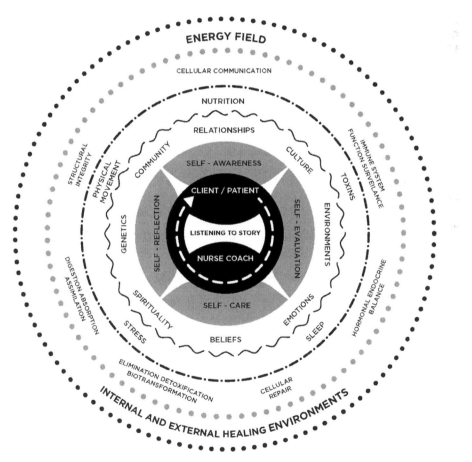

Figure 7-1 Integrative Lifestyle Health and Wellbeing Model.
Source: Copyright © 2014 by the International Nurse Coach Association. www.inursecoach.com

- **Health on a wellness continuum:** Views health as a dynamic balance on multiple levels and trusts that our human capacity seeks to identify, restore, and support our innate resilience and reserve to enhance wellbeing and healing throughout the life cycle (as seen in **Figure 7-1**).

Global Patterns of Lifestyle Health

As humans, we process and filter our perceptions through a unique lens that is colored by the complexity of each unique life story that holds the key to wellbeing. In 2006, the World Health Organization (WHO) defined wellness as the optimal state of health of individuals and groups with two focal concerns:

- Realization of the fullest potential of an individual physically, psychologically, socially, spiritually, and economically, and
- Fulfillment of one's role expectations in the family, community, workplace, place of worship, and other settings (Smith, Tang, & Nutbeam, 2006).

Lifestyle factors are a bigger threat today than communicable diseases, according to the World Health Organization (WHO), which has developed the 2008–2013 Action Plan for the Global Strategy on Diet, Physical Activity and Health for the Prevention and Control of Noncommunicable Diseases (WHO, 2011). In 2013, the World Health Assembly endorsed the Global NCD Action Plan 2013–2020, which includes a set of actions for member States, international partners, and the WHO Secretariat to promote healthy diets and physical activity, and to attain nine voluntary global targets to be achieved by 2025 (WHO, 2013). According to WHO, obesity, and related noncommunicable diseases, is largely preventable. A recent WHO report estimates that childhood obesity is one of the most serious public health challenges of the 21st century. Globally, in 2010, the number of overweight children under the age of five was estimated to be over 42 million. Close to 35 million of these children are living in developing countries. Overweight and obese children are likely to develop diabetes and cardiovascular diseases at a younger age, and this epidemic is largely preventable according to the report.

Envisioning a culture that promotes healthy lifestyles, a bigger perspective beyond individual health issues and goals is needed. How we alter the health of our outer environment governs our individual health and reflects in the challenges to our most basic needs for survival including the food we eat, the air we breathe, the water we drink, and the multiple stressors and environmental assaults experienced daily As a global community, we need to rethink the way communities are designed and built; the need for access to clean air and water; the production of real food; how our workplace environments must support the health of workers; and how our health policies must reflect the wellbeing of all citizens.

In the history of humankind, the story of survival as a species had remained constant until recent times. It has been said that as humans we could be the first species to cause our own extinction if we do not change our behaviors. If we reflect back to our roots, our ancestors were connected to the natural environment, in search of food to bring back to the community, sharing the hunt or the ripened berries found while foraging. Survival was interdependent on the "we" as one unit. Shared values, beliefs, and rituals were essential for the survival of the group as a whole. As we explore our modern lifestyle choices, we see how most communities have drifted far from a deeper connection of what it is to be human including connection to community, nature, and a healthy environment. *What has replaced the shared rituals in modern times? Do they support the health of the individual and the community? What could be new ways to create rituals to support a healthy lifestyle?*

A Nurse Coach Model for ILHWB

Everyone has their explanatory narrative that encompasses the multidimensional layers of being human. Listening to our own story and the story of others reveals one's beliefs and worldview for further exploring and expanding possibilities for growth and change in our movement toward wholeness. Foundational to nurse coaching is listening to the client/patient story as a key for opening doors. Introducing coaching questions, reframing one's medical diagnosis, and exploring the personal meaning of health, illness, dying, and healing, offers new insights into imbalances and brings awareness to one's vulnerability as part of the human condition. Balance is attained through a dynamic interaction and inter-connectedness between the individual and her/his environment within a complex web of physiological, cognitive/emotional, and physical processes. Grounded in scientific princi-ples and information widely available in our current medical and nursing literature today, this model embraces the Theory of Integrative Nurse Coaching (see Chapter 2) and addresses the totality of the individual, weaving the internal and external environment within the context of community and culture.

Integrative Lifestyle Health (ILH) Model

Healthcare providers and the public are seeking new explanatory models for promoting health and wellbeing. Our current disease-focused medicine model is being challenged and transformed by a new paradigm that explores and examines the underlying causation of ill health and disease. Functional medicine and personalized lifestyle medicine have emerged to bring about a new healthcare movement that emphasizes nutritional, environ-mental, and lifestyle interventions. An ILH model shares many of the tenets of functional medicine. In addition, an ILH model integrates the art and science of nursing, building on holistic nursing philosophy, nursing theory, nursing practice, and nursing process. The cor-nerstone of both models is patient-centered and views health through a dynamic inter-action and interconnectedness between the individual and her/his environment. Health is viewed as a positive vitality, representing more than the absence of disease. The ILH model views the Nurse Coach relationship as a therapeutic partner, understanding the energetic presence and use of self in relationship-centered care. Coaching strategies for a healthy lifestyle become an opportunity for nurses to bring new skills, tools, and modalities to the art and science of nursing. In this model, Nurse Coaches view health, energy, and balance through an expanded holistic, integral, and integrative perspective.

A Nurse Coach assesses and explores with the client the physical and social envi-ronment in which he or she lives and works, the dietary habits and patterns (present and past), the culture and beliefs about one's health, illness, or diagnosis, and the combined impact of lifestyle factors on social, physical, and psychological function. It is in the dis-covery of factors that can aggravate or ameliorate symptoms, and that can predispose one to illness or facilitate recovery, that provides the greatest possibilities for co-creating one's integrative care plan, establish realistic goals, and explore new possibilities for heal-ing and wellbeing. A nurse coaching collaborative partnership recognizes the individual's experience and explanatory model as key, and it is within this larger context where insights and strategies for changing behaviors occur.

In the ILHWB model (see Figure 7-1), the Nurse Coach process begins by deeply listening to the story to uncover the antecedents, triggers, and mediators that underlie symptoms, signs, and behaviors or what may have been labeled as disease pathology. This approach is collaborative, flexible, and focused on each person's unique constellation of perceptions, beliefs, and circumstances. In this patient-centered care model, it is the Nurse Coach's opportunity to understand not just the ailments and diagnoses from a medical

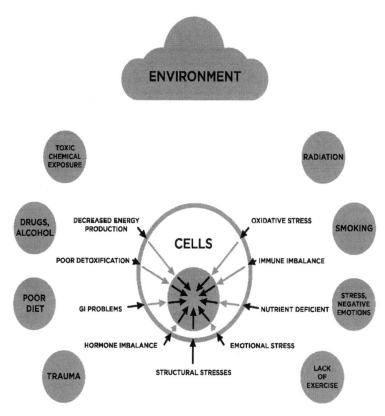

Figure 7-2 Lifestyle Influences on Health and Wellbeing.
Source: Copyright © 2014 by the International Nurse Coach Association. www.inursecoach.com

construct but through an expanded holistic lens that includes the physical, cultural, and social environment in which symptoms occur; the dietary habits of the person (present and past); the environment in which one lives; and one's beliefs about her/his health, illness, or diagnosis, weaving a timeline to document the story told. Nurse Coach conversations include exploring lifestyle variables that impact both short- and long-term health.

LIFESTYLE INFLUENCES ON PATTERNS AND BEHAVIORS

Most chronic conditions today are preventable and much appears to be reversible (**Figure 7-2**). The WHO reports hypertension as the leading cause of global mortality annually with over 7 million deaths (about 15% of all deaths). Prevention of hypertension is essential to improving health and preventing morbidity and mortality, both in developing and developed countries. A recent large prospective population-based cohort study in Finland included 9,637 men and 11,430 women (ages 25 to 74). It found that the following healthy lifestyle behaviors can reduce hypertension risk by two-thirds (Wang et al., 2013):

- not smoking,
- alcohol consumption less than 50 g per week,
- physical activity at least 3 times per week,

- daily consumption of vegetables, and
- normal weight (BMI < 25 kg/m^2).

Nurse Coaches inspire individuals, families, and communities to move beyond self-limiting expectations to connect with their hope, resiliency, and new possibilities for improving their health and recovery in times of illness or crisis. After surgery, or trauma, *how does one achieve a level of autonomy necessary to engage in health-promoting activities and a commitment to an improved quality of life? How do patients become motivated to increase their capacity to heal?* In a Nurse Coach relationship, drawing on the client/patient's desire toward hopefulness allows an individual to take action, shifting her or his self-limiting beliefs and perceptions to create new possibilities. Empowering the client/patient to mobilize her or his inner strengths is reflected in the emerging science of neuroplasticity and the capacity to grow new neuronal networks as demonstrated in the research with stroke survivors (Wahl & Schwab, 2014).

Neuroplasticity is a new frontier in reassessing our human potential and expanding scientific inquiry with emerging studies ranging from children with disabilities, to strength training and building new muscle fibers, to rehabilitation post-stroke (Nahum, Lee, & Merzenich, 2013). Lifestyle research on the scientific data on nutrition, exercise and yoga, and stress management, meditation, and mindfulness practices for improving health outcomes can no longer be considered "alternative medicine." Integrating new modalities and skills into daily practice can improve health outcomes while being cost-effective. This approach builds upon the human experience and will to move from helplessness to hopefulness and resilience as key to accessing and connecting to one's innate healing capacity and healing potential.

Hope is important because it can make the present moment less difficult to bear. If we believe that tomorrow will be better, we can bear a hardship today.
Thích Nhât Hạnh (1992)

Nurse Coaches work with patients/clients to discover new meaning in their illness and in their ability to learn new behaviors to support future health goals that can range from lowering blood pressure to coping with post-traumatic stress disorder (PTSD), and cancer survivorship. The Nurse Coach listens to the story on multiple levels, noticing interconnections between the patient's physiological, psychosocial, environmental, and energetic dynamics. Our professional nursing orientation, in providing relationship-centered care to effectively improve health outcomes, offers the Nurse Coach the ability to adapt change theory models in assisting patients in finding new meaning in their illness and in supporting future health goals.

Theoretical models of behavior change consider psychological constructs such as intention, self-efficacy, and resiliency and include the role of stress and psychological distress in developing new coping strategies. As the Nurse Coach assists the client/patient in recognizing existing patterns she/he can provide tools and guidance to moderate the impact of external stressors. Introducing awareness and mindfulness-based practices, we expand our scope of nursing practice. Nurse Coaches are uniquely positioned to bring these skills to our work with patients/clients, families, and communities.

WELLBEING

Concepts of wellbeing have been explored by many disciplines and cultures. Embedded in *wellness* is the concept of wellbeing often defined clinically as the absence of negative conditions while the psychological perspective defines wellbeing as the prevalence of positive attributes. Positive psychological definitions of wellbeing have been associated with:

- Self-perceived health
- Longevity
- Healthy behaviors
- Social connectedness
- Productivity

A sense of wellbeing encompasses the presence of positive emotions and moods including: contentment and happiness; the absence of depleting emotions including prolonged depression and anxiety; satisfaction with life; and fulfillment and positive functioning. In a holistic assessment of wellbeing, physical wellbeing and experiencing vitality and energy are viewed as essential to overall wellbeing. Researchers from different disciplines have examined different aspects of wellbeing to include:

- Physical wellbeing
- Economic wellbeing
- Social wellbeing
- Emotional wellbeing
- Psychological wellbeing
- Life satisfaction
- Meaningful activities and work
- Spiritual wellbeing

Higher levels of wellbeing are associated with decreased risk of disease, illness, and injury; better immune functioning; speedier recovery from illness; and increased longevity. Individuals with high levels of wellbeing are more productive at work and are more likely to contribute to their communities. This has major implications for healthcare policy and incentives for wellness initiatives in the workplace. McAllister and McKinnon (2009) defined wellbeing as more than the absence of illness or pathology with subjective (self-assessed) and objective (ascribed) dimensions. Health and sense of wellbeing are inextricably intertwined.

A Nurse Coach explores the wellbeing of each individual and may ask the client to reflect on the following questions, *"What does wellbeing mean for me?" "How can I enhance my wellbeing?"*

When we reflect on what we need beyond security and material comfort, it appears that universally we all seek meaning and purpose and connections to families, culture, communities, and our environment, according to Centers for Disease Control and Prevention (CDC) research, which has been studying and monitoring *wellbeing* using various instruments and surveys for several years. The CDC defines wellbeing as a positive outcome that is meaningful for people across many sectors of society because it informs that people perceive that their lives are going well. Living conditions, including housing, employment, and access to food, appear to be fundamental to wellbeing. Tracking these conditions is important for public policy. Wellbeing generally includes global judgments of life satisfaction and feelings ranging from depression to joy.

The CDC's Health-Related Quality of Life Program has led an effort to examine how wellbeing can be integrated into health promotion and how it can be measured in public health systems (CDC, n.d.). Currently the CDC and three states (Oregon, Washington, and New Hampshire) are collecting data using the Satisfaction with Life Scale on the 2010 Behavioral Risk Factor Surveillance System. The CDC also is leading the development of overarching goals related to quality of life and wellbeing for the Healthy People 2020 initiative (CDC, 2013). Embedded in these wellbeing models is the concept of *happiness*.

Happiness

Attaining happiness has been a human quest that philosophers have pondered throughout the ages. Aristotle believed that "happiness is that activity of the soul which functions in accord with excellence. Happiness is the highest good since it is desired (or ought to be desired) for its own sake and is the end toward which all other goods strive."

Nurse Coaches explore these concepts as part of one's self-discovery process. Having a sense of wellbeing, being happy, and finding life meaningful may overlap yet are distinct. A feeling described as *happiness* is often associated in the literature with good health. Many studies have noted the connection between a happy mind and a healthy body. In a meta-analysis of 150 studies on this topic, researchers summarized as follows: "Inductions of wellbeing lead to healthy functioning, and inductions of ill-being lead to compromised health" (Howell, Kern, & Lyubomirsky, 2007). According to a new report released by the CDC, January, 2014, a large survey revealed multiple differing predictors of happiness (controlling for meaning) and meaningfulness (controlling for happiness). Satisfying one's needs and wants increased happiness but was largely irrelevant to meaningfulness. Happiness was largely present-oriented, whereas meaningfulness involves integrating the past, present, and future. For example, thinking about the future and the past was associated with high meaningfulness but low happiness. Happiness was linked to being a taker rather than a giver, whereas meaningfulness was linked with being a giver rather than a taker. Higher levels of worry, stress, and anxiety were linked to higher meaningfulness but lower happiness. Concerns with personal identity and expressing the self contributed to meaning but not happiness.

Meaningfulness is presumably both a cognitive and an emotional assessment of whether one's life has purpose and value. People may feel that life is meaningful if they find it consistently rewarding in some way, even if they cannot articulate just what it all means. Happiness may be rooted in having one's needs and desires satisfied, including being largely free from unpleasant events. Meaningfulness may be considerably more complex than happiness, because it requires interpretive construction of circumstances across time and includes present events that draw meaning from past and future events according to abstract values and other culturally mediated ideas.

In a Nurse Coach model, exploring meaningfulness and the meaning of life without imposing external definitions is a reflective practice. Often, when one is recovering from illness, moving toward end of life, or hoping for staying healthy with aging, this contemplative exploration becomes an opportunity to deepen the meaning of one's life as a path to inner peace and healing. The skillful Nurse Coach in supporting the process of self-discovery and self-exploration may ask deeper questions about "What is meaningful for you in your life journey at this time?"

Healthy Aging

Quality of life is a broad-ranging concept affected by the complexity of a person's physical health, psychological state, personal beliefs, social relationships, and relationship to her or his environment. Americans today are living longer than ever, and their life expectancy is increasing every year. A recent analysis by the Institute of Medicine (2013) suggests that increases in life span in the United States are not matched by increases in "health span"—time spent living in good health. Life expectancy is greatly influenced by advances in medicine and the public health system, while the health span is most affected by lifestyle practices. "The next chapter in medical advance will need to be as much about lifestyle as medicine if we are to add life to years along with years to life," according to David Katz, Director, Yale University Prevention Research Center, U.S. National Center for Health Statistics (Katz, 2014).

Small, healthy lifestyle changes and involvement in meaningful activities are critical to healthy aging according to a recent study (Clark, 2011). The Well Elderly 2 trial was performed between 2004 and 2009. Seniors participating in the study made small, sustainable changes in their routines (such as visiting a museum with a friend once a week) that led to measurable gains in quality of life, including lower rates of depression and better reported satisfaction with life. Quality of life was measured using a variety of indicators, including physical health, mental health, social wellbeing, and life satisfaction. The program participants were compared to a control group that did not receive the intervention. Though the two groups started out roughly equivalent, the intervention group showed significant improvement in lessening bodily pain and depression while improving vitality, social function, mental health, and overall life satisfaction.

Making positive changes in how one lives each day, and sustaining those changes over the long term, appears critical for maintaining independence and preventing health decline. Current trends in public health strategies focus on preventing illness and disability, as opposed to treating issues once they already have begun to negatively impact health. The goal of prevention and wellness is really a key to healthcare reform, and results in cost savings to society. "There are non-pharmacologic interventions that work," reported Dr. Clark, professor and associate dean in the Division of Occupational Science and Occupational Therapy at the Herman Ostrow School of Dentistry of the University of Southern California. "The emphasis now is prevention." This research demonstrated that small, healthy lifestyle changes and involvement in meaningful activities going beyond just diet and exercise are critical to healthy aging. "What is critical is that as we age, we continue to be engaged in life through a sustainable mix of productive, social, physical and spiritual activities," she concluded (Clark, Jackson, & Carlson, 2004).

Another recent study demonstrated that a program that integrates functional movement and mindful body awareness can improve cognitive and physical function and quality of life while reducing caregiver burden compared with usual care (Barnes, Mehling, Yaffe, Flores, & Chesney, 2013). According to the investigators, traditional exercise programs have been shown to improve physical function in individuals with dementia, but little is known about the effect of exercise that integrates functional movements with mindful body awareness, which may also affect cognitive function. Known as Preventing Loss of Independence through Exercise (PLIÉ), the program "combines the best elements of eastern and western exercise traditions including yoga, *tai chi*, Feldenkrais, physical therapy, occupational therapy, mindfulness, and dance movement therapy," said Barnes. The study worked with practitioners from various traditions to determine the elements that would work best in individuals with dementia. As Nurse Coaches expand their knowledge of the research in the fields of healthy aging, opportunities arise to guide coaching questions and introduce new integrative skills with individuals, groups, and communities.

Vignette: Mary

Mary, 88 years old, lives alone and rarely leaves her house. She has three grown children, all who live in other parts of the country. She has felt alone since her husband died over a decade ago and she sees her family infrequently for their holiday visits. She remains mobile but uses a walker for balance and recently experienced spells of "forgetfulness." Local church members look in on Mary and provide a part-time companion for her five days a week to shop, clean, and take her to doctor appointments. A Nurse Coach in the community who attends her church and who has known Mary over the years offered to visit Mary at her home and assess her ability to live independently.

Telomeres: Markers of Healthy Aging

A telomere is the segment of DNA that occurs at the ends of chromosomes (**Figure 7-3**). Multiple factors have been shown to affect telomere length, the parts of chromosomes that influence aging. Telomere shortening is a predictor of aging and part of life's natural process. A recent review of the research on telomeres suggests that there is a relationship between psychosocial, environmental, and behavioral factors that influence changes in telomere length. These factors need to be considered in aging and healthy aging (Stark-weather et al., 2014). Recent research demonstrated for the first time that changes in diet, exercise, stress management, and social support may result in longer telomeres. Dean Ornish, founder of the Preventive Medicine Research Institute and researcher on the study (Ornish et al., 2013), observed, "Our genes, and our telomeres, are not necessarily our fate. These findings indicate that telomeres may lengthen to the degree that people change how they live. Research indicates that longer telomeres are associated with fewer illnesses and longer life." Thirty-five men with localized, early-stage prostate cancer were followed to explore the relationship between comprehensive lifestyle changes, telomere length, and telomerase activity. All the men were engaged in active surveillance, which involves closely monitoring their condition through screening and biopsies. Ten of the patients embarked on lifestyle changes that included: a plant-based diet (high in fruits, vegetables, and unrefined grains, and low in saturated fats and refined carbohydrates); moderate exercise

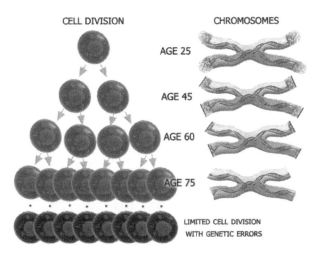

Figure 7-3 Telomeres.
Source: Copyright © 2014 by the International Nurse Coach Association. www.inursecoach.com

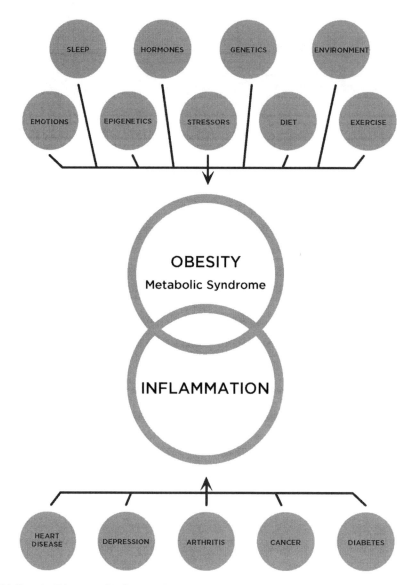

Figure 7-4 Lifestyle Triggers of Inflammation.
Source: Copyright © 2014 by the International Nurse Coach Association. www.inursecoach.com

(walking 30 minutes a day, six days a week); and stress reduction (gentle yoga-based stretching, breathing, and meditation). They also participated in weekly group support. They were compared to the other 25 study participants who were not asked to make major lifestyle changes. The group that made the lifestyle changes experienced a "significant" increase in telomere length of approximately 10%. The study concluded that the more people changed their behavior by adhering to the recommended lifestyle program, the more dramatic their improvements in telomere length, the scientists learned. These studies open new doors for Nurse Coach directions and interventions.

In an integrative Nurse Coach model, lifestyle assessment of stress, sleep, lack of nutrients, and environmental exposures can trigger a multitude of inflammatory responses. Multiple systems can be affected, including cardiovascular, neurological, immune, and hormonal systems. Inflammatory triggers (**Figure 7-4**) can be assessed and identified, and through the coaching process, increasing awareness and choices can lower the inflammatory response and improve symptoms and health outcomes. Identifying and removing inflammatory triggers is part of the exploration of lifestyle strategies to "put out the fire." (See Chapter 8 for details.)

Stress

Stress originates from both internal and external sources and can impact all aspects of one's health and sense of wellbeing. On a physiological level, stress triggers a cascade of chemicals and inflammatory processes that impact immune, neurological, and hormonal balance. An individual's emotions, attitudes, beliefs, and predispositions influence the way stimuli is perceived and responded to. Anticipation of stressors, often based on previous experiences, influences the way of processing stress and the physiological stress response that follows. Primary appraisal is the perception of a threat, and this perception is often in anticipation of something happening, most frequently based on a previous experience, perhaps in a similar surrounding. After consideration of the individual's resources, including includes social variables, psychological and constitutional resources, a decision occurs (with or without awareness) of what kind of coping strategy is of use, and implementation takes place, both mentally and physically. Secondary appraisal processes are already part of the coping strategy to internal and environmental demands to reestablish equilibrium. The initial stress response may be adaptive, producing an "emergency reaction" that is an arousal process of the sympathetic nervous system and may allow more effective coping with the stressful situation.

According to current research, psychological stress is linked with impaired glycemic control in diabetics and increased risk of diabetes mellitus. Physiological responses to stress, including increased glucose production, glucose mobilization, and insulin resistance could influence future diagnoses and health outcomes and lowering the stress response through learned practices can mediate this risk.

The Nurse Coach and client explore the individual's stress response physiologically and psychologically. Introducing awareness practices in the initial arousal phase can recalibrate and rebalance the impact on biochemical stress responses that long term can bathe the body in hormones and inflammatory cytokines that can impact all systems, especially the endocrine, nervous, and immune systems. According to the seminal work by Hans Selye (1976–1984), the process of arousal has three stages: the alarm reaction, the stage of resistance, and the stage of exhaustion. In the alarm reaction, the adrenal gland releases adrenaline, which makes one more aware of one's surroundings as well as prepares the body to take action (fight or flight). When the body and mind begin to cope with the stressor, the stage of resistance is at work, and if coping with the stressor is unsuccessful the stage of exhaustion sets in because the adrenal gland can no longer produce adrenaline. In adapting to stress, cortisol is dysregulated along with stress to the HPA (hypothalamus-pituitary-adrenal) axis that can impact sleep, endocrine and immune function, metabolism, and cause fatigue, mood disorders, and weight gain (Selye, 1984).

As part of the client intake, the Integrative Health and Wellness Assessment (IHWA) (Chapter 6) can deepen the connection to ones unique stress responses. A meaningful question to ask a client is, *"When you experience stress, where do you notice it in your body?"* (See Appendix F for different awareness practices). Meditation and mindfulness programs have been shown to reduce multiple negative dimensions of psychological behavioral stress (Goyal et al., 2014). According to recent research published in the *Journal of Internal Medicine* (Goyal et al., 2014), meditation programs can result in small-to-moderate reductions of multiple negative dimensions of psychological stress in cancer patients, and clinicians should be prepared to talk with their patients about the role that a meditation program could have in addressing psychological stress.

As Nurse Coaches offer patients/clients mindfulness and awareness practices as part of their coaching process, the client/patient is encouraged to record her/his experience and observe the impact of how reducing stress can shift her/his sense of wellbeing and quality of life. Strategies for the client/patient to implement these practices include creating a "relaxation ritual":

- Developing a consistent routine: practice at the same time and in the same space daily.
- Discovering a quiet space or creating a healing environment.
- Exploring a variety of relaxation tools and techniques to find which one resonates with the client/patient.
- Inviting client/patient to write or record the images and words that hold meaning for her or him.

The Nurse Coach uses this practice for her/his own self-development and in integrating these tools into daily practice.

Smoking

Smoking can be a stress-coping behavior as well as a cultural phenomenon. If smoking cessation is part of why a client seeks out a Nurse Coach or is referred to a Nurse Coach for behavioral modification, it is meaningful to explore all of the reasons why an individual chooses to smoke. Most people are already aware of the health risks associated with smoking. What are the benefits to continuing in a behavior knowing the risks? What are the challenges in stopping smoking?

The 2014 Surgeon General's report commemorates the 50th anniversary of the 1964 report. The evidence on the health consequences of smoking has been updated many times in the Surgeon General's reports since the first one in 1964. These reports have summarized our evolving understanding of the broad spectrum of deleterious health effects resulting from exposure to tobacco smoke and second-hand smoke. In turn, this evidence has been translated into tobacco control strategies implemented to protect the public's health. The Surgeon General's report and the progress made is an enduring example of evidence-based public health policy in practice although cigarette smoking remains one of the most pressing global health issues of our time (Alberg, Shopland, & Cummings, 2014). The CDC has declared reducing tobacco use a "winnable battle" in a new report, January, 2014. The CDC supports comprehensive efforts to prevent the initiation of tobacco use, promote quitting, and ensure smoke-free environments. This report documents recent decreases in lung cancer incidence during 2005–2009 in the United States, with lung cancer incidence declining more rapidly among men compared with women in all age groups except age <35 years.

Smoking is associated with elevated blood pressure, increased lipids, sticky platelets, and raising the risk of clots. Although heavy cigarette smokers are at greatest risk, people who smoke as few as three cigarettes a day are at higher risk for blood vessel abnormalities that endanger the heart. Regular exposure to passive smoke also increases the risk of heart disease in nonsmokers. Cigarette smoke contains at least 20 chemical carcinogens. Due to a wide spectrum of harmful effects of smoking, the common recommendations for cancer prevention in almost all lifestyle studies is no smoking as part of a comprehensive preventive lifestyle approach. In addition, smoking influences body weight such that smokers weigh less than nonsmokers and smoking cessation often leads to weight increase.

The relationship between body weight and smoking is partly explained by the effect of nicotine on appetite and metabolism (Thorgeirsson et al., 2013). However, the brain reward system is involved in the control of the intake of both food and tobacco. There is a common biological basis of the regulation of our appetite for tobacco and food, and thus the vulnerability to nicotine addiction and obesity leads the innovative Nurse Coach to offer integrative approaches for lifestyle change. Introducing "eating with awareness" tools (Appendix E) can guide the client in learning new patterns of eating to support the body and mind during cessation of nicotine.

Alcohol

Alcohol is a social and cultural choice as well as a stress reduction and coping strategy for many people. If a client/patient reveals that her/his alcohol intake is affecting her/his life, it is often an indicator for motivation and an opportunity for the Nurse Coach to explore the client/patient's readiness for changing behavior. Alcohol is also addicting, and some people have genetic predispositions in the way they metabolize and detoxify alcohol, making it a more deleterious substance to some people while others can drink moderately without notable effect. The Nurse Coach explores drinking patterns that might reveal biochemical, physical, and psychological contributors to health issues. Nurse Coaches recognize health risk factors and challenges for the client/patient if alcohol is identified by the client/patient as impairing quality of life and wellbeing. Identifying readiness for change and exploring patterns of alcohol use and triggers with the client is a first step for the client and the Nurse Coach.

Sleep

Monitoring sleep and strategies to improve sleep are essential to long-term health and healthy aging. It is estimated that 30–40% of American adults sleep less than six hours per night. Endocrinologists and cardiologists recognize that poor sleep habits and sleep loss may be risk factors for obesity and diabetes. According to research, individuals who sleep less than five hours a night increase their risk of developing diabetes by 46% compared with those who sleep seven hours or more. In addition, up to 30% of our genes function according to our circadian rhythm cycle. Many of these genes control some aspect of our metabolism, such as fat and sugar burning.

Many of the hormones the body needs to repair itself are released during sleep, with the deepest and most regenerative sleep occurring between 10 p.m. and 2 a.m. "Sleep is an important modulator of neuroendocrine function and glucose metabolism and sleep loss has been shown to result in metabolic and endocrine alterations, including decreased glucose tolerance, decreased insulin sensitivity, increased evening concentrations of cortisol, increased levels of ghrelin, decreased levels of leptin, and increased hunger and appetite" (Beccuti & Pannain, 2011). Recent epidemiological and laboratory evidence confirm previous findings of an association between sleep loss and increased risk of obesity. The Nurse Coach assesses sleep patterns as nocturnal sleep can reveal triggers to weight gain, inflammation, and immune and hormonal health. Since sleep and wakefulness are influenced by different neurotransmitter signals in the brain, foods and medicines that change the balance of these signals affect whether we feel alert or drowsy and how well we sleep. (See Appendix E-17.)

Vignette: Andy

Andy, a diabetic patient showing periodic spikes in blood sugar, was evaluated via lab tests, and an additional medication was prescribed. It was assumed that he "cheated" on the dietary guidelines and food exchange lists he was handed at his last appointment. He sought out a Nurse Coach in his community as he intuitively know that something else was triggering his sugar spikes and was curious to understand more.

As healthcare providers, we often make quick and easy assumptions but do not ask the questions that will inform us to see more clearly. What if Andy was asked what he believed triggered the fluctuations in blood sugar, before the physician automatically prescribed additional medication? "What other contributing factors may have triggered your spike in blood sugar, unique to your situation?" What were Andy's sleep patterns? As it turned out, Andy was under a lot of personal stress, recently losing his job, and finding it almost impossible to sleep due to the worry of having no income.

Lifestyle factors including stress, exercise, sleeping patterns, and environmental exposures (see Chapter 9) may be influencing blood sugar levels and drive obesity when we explore the client/patient's story. When patients are asked and report that they did not consume additional carbohydrates or sugar, how can we explore other lifestyle factors, ask additional meaningful questions, and engage the client in discovering possible triggers as a first step in becoming aware of possible cofactors. When the Nurse Coach explores the patient's story and the client/patient responds "I have been under stress," what is that we, as nurses might offer in our brief encounter at the office in the expanded role as Nurse Coach? Could we ask the client to become aware of her/his stress response patterns and support her/him in learning more about his/her unique responses to stress? At the appropriate moment, can we offer an awareness or relaxation practice to do at home? We can invite the client/patient to explore her/his evening habits that might contribute to sleep disturbances and elevated cortisol levels at night, which can also impact blood sugar regulation.

Environmental Exposures

In the home, workplace, and community, the impact to our health on a daily basis as environmental inputs are ubiquitous and omnipresent. Environmental inputs may include noise; chemicals in food, air, and water; temperature; light, both artificial and natural; electromagnetic fields; and more (see Table 9-1 and Chapter 9).

Nutrition

Nutrition is integral to maintaining health throughout the life cycle and has a profound influence on disease prevention, health maintenance, and the aging process (see Chapter 8).

PHYSICAL ACTIVITY AND MOVEMENT

Activity and movement are vital to health promotion and wellbeing throughout the life cycle. Physical activity has always been part of our human behavior until recent times. The emerging research health benefits are striking, including the impact on:

- Cardiovascular disease and circulation
- Control of blood sugar regulation, metabolic syndrome, and diabetes

- Cancer prevention and survivorship
- Enhancement of cognitive function and healthy aging
- Improvement in mood and sleep
- Balance of hormones
- Extending telomere length and healthy aging
- Improving joint diseases and daily mobility

Nurse Coaches, as part of the coaching process, assess the client/patient's motivation to include physical activity in her/his lifestyle plan and evaluate her/his willingness to engage in physical activities that are meaningful. Listening to a client's choices, or their resistance to change, is meaningful in exploring what are the possible options for clients to discover. The value of choice and responsibility in self-motivation is critical for creating a personal plan and goals. Clear SMART goals (Specific, Measurable, Achievable, Realistic, Time-lined) act as a guide for achieving success when discovering exercise and movement patterns and creating new routines (see Chapter 15). As nurses, we can evaluate and collaborate with the client's medical team to clarify physical activity limitations while offering new possibilities, whether on a physical level or using the mind and positive imagery to visualize strengthening new muscles and fibers if physical activity is not possible. Based on new research on telomeres and neuroplasticity and connecting new neuronal networks, mindfulness-based practice may lead to new biochemical-electrical circuitry in those unable to participate in physical activity.

Research and Review

An essential advantage of being a Nurse Coach is that we have the science and knowledge to assess our client/patient's health and also wear the hat of nurse educator and advocate at appropriate times. As part of our role, we can share information to demonstrate the benefits documented in the research. Information can be a tool that assists in motivating the client/patient toward positive lifestyle change while setting realistic goals. In reviewing the client's physical health assessment, in many conditions, exercise and movement can be challenging including those with obesity and structural problems. Exploring the meaning of improving health outcomes and creating small steps are recommended to promote sustainable change (see Appendices E-12 and E13).

The American Heart Association recently recommended motivational strategies as an effective approach to engage patients in low-intensity interventions (exercise and diet) to promote health-related outcomes for improving cardiovascular health. A review of the research indicates coaching as an effective strategy and a collaborative component, drawing on the client's personal motives for behavioral change and personal choice leading to health-promoting behaviors and enhancing self-efficacy. As the Nurse Coach assesses the client's readiness to change and realistic goals, the personal meaning of the client's limitations and of her/his hopes for renewed capacity connects the client with her/his innate wisdom and potential. As the Nurse Coach and client/patient engage in change talk, the motivation to engage in changing behaviors increases and promotes long-lasting, sustained change.

According to recent research, exercise can be as effective as many frequently prescribed drugs in treating some of the leading causes of death.

- A new study raises important questions about whether our healthcare system focuses too much on medications and too little on activity to combat physical ailments. Researchers compared how well various drugs and exercise succeed in reducing deaths among people who have been diagnosed with several common and serious conditions, including heart disease and diabetes. The Stanford Prevention Research Center at the Stanford University School of Medicine decided to create a comprehensive comparison of the effectiveness of drugs and exercise in lessening mortality among people who had been diagnosed with one of four diseases: heart disease, chronic heart failure, stroke, or diabetes. They chose these particular conditions because those were the only ones for which they could find studies that had examined whether exercise lessened the risk of death among patients with these diseases.

The researchers gathered all of the recent randomized controlled trials, as well as previous reviews and meta-analyses of older experiments relating to mortality among patients with those diseases, whether they had been treated with drugs or exercise. The data analyzed over 305 past experiments that, collectively, involved almost 340,000 participants. The lead researcher said, "Our results suggest that exercise can be quite potent" in treating heart disease and the other conditions, equaling the lifesaving benefits available from most of the commonly prescribed drugs, including statins. The results also underscore how infrequently exercise is considered or studied as a medical intervention. Intensive lifestyle changes have been shown to reverse atherosclerosis, improve cardiovascular risk profiles, and decrease angina pectoris and cardiac events (Daubenmier et al., 2007).

- Diabetes mellitus is a growing health concern projected to affect 366 million people worldwide by around 2030. Multiple approaches to address this health concern are documented, amongst which increased habitual physical activity has been shown to be beneficial. Various mechanisms demonstrated show improvement of cellular insulin sensitivity. The interplay between insulin sensitivity and insulin resistance plays a key role in development and persistence of the diabetic state, which can be directly linked to the levels of physical activity. Regulation of adiponectin and leptin levels is also linked to physical activity via reduction of central obesity. Inflammatory markers, free radical reduction, and up-regulation of physiological antioxidant processes are also observed in subjects with increased physical activity schedules, all of which play a significant role in the pathogenesis of diabetes mellitus.

  Multiple approaches to address this health concern have been documented in the research; notably, increased habitual physical activity has been shown to be beneficial. Various mechanisms show improvement on cellular insulin sensitivity (Venkatasamy, Pericherla, Manthuruthil, Mishra, & Hanno, 2013). Life-long physical activity restores metabolic and cardiovascular function in type 2 diabetes (T2DM) and provides evidence that a life-long active lifestyle even in T2DM may be able to effectively normalize cardiovascular risk. Short-to-moderate duration exercise training improves fitness and lowers cardiovascular risk in T2DM. This study examined the impact of a life-long active lifestyle by comparing physical fitness, cardiovascular risk, and vascular function between long-term physically active T2DM patients versus sedentary T2DM patients and controls. Exercise has also been shown to improve cholesterol and lipid levels and maintain weight control. People who are sedentary are almost twice as likely to suffer heart attacks as are people who exercise regularly.

- Researchers identify that exercise can help prevent cancer, slow the disease progression, enhance recovery, and prevent recurrence. Exercise also appears to regulate the levels of insulin, the hormone that causes most of the body's cells to take up glucose from the blood and triggers faster cell growth, boosting women's risk of breast cancer and recurrence of the disease. Current consensus in the discipline of exercise oncology is that both regular physical activity and exercise training exert some protective effect against breast cancer risk, and may reduce morbidity even in some advanced cases (Goh, Kirk, Lee, & Ladiges, 2012). Exercise also cuts blood levels of estrogen and testosterone, two sex hormones produced in both men and women that have been associated with uterine lining, prostate, and breast cancers. Exercise burns fat, which can hoard additional amounts of estrogen. Thus, by decreasing obesity, exercise can diminish the risk of a series of cancers. Scientists also found that when people sleep less than seven hours a night, the benefits of regular exercise may disappear. In some cases, the risk of developing cancer may actually double.

Many healthcare providers are recommending exercise programs to their patients, as a part of the therapy. Everyday movement on top of working out is also important for maintaining health. These findings are part of the national women's health initiative study, the largest and most ethnically diverse of its type, of women, ages 50–79, who were followed over 12 or more years (Seguin et al., 2014). The study of 93,000 postmenopausal American women found those with the highest amounts of sedentary time—defined as sitting and resting, excluding sleeping—died earlier than their most active peers. The association remained even when controlling for physical mobility and function, chronic disease status, demographic factors and overall fitness—meaning that even habitual exercisers are at risk if they have high amounts of idle time. Excess sedentary time tends to make it harder to regain physical strength and function. When people sleep less than seven hours a night, the benefits of regular exercise may disappear (McLain, Lewin, Laposky, Kahle, & Ladiges).

- Health communication around physical activity is critical in supporting behavioral change with cancer patients. A recent study suggests that narratives may be more effective than in just providing information and education in improving perceived physical abilities, self-efficacy, and involvement in physical activity. This provides an opportunity for the Nurse Coach to explore the meaning and beliefs around physical activity from the patient/client perspective (Falzon, Radel, Cantor, & d'Arripe-Longueville).

Nurse Coach Exercise and Movement Tips

- Engage client with the Integrative Health and Wellness Assessment and Exercise component (see Chapter 6).
- Use the Exercise and Movement Survey to open the conversation (see Appendix E-11).
- Explore client interests in engaging in a new exercise program and motives for engaging in a movement/exercise plan.
- Explore clients' relationship and interest in improving—flexibility, muscle strength, postural improvement, balance, relaxation, cardio endurance, body weight, relaxation, or stress release through activity...be aware that some patients/clients react to the term "exercise" and "movement" or "physical activity" may be more therapeutic.
    What have you done in the past that worked for you?
    What was your best experience?
    What are your current challenges or current limitations?
    Where might you begin?

Movement and Exercise Tips

- Establish goals
- Plan activity
- Affirmation/agreement/commitment (see Appendix E-13)

Vignette: Jake

Jake is a 56-year-old executive who travels to different cities three days a week for business. He is divorced and has a good relationship with his two adult children and had isolated himself from old friends since his divorce. He has gained 25 pounds in the past two years, mostly around his abdomen. He describes his work as "a high-stress job." Jake scheduled a visit for guidance in changing his "lifestyle" following his annual physical and his doctor's concerns.

Jake shared the comfort of eating a large meal at the end of a long day along with a few drinks with associates several times a week. He described his main physical activity was "running through the airport to catch a flight...and always short of breath." He had elevated lipids along with the inflammatory marker C reactive protein and hemoglobin A1C. His blood pressure was borderline elevated. He reported that his doctor told him that he had "a classic case of metabolic syndrome" and expressed fear of having a heart attack and dying like his father. Lifestyle triggers to explore include: Diet, stress, inactivity, social isolation. (See Chapter 8.)

Healthy Lifestyle and Breast Cancer Prevention

Lifestyle risk factors for breast cancer appear to play a major role in breast cancer prevention. Breast cancer research has long associated lifestyle risks including lack of physical activity, alcohol use, ingestion of a high saturated-fat/low-fiber diet, and lack of sleep and provides a model for how lifestyle factors contribute to epigenetic changes. Family history and the BRCA 1&2 genetic polymorphism appear to account for only 5–10% of breast cancers in today's world. A growing body of research points to a gap in breast cancer prevention, education, and lifestyle strategies essential for reducing risks throughout a woman's life cycle. Nurse Coaches are increasingly working with breast cancer patients/clients in supporting lifestyle changes for both prevention and survivorship.

Vignette: Sally

Sally is employed as a nurse working the night shift at a busy metropolitan hospital. She reports being highly stressed at work. She has erratic eating and sleeping patterns and has experienced recent weight gain. Married eight years, she has had two miscarriages... Her mother had premenopausal breast cancer and Sally is fearful of the same fate. She sought out the Nurse Wellness Coach through her hospital wellness program as a last resort before leaving her job. Sally arrived at her session tearful, fearful, and overwhelmed with events in her life.

Review of the Breast Cancer Research

A recent study assessed a healthy lifestyle index in relation to the risk of breast cancer. "Healthy lifestyle is associated with a reduction in risk for breast cancer. Primary prevention should be promoted in an integrated manner. Effective strategies need to be identified to engage women in healthy lifestyles" (Sánchez-Zamorano et al., 2011). A growing number of studies show that diet and environmental exposures including prenatal, and stress can influence DNA expression and have an effect on health outcomes later in life. Research also identifies healthy lifestyle habits as mediating epigenetic changes and one's ability to lower risks through diet, exercise, social support, stress reduction and relaxation techniques, including yoga and mindfulness-based practices.

As part of the women's health initiative, Thompson et al. (2014) looked at the impact of nutrition and physical activity on overall cancer risk with aging of 65,838 postmenopausal women enrolled in the Women's Health Initiative Observational Study. The conclusion of this large study was that healthy lifestyle behaviors reduce cancer risk and overall mortality. Cancer-preventive health behaviors were associated with lower risk of total breast and colorectal cancers and lower cancer-specific mortality in postmenopausal women.

A recent publication, *The Ecology of Breast Cancer: the Promise of Prevention and the Hope for Healing* (Schettler, 2014), addresses cancer patterns that must include features woven into our lives and communities: the agriculture and food system, many aspects of the built environment, and pervasive hazardous chemicals that all play a role in breast cancer. This analysis emphasizes the importance of taking a life course approach throughout the life cycle.

Nurse Coaches have an opportunity to impact women's health on multiple levels including, coaching, education, and advocacy for healthier communities. An expanded Nurse Coach role includes supporting and empowering communities to seek solutions for local health risk factors impacting health and the quality of life including access to healthier foods and a cleaner environment.

The Nurse Coach explores and listens to where the client/patient is with readiness for lifestyle change cues:

- Ambivalence (I should)
- Desire (I wish)
- Ability (I could, I can)
- Need (I must)
- Commitment (I will, I am ready)

Guidelines for Lifestyle Change

- Explore client's list of concerns and benefits to each aspect of her/his lifestyle behaviors.
- Explore what the client sees as her/his options for changing behaviors.
- Explore core values, strengths, motivators, reasons for change.
- Identify throughout process, where client is in stages of change.
- Explore challenges, obstacles, and beliefs that may interfere with behavioral change.
- Co-create strategies for possible solutions for behavioral change.
- Co-identify appropriate behavioral lifestyle goals.
- Elicit client to commit willingness to change and set one reachable goal.

Nurse Coach Questions to Guide Client Conversation for Lifestyle Change

- What concerns do you have about your current health?
- How might your current behaviors influence your health or future health concerns?
- Do you believe that your current lifestyle supports your health and wellbeing?
- What are the benefits of change?
- What are the benefits of staying the same?
- What changes would you like to make in your current patterns or behaviors?
- What do you believe are your challenges or obstacles (standing in your way) for moving forward?

Integrative Nurse Coach Process

- Create a wellness vision
- Connect with life goals
- Client connects to strengths and motivators
- SMART goals realistic for change (break down large goals)
- Readiness for change indicators
- Self efficacy-potential for success

- Value to self (not imposed from the outside)
- Identify specific action steps
- Time frame for realistic achieving goals

SUMMARY

- Nurse Coaches are uniquely positioned to coach and engage individuals, families, and communities in the process of meaningful and health-promoting strategies for behavioral change.
- With a renewed focus on wellness promotion in healthcare reform, it is an important moment for nurses to expand their skills and scope of practice.
- Lifestyle factors, including nutrition, environmental influences, and physical activity, all impact health and wellbeing throughout the life cycle and are central to an integrative Nurse Coach assessment and coaching process.

NURSE COACH REFLECTIONS

After reading this chapter, the Nurse Coach will be able to bring awareness and personal insight to the following questions:

- What changes can I make to enhance my wellbeing?
- What lifestyle patterns do I recognize that might interfere with my wellbeing?
- What new awareness practice can support healthier lifestyle choices and behaviors?
- What new practices am I willing to bring into my life to encourage my wellbeing?
- Who are the people in my life who would support me in making healthy changes?
- How does a Nurse Coach co-create and promote a culture of health and wellbeing to build healthier communities?
- How do we integrate these concepts of wellbeing into our work within the current health paradigm?

REFERENCES

Alberg, A., Shopland, D., & Cummings, K. (2014, January 15). The 2014 Surgeon General's Report: Commemorating the 50th anniversary of the 1964 report of the advisory commitee to the US Surgeon General and updating the evidence on the health consequences of cigarette smoking. *American Journal of Epidemiology.* doi:10.1093/aje/kwt335

Barnes, D., Mehling, W., Yaffe, K., Flores, C., & Chesney, M. (2013, March 20). Preventing loss of independence through exercise (PLIÉ): An integrative exercise program for individuals with dementia. American Academy of Neurology (AAN) 65th Annual Meeting, S24.077.

Beccuti, C., & Pannain, S. (2011). Sleep and obesity. *Current Opinion Clinical Nutritional Metabolic Care 14*(4), 402–412. doi:10.1097/MCO.0b013e3283479109

Centers for Disease Control and Prevention (CDC) (n.d.). Health Related Quality of Life Surveillance Program. Retrieved from http://www.cdc.gov/hrqol/concept.htm

Centers for Disease Control and Prevention (CDC) (2013, December 20). Retrieved from www.cdc.gov/obesity/index.html www.cdc.gov/hrqol/wellbeing.htm

Clark, F. A. (2011). Occupation embedded in a real life: Interweaving occupational science and occupational therapy [1993 Eleanor Clarke Slagle Lecture]. In R. Padilla & Y. Griffiths (Eds.). *A professional legacy: The Eleanor Clarke Slagle lectures in occupational therapy, 1955–2010* (3ʳᵈ ed.). Bethesda, MD: AOTA Press. http://myaota .aota.org/shop_aota/prodview.aspx?TYPE=D&PID=978&SKU=1234A

Clark, F. A., Jackson, J. M., & Carlson, M. E. (2004). Occupational science, occupational therapy and evidence-based practice: What the Well Elderly Study has taught us. *Occupation for occupational therapists* (pp. 200–218). Oxford, UK: Blackwell Publishing.

Daubenmier, J., Weidner, G., Sumner, M. D., Mendell, N., Merritt-Worden, T., Studley, J., & Ornish, D. (2007). The contribution of changes in diet, exercise, and stress management to changes in coronary risk in women and men in the multisite cardiac lifestyle intervention. *Annals of Behavioral Medicine, 33*(1), 57–58.

Falzon, C., Radel, R., Cantor, A., & d'Arripe-Longueville, F. (2014, September 4). Understanding narrative effects in physical activity promotion: The influence of breast cancer survivor testimony on exercise beliefs, self-efficacy, and intention in breast cancer patients. *Support Care Cancer.*

Goh, J., Kirk, E. A., Lee, S. X., & Ladiges, W. C. (2012). Exercise, physical activity and breast cancer: The role of tumor-associated macrophages. *Exercise Immunology Review 18*, 158–176.

Goyal, M., Singh, S., Sibinga, E. M., Gould, N. F., Rowland-Seymour, A., Sharma, R., & Haythornthwaite, J. A. (2014). Meditation programs for psychological stress and well-being: A systematic review and meta-analysis. *JAMA Internal Medicine.* doi:10.1001/jamainternmed.2013.13018

Howell, R. T., Kern, M. L., & Lyubomirsky, S. (2007). Health benefits: Meta-analytically determining the impact of well-being on objective health outcomes. *Health Psychology Review 1*(1), 83–136. doi:10.1080/17437190701492486

Institute of Medicine (IOM) (2013). U.S. Health in International Perspective: Shorter Lives, Poorer Health. Retrieved from http://www.iom.edu/~/media/Files/Report%20Files/ 2013/US-Health-International-Perspective/USHealth_Intl_PerspectiveRB.pdf

Katz, D. (2014). U.S. National Center for Health Statistics, Jan. 6, 2014. Yale University Prevention Research Center.

McAllister, M., & McKinnon, J. (2009). The importance of teaching and learning resilience in the health disciplines: A critical review of the literature. *Nurse Education Today, 29*(4), 371–379.

McClain, J., Lewin, D., Laposky, A., Kahle L., & Berrigan, D. (2014, September). Associations between physical activity, sedentary time, sleep duration and daytime sleepiness in US adults. *Preventive Medicine 66*, 68–73.

Nahum, M., Lee, H., & Merzenich, M. M. (2013). *Progressive Brain Research 207*, 141–171. doi: 10.1016/B978-0-444-63327-9.00009-6

Nightingale, F. (1860). *Notes on nursing: What it is and what it is not* (p. 1). London, UK: Harrison.

Ornish, D., Lin, J., Chan, J., Epel, E., Kemp, C., Weidner, G., & Blackburn, E. (2013). Effect of comprehensive lifestyle changes on telomerase activity and telomere length in men with biopsy-proven low-risk prostate cancer. *The Lancet Oncology, 14*(11), 1112–1120. doi:10.1016/S1470-2045(13)70366-8

Sánchez-Zamorano, L., Flores-Luna, L., Angeles-Llerenas, A., Romieu, I., Lazcano-Ponce, E., Miranda-Hernández, H., … Torres-Mejia, G. (2011). Healthy lifestyle on the risk of breast cancer. *Cancer Epidemiology, Biomarkers & Prevention, 20*(5), 912–922. doi:10.1158/1055-9965.EPI-10-1036

Schettler, T. (2014). *The ecology of breast cancer: The promise of prevention and the hope for healing.* Science for Health and the Environment Network. California. Online publication http://www.sehn.org/emandeh.html

Seguin, R., Buchner, D., Liu, J., Allison, M., Manini, T., Wang, C., … LaCroix, A. (2014). Sedentary behavior and mortality in older women: The women's health initiative. *American Journal of Preventive Medicine, 46*(2), 122–135. doi:10.1016/j.amepre.2013.10.021

Selye, H. (1984). *The stress of life,* New York, NY: McGraw-Hill.

Smith, B. J., Tang, K. C., & Nutbeam, D. (2006). WHO health promotion glossary: New terms *Health Promotion International, 21*(4), 340–345. doi: 10.1093/heapro/dal033

Starkweather, A. R., Alhaeeri, A. A., Montpetit, A., Brumelle, J., Filler, K., Montpetit, M., Mohanraj, L., Lyon, D. E., & Jackson-Cook, C. K. (2014). An integrative review of factors associated with telomere length and implications for biobehavioral research. *Nursing Research, 63*(1), 36–50. doi:10.1097/NNR.0000000000000009

Thompson, C., McCullough, M., Wertheim, B., Chlebowski, R., Martinez, M., Stefanick, M., … Neuhouser, M. (2014). Nutrition and physical activity cancer prevention guidelines, cancer risk, and mortality in the women's health initiative. *Cancer Prevention Research, 7*(1), 42–53. doi:10.1158/1940-6207.CAPR-13-0258

Thorgeirsson, T., Gudbjartsson, D., Sulem, P., Besenbacher, S., Styrkarsdottir, U., Thorleifsson, G., … Stefansson, K. (2013, July). A common biological basis of obesity and nicotine addiction. *Translational Psychiatry, 3.*

Venkatasamy, V. V., Pericherla, S., Manthuruthil, S., Mishra, S., & Hanno, R. (2013). Effect of physical activity on insulin resistance, inflammation and oxidative stress in diabetes mellitus. *Journal of Clinical Diagnosis Research, 7*(8), 1764–1766. doi:10.7860/JCDR/2013/6518.3306. Epub 2013 Jul 17.

Wahl, A., & Schwab, M. (2014, January 9). Finding an optimal rehabilitation paradigm after stroke: enhancing fiber growth and training of the brain at the right moment. *Frontiers in Human Neuroscience, 7,* 911. doi:10.3389/fnhum.2013.00911

Wang, Y., Tuomilehto, J., Jousilahti, P., Antikainen, R., Mähönen, M., Katzmarzyk, P. T., & Hu, G. (2013). Healthy lifestyle status, antihypertensive treatment and the risk of heart failure among Finnish men and women. *Journal of Hypertension, 31*(11), 2158–2164. doi: 10.1097/HJH.0b013e328364136d

World Health Organization (WHO) (2011). *Noncommunicable diseases country profiles 2011.* Geneva, Switzerland: WHO Press.

World Health Organization (WHO) (2013). *Global action plan for the prevention and control of non-communicable diseases, 2013–2020.* Geneva, Switzerland: WHO Press.

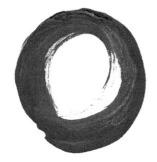

CHAPTER **8**

Nutritional Health

Susan Luck

No amount of medical knowledge will lessen the accountability for nurses to do what nurses do; that is, manage the environment to promote positive life processes.

Florence Nightingale, 1860

LOOKING AHEAD...

After reading this chapter, you will be able to:

- Expand understanding of nutrition as an energy model.
- Explore the role of the Nurse Coach in promoting nutritional behavioral change.
- Explore nutrition beliefs and patterns using a bio-psycho-social-cultural-spiritual framework.
- Deepen understanding of the role of food and nutrition in maintaining health throughout the life cycle.
- Explore awareness practices for promoting healthy eating behaviors.

DEFINITIONS

Adinopectin: A protein hormone produced and secreted exclusively by adipocytes (fat cells) that regulates the metabolism of lipids and glucose.

Diabesity: A popular concept for the clinical association of type 2 diabetes mellitus and obesity.

Free radicals: Electrically charged molecules with an unpaired electron capable of attacking healthy cells in the body, causing them to lose their structure and function.

Glycemic index: An index that classifies carbohydrate foods according to their glycemic response (effect on blood glucose levels), which varies with fiber content, starch structure, food processing, and presence of proteins and fats.

Gluten: A mixture of proteins found in wheat and other grains that are not soluble in water and that give wheat dough its elastic texture.

Inflammation: The body's attempt at self-protection; the aim being to remove harmful stimuli, including damaged cells, irritants, or pathogens.

Leptin: A protein hormone that is produced by fat cells and plays a role in body weight regulation, eating behavior, and appetite.

Metabolic syndrome: A collection of risk factors that increase the chance of developing heart disease, stroke, and diabetes. The condition is also known as syndrome X cardio-metabolic syndrome, and insulin resistance syndrome.

Metabolomics: The study of all the metabolites present in cells, tissues, and organs.

Microbiome: The collective genomes of the microbes that live inside and on the human body.

Nutrigenomics: A branch of nutritional genomics and the study of the effects of foods and food constituents on gene expression.

Obesogens: Chemicals that disrupt the endocrine system and promote weight gain and obesity.

OPTIMIZING NUTRITION FOR WELLBEING

Through an evolutionary perspective, our modern-day food supply has been dramatically altered although our human biological nutrient needs have not changed. In today's world, optimizing nutrition is critical to maintaining health and wellbeing. Nutrition has a profound influence on healing and longevity and in preventing disease throughout the life cycle.

Nutrition Strategies in Nurse Coaching

In an expanded holistic and integrative Nurse Coach model, the discovery of the complex relationship of nutrition and the meaning of food in one's life acknowledges and honors the complexity and totality of the individual. Each person's worldview comprises a unique constellation of perceptions and circumstances that influence health behaviors.

The Nurse Coach explores how beliefs, attitudes, eating patterns, food choices, and culinary styles are influenced by one's cultural, physiological, psychological, emotional, spiritual, genetic, socioeconomic, and environmental dimensions that guide choices and behaviors.

In a Nurse Coach personalized care model, eliciting the client/patient's story reflects the relationship to food, eating behaviors, preferences, and the many unique factors influencing one's current choices and future goals. A Nurse Coach strategy includes uncovering antecedents, triggers, and mediators that provide a map of one's life and that can reveal patterns, symptoms, and disease processes. The discovery of the factors that can aggravate or ameliorate symptoms, and that can predispose one to illness or facilitate recovery, provides possibilities for creating lifestyle and behavioral change.

Central to this process is raising awareness for both the Nurse Coach and the client/patient and assessing stages of change (see Chapter 15) and one's readiness for establishing realistic attainable and sustainable goals around food and eating behaviors for improving health outcomes.

This chapter will explore how food choices play a central role in many common conditions, including inflammation and pain, digestive and gastrointestinal disturbances, allergies and food sensitivities, fatigue, mood disorders, and immune dysfunction. For Nurse Coaches, this chapter provides a map for navigating new directions in the process of awareness and change for improving health and wellbeing. In summary, the Nurse Coach begins the exploration process through deepening awareness of:

- eating patterns and habits (present and past);
- beliefs about the influence of food choices on present health concerns;
- the impact of eating behaviors on social, cultural, psychological, and physical function;
- the economics and availability of food choices and options; and
- nutritional factors that influence health and wellbeing.

The Nurse Coach conversation can be guided by the Integrative Health and Wellness Assessment (see Component 6, Nutrition, Appendices C-1 [short form] and C-2 [long form]) to deepen one's awareness of food choices, preferences, and challenges. Nutrition guidelines (Appendices E-4 to E-11) can assist the client/patient in developing realistic goals for wellness promotion and lifestyle change.

In a comprehensive nutrition and lifestyle assessment, there are multiple factors to explore that can affect digestion, absorption, transport, assimilation, and storage of nutrients, including stress, toxins, hormones, exercise and movement, sleep, medications, and genetic influences. Integrating nutrition concepts, including portion size, meal planning, food intolerances, and cravings, are all considered along with education tools as part of the Nurse Coach expanded role in guiding the client/patient to develop a personalized nutrition plan and setting realistic goals and strategies for success.

FOOD AS ENERGY

Food and nutrients are no longer viewed merely as providing substances whose absence would produce disease, but as having a positive impact on an individual's health, physical performance, healthy aging, and frame of mind. It has become common knowledge that many foods produced today are processed and denatured, depleted of nutrients, and often contain toxic chemicals, including additives, preservatives, pesticides, residues, and genetically modified ingredients.

Food composition and macronutrients are essential for biochemical processes that work synergistically to produce energy on a cellular level. Without adequate nutrients and healthy cellular communication, the end result is diminished function, decreased energy output, inflammation, and lowered immune response. Essential macronutrients and micronutrients include complex carbohydrates, proteins, fats, vitamins, and minerals (Luck, 2013).

The fundamental physiological processes of nutrition are grounded in bioenergetics and energy production, communication both outside and inside the cell, and the transformation of food into energy. Overt symptoms of nutrient deficiency are the result of a long chain of reactions in the body. When an individual consumes a nutrient-deficient diet, the initial reactions are on a molecular level. Deficiencies may continue for many years until the body can no longer carry out its functions. Eventually, overt signs and symptoms appear, even though the deficiency may still be considered subclinical and routine laboratory tests may not test for nutrient deficiencies. Over time, a broad range of nonspecific symptoms and conditions that can diminish an individual's overall quality of life emerge, and over many years, the body becomes more vulnerable to illnesses to which the individual may be genetically predisposed. As resilient beings, even when health is compromised, we can reprogram and regenerate cells and create an internal and external healing environment to restore health and balance.

Energy Field Principles in Nursing

Nurse Coaches address the underlying key imbalances and energetic dynamics that can impact vitality, a sense of wellbeing, and quality of life. The unique contribution of holistic nursing theory and practice and the extensive clinical research and application from integrative health, functional medicine, neuroscience, spiritual traditions, cognitive psychology, sociology, and diverse cultural healing systems all provide an expanded framework for health and healing the whole person and recognize the nutritional qualities necessary to the healing process through:

- *Supporting* indivisible interconnectedness—mind–body–spirit continuum
- *Optimizing* multidimensional cellular communication and function—energy dynamics

- *Connecting* the circuits—psychoneuroimmunology
- *Nurturing* our roots—culture, beliefs, and tradition

Understanding nutrition as an energy model, core imbalances are viewed as multifactorial and interconnected and are addressed from within the complexity of the multidimensional aspects of the individual. Nutrient energy field disturbances in the internal and external environment impact:

- mind-body/body-mind communication;
- digestion, absorption, and assimilation of nutrients;
- inflammatory triggers and immune dysregulation;
- elimination, detoxification, and biotransformation;
- hormonal and neurotransmitter communication;
- oxidative stress, cellular energy, and mitochondrial dysfunction; and
- structural integrity.

For the Nurse Coach, nutrition research and its clinical implications and applications along with a comprehensive whole foods-based approach, deepens the connection between food choices, eating patterns and behaviors, health risks, and health goals. Health-promoting behaviors often lead to positive outcomes for the most common symptoms, including: alleviating pain, improving digestion, and lessening the need for conventional medical treatment protocols. Energy imbalance can also be considered as contributing to the obesity epidemic and other chronic conditions: a combination of excess empty dietary calories and a lack of physical activity, along with environmental obesogenic chemicals (see Chapter 9). Biochemically, metabolically, and energetically, excess consumption of highly refined carbohydrates can interfere with cell signaling messengers that control feelings of satiety after eating.

The Nurse Coach often engages clients/patients in self-reflection about their eating styles and behaviors as they transition from mindless eating to mindfulness eating practices (see Appendix F). Increased awareness of food patterns and choices begins the change process around food and opens the possibilities for:

- regulating metabolism and healthy fat cell signaling;
- supporting healthy energy exchange inside the cell;
- promoting healthy weight loss;
- reversing insulin resistance and balancing blood sugar control mechanisms and regulation; and
- lowering inflammation and inflammatory triggers—all to attain and sustain long-term health goals.

Effective nutrition programs integrate coaching skills into a process that is gradual and a highly individualized approach for reversing long-term patterns and for learning new behaviors. Effective health promotion strategies include awareness practices, movement and exercise, behavioral motivation, and nutrition education.

Restoring balance throughout the life cycle will impact the aging process, including physical and cognitive function, by addressing the modifiable risk factors to support the body's ability to:

- reverse nutrient deficiencies;
- ensure adequate energy intake, production, and storage;
- optimize nutrient absorption;
- maintain healthy immune response;

- support elimination and detoxification pathways;
- avoid toxic compounds in the environment; and
- increase activity and exercise to increase metabolism.

Food as Information

Foods manufactured today and available on the global market contribute to a rising number of health problems throughout the life cycle, including learning disabilities, cognitive impairment, obesity, diabetes, atherosclerosis, heart disease, hypertension, immune and autoimmune diseases, and various cancers. Current nutrient standards and guidelines do not take into account individual lifestyle and health needs. The government's Recommended Daily Allowance (RDA) addresses the basic nutrients to prevent overt deficiencies but does not consider levels needed for the optimal health potential of the individual or the stress and toxic body burden of living in today's world. Our ancestors would not recognize the "foods" consumed today. The standard American diet (SAD) leads to metabolic and functional imbalance responsible for diminished health and illness across the life cycle.

Current research supports Nurse Coaches in all healthcare settings to coach individuals and communities in nutrition and lifestyle change to impact health in both prevention and in offering possibilities to reverse chronic health conditions through attainable nutrition interventions to reach long-term goals and impact health outcomes. Several recently published studies demonstrated consistent results using lifestyle and healthy nutrition as a primary preventive intervention to be recommended before conventional treatment protocols are considered. The evidence-based science of nutrition and lifestyle interventions for preventing or treating chronic disease demonstrates the powerful, cost-effective, and critical role nutrition plays in the promotion and restoration of health. Multiple studies demonstrate that healthful dietary patterns as demonstrated by a Mediterranean style food plan that includes whole grains, legumes, nuts, vegetables, fruits, olive oil, and fish, is associated with a decrease in chronic disease and death from all causes. The harmful effects of trans and certain saturated fats, refined carbohydrates, and other food additives or toxins are well documented throughout the medical literature (Michas, Micha, & Zampelas, 2014).

Global Health

A study published in the *Bulletin of the World Health Organization* (De Vogli, Kouvonen, & Gimeno, 2014) suggests that if governments took firmer action, they could start to prevent people becoming overweight and obese—conditions with serious long-term consequences such as diabetes, heart diseases, and cancer. Governments could slow or even reverse the growing obesity epidemic if they introduced more regulation into the global market for fast foods such as burgers, chips, and fizzy drinks, researchers report. WHO is urging governments to do more to try to prevent obesity happening in the first place, rather than risking the high human and economic costs when it does (De Vogli et al., 2014). Suggested policies include economic incentives for growers to sell healthy, fresh foods; disincentives for industries to sell ultra-processed foods and soft drinks; cutting subsidies to growers and companies who use large amounts of fertilizers, pesticides, chemicals, and antibiotics; and tighter regulation of fast-food advertising, especially to children.

New research in the *Proceedings of the National Academy of Sciences* suggests that our growing global reliance on a handful of food crops may also accelerate the worldwide rise in obesity, heart disease, and diabetes. A detailed study of global food supplies confirms for the first time what experts have long suspected: human diets around the world have grown ever more similar and the trend shows no signs of slowing, with major consequences for human nutrition and food supply reliability. A massive decline in food crop diversity threatens global food security (Khoury et al., 2014).

Changes in global foods and nutrition can be attributed to several factors, including:

- Rising incomes in developing countries have allowed more consumers to include larger quantities of animal products, oils, and sugars in their diets.
- Urbanization has encouraged greater consumption of processed and fast foods.
- Trade has improved commodity transport. Multinational food industries and food safety standardization have further reinforced these trends.
- Loss of land and poor soil quality are caused by overuse of fertilizers and pesticides.

Data from the Food and Agriculture Organization of the United Nations looked at more than 50 crops and over 150 countries (accounting for 98% of the world's population) for the period 1961–2009. "International agencies have hammered away in recent years with the message that agriculture must produce more food for over 9 billion people by 2050," researcher Andy Jarvis said. "Just as important is the message that we need a more diverse global food system. This is the best way, not only to combat hunger, malnutrition, and over-nutrition, but also to protect global food supplies" (Khoury et al., 2014). The researchers single out five actions that are needed to foster diversity in food production and consumption and thus improve nutrition and food security:

- Actively promote the adoption of a wider range of varieties of the major crops worldwide to boost genetic diversity and thus reduce the vulnerability of the global food system in the face of challenges that include climate change, rising food demand, and increased water and land scarcity. This action is especially important for certain crops.
- Support the conservation and use of diverse plant genetic resources—including farmers' traditional varieties and wild species related to crops—which are critical for broadening the genetic diversity of the major crops.
- Enhance the nutritional quality of the major crops on which people depend—for example, through crop breeding to improve the content of micronutrients like iron and zinc—and make supplementary vitamins and other nutrient sources more widely available.
- Promote alternative crops that can boost the resilience of farming and make human diets healthier; specifically, identify and conserve nutritious locally grown "neglected and underutilized" crops.
- Foster public awareness of the need for healthier diets, based on better decisions about what and how much we eat as well as the forms in which we consume food.

Policies targeting food and nutrition are needed across several sectors, including agriculture, industry, health, social welfare, and education. Many countries that are transitioning from a traditional diet to one that is high in fat, sugar, and processed foods need to take action to align the food supply with the health needs of the population. The new study echoes a growing body of literature providing evidence for measures that governments could take to reverse the obesity epidemic by hindering the spread of ultra-processed foodstuffs. According to the recent *Bulletin of the World Health Organization*, measures include:

- economic incentives for growers to sell healthy and fresh food items rather than ultra-processed foods and subsidies to grow fruit and vegetables;
- economic disincentives for industries to sell fast foods, ultra-processed foods, and soft drinks, such as an ultra-processed food tax and/or the reduction or elimination of sub-

sidies to growers/companies using corn for rapid tissue growth and excessive amounts of fertilizers, pesticides, chemicals, and antibiotics;

- zoning policies to control the number and type of food outlets;
- regulation of the advertising of fast food and soft drinks, especially to children;
- trade regulations discouraging the importation and consumption of fast food, ultra-processed foods, soft drinks, and highly processed sugar foods;
- advocacy for new food policy and a reevaluation of food subsidies from high-glycemic foods that are fueling the obesity and diabetes epidemics; and
- access to fresh produce and "real" food as part of societal change.

Reprioritizing global food policy is now viewed as a human rights issue, essential to promote health for all. Nurse Coaches are in a strategic role to guide and motivate individuals and communities toward advocating for healthier food availability and choices while supporting individual health goals for changing behaviors (De Vogli et al., 2014).

Nurse Coaches in New Community Models

Community members along with healthcare workers are seeking new models of self-sufficiency and sustainability, local to global. Nurse Coaches provide the guidance and support needed to create healthy communities. In urban environments, urban farms are being created in empty spaces, in school yards, and on rooftops. Communities are learning and participating in permaculture, sustainability, and growing their own food "from urban farm to table."

Nurse Coach Profiles in Community Health

Nurse Coaches are joining the movement advocating for creating healthier communities and are bringing people together to take back their health as part of community health and public health initiatives to bring real food home to nourish their body, mind, spirit, culture, and economic needs.

- Carla, a nurse practitioner and an Integrative Nurse Coach in rural Kentucky, invites community members to her family farm to share local farming practices along with nutrition information for improving her community's health.
- Tom, a nurse practitioner working with the homeless in an urban environment, works with the local homeless shelter to build a community garden for homeless members to grow their food and to feel a connection to the Earth, which offers hope and new possibilities.
- Tina, a public health nurse, works in an urban environment where community residents are mostly from the Caribbean and Central America and often express their longing for the tropical foods they knew in their homeland to be available in their neighborhood. In a community support group organized at the local clinic for those with obesity and related health issues, Tina engaged the community in a group coaching process and began with asking, "What foods do you recall in your childhood?" This conversation led to deeper questions on what steps could the community take to bring more "real" food into their neighborhood to improve their health and that of their families.

    A group of residents, both young and elderly, came up with a strategy and a plan for bringing better food choices into their community. They asked for a meeting at their local clinic and invited local community leaders along with the clinic's healthcare providers. They shared their cultural roots and their community's story about their lack of access to fresh food. They described their diet of packaged and canned food choices available in their local market. The group created a list of foods most available and foods that they wanted to see in their corner "bodega."

Tina coached and supported their process and offered information on healthy eating to build on their initiative and advocacy for change. The organizers gathered signatures and presented them to two local bodegas. At the same time, they reached out to a food cooperative in another part of the city that delivered fresh produce from regional farms at affordable prices. Within a few months, the local clinic served as the drop off and pick up for food packages that included avocados, tomatoes, sweet potatoes, papayas, mangos, and other vegetables, all part of their indigenous diet. Community participants decided to continue to meet weekly and share recipes and stories about their memories of food in their childhood and culture. As they came together to create a community they became aware of how the processed modern foods were creating many of their health issues. As they begin to integrate the "new" foods, Tina began to see improvements in their symptoms, weight, and quality of life.

These stories of Nurse Coaches reflect how nurses globally, in all healthcare settings, coach individuals and advocate for healthy food choices and eating behaviors that impact health and wellbeing. Integrating lifestyle coaching and nutrition education into clinical practice has become a new direction in nurse coaching as part of a comprehensive approach in individual and community health today.

KEY NUTRITION CONCEPTS

Inflammation

Inflammation is part of the body's natural response to infection, injury, allergens, and other foreign substances in the body including chemicals in our environment. Identifying and removing inflammatory food triggers for restoration of wellbeing becomes part of the Nurse Coach exploration of lifestyle and nutritional strategies to "put out the fire." White blood cells, immune proteins, or other inflammatory chemical signaling mechanisms may be dispatched as part of our innate defense system. This immune-system response may be exhibited through signs of swelling, redness, and heat, often resulting in pain, and is involved in most disease processes. If thrown out of balance, the immune system can begin to attack healthy tissue. This may cause low-grade, chronic inflammation, and aches and pains, and may also contribute to autoimmune conditions, including psoriasis, lupus, multiple sclerosis, and rheumatoid arthritis. Inflammatory processes increase the risk of heart disease, Alzheimer's, diabetes, and certain cancers. Many research articles and books have been written on food elimination programs and on the "anti-inflammatory diet." The anti-inflammatory diet is "probably very close to the Mediterranean diet," says Christopher Cannon, MD, associate professor of medicine at Harvard Medical School and a cardiologist at Brigham and Women's Hospital, Boston (see Appendix E-9). The Mediterranean diet plan is rich in omega-3 essential fatty acids (Das, 2008) and anti-inflammatory phytochemicals found in the plant foods that reduce inflammation.

Dietary inflammatory triggers that can be identified and eliminated as part of a Mediterranean plan can resolve symptoms and become a biofeedback mechanism to reinforce how new choices can improve one's health and wellbeing.

Lifestyle strategies as mediators to "put out the fire" include:

- Mediterranean anti-inflammatory food plan (see Appendix E-10);
- relaxation techniques (see Appendices F-1 to F-9);

- mindfulness/relaxation practices;
- exercise and movement (see Appendices E-11 to E-13);
- social support and connection;
- adequate restful sleep (see Chapter 7); and
- elimination of environmental chemicals (see Appendices E-14 and E-15).

Gut Microbiome

Dietary factors and their interactions with the gut microbiome have important implications and clinical applications. The recent flood of research indicates that it is essential to support our living world within. Chronic conditions, including inflammatory bowel disease, migraine headaches, mood disturbances, digestive problems, weight gain, and obesity, may be attributed to an imbalance of healthy gut flora.

Billions of friendly bacteria live in the gastrointestinal tract, offering multiple beneficial effects on overall health. These microorganisms must be present to assist in synthesizing B vitamins, digesting proteins, regulating neurotransmitters, balancing intestinal pH, reducing serum cholesterol, maintaining the immune system in the gut and overall immune health, preventing parasites and overgrowth of yeast, maintaining bowel regularity, modulating weight gain, and much more that science is discovering. The most common reason for the destruction of friendly bacteria in the gastrointestinal tract is the use of antibiotics from ingestion of antibiotic-treated animal products. Studies indicate that beneficial bacteria must be replaced (probiotic supplementation) following antibiotic therapy to prevent symptoms of dysbiosis that often appear as fatigue, bloating, gas, diarrhea, constipation, and food allergies (Goldsmith & Sartor, 2014). The Nurse Coach listens to the story and the antecedents, mediators, and triggers that can reveal complicity of the gastrointestinal system in many symptoms presented.

Gluten and Elimination Food Plans

The complex issues of digestion need to also include the balance of microorganisms and food sensitivities. Fifty-eight million Americans suffer from irritable bowel syndrome, a chronic disease of bowel inflammation with symptoms ranging from diarrhea to constipation, pain, and food intolerance.

There is a growing body of research indicating that the ingestion of gluten proteins found in wheat, barley, and other grains can affect normal gut function. Digestive system dysfunction, whether genetic as in celiac disease; the result of food intolerance, food allergies, or gut permeability; or from the inability to digest the increasing concentration of gluten proteins in our food supply, is reported to be on the rise. When small protein chains absorb into the blood stream in sensitive individuals, a satellite of symptoms occur, including altered brain function to immunological and intestinal symptoms (Kabbani et al., 2014).

A gluten-free diet is based on the elimination of all foods containing gluten to allow the body to function in the absence of this potent inflammatory trigger (see Appendix E-8).

Each person has a unique relationship with food and the multitude of chemical properties. Therefore, a nutritional assessment and dietary recommendations are based on biochemical individuality. Self-assessment and -awareness tools draw upon the strengths of the individual to become aware of her/his physiologic responses to foods and to her/his symptoms and triggers often missed in traditional medicine.

Many people are now searching for patterns of how food is affecting their health. In a gluten elimination plan, it is recommended that the individual eliminate all gluten products for a minimum of three weeks. It is important to guide the awareness through keeping a food journal and becoming aware of any changes experienced, including digestion, mood, energy, weight changes, pain, food cravings, or any other symptoms unique to the individual.

A food journal becomes a reflective practice as the Nurse Coach and client/patient explore food intake, challenges, and new choices as a key to understanding what foods may be affecting one's energy, mental function, digestion, headache, pain, or any other symptoms unique to the individual.

Vignette: Jake

Jake is a 56-year-old executive who travels to different cities three days/week for business. He is divorced and has a good relationship with his two adult children. He has gained 25 lbs in the past two years, mostly around his abdomen. He describes his work as "a high-stress job." Jake scheduled a visit for guidance in changing his health and eating habits following his annual physical and his doctor's concerns. Jake shared the comfort of eating a large meal at the end of a long day along with a few drinks with associates several times a week. He said he always had pills for his "indigestion." He craved carbohydrates, especially bread and pasta. He described his main physical activity was "running through the airport to catch a flight...and always short of breath." He had elevated lipids along with the inflammatory marker C reactive protein and hemoglobin A1C. He reported that his doctor told him that he had "a classic case of metabolic syndrome," and he expressed fear of having a heart attack and dying like his father.

Obesity and Diabetes: A Global Epidemic

Obesity is on the minds of health policy analysts and healthcare providers globally. Obesity reduces life expectancy while increasing the risk of illness and death from a range of other diseases. It is now so common in adults and children that WHO characterizes the condition as an *epidemic.* It is estimated that 48 million Americans are overweight and 50 million are obese, which calculates to over one-third of adults and 17% of youth in the United States (Ogden, Carroll, Kit, & Flegal, 2014).

According to a recent Centers for Disease Control (CDC) report (2010), "Obesity is a complex problem that requires both personal and community action." The report states that obesity is a contributing cause of many health problems, including heart disease, stroke, diabetes, and some types of cancer. It mandates that people in all communities should be able to make healthy choices and that a national strategy and changes in current health policy to promote lifestyle behavioral change are needed to lower the burden of chronic illness on individuals and society. Nurse Coaches working in diverse community settings, with individuals and groups, are reporting that lifestyle changes and nutritional strategies are impacting the health of their patient population. A study published earlier this year in the *American Journal of Preventive Medicine* found that by 2030, 42% of U.S. adults could be obese, adding $550 billion to healthcare costs over that period (Finkelstein et al., 2012). State-by-state obesity data released by the CDC in August, 2013, projects obesity rates of at least 44% in every state and over 60% in 13 states. Other health risks attributed to obesity include sleep apnea, asthma and breathing problems, limited mobility, pain, and early deterioration of joints, leading to arthritis and osteoporosis.

In 2012, the Institute for Health Metrics and Evaluation, funded by The Bill and Melinda Gates Foundation, published a report on the "Global Burden of Disease 2010 Project." The results indicate that changes in cause of death in adults are related to chronic diseases and associated changes in lifestyle risk factors. Globally, this presents a new challenge to "the rising burden from mental and behavioral disorders, musculoskeletal disorders, obesity and diabetes" (Gore et al., 2011).

Obesity Defined

Obesity is defined as weighing in excess of 40 pounds above ideal body weight and a body mass index (BMI) above 30. Overweight means a BMI of 25 to 29.9. BMI is calculated by taking weight in pounds and dividing it by the square of height in inches, and multiplying the result by 703. For instance, someone who is 5 feet, 5 inches (1.6 meters) tall and weighs 185 pounds (84 kg) has a BMI of 30.8 (see Appendix C-4). One word of caution on the BMI: Some "normal weight" individuals also have metabolic syndrome and can be known as "skinny fat." Normal weight obesity carries risks similar to being overweight or obese, specifically a low muscle mass and bone density. The Mayo Clinic study revealed that people with normal weight obesity are also more likely to have metabolic syndrome (Romero-Corral, 2010). As noted, lifestyle interventions can mediate all of these health issues.

Research on the relationship between BMI and breast cancer diagnosis and prognosis has offered insight into the impact of obesity on hormones and inflammatory markers in breast cancer. Obesity has been correlated to increased risk of post-menopausal breast cancer (Khan, Shukla, Sinha, & Meeran, 2013).

Two recent studies have focused on how BMI might affect breast cancer treatment outcomes in patients receiving chemotherapy as a first treatment option before any surgery for their cancer. Another study considered how type 2 diabetes might affect outcomes for these patients. The researchers found that breast cancer patients with obesity and diabetes were more likely to be diagnosed with more advanced tumors and advanced-stage cancer (Fontanella et al., 2014). In the most recent women's health initiative study on nutrition and physical activity, cancer prevention guidelines, cancer risk, and mortality, healthy lifestyle behaviors are recommended to reduce cancer risk and overall mortality (Thomson et al., 2014).

Vignette: Maria

Maria, a 50-year-old woman, was concerned about her health and sought an integrative Nurse Coach to guide her in lifestyle changes. Maria's mother had been diagnosed with breast cancer when she was Maria's age. Maria was tested for the BRCA genes and tested negative. Although relieved by these results, she was motivated to lower her risk as she had two young daughters and hoped to live to see her grandchildren some day. She worked at a high-stress job, had difficulty sleeping, and had gradually gained weight over the past 10 years and reported having great difficulty following a "diet." After her recent checkup, she was referred to a Nurse Coach by her nurse practitioner who managed her care and suggested that she could lower her risk by losing weight, improving her food choices, and implementing some new lifestyle behaviors.

Leptin Resistance

The role of leptin in fat cells is to reduce appetite and stimulate fat burning. Leptin appears to be blocked in chronically overweight individuals, who often develop leptin resistance, and losing weight becomes increasingly difficult if not impossible. Fat also regulates the processes by which the body burns fuel for energy, especially in muscle. Adiponectin, another hormone-like chemical, also plays a central role in the biology of fat and is normally produced to curb appetite and spark the burning of fat. Unlike leptin, it remains present but stops functioning. Chronically overweight individuals have an adinopectin deficiency. Secretion of adinopectin improves following a weight loss program combined with exercise (Kelly et al., 2014).

For healthy fat metabolism, leptin, an adipocyte-derived hormone, plays an essential role in the maintenance of normal body weight and energy expenditure, as well as glucose homeostasis. Since many of these chemical processes can also act as mediators of inflammation and promote and encourage the inflammatory response, weight loss is associated with reduced inflammation systemically. Routine exposures to man-made chemicals may also be increasing an individual's risk of obesity. The "obesogen hypothesis" proposes that perturbations in metabolic signaling, resulting from exposure to environmental chemicals, may further exacerbate the effects of imbalances, resulting in an increased susceptibility to obesity and obesity-related disorders.

Metabolic Syndrome

Metabolic syndrome is described as a cluster of health issues including high blood pressure, blood sugar and triglyceride elevations, insulin resistance, and low HDL cholesterol, all precursors to diabetes and cardiovascular disease.

Metabolic syndrome is diagnosed when three of the following are present:

- abdominal obesity (fat around the waist)
- low HDL ("good") cholesterol
- high triglyceride levels
- high blood pressure
- insulin resistance

Obesity increases the risk of metabolic syndrome and cardiovascular disease. According to the American Heart Association (AHA), a healthy diet and lifestyle are your best weapons to fight cardiovascular disease. Atherosclerotic changes associated with dyslipidemia and increased cardiovascular disease risk are believed to begin in childhood. This heightened emphasis on preventing disease throughout the life cycle includes lowering sugar consumption in adolescence to prevent obesity in adulthood. Addressing healthy lifestyle behaviors and changing unhealthful behaviors appears to be essential early in life (Lee et al., 2014). According to Mark Houston, MD, cardiologist and director of research at the Hypertension Institute in Nashville, macronutrient and micronutrient deficiencies are frequently found in subjects with cardiac disease, vascular problems, hypertension, and dyslipidemia. Food patterns and behaviors that often begin in childhood, combined with genetic–environmental interactions, along with prescription and over-the-counter drug use can interfere with nutrients.

To promote healthy eating patterns, a review of the current AHA (Eckel et al., 2013) guidelines includes:

- Balance calorie intake and physical activity to achieve or maintain a healthy body weight.
- Consume a diet rich in a variety of vegetables and fruits.
- Choose whole-grain, high-fiber foods. These include fruits, vegetables, and legumes (beans). Good whole-grain choices include whole wheat, oats/oatmeal, rye, barley, brown rice, buckwheat, bulgur, millet, and quinoa.
- Consume fish, especially oily fish, at least twice a week (about 8 ounces/week). Oily fish such as salmon, mackerel, and sardines are rich in the omega-3 fatty acids eicosapentaenoic acid (EPA) and docosahexaenoic acid (DHA). Consumption of these fatty acids is linked to reduced risk of sudden death and death from coronary artery disease. People with existing heart disease should consider taking fish oil supplements of 850–1,000 mg EPA and DPA.
- Limit daily intake of saturated fat (found mostly in animal products) to less than 7% of total calories, trans fat (found in hydrogenated fats, commercially baked products, and many fast foods) to less than 1% of total calories, and cholesterol (found in eggs, dairy

products, meat, poultry, fish, and shellfish) to less than 300 mg per day. Choose lean meats and vegetable alternatives (such as soy). Select fat-free and low-fat dairy products. Grill, bake, or broil fish, meat, and skinless poultry.

- Use little or no salt in your foods. Reducing salt can lower blood pressure and decrease the risk of heart disease and heart failure.
- Cut down on beverages and foods that contain added sugars (corn syrups, sucrose, glucose, fructose, maltrose, dextrose, concentrated fruit juice, and honey).
- If you drink alcohol, do so in moderation. The AHA recommends limiting alcohol to no more than two drinks per day for men and one drink per day for women.

Prediabetes

Worldwide, the number of adults with diabetes will rise from 285 million in 2010 to 439 million in the year 2030 (Shaw, Sicree, & Zimmet, 2010). Nurse Coaches have the ability to directly impact the prevention of diabetes. It is estimated that 57 million adults have "prediabetes." Research repeatedly shows that changes in weight, exercise, and diet can not only prevent prediabetes from becoming diabetes, but can also return blood glucose levels to the normal range. Whether prediabetes progresses to full-blown type 2 diabetes is largely up to the individual's lifestyle choices. Although the genes one inherits may influence the development of type 2 diabetes, they take a back seat to behavioral and lifestyle factors. Type 2 diabetes can be prevented. A recent study in mid-age women demonstrated that lifestyle Interventions integrated into care can prevent weight gain and lower blood pressure and the risk of metabolic syndrome (Williams et al., 2014).

In a recent study to assess the long-term effects of a Mediterranean food plan for glycemic control, the need for diabetes medications, and remission of type 2 diabetes for people recently diagnosed with type 2 diabetes, eating lots of olive oil, fish, and whole grains was shown to slow progression of the disease more than restricting fat, according to a new analysis published in the journal *Diabetes Care* (Esposito, Maiorino, Petrizzo, Bellastella, & Giugliano, 2014). Participants were followed for more than eight years. Those following a Mediterranean type diet went significantly longer before needing diabetes medication and more of them had their diabetes go into remission, compared to those on a low-fat diet. "There's been lots of epidemiology suggesting that a Mediterranean diet was beneficial with metabolic syndrome and diabetes," according to lead researcher Esposito. This approach has important implications for Nurse Coaches when guiding clients and patients with metabolic syndrome and prediabetes to healthier food choices. With a variety of foods available, individuals can create an individualized meal plan that can offer multiple health-promoting benefits.

Vignette: John

John, a 40-year-old male, was diagnosed as "prediabetic" by his physician. He had occasional spikes in blood sugar and an elevated hemoglobin A1C. The doctor assumed that John had "cheated" on the hypoglycemic food guidelines he was given. John said he was following the "plan" as given. He was prescribed more oral medication. John wondered what other contributing factors may have triggered his spike in blood sugar. When he went to see a Nurse Coach at a friend's recommendation, he appeared frustrated. He said that he was following the nutritionist's guidelines. He also felt that just prescribing more medicine was not addressing what might be triggering the spikes, and he wanted to understand as he was motivated to eat well and get healthy for his retirement as he hoped to travel the world.

As a Nurse Coach, we listen to our client/patient's story or explanatory model. The first question a Nurse Coach would ask is "What did John believe might be triggering the fluctuations in his blood sugar?" As part of the Nurse Coach process, we assess other contributing factors, including stress, exercise, sleeping patterns, or environmental exposures that may be influencing symptoms, and, in John's situation, his blood sugar levels. According to current research, psychological stress is linked with impaired glycemic control in prediabetics and increased risk of diabetes mellitus. Physiological responses to stress, including increased glucose production, glucose mobilization, and insulin resistance, can all potentially influence outcomes. Could lowering John's stress response through learned practices mediate the spikes in blood sugar while John continued to focus on a hypoglycemic whole food plan? (See Appendix E-10.)

Exercise

Exercise has a number of effects that benefit the heart and circulation, including improving cholesterol and lipid levels and maintaining weight control. People who are sedentary are almost twice as likely to suffer heart attacks as are people who exercise regularly. A recent study published in the *Journal of the American Heart Association* demonstrated that interventions by healthcare providers supporting changes in diet and/or diet plus physical activity, given soon after diagnosis of diabetes and risk of cardiovascular disease in real-world healthcare settings, improved markers of inflammation and cardiovascular risk in patients with type 2 diabetes (Thompson et al., 2014). This is another model for Nurse Coach interventions in healthcare settings where coaching skills can be integrated into care.

Regular exercise improves glucose control in diabetes. Physical activity has been shown to bring down HBA1c levels; structured exercise training that consists of aerobic exercise, resistance training, or both combined is associated with HBA1c reduction in patients with type 2 diabetes. The HBA1C test result reflects the average blood sugar level for the past two to three months. Specifically, the A1C test measures what percentage of hemoglobin—a protein in red blood cells that carries oxygen—is coated with sugar (glycated). The higher the A1C level, the poorer the blood sugar control and the higher one's risk of diabetes.

Physical activity is associated with lower HBA1c, when combined with nutritional changes. By implementing lifestyle changes, one can lower A1C, and this improvement can act as biofeedback to motivate clients that their hard work has been rewarded (Umpierre et al., 2011). A Nurse Coach explores movement, physical activities, and exercise for the client to come up with a realistic plan that she or he will follow (see Appendices E-11 to E-13).

The overall pattern of behaviors and choices around food bring nurse coaching to the forefront in a new direction for health promotion and disease management. Key to changing behaviors and improving one's health is self-assessment and increasing self-awareness to deepen the connections between food triggers and choices that can impact one's energy, cognitive function, pain, digestion, moods, and other symptoms. Coaching provides an added dimension to the role of the nurse in providing guidance and support for behavioral change, weaving our role as nurse as advocate and educator for promoting health through lifestyle change.

SUMMARY

- Nurse Coaches are uniquely positioned to coach and engage individuals, families, and communities in the process of meaningful and health-promoting nutritional strategies.
- Increasing awareness of how foods affect health and wellbeing is the key to healthy behavioral change.
- As Nurse Coaches expand their skills and competencies for wellness promotion, nutrition is an essential component in the Nurse Coach process.

NURSE COACH REFLECTIONS

After reading this chapter, the Nurse Coach will be able to bring awareness and personal insight to the following questions:

- What changes can I make to enhance my nutrition?
- What nutrition patterns and behaviors do I recognize that might interfere with my wellbeing?
- What new awareness practice can support healthier eating choices and behaviors?
- How can I integrate new nutritional practices at home?
- Who are the people in my life who support me in making healthy nutrition changes?

REFERENCES

Centers for Disease Control (CDC) (2010). Vital signs: State-specific obesity prevalence among adults—United States, 2009. *Morbidity and Mortality Weekly Report*, 59, 1.

Das, U. N. (2008). Can essential fatty acids reduce the burden of disease(s)? *Lipids in Health and Disease*, 7, 9. doi:10.1186/1476-511X-7-9

De Vogli, R., Kouvonen, A., & Gimeno, D. (2014). The influence of market deregulation on fast food consumption and body mass index: A cross-national time series analysis. *Bulletin of the World Health Organization*, *92*(2), 99–107A. doi:10.2471/BLT.13.120287

Eckel, R., Jakicic, J. M., Ard, J. D., Miller, N. H., Hubbard, V. S., Nonas, C. A., de Jesus, J. M., … Yanovski, S. (2013). 2013 AHA/ACC guideline on lifestyle management to reduce cardiovascular risk: A report of the American College of Cardiology/American Heart Association Task Force on Practice Guidelines. *Journal of the American College of Cardiology*, Advance online publication. doi:10.1016/j.jacc.2013.11.003

Esposito, K., Maiorino, M., Petrizzo, M., Bellastella, G., & Giugliano, D. (2014). The effects of a Mediterranean diet on need for diabetes drugs and remission of newly diagnosed type 2 diabetes: Follow-up of a randomized trial. *Diabetes Care*, Advance online publication, April 10, 2014, 1935–5548. doi:10.2337/dc13-2899

Finkelstein, E., Khavjou, O., Thompson, A., Trogdon, J. G., Pan, L., Sherry, B., & Dietz, W. (2012) Obesity and severe obesity forecasts through 2030. *American Journal of Preventive Medicine*, *42*, 563–570. http://dx.doi.org/10.1016/j.amepre.2011.10.026

Fontanella, C. L., Slaets, P., Neven, S., Loibl, M., Vanoppen, J., Bogaerts, G., von Minckwitz, D., & Cameron, M. (2014). Influence of body mass index on long-term outcome of breast cancer patients receiving neoadjuvant therapy - Combined results from the GBG (German Breast Group) and the EORTC cohorts. Poster presented at the European Breast Cancer Conference, Glasgow, Scotland.

Goldsmith, J. R., & Sartor, R. B. (2014, March 21). The role of diet on intestinal microbiota metabolism: Downstream impacts on host immune function and health, and therapeutic implications. *Journal of Gastroenterology.* doi:10.1007/s00535-014-0953-z

Gore, F., Bloem, P., Patton, G., Ferguson, J., Joseph, V., Coffey, C., Sawyer, S., & Mathers, C. (2011). Global burden of disease in young people aged 10–24 years: A systematic analysis. *The Lancet, 377*, 2093–2102.

Kabbani, T. A., Vanga, R. R., Leffler, D. A., Villafuerte-Galvez, J., Pallav, K., Hansen, J., ... Kelly, C. P. (2014). Celiac disease or non-celiac gluten sensitivity? An approach to clinical differential diagnosis. *The American Journal of Gastroenterology*, Advance online publication. doi:10.1038/ajg.2014.41

Kelly, K. R., Navaneethan, S. D., Solomon, T. P., Haus, J. M., Cook, M., Barkoukis, H., & Kirwan, J. P. (2014). Lifestyle-induced decrease in fat mass improves adiponectin secretion in obese adults. *Medical Science Sports Exercise, 46*(5), 920–926.

Khan, S., Shukla, S., Sinha, S., & Meeran, S. M. (2013). Role of adipokines and cytokines in obesity-associated breast cancer: Therapeutic targets. *Cytokine & Growth Factor Reviews, 24*(6), 503–513. doi:10.1016/j.cytogfr.2013.10.001

Khoury, C. K., Bjorkman, A. D., Dempewolf, H., Ramirez-Villegas, J., Guarino, L., Jarvis, A., & Struik, P. C. (2014). Increasing homogeneity in global food supplies and the implications for food security. *Proceedings of the National Academy of Sciences of the United States of America, 111*(11), 4001–4006. doi:10.1073/pnas.1313490111

Lee, A. K., Binongo, J. N., Chowdhury, R., Stein, A. D., Gazmararian, J. A., Vos, M. B., & Welsh, J. A. (2014). Consumption of less than 10% of total energy from added sugars is associated with increasing HDL in females during adolescence: A longitudinal analysis. *Journal of the American Heart Association, 3*(1), e000615. doi:10.1161/JAHA.113.000615

Luck, S. (2013). Nutrition. In B. M. Dossey & L. Keegan (Eds.), *Holistic nursing: A handbook for practice* (6th ed., pp. 261–293). Burlington, MA: Jones & Bartlett Learning

Michas, G., Micha, R., & Zampelas, A. (2014). Dietary fats and cardiovascular disease: Putting together the pieces of a complicated puzzle. *Atherosclerosis, 234*(2), 320–328. doi: 10.1016/j.atherosclerosis.2014.03.013

Nightingale, F. (1860). *Notes on nursing: What it is and what it is not.* London, UK: Harrison.

Ogden, C. L., Carroll, M. D., Kit, B. K., & Flegal, K. M. (2014). Prevalence of childhood and adult obesity in the United States, 2011–2012. *JAMA: The Journal of the American Medical Association, 311*(8), 806–814. doi:10.1001/jama.2014.732

Romero-Corral, A. (2010). Normal weight obesity: A risk factor for cardiometabolic dysregulation and cardiovascular mortality. *European Heart Journal, 31*, 737–746.

Shaw, J. E., Sicree, R. A., & Zimmet, P. Z. (2010). Global estimates of the prevalence of diabetes for 2010 and 2030. *Diabetes Research and Clinical Practice, 87*(1), 4–14. doi:10.1016/j.diabres.2009.10.007

Thompson, D., Walhin, J. P., Batterham, A. M., Stokes, K. A., Cooper, A. R., & Andrews, R. C. (2014). Effect of diet or diet plus physical activity versus usual care on inflammatory markers in patients with newly diagnosed type 2 Diabetes: The Early ACTivity in Diabetes (ACTID) Randomized, Controlled Trial. *Journal of the American Heart Association, 3*(3), e000828. doi:10.1161/JAHA.114.000828

Thomson, C., McCullough, M., Wertheim, B., Chlebowski, R. T., Martinez, M. E., Stefanick, M. L., Rohan, T. E., ... Neuhouser, M. L. (2014). Nutrition and physical activity cancer prevention guidelines, cancer risk, and mortality in the women's health initiative. *Cancer Prevention Research (Philadelphia)*, *7*(1), 42–53. doi:10.1158/1940-6207.CAPR-13-0258

Umpierre, D., Ribeiro, P. A., Kramer, C. K., Leitao, C. B., Zucatti, A. T., Azevedo, M. J., ... Schaan, B. D. (2011). Physical activity advice only or structured exercise training and association with HbA1c levels in type 2 diabetes: A systematic review and meta-analysis. *JAMA: The Journal of the American Medical Association*, *305*(17), 1790–1799. doi:10.1001/jama.2011.576

Williams L. T., Hollis, J. L., Collins, C. E., & Morgan, P. (2014). Can a relatively low-intensity intervention by health professionals prevent weight gain in mid-age women? 12-Month outcomes of the 40-Something randomised controlled trial. *Nutrition & Diabetes*, *4*, e116. doi:10.1038/nutd.2014.12

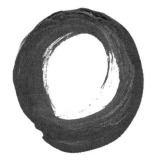

CHAPTER 9

Environmental Health

Susan Luck

The incidence of disease is related to...the want of fresh air, or of light, or of warmth, or of quiet or of cleanliness...

Florence Nightingale, 1860

LOOKING AHEAD...

After reading this chapter, you will be able to:

- Explore our inner environment as a microcosm of our outer world.
- Increase knowledge of the relationship between health and the environment.
- Analyze how the environment plays a critical role in the health of present and future generations.
- Examine the role of a Nurse Coach in assessing the client/patient environment as part of exploring lifestyle health and wellbeing.
- Expand the role of a Nurse Coach as environmental educator and environmental health advocate.
- Explore possibilities for creating healthier home and workplace environments.

DEFINITIONS

Endocrine disruptors (xenoestrogens): Synthetic hormone-mimicking compounds that interfere with the synthesis, secretion, transport, binding action, or elimination of natural hormones in the body.

Environment: Everything that surrounds an individual or group of people: physical, social, psychological, cultural, or spiritual characteristics; external and internal features; animate and inanimate objects; climate; seen and unseen vibrations, frequencies, and energy patterns.

Environmental ethics: A division of philosophy concerned with valuing the environment, primarily as it relates to humankind, secondarily as it relates to other creatures and to the land.

Epigenetics: The study of heritable changes in gene activity and gene expression caused by mechanisms other than changes in the underlying DNA sequence.

Exposome: A measure of the effects of life-long environmental exposures on health.

Obesogens: Foreign chemical compounds that disrupt normal development and balance of lipid metabolism, which in some cases can lead to obesity.

ENVIRONMENTAL HEALTH IN TODAY'S WORLD

At the heart of Florence Nightingale's (1820–1910) legacy is a knowing that our external environment is inextricably interconnected to the health and wellbeing of all species and ecosystems. Nurse coaching follows in Nightingale's footsteps and expands both the urgency and opportunity to address environmental factors that affect the lives of our clients/patients, families, and communities. In its broadest sense, the term "environment" can mean everything, both within and external to each person. When considering the environment, it is imperative to listen and respond to a larger story, not only as practitioners, but also as members of communities, cultures, and humankind.

As Nurse Coaches we hold a worldview and awareness of our place in nature. Our holistic philosophy embraces that we are the microcosm of the macrocosm within in the vast complexity and unpredictability of life and that our health is also determined by the health of our external world. Part of our role as a Nurse Coach is to empower individuals and families in creating healthier communities through personal and community advocacy and change. Nurse Coaches promote practices that create healing environments in our home, workplace, and community. As Nurse Coaches, we recognize that environmental health supports wellbeing and freedom from illness or injury related to exposure to toxic agents and other environmental conditions that are potentially detrimental to all.

In today's world, we all face many new challenges for maintaining health and preventing disease. Globally, exposure to environmental toxins and pollution is contributing to many of the growing health challenges throughout the life cycle, including immune dysfunction, hormonal imbalances, inflammatory conditions, and neurological problems. The World Health Organization (WHO) declared that "environmental health comprises those aspects of human health, including quality of life, that are determined by interactions with physical, chemical, biological and social factors in the environment." It also refers to the theory and practice of assessing, correcting, controlling, and preventing those factors in the environment that may adversely affect the health of present and future generations. The evidence shows that environmental risk factors play a role in more than 80% of the diseases regularly reported by WHO (Prüss-Üstün & Corvalán, 2006).

In 2012, WHO warned that chronic, noncommunicable diseases are rapidly becoming epidemic worldwide. Escalating rates of neurocognitive, metabolic, autoimmune, and cardiovascular diseases are no longer ascribed only to genetics, lifestyle, and nutrition; environmental exposures can be passed down through generations and often begin in utero during this critical window of development. Ongoing exposures are bioaccumulated, increasing toxic body burden and implicated as potential contributors to chronic disease later in life (WHO, 2013). Environmental contributors to ill health are summarized from multiple perspectives—biological effects of classes of toxicants, mechanisms of toxicity, and a synthesis of toxic substances as cofactors in most major diseases.

Healthcare practitioners have wide-ranging roles in addressing environmental factors in policy and public health as well as in clinical practice. Public health initiatives include risk recognition and chemical assessment, exposure reduction, remediation, monitoring, and avoidance. The complex web of disease and environmental contributors is amenable to some straightforward clinical approaches addressing multiple toxicants. How much disease could be prevented through increasing awareness and through better management of our environment? More than 100 experts were consulted for their estimates of how much environmental risk factors contribute to the disease burden of 85 diseases globally. The evidence concluded that environmental risk factors play a role in more than 80% of the diseases regularly reported by WHO. Globally, nearly one-quarter of all deaths and of the total disease burden can be attributed to the environment. These findings have important policy implications because the environmental risk factors that were studied largely can be modified by established, cost-effective interventions. The interventions promote equity by benefiting everyone in the society, while addressing the needs of those most at risk (WHO, 2012).

Environmental Health: A Nurse Coach Model

Nightingale knew that putting the patient in the healthiest environment was essential for healing to occur. Nurse leadership in environmental coaching, education, and advocacy in healthcare is rooted in our history. An expanded role within nurse coaching is to assist clients and patients to discover and uncover the environmental cofactors contributing to symptoms, conditions, disease patterns, and daily quality of life. Environmental exposures can contribute to one's health challenges including cognitive impairment, immune dysfunction, hormonal imbalances, impaired digestive processes, weight management, and a host of often unexplained symptoms (Luck & Keegan, 2013).

Nurse Coaches integrate environmental assessment tools (see Integrative Health and Wellness Assessment (IHWA), Appendix C-1 (long form), Appendix C-2 (short form), and Appendix E-14) in their inquiry to increase awareness of potential environmental influences impacting one's health. Nurse Coaches provide opportunities for clients/patients to consider how their environment affects their wellbeing, identify exposures, and develop new strategies and choices leading to improving health outcomes. For example, Nurse Coaches working with young women can explore the environmental lifestyle factors that are potential future determinants of a healthy pregnancy outcome. Nurse Coaches working with breast cancer survivors can explore the relationship between their client/patient's environment and potential carcinogens and estrogen-disrupting chemicals in their home and workplace, including pesticides, food additives, plastics, and personal care products.

Precautionary Principle

The essence of the precautionary principle states that "when an activity raises threats of harm to human health or the environment, precautionary measures should be taken even if some cause and effect relationships are not fully established scientifically" (Raffensperger, 1998). Dossey (2005) describes Nightingale as an environmentalist and one of the early proponents of the precautionary principle. She understood that nurses have an ethical and moral responsibility to take anticipatory actions to prevent harm.

The International Council of Nurses (ICN), in a Position Statement on *Reducing Environmental and Lifestyle Related Health Risks* (2011), states that it is concerned about the enormous human suffering caused by the growing burden of environmental and lifestyle-related noncommunicable diseases, which are largely preventable. The Council asks that nurses and national nurses associations play a strategic role in helping reduce environmental and lifestyle health risks related to non-communicable diseases. According to the ICN, "The concern of nurses is for people's health—its promotion, its maintenance, its restoration. The healthy lives of people depend ultimately on the health of Planet Earth—its soil, its water, its oceans, its atmosphere, its biological diversity—all of the elements which constitute people's natural environment."

The American Nurses Association (ANA), in their landmark document *Principles of Environmental Health for Nursing Practice with Implementation Strategies* (2007), put forth a call to action, encouraging nurses to gain a working understanding of the relationships between human health and environmental exposures and to integrate this knowledge into all nursing practice. It is foundational that human health is linked to the quality of the environment and that air, water, soil, food, and products should be free of potentially harmful chemicals. The following principles of environmental health in nursing practice are listed in **Table 9-1**. These principles are applicable in all settings where registered nurses practice and are intended to protect nurses themselves, patients and their families, other healthcare workers, and the community and to recognize our role as environmental health leaders.

TABLE 9-1 American Nurses Association (ANA) Principles of Environmental Health in Nursing Practice.

- Knowledge of environmental health concepts is essential to nursing practice.
- The precautionary principle guides nurses to use products and practices that do not harm human health or the environment and to take preventive action in the face of uncertainty.
- Nurses have a right to work in an environment that is safe and healthy.
- Healthy environments are sustained through multidisciplinary collaboration.
- Choices of materials, products, technology, and practices in the environment that impact nursing practice are based on the best evidence available.
- Approaches to promoting a healthy environment respect the diverse values, beliefs, cultures, and circumstances of patients and their families.
- Nurses participate in assessing the quality of the environment in which they practice and live.
- Nurses, other healthcare workers, patients, and communities have the right to know relevant and timely information about the potentially harmful products, chemicals, pollutants, and hazards to which they are exposed.
- Nurses participate in research of best practices that promote a safe and healthy environment.
- Nurses must be supported in advocating and implementing environmental health principles in nursing practice.

Source: Copyright © 2014 by Susan Luck. Adapted from the American Nurses Association (2007). *Principles of environmental health for nursing practice with implementation strategies.* Silver Spring, MD: Author.

CREATING HEALTHY ENVIRONMENTS

Workplace Environment

In Nightingale's *Notes on Hospitals* the preface begins as follows: "It may be a strange principle to enunciate as the very first requirement in a Hospital that it should do the sick no harm. It is quite necessary nevertheless to lay down such a principle, because the actual mortality in hospitals, especially in those of large crowded cities, is very much higher than any calculations founded on the mortality of the same class of patient treated out of hospitals would lead us to expect" (Nightingale, 1863, Preface, p. 1).

As an environmental advocate and educator, Nightingale observed and used the precautionary principle as previously discussed, and wrote in *Notes on Nursing* "If you think a patient is being poisoned by a copper kettle, cut off all possible connection to avoid further injury; it has actually been made a question of medical ethics, what should a medical man do who suspects poison?" (Nightingale, 1860, p. 70). In today's hospital environment, healthcare workers face new environmental challenges as seen in the following vignette. As Nurse Coaches, how do we increase awareness, create opportunities, and advocate for a healthier workplace to transform hospitals into sustainable environments for patients and for all who work there? Begin to notice your workplace environment. Are there chemicals you are exposed to daily that might be affecting your health? Are your co-workers affected by cleaning products used? What are other choices or options? How can nurses create a healthier workplace environment?

Vignette: Jenny

Jenny, a young nurse working on a medical surgical unit, recently experienced headaches and weight gain and became concerned. She hoped to begin a family but had not been able to get pregnant. She was curious about what might be the triggers and began to explore if her symptoms might be related to her work environment. She found research on triclosan, an antibacterial and antifungal agent, that peeked her interest. At work, Jenny compulsively washed her hands approximately 50 times daily with the dry powder in the containers on the wall found in-between patient rooms. She began to wonder if this could be contributing to her recent health-related issues and her infertility. Jenny worked the evening shift and was also aware of the strong odor of the chemical disinfectants used to clean the unit as she began experiencing a burning sensation in her throat and eyes.

As Jenny increased her awareness, she began to speak with other nurses on her team. Together, they decided to write a letter to their hospital administration and advocated for the creation of an environmental health committee, as they took a leadership role for developing innovative strategies that included safer products on the units, waste management, energy reduction, recycling, and environmental health education. Jenny, along with other representatives on the committee, attended a local Greener Hospitals meeting (part of the national Healthier Hospitals Initiative) and brought back information to hospital administration. Changes in the workplace environment were implemented over time, including nonfragrant disinfectants on the unit, safe disposal of pharmaceuticals, and healthier food choices in the hospital cafeteria. To stay informed of the latest research, they stayed abreast of specific research by Health Care without Harm (http://www.noharm.org), Healthier Hospitals Initiatives (http://healthierhospitals.org), and Clean Med (http://www.cleanmed.org).

Creating Healthier Communities

In the spirit of Nightingale, nurses continue to take a leadership role in public awareness campaigns, carrying our legacy forward in today's world—in communities and in the greening of healthcare within hospitals. Nurses are uniquely positioned to identify and reduce health risks associated with exposures and potential hazards in the workplace, community, and home environment. Today, nurses are engaged in efforts to raise awareness and to educate and advocate on environmental issues at local, state, national, and global levels.

What are the "greening" behaviors or activities that Nurse Coaches can engage their communities in to improve their environment and health outcomes? How can Nurse Coaches educate their colleagues and initiate greening programs in their communities and healthcare organizations? **Table 9-2** provides guidelines for environmental lifestyle change.

Table 9-2 Guidelines for Environmental Lifestyle Change.

- Explore client's list of concerns and benefits to each aspect of her/his lifestyle behaviors.
- Explore what the client sees as her/his options for changing behaviors.
- Explore core values, strengths, motivators, reasons for change.
- Identify throughout process, where client is in stages of change.
- Explore challenges, obstacles, and beliefs that may interfere with behavioral change.
- Co-create strategies for possible solutions for behavioral change.
- Co-identify appropriate environmental behavioral lifestyle goals.
- Elicit client to commit willingness to environmental change and set one reachable goal.

Source: Copyright © 2014 by the International Nurse Coach Association. www.inursecoach.com

The emerging Nurse Coach role is perfectly positioned to increase awareness that supports clients, patients, and communities in exploring healthier environmental choices to protect the health of present and future generations. Nurse Coaches advocate for and inspire communities to create new possibilities and solutions while continuing our nursing legacy of caring for all of life and for creating healing environments. Informing and empowering individuals and families and creating healthier communities can lead to personal and community advocacy and change.

Nurse Coaching Process

Integral to the nurse coaching process is viewing the environment within which all living systems participate and interact, including the physical body and its habitat along with cultural, psychological, social, and historical influences. The environment includes both the external physical space and the person's internal physical, mental, emotional, social, and spiritual experience. Wellbeing is possible for all. Illness and imbalance provides opportunities and possibilities for movement towards change to enhance wellbeing (Hess et al., 2013).

Nurse Coaches engage the client/patient in identifying potential environmental exposures that can impact health and wellbeing. Listening to the story includes inquiry into family history, including a timeline that spans parent occupation; family migration patterns; hobbies, both past and present; work history; and current daily routines and personal habits. Discovering the antecedents, mediators, and triggers of symptoms is essential to recognize that each person's story spans generations, begins before conception, and is mediated by one's lifestyle choices and consequent epigenetic expression. Along one's health continuum throughout the life cycle, there are critical windows of development when environmental exposures may have greater impact. Critical Windows of Development is a timeline of how the human body develops in the womb, with animal and human research showing when low-dose exposure, for example, to endocrine-disrupting chemicals during development results in altered health outcomes (Goncalves, Cunha, Barros, & Martinez, 2010). The interplay and influence of multiple environmental factors contributing to health and disease patterns is essential for all clinicians to recognize and meaningful in a Nurse Coach model.

Integrative Nurse Coaches introduce environmental health assessment tools (see Appendices C-1, C-2, and E-14) with a client/patient to increase awareness of potential environmental cofactors and begin to connect the dots about exposures, risks, consequences, and choices that are critical to deepening the connection between one's symptoms or pathology and for restoration of health and wellbeing. Assessing risks and offering strategies expands our role as educators and advocates. How do Nurses Coaches ask questions that might offer insight and information about a client/patient's exposome?

Environmental nurse coaching expands the Nurse Coach role as nurse educator and nurse advocate for impacting the external environment for lasting change. How do Nurse Coaches partner with the client/patient to identify, address, and change common exposures in the home or workplace environment? As Nurse Coaches, we listen to all possible influences in the client/patient's life story that might be contributing to her/his current challenges, asking coaching questions to increase awareness of the connection of how the environment affects the client/patient's health and quality of life. It is this opportunity for Nurse Coaches in a comprehensive assessment to begin to increase client awareness in the coaching process towards change. Expanding our nursing knowledge of the potential links to many of the issues seen in healthcare is essential as Nurse Coaches also connect the dots when listening to the story.

Vignette: Marge

Marge, a 26-year-old woman, recently began experiencing respiratory problems and was diagnosed with adult onset of asthma. She was referred to a Nurse Coach by a friend who was concerned that her symptoms could be "psychological" and related to her new high-stress, demanding job in a busy advertising agency. Marge came to her first coaching session hoping to learn new tools to help her to relax and better cope with her new fast-paced work environment. After listening to her story, Marge was introduced to an awareness practice that she could integrate into her daily routine. Although her Nurse Coach was aware that Marge came to learn new stress-coping skills, she knew that the environment can in turn trigger symptoms.

As the Nurse Coach explored Marge's beliefs about her symptoms, she looked for opportunities to address the added environmental component when Marge mentioned her "newly renovated office." At the end of the session, her Nurse Coach asked her if she would be willing to fill out an environmental assessment form and bring it to the next session. Marge responded positively and shared that she had not considered the role of the environment in explaining her symptoms as she convinced herself that it was "all in her mind."

LIVING IN THE MODERN WORLD

Children's Health and the Environment

The prevalence of autism, asthma, attention-deficit hyperactivity disorder (ADHD), obesity, diabetes, and birth defects has grown substantially among children around the world. Not coincidentally, more than 80,000 new chemicals have been developed and released into the global environment during the past 40 years.

Children are exquisitely sensitive to their environment. Exposure during their developmental "windows of susceptibility" can trigger cellular changes that lead to obesity, disease, and disability across the life span.

Environment chemical exposures interacting with our human genome can trigger health responses based on each individual's unique predisposition, vulnerability, and susceptibility. It was recently estimated that costs in the United States of environmental disease in children alone amounted to $76.6 billion just from "lead poisoning, prenatal methylmercury exposure, childhood cancer, asthma, intellectual disability, autism, and attention deficit hyperactivity disorder" (Winneke, 2011). The widespread implications are vividly illustrated by considering neurocognitive disorders across society and cultures. According to a recently published *Lancet Neurology* study (Grandjean & Landrigan, 2014), neurodevelopmental disabilities, including autism, ADHD, dyslexia, and other cognitive impairments affect millions of children worldwide, and some diagnoses seem to be increasing in frequency. Industrial chemicals that injure the developing brain are among the known causes for this rise in prevalence. The analysis in *Lancet Neurology* concludes that current chemical regulations worldwide are woefully inadequate to safeguard children whose developing brains are uniquely vulnerable to toxic chemicals in the environment. To control the pandemic of developmental neurotoxicity, the authors propose a global prevention strategy. While global efforts on new environmental health policies for untested chemicals are being discussed by scientists and health policy experts, the role of a Nurse Coach working in diverse communities can have a long-lasting impact on the health of present and future generations.

There is strong evidence that the role of early life influences, including environmental exposures, can have an effect on the occurrence of different cancers and communicable diseases, according to the recent *World Cancer Report* (Stewart & Wild, 2014).

The National Institute of Environmental Health Sciences (NIEHS), part of the National Institutes of Health, supports expanding scientific understanding to include endocrine effects not only on traditional endocrine glands, their hormones, and receptors (such as estrogens, anti-androgens, and thyroid hormones), but also all other hormones and signaling cascades that affect the body's systems and processes, including reproductive function, fetal development, the nervous system and behavior, the immune and metabolic systems, and gene expression. Prenatal exposures to hundreds of toxic compounds via cord blood include numerous toxic compounds present during the critical stages of hormonal, immunological, and neurological development. Outcome studies have shown that animal and human offspring who are so exposed can not only be born with birth defects, but suffer from life-long health problems, including obesity and behavioral challenges. According to the TEDX Endocrine Disruptor Exchange database (2012), there are nearly 1,000 endocrine disruptors in our daily lives.

The National Cancer Institute (NCI) recently reported that the link between exposure to everyday chemicals and cancer risk has been "grossly underestimated" (NCI, 2010). NCI urges the U.S. Administration to identify and eliminate environmental carcinogens from workplaces, schools, and homes. It estimates there are nearly 80,000 "largely unregulated" chemicals on the market. The knowledge that environmental factors play a role in carcinogenesis dates back centuries. According to a report by the Harvard School of Public Health, Dr. Percival Pott described scrotal tumors in young chimney sweeps of 18th-century London, demonstrating that cancer could be caused by environmental factors. "We need a new national cancer-prevention strategy emphasizing primary prevention that redirects both research and policy agendas and sets tangible goals for reducing or eliminating environmental exposures implicated in cancer causation" (Christiani, 2011).

Endocrine-Disrupting Chemicals (EDCs)

The endocrine system is the exquisitely balanced system of glands and hormones that regulates such vital functions as body growth, response to stress, sexual development and behavior, production and utilization of insulin, rate of metabolism, intelligence and behavior, and the ability to reproduce. Categories of EDCs listed in **Table 9-3** are substances that interfere with the release, transport, metabolism, binding, action, or elimination of the body's natural hormones. EDCs appear to interfere with the body's endocrine system and produce adverse developmental, reproductive, neurological, and immune effects in both humans and wildlife. Endocrine disruptor compounds are ubiquitous in our environment, according to the WHO's *State of the Science of Endocrine Disrupting Chemicals* (2013).

Research on the hormone-like effects of environmental chemical exposures such as industrial chemicals and pesticides found in wildlife and humans warrants strong scientific inquiry into the multitude of exposures leading to a new wave of health issues from autism and neurological problems to infertility in both men and women, thyroid dysfunction, and an increase in breast, thyroid, and prostate cancer globally. The endocrine effects of these chemicals are believed to be a result of their ability to:

- mimic the effect of endogenous hormones,
- antagonize the effect of endogenous hormones,
- disrupt the synthesis and metabolism of endogenous hormones, and
- disrupt the synthesis and metabolism of hormone receptors.

A comprehensive literature search found 91 studies linking bisphenol (BPA) to human health; 53 studies were published within the last year (Rochester, 2013). EDCs can cause harmful health effects in both adults and children. Pregnant women can transfer chemicals to the developing child in the womb. Even very low doses can have life-long, irreversible effects, limiting a child's full potential development. Nurse Coaches assess environmental exposures when working with clients/patients to identify EDCs. The precautionary principle as previously discussed is woven into our role as Nurse Coaches to explore the following questions with our clients/patients:

- What are the implications of constant everyday low-dose exposures that increase our "toxic body burden" for one's health and for public health and safety?
- How do prenatal exposures affect future generations and the health of our communities?

The following discussion reviews the common EDC categories that we encounter in our daily lives. See Appendix E-15 for a list of common EDCs, health risks, and prevention tips.

Table 9-3 Categories of Endocrine Disruptor Chemicals (EDCs).

Household product ingredients	**Industrial additives**
Chemicals found in items such as appliances, vehicles, building materials, electronics, crafts, textiles, furniture, and household cleaning products.	Chemicals such as preservatives, antioxidants, and surfactants used in such things as glue, plastic, rubber, paint, and wood products.
	Solvents
	Chemicals used to dissolve other chemicals. Common in cleaning products in the home.
Personal care products/cosmetic ingredients	**Food additives**
Chemicals found in products such as cosmetics, shampoos, lotions, soaps, deodorants, fragrances, and shaving products.	Dyes, preservatives, and many compounds used in food processing and as components in food packaging.
Pesticide ingredients	**Metal/metallurgy**
Insecticides/acaricides (miticides), herbicides, fungicides, rodenticides, and other biocides, including chemicals described as "inert".	Elements or chemicals used in the extraction, processing, or manufacturing of a metal or metal-containing product, including welding.
Flame retardants	**Medical/veterinary/research**
Chemicals used to prevent fires. Applied to clothing, mattresses, and furniture.	Chemicals used in hospitals, medical supplies, and equipment, in laboratories or as reagents, and pharmaceuticals.
Plastics/rubber	**Antimicrobials**
Components, reactants, or additives used in the manufacturing of rubbers or plastics.	Chemicals that prevent the growth of and/or destroy microorganisms including hand washing products.

Source: Copyright © 2014 by the International Nurse Coach Association. www.inursecoach.com

Bisphenol A (BPA)

One of the most studied and ubiquitous EDCs, BPA, is used in the manufacturing of various plastics and resins for food packaging and consumer products and mainly enters the human body as a result of leaching from the packaging into food and drink. In 2013, nearly 100 researchers studying the health effects of BPA gathered at NIEHS to provide an update on their findings. They presented research that BPA exposure during fetal mammary gland development, even at low doses, has resulted in significant alterations in the gland's morphology that varied from subtle ones observed during the exposure period to precancerous and cancerous lesions manifesting in adulthood. "Exposure in utero is extremely important because that's the time organs are being formed," observed Dr. Ana Soto, a professor at Tufts University School of Medicine and one of a team of scientists who worked on the new research. "The risk of breast cancer starts in the womb" and thus could be a critical factor in understanding why so many women without known risks are developing breast cancer (Soto et al., 2013).

A growing number of synthetic chemicals, including BPA and phthalates, have been used in the production of almost everything we purchase. Recent extensive literature has raised concerns about its possible implication in the etiology of some human chronic diseases such as diabetes, obesity, reproductive disorders, cardiovascular diseases, birth defects, chronic respiratory and kidney diseases, and breast cancer (Rezg, El-Fazaa, Gharbi, & Mornagui, 2014) These chemicals have become a part of our indoor environment, found in cosmetics, cleaning compounds, baby and children's toys, food storage containers, furniture and carpets, computers, phones, and appliances.

We encounter these compounds as plastics and resins every day in our cars, trucks, planes, trains, sporting goods, equipment, medical equipment, dental sealants, and pharmaceuticals. Instead of steel and wood, plastics and resins are now being used to build our homes, offices, and schools. BPA was evaluated in first- and second-trimester human fetal liver samples to evaluate gene expression specific for BPA metabolism. This research provides new evidence that when there is considerable exposure to BPA during human pregnancy, the capacity for BPA metabolism and biotransformation is altered in various enzymatic pathways in the human fetal liver. This research continues to examine potential health risks of in utero BPA exposure on future breast cancer risk.

Obesogens

Obesity has become one of the major threats for public health in both the industrialized and developing world, in both children and adults. Obesity is influenced by an interaction of genes, nutrition, environment, and lifestyle risk factors. A major focus in research is the environmental and chemical exposures beginning in utero. Removing or limiting chemical exposures appears to be an important contributor that needs to be addressed in all weight loss programs. Avoiding potential obesogens throughout life is essential for the management of obesity and the health-related consequences (Bašić, Butorac, Landeka Jurčević, & Bačun-Družina, 2012). The "obesogen hypothesis" proposes that perturbations in metabolic signaling, resulting from exposure to environmental chemicals, may further exacerbate the effects of imbalances in diet and exercise, resulting in an increased susceptibility to obesity and obesity-related disorders (Grün & Blumberg, 2009).

A study published in the *American Journal of Preventive Medicine* found that by 2030, 42% of U.S. adults could be obese, adding $550 billion to healthcare costs over that period. Current guidelines focus on nutrition and dietary guidelines, a missing component includes the role of chemicals interfering with fat cell metabolism (Wang, Sun, Hou, Pan, & Li, 2013).

As Nurse Coaches, knowing that compounds in the environment increase an individual's risk of obesity, beginning in childhood, how can we coach our clients/patients, families, and communities to begin to consider this aspect of health in their lifestyle changes and behaviors? With the growing body of research on childhood obesity fueled by environmental triggers that begin in utero and program children for weight gain challenges throughout their lives (Brennan, Brownson, & Orleans, 2014). This becomes a Nurse Coach opportunity to bring awareness and choice into all coaching conversations that include weight loss goals.

Pesticides

Hundreds of pesticides and herbicides are used on lawns, gardens, and our bodies to "protect" us and our food supply. Of particular concern related to pesticides is that they have been designed to disrupt biological systems, causing death to target organisms such as insects or plants by acting on their hormonal and neurological systems. Since the biochemistry of most living things is similar enough in humans, wildlife, and plants, it is observed through animal and human studies that we can also be adversely affected by pesticides, especially during critical windows of development, as they are both neurotoxic as well as classified as endocrine disrupting (see Table 9-3). In the past, much of the human and wildlife health-related research on pesticides has dealt with more or less immediate toxicity at relatively high doses, or has been concerned only with the primary mode of action of a single active ingredient in the pesticide product. In recent years, these concerns have broadened to include other possible actions of the ingredients and testing at exposure levels more relevant to what may be in the environment. Multiple studies on pesticide exposure and childhood illnesses are in the literature, including increases in neurodevelopmental and behavioral deficits from prenatal and postnatal exposures (Winneke, 2011).

Nurse Coaches work with clients/patients in the prevention of cancer, with those who are diagnosed with cancer and seeking support, and with those who are post-treatment and hope for recovery and long-term survivorship. According to a study on lifestyle behaviors associated with exposures to EDCs, identifying and characterizing sources of exposure to EDCs, including phthalates and BPA, have proved challenging due to the presence of multiple co-exposures resulting from a wide variety of home environments and lifestyles (Martina, Weiss, & Swan, 2012). There is much evidence that demonstrates that by optimizing nutrition and avoiding chemical exposures in our daily lives, we can support detoxification of environmental toxins through elimination pathways, thus lowering the toxic body burden (Sears & Genuis, 2012). Nurse Coaches, we guide our clients/patients in healthy lifestyle behaviors and support their resilient innate healing potential. The challenge remains to identify how exposures may be impacting one's quality of life and follow the precautionary principle. Willingness to avoid or eliminate potential environmental triggers is part of the Nurse Coach role and nurse coaching process towards healthy people and communities.

SUMMARY

- Nurse Coaches are uniquely positioned to coach and engage individuals, families, and communities in the process of meaningful and environmental health-promoting strategies for behavioral change.
- With a renewed focus on wellness promotion in healthcare reform, nurses are expanding their skills and scope of practice as environmental leaders.
- Lifestyle factors, including nutrition, environmental influences, and physical activity, all impact health and wellbeing throughout the life cycle and are central to an integrative Nurse Coach assessment and coaching process.

NURSE COACH REFLECTIONS

After reading this chapter, the Nurse Coach will be able to bring awareness and personal insight to the following questions:

- What concerns do I have about my current health?
- How does my current environment influence my health?

- What changes can I make in my personal environment to enhance my wellbeing?
- What do I see as my challenges in creating a healthy workplace environment?
- What environmental lifestyle patterns do I recognize that might influence my health and the health of my family and community?
- How can I become more aware of my environmental choices and behaviors?
- What steps can I take to create a healthier home and workplace environment?
- What new environmental practices am I willing to bring into my life to support my wellbeing?
- Who are the people in my life who would support me in making healthy changes?

REFERENCES

American Nurses Association (2007). *Principles of environmental health for nursing practice with implementation strategies*. Retrieved from http://www.nursingworld.org/MainMenuCategories/ThePracticeofProfessionalNursing/NursingStandards/ANAPrinciples/ANAsPrinciplesofEnvironmentalHealthforNursingPractice.pd

Bašić, M., Butorac, A., Landeka Jurčević, I., & Bačun-Družina, V. (2012). Obesity: Genome and environment interactions. *Arh Hig Rada Toksikol, 63*(3), 395–405. doi:10.2478/10004-1254-63-2012-2244

Brennan, L. K., Brownson, R. C., & Orleans, C. T. (2014). Childhood obesity policy research and practice: Evidence for policy and environmental strategies. *American Journal of Preventive Medicine, 46*(1), e1–16. doi:10.1016/j.amepre.2013.08.022

Cannon, C. (2006). *The complete idiot's guide to the anti-inflammation diet*. New York, NY: Alpha Books.

Christiani, D. (2011). Combating environmental causes of cancer. *New England Journal of Medicine, 364*, 791–793.

Dossey, B. M. (2005). Florence Nightingale's tenets: Healing, leadership, global action. In B. M. Dossey, L. C. Selanders, D. M. Beck, & A. Attewell (Eds.), *Florence Nightingale today: Healing, leadership, global action* (pp. 21–24). Silver Spring, MD: Nursesbooks.org.

Goncalves, C. R., Cunha, R. W., Barros, D. M., & Martinez, P. E. (2010). Effects of prenatal and postnatal exposure to a low dose of bisphenol A on behavior and memory in rats. *Environmental Toxicology Pharmacology, 30*(2), 195–201.

Grandjean, P., & Landrigan, P. J. (2014). Neurobehavioural effects of developmental toxicity. *Lancet Neurology, 13*(3), 330–338. doi:10.1016/S1474-4422(13)70278-3

Grün, F., & Blumberg, B. (2009). Minireview: The case for obesogens. *Molecular Endocrinology, 23*(8), 1127–1134. doi:10.1210/me.2008-0485

Hess, D. R., Dossey, B. M., Southard, M. E., Luck, S., Schaub, B. G., & Bark, L. (2013). *The art and science of nurse coaching: The provider's guide to coaching scope and competencies*. Silver Spring, MD: Nursesbooks.org.

International Council of Nurses (ICN) (2011). *Position Statement*: Reducing environmental and lifestyle related health risks. Geneva, Switzerland.

Luck, S., & Keegan, L. (2013). Environmental health. In B. M. Dossey & L. Keegan (Eds.), *Holistic nursing: A handbook for practice* (6th ed., pp. 663–676). Burlington, MA: Jones & Bartlett Learning.

Martina, C. A., Weiss, B., & Swan, S. H. (2012). Lifestyle behaviors associated with exposures to endocrine disruptors. *Neurotoxicology, 33*(6), 1427–1433. doi:10.1016/j.neuro.2012.05.016

National Cancer Institute (NCI) (2010). *Reducing environmental cancer risk: What we can do now*. Retrieved from http://www.cancer.gov/cancertopics/understanding-cancer/environment/

National Institute of Environmental Health Sciences (NIEHS) (n.d.). *Endocrine disruptors*. Retrieved from http://www.niehs.nih.gov/health/topics/agents/endocrine

Nightingale, F. (1860). *Notes on nursing: What it is and what it is not*. London, UK: Harrison.

Nightingale, F. (1863). *Notes on hospitals* (3rd ed.). London, UK: John W. Parker.

Prüss-Üstün, A., & Corvalán, C. (2006). *Preventing disease through healthy environments: Towards an estimate of the environmental burden of disease*. Geneva, Switzerland: WHO Press.

Raffensperger, C. (1998). *The precautionary principle, science and environmental health network*. Retrieved from http://www.sehn.org

Rezg, R., El-Fazaa, S., Gharbi, N., & Mornagui, B. (2014). Bisphenol A and human chronic diseases: current evidences, possible mechanisms, and future perspectives. *Environment International, 64*, 83–90. doi:10.1016/j.envint.2013.12.007

Rochester, J. R. (2013). Bisphenol A and human health: A review of the literature. *Reproductive Toxicology, 42*(12), 132–155.

Sears, M. E., & Genuis, S. J. (2012). Environmental determinants of chronic disease and medical approaches: Recognition, avoidance, supportive therapy, and detoxification. *Journal of Environmental and Public Health*, article ID 356798. doi:10.1155/2012/356798

Soto, A. M., Brisken, C., Schaeberle, C., & Sonnenschein, C. (2013). Does cancer start in the womb? Altered mammary gland development and predisposition to breast cancer due to in utero exposure to endocrine disruptors. *Journal of Mammary Gland Biology Neoplasia, 18*(2), 199–208. doi:10.1007/s10911-013-9293-5

Stewart, B. W., & Wild, C. P. (2014). *World Cancer Report 2014*. Lyon, France: International.

TEDX (2012). The endocrine exchange. Retrieved from http://endocrinedisruption.org

Wang, J., Sun, B., Hou, M., Pan, X., & Li, X. (2013). The environmental obesogen bisphenol A promotes adipogenesis by increasing the amount of 11β-hydroxysteroid dehydrogenase type 1 in the adipose tissue of children. *International Journal of Obesity (London), 37*(7), 999–1005. doi: 10.1038/ijo.2012.173

Winneke, G. (2011). Developmental aspects of environmental neurotoxicology: Lessons from lead and polychlorinated biphenyls. *Journal of Neurology Science, 308*(1-2), 9–15. doi:10.1016/j.jns.2011.05.020

World Health Organization (WHO) (2012*)*. Enhancing nursing and midwifery capacity to contribute to the prevention, treatment and management of noncommunicable disease in practice: Policy and advocacy, research and education. *Human Resources for Health Observer, 12*, Retrieved from http://www.who.int/hrh/resources/observer12/en/

World Health Organization (WHO) (2013). *Global action plan for the prevention and control of non-communicable diseases, 2013–2020*. Retrieved from http://www.who.int/nmh/events/ncd_action_plan/en/

World Health Organization and the United Nations Environmental Programmes (2013). *State of the science of endocrine disrupting chemicals.* Geneva, Switzerland: WHO Press.

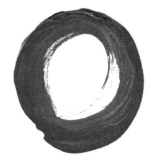

CHAPTER 10

Case Studies: Integrative Lifestyle Health and Wellbeing (ILHWB)

Susan Luck

The reparative process which Nature has instituted and which we call disease has been hindered by some want of knowledge or attention, in one or in all things, and pain, suffering, or interruption of the whole process sets in.

Florence Nightingale, 1860

LOOKING AHEAD...

After reading this chapter, you will be able to:

- Listen to the client/patient story through a multidimensional nonlinear bio–psycho–social–spiritual–cultural–environmental model of health and wellbeing.
- Introduce the Integrative Health and Wellness Assessment (IHWA) into an Integrative Lifestyle Health and Wellbeing (ILHWB) model for guiding the coaching conversation.
- Support the client/patient in developing self-awareness practices and choices for behavioral change.
- Listen to the client/patient story through appreciation of her/his strengths, resilience, and innate capacity for healing.
- Support the client/patient in her/his journey and exploration of beliefs, perceptions, and values.
- Deepen understanding of energy and balance in the ILHWB model.

DEFINITIONS

See Chapters 7, 8, and 9 definitions related to the following case studies.

COACHING CLIENTS/PATIENTS: EXPLORING INTEGRATIVE LIFESTYLE HEALTH AND WELLBEING

Changing lifestyle behaviors, while challenging, presents opportunities to increase aware-ness, change, and transformation in an individual's health and sense of wellbeing, and this requires the art and science of nurse coaching. In an authentic Nurse Coach relationship, the client/patient guides the coaching conversation while the Nurse Coach deeply listens to the story and skillfully asks open-ended questions.

The Theory of Integrative Nurse Coaching (TINC) and the TINC Component 5 Lis-tening with HEART (see Chapter 2) weave the Integrative Health and Wellbeing Assess-ment (IHWA) tools [see Chapter 6 and Appendix C-1 (IHWA short form) and Appendix C-2 IHWA (long form)] into the coaching process while exploring each person's unique story through a multidimensional and interconnected framework. The following case studies bring to life the Nurse Coach process and demonstrate the client/patient challenges, strengths, and possibilities in supporting lifestyle health and behavioral change.

CASE STUDY 1: ANDY—COACHING THE DIABETIC PATIENT

Client's Presentation

Setting: Community healthcare center

Andy's narrative: Andy is 52 years old and has been diagnosed with prediabetes for several years, having persistent elevated triglycerides and hemoglobin A1c and a steady weight gain of 30 pounds over a 20-year period. One year ago, following the death of his wife, he was diagnosed with diabetes and placed on oral medication. For the past six months, he has been following the recommended food plan given to him by the diabetic educator at his community health center. Andy was advised to see the Nurse Coach by his primary care physician after "unexplained" spikes in his blood sugar. He was scheduled for an initial intake with follow-up visits as needed. He reported on the first visit with the Nurse Coach that he was following the prescribed medication and food plan and it had been a struggle to shed weight. He also shared that he was trying to implement better lifestyle choices and was not sure what he needed to do as did not understand why his blood sugar was still not under control. He was frustrated that he had periodic spikes when self-testing at home. At a recent appointment with his primary care physician, a new medication was prescribed to control his blood sugar. He refused to take another medication and expressed concern that his physician suspected him of cheating on the dietary guidelines and food exchange lists he said that he had been strict in following.

Triggers: Elevated blood sugar with accompanied fatigue and anxiety.

Antecedents: Lifetime history of high sugar intake and family history of diabetes.

Mediators: Life stress events including death of spouse and recent financial problems.

Nurse Coach narrative: As healthcare providers, we often make assumptions based on our professional knowledge and beliefs about what is going on with a client/patient. Listening to the client/patient story and asking questions can reveal new information and insight for exploring potential triggers related to symptoms and health conditions. For example, asking Andy what he believed triggered the fluctuations in blood sugar before being prescribed an additional medication. Were there other health promoting interventions that could have mediated his physiological responses?

Session 1 with Nurse Coach (NC)

Andy had filled out an initial clinic health intake form describing why he has a prescription to see the Nurse Coach. At the initial session (one half-hour on clinic schedule), Andy appeared tense, shifting in the chair and making poor eye contact.

NC: *Thank you for scheduling an appointment. Thank you for completing the intake form. You shared that your doctor suggested that we meet to explore your health concerns. What do you believe is your biggest health concern?*

Andy: My doctor referred me because honestly I do not know what else to do to control my blood sugar. Sometimes it feels like I have no control over it. Other times it is okay. I was just put on another medication and I do not want to take it and I do not like how medication makes me feel. I guess that is why I am here. That is my biggest concern.

NC: *I hear that you have some challenges controlling your blood sugar and that is what you want to focus on today?*

Andy: Yes. I eat the same thing every day just as I was told to do by the dietician and sometimes it is normal and sometimes it is not.

NC: Tell me more about what normal is for you. Is there anything you notice?

Andy: I don't know anymore...(appears agitated with shallow breathing noted). I just know that I do not want to become diabetic and shoot insulin every day like my dad did.

NC: That must have been very difficult for you. Let's take a look at what is working for you. Tell me about a good day. What is going on when you are feeling well and your blood sugar is normal?

Andy: Well, I know if I eat consistently, it helps.

NC: Say more about how it helps you to eat more regularly...

Andy: I have more energy and also notice I am not irritable at work.

NC: So I hear you saying that if can eat more regularly, it can control how you feel and control your blood sugar?

Andy: At work, I have a lot of pressure with downsizing in my company, and week to week I don't know if I will have to lay off employees...or be laid off. Sometimes I don't have time to eat. I am also stressed a lot of the time and just feel overwhelmed and overwound.

NC: Can you describe what overwound feels like?

Andy: Tight. Sometimes my chest feels tight. Sometimes my neck is stiff.

NC: Are you feeling that now? (Andy appears "stiff.")

Andy: I guess so (shifts in chair).

NC: Would you be willing to try something?

Andy: I am willing to try whatever can help me.

NC: Have you ever experienced doing a relaxation technique?

Andy: You mean like when my friend took me to a yoga class at the gym once? He said I needed to learn to relax.

NC: What was that like for you?

Andy: I remember that I liked the part about slowing down.

NC: Since you are familiar with a technique to relax, I am going to ask if you can take a moment to focus on your breath...perhaps as you did in your yoga class. You can close your eyes if you choose...or you can find a comfortable way to rest them. Become aware of any areas that feel tight in your body...beginning with your neck and shoulders...and make any adjustments in your chair that is supporting you (Andy closes his eyes and begins to shift his body and sit back in his chair...he sighs deeply). Focus on your body relaxing...whenever you are ready, open your eyes.

Andy: (after a few deep breaths, he opens his eyes) I enjoyed that. Can't say I feel relaxed very often these days.

NC: Can you recall when you have felt relaxed?

Andy: I feel relaxed after I go to the gym and being on the treadmill and doing some stretching.

NC: What else can you notice?

Andy: I remember that when I tested my blood sugar it was a perfect 82. I had this belief that working out would mess up my blood sugar and raise my blood pressure, which is borderline high, but instead I remember thinking that maybe it helps to control both.

NC: Can you describe more about what happens when you go to the gym?

Andy: I hadn't exercised in years and had gained 30 pounds over 20 years and my doctor told me that I had to lose weight. He really scared me. You know, my dad died of complications from diabetes in his sixties (drifts into thought for a moment). Anyway, a friend bought me a membership to a neighborhood gym.

NC: Sounds like a really good friend.

Andy: After my wife died, I felt so alone and my old buddy John bought me a one-year membership and I was so grateful for his kindness and because financially I could not have bought it for myself. Sometimes we work out together.

NC: Sounds like your buddy is a wonderful support for you. I heard you say that you notice that after the gym, your blood sugar becomes normal. What do you believe might be going on?

Andy: Well you know I am very anxious these days. The doctor asked me if I wanted to go on an anti-anxiety medication but I refused. Like I said, I do not like medications. Ever see all of those ads and the side effects on television?

NC: Anything else come to mind about how exercise makes you feel?

Andy: I definitely feel more relaxed. I also feel good because I lost 10 pounds since I started at the gym a few months ago.

NC: I want to acknowledge you for your success. So you describe feeling more relaxed after exercising. Do you think that could have an effect on your blood sugar?

Andy: Everyone always says just focus on what you eat and exercise for losing weight.

NC: Yes, what you eat is very important. Exercise is important...and your hunch is a good one...stress can affect your blood sugar as well.

Andy: I was right!

NC: Yes, you were. How did you feel after we did a brief breathing practice at the beginning of our session?

Andy: I did feel that it helped me to relax as I was really nervous coming to this appointment not knowing what to expect.

NC: Would you be willing to try this practice during the week, knowing that when you relax, you are supporting healthy blood sugar and your overall health?

Andy: I would be willing to try this especially if it will prevent me from taking more medication.

NC: You sound like you are ready to try something new and on your terms. Can you see practicing a simple breathe in and breathe out daily?

Andy: I can do that especially if I can prove to my doctor that I can control my blood sugar.

NC: What would be realistic for you?

Andy: I can manage to find 15 minutes every day.

NC: Is there a time of day that would work best for you?

Andy: Maybe on my afternoon break, which is when I usually feel tension build from my day.

NC: Sounds like a good plan...and to see how you might be able to control your blood sugar...maybe without medication as time goes on.

Andy: I have been looking for something new to get a handle on this problem I just didn't know what or how. I do believe I am the captain of my ship.

NC: Can you tell me what "captain of my ship" means to you?

Andy: Well I think I have more control over my body and mind than I know if that makes sense. I think that the relaxation is a good beginning because if I feel more relaxed, my blood sugar can improve.

NC: You sound like you have a strong will...and you are motivated to be successful. Is there anything else before our session is over?

Andy: I am just thinking that I also get anxious when I come home and I am alone in the evening and maybe this will help...maybe I can do this again in the evening. I used to have a few drinks to unwind but can't do that anymore.

NC: Sounds like a perfect time to do this practice. So let me review with you what I hear you say that you are agreeing to do. You are going to practice focusing on your breath for 10–20 minutes on your break and again in the evening?

Andy: I am willing to try. Did I tell you that I am going to see my daughter and new grand-child in a few months?

NC: *That is wonderful. I would love to hear more about your family. Our time is up for today. Shall we set up another appointment?*

Andy: How about next week? I really want to review what I am eating as there are some things I am not sure about like diet soda because sometimes I think it also raises my blood sugar.

NC: *Let's explore this the next time. Can I give you a food journal form where you can write down everything you eat and drink and you can bring it to our next appointment and we can review it together? There is also a column to describe how you feel after eating, and this will help to identify if any foods or drinks, including diet soda, may affect how you feel. [The NC gives Andy a form to bring to the next session (Appendix E-5)]. Also, I notice that you didn't fill out the Integrative Lifestyle Health and Wellness Assessment (IHWA) yet that you were given as part of your intake packet. If you can fill it out and bring to our next session, we can explore other factors that might be influencing your overall health and wellbeing.*

Andy: I will fill it out and bring it with me.

NC: *It is wonderful to see how open you are to new possibilities for improving your health. I enjoyed our time together and look forward to seeing you next week.*

Andy's Action Plan

- Maintain a Food Awareness Journal (Appendix E-5) for one week.
- Integrate Connecting with Breath Awareness (Appendix F-5) and breath practice into routine, twice daily.
- Continue to monitor his blood sugar with home kit.
- Continue gym routine.
- Complete IHWA (long form) (see Chapter 6 and Appendix C-2) and bring to next session.

Nurse Coach Summary Notes

As Nurse Coaches, we consider how multiple lifestyle factors, including stress, exercise, sleeping patterns, and environmental exposures (see Chapter 9), may be influencing physiological processes, including blood sugar levels. When we explore the client/patient story, how do we include other lifestyle factors, ask meaningful questions, and engage the client in self-discovery about possible triggers and increase awareness of contributing cofactors? When the Nurse Coach explores the story and the client/patient responds "I have been under stress," what is it that we, as nurses, might offer in our brief encounter at the office as a Nurse Coach? Could we ask the client to become aware of her/his stress response patterns, support her/him in learning more about her/his unique response to stress, and offer an awareness or relaxation practice to integrate into her/his daily routine?

Session 2 (one week later)

Andy returns at his scheduled appointment one week later and appears more relaxed.

NC: *Good to see you again. What have you discovered since we met last week?*

Andy: I couldn't wait to come and tell you that my sugar has been stable all week and I did not need to start the new medication!

NC: *Wonderful news. Tell me more.*

Andy: I notice that I have been more relaxed and I have been practicing the relaxation you did with me, twice daily. I was with my buddy, and we went to my local health food market as he is a health nut. He bought me a relaxation tape for my birthday with beautiful images that I can listen to on my iPod...and it has helped me fall asleep. Did I tell you that I had trouble sleeping since my wife died?

NC: *Wonderful that you are sleeping better. Can you describe how your sleep has changed?*

Andy: Well, I had trouble falling asleep and then would wake up in the night sometimes with my chest pounding...and I didn't feel rested in the morning. Now I am wondering if that affected my sugar as well.

NC: *And what was your sleep experience this past week?*

Andy: I think that listening to the relaxation tape puts my mind and body at ease before sleep. As the tape says "begin to quiet your thoughts..."

NC: *Your intuition is right again. You know your body. Not sleeping well can affect your blood sugar. It sounds like you have discovered a powerful natural support for your body and mind.*

Andy: I am beginning to feel more like my old self, and I haven't in a long time.

NC: *Can you describe what your "old self" feels like?*

Andy: More enthusiasm for life...more hopeful for my future...(pause). I really want to discuss food. I brought the food journal with me.

NC: *And what did you notice keeping the journal?*

Andy: I notice that I eat a lot...(pause)...probably more than my body needs and not necessarily healthy foods. Since I take medication, I have to eat and when I don't eat, my blood sugar can drop.

NC: *What do you feel that your body needs?*

Andy: As I exercise, I am more tuned in to when I am feeling full. I think that I need to cut back on portion size.

NC: *How might you do that?*

Andy: This will sound weird but maybe if I use a smaller plate? When I use a big plate, I fill the whole plate with food and then eat it all.

NC: *This sounds like it will be a good cue for you for remembering portion size.*

Andy: I come from a home where there wasn't enough food. We were poor. So I think that when I grew up, I overcompensated and over ate. And that includes pastries and sugars...and that is what got me into this mess.

NC: *Well, it sounds like you are becoming more aware and thinking on how to make new choices. (Andy appears to be wandering off.)*

NC: *Are you able to share what just happened? [Something triggered a memory. Over the next 10 minutes, Andy shared his life story and the Nurse Coach listened. Andy spoke about his family life, where he grew up, his Irish culture, the family foods including lots of potatoes, sweets, and alcohol. He remembered his father (teary-eyed as he imitated his tough Irish brogue). He began to connect to his roots and some of the old patterns including overeating and drinking, and said that it didn't serve him at this time in his life. He realized his patterns. He spoke again of his daughter and grandchild he was hoping to visit in a few months and how he wanted to be healthy when he visited them.]*

NC: *I appreciate your sharing your life story. It sounds like you have a lot of insight into your family and yourself.*

Andy: I haven't shared my story or talked about my father in a long time (teary-eyed, long pause).

NC: *May I suggest that you consider writing and keeping a journal and write your thoughts and memories. It sounds like you have an important story.*

Andy: My daughter might be interested to know more about me. I am a private person, and I know it has kept us at a distance. I would like to know her also.

NC: It sounds like you are learning a lot about yourself and that you want to be closer to your daughter and grandchild. Perhaps this is a new beginning. (Andy nods his head in agreement.)

NC: Since you are exploring changing the way you eat, would you be willing to try an Eating with Awareness practice at home this next week?

Andy: Sure.

NC: Here is an Eating with Awareness Practice Worksheet (Appendix E-6). If you can fill this out and try some of the practices over the next few weeks you can continue to notice your eating style and choices and what you might want to change. Along with your food journal, you can list a few changes that you can begin to make that works for you. How does that sound?

Andy: Just what I had been hoping for. I want to come back in three weeks.

Andy's Action Plan

- Use the Eating with Awareness Review (Appendix E-7).
- Continue with daily Relaxation Breath Practices (Appendices F-1 and F-5).
- Engage in an evening relaxation practice and observe sleeping patterns.
- Continue with the gym routine.
- Continue to monitor blood sugar.
- Begin to keep a story journal.

Nurse Coach Summary Notes

In this 30-minute session, Andy openly shared his family story, his personal history, and his hopes for healing a relationship with his daughter. He described his sleep patterns and explored his eating patterns and behaviors that might have contributed to some health issues, including sleep disturbances at night. He became aware that poor sleep may also impact blood sugar regulation. Andy experienced the benefits of relaxation techniques and discovered what time and type of relaxation practice worked best for him. He is becoming more aware of how stress affects not only his blood sugar but his overall sense of wellbeing. He is interested in the foods he is eating. He is beginning to connect the dots. The Nurse Coach with full presence was able to bear witness to his story.

Session 3 (three weeks later)

Andy came in to the office noticeably more relaxed and lighter.

NC: How have you been since last we met?

Andy: That Eating with Awareness Review was an eye opener.

NC: Can you share more about how that was an eye opener?

Andy: I used the review a few times, and each time I noticed more. I started to pay attention to how I eat and that most of the time I am not very aware of how what I eat affects me. I realize that I can bring a better lunch to work than depending on fast food in the neighborhood...or not eating and then devouring chips or pizza. A few times I brought a chicken wrap that I picked up at a local take-out on the way to work, and I really enjoyed it.

NC: Anything else you noticed?

Andy: I noticed that when I eat while watching television at night I never taste my food... or chew it.

NC: It sounds like you have really increased your awareness about the foods you eat and the choices you make.

Andy: And I decided to try to make some changes these past two weeks.

NC: Tell me more...

Andy: I am eating smaller portions with my new plate...and I even tried shutting off the TV when I eat so I can concentrate on my food. This is a whole new experience for me... and not easy to break this habit.

NC: Can you describe the experience?

Andy: Well, using a smaller plate and eating less at night is part of the eye opener. I think it has helped my digestion. Usually I need to go to bed feeling full, and that probably affected my sleep as well.

NC: So changing the way you eat in the evening has affected your sleep?

Andy: I slept the whole night twice this past week and haven't done that in years.

NC: So I hear you saying that eating smaller meals at night has helped your sleep?

Andy: Definitely.

NC: Sounds like this awareness can affect you in many positive ways.

Andy: I am listening to the relaxation tape instead of watching TV and the evening news to zone out and fall asleep, and I think this helps.

NC: You have really made some important lifestyle changes.

Andy: I think that focusing on what I am eating has also helped me lose five more pounds... and my sugar spiked only one time when I had a very stressful day and I didn't eat and then needed carbs and sugar to get me through it. And, I decided that I really need to learn how to cook. My wife did all of the cooking, and I never paid attention.

NC: You sound excited about the changes you are making and the many new possibilities.

Andy: I am. At the health food store in the area that I mentioned earlier, they have cooking classes and I am going to sign up for the next series...it will give me something to do at night.

NC: I look forward to your sharing some recipes. What do you think about scheduling our next appointment in a few months as you have a plan that sounds like it is working for you. Also, you will be repeating your labs in the next few months, and let's see how your positive lifestyle changes have influenced your results. Before you leave, can you review your action plan and goals for the next three months?

Andy: I am going to continue at the gym...and maybe even try the yoga class there. I will continue to monitor my portions...and chew my food. I plan to start a cooking class and begin to prepare food at home probably on weekends when I have time. And I will continue to practice relaxing and listening to the tapes at night to sleep better.

NC: This sounds like a wonderful plan with many positive changes. I just want to ask if it is realistic for you so you can attain your goals.

Andy: I am in a different frame of mind than when we first met. I am ready.

NC: I believe you will see many positive changes as you continue. I look forward to seeing you in three months. Since we did not have time to review your assessment tool, fill it out again before your next visit. It will be helpful for you to see what has changed in your perception of your health and wellbeing since you did the IHWA before our first visit.

Andy: I have an appointment with the doctor next week and am hoping I can wean off of the medication I am on. I know he will be surprised and pleased with my progress.

NC: I look forward to hearing the good news.

Nurse Coach Summary Notes

Following three sessions over five weeks, Andy demonstrated that he was ready to change old patterns and he was motivated to improve his quality of life.

- The client established his SMART goals (see Chapter 15) for himself.

- The client demonstrated a willingness and openness to new possibilities.
- The client expressed being hopeful about his future.

Andy contacted the Nurse Coach one month later to report that he felt that he needed ongoing support for sustaining his goals. He was referred to a monthly diabetic support group at his community health center that was facilitated by the community health nurse who is also a skilled Integrative Nurse Coach.

Group Coaching offered the client a supportive community and connection with others who shared both his hopes and his challenges and who identified with his vulnerabilities and his resilience. The Nurse Coach guided the process while the group guided the conversation. See Group Coaching Guidelines, Appendix B-2.

CASE STUDY 2: GAIL—COACHING THE BREAST CANCER SURVIVOR

Client's Presentation

Setting: Integrative Nurse Coach's office in an integrative interdisciplinary practice

Gail's narrative: Gail is a 44-year-old woman diagnosed three months earlier with ER+ breast cancer after she had a dream where she saw something in her breast. She made an appointment following her intuition, and a small nodule that was seen on her ultrasound and followed up with mammography. She had a lumpectomy and came to see the Nurse Coach contemplating whether to move forward with the suggested medical treatment options of radiation and chemotherapy since one positive lymph node was removed.

Her health history includes 20-pound weight gain in adulthood and a long history of stressful life events, including diagnosis and difficult treatment for lymphoma at age 21. She has been divorced for over a decade and lives alone. She has a good relationship with her two children, both in college in another state. She scheduled a visit to meet with an Integrative Nurse Coach to discuss her options and her ambivalence about going the medical route for follow-up treatment and has been weighing her choices using alternative therapies.

Triggers: Fear and stress over recent diagnosis and need to make decisions about treatment.

Antecedents: History of lymphoma at 21 years of age and residual trauma.

Mediators: Gail is thoughtful and informed and hopes to gain clarity moving forward.

Session 1 with Nurse Coach (NC)

Gail had been sent via email a set of forms to fill out to reflect on her health before meeting with the Integrative Nurse Coach and setting her intention for the session (see Integrative Lifestyle Health and Wellbeing Nurse Coach Intake, Appendix E-1).

NC: *Thank you for coming in today and for filling out the intake questionnaire in advance. (The NC noticed Gail seemed distracted and had rushed to the appointment, arriving a few minutes late.) Would you be willing to take a moment to focus on what you are hoping for in coming in today? Will you join me in a moment of taking a few slow deep breaths so we can both be present together...(a few moments later...)?*

Gail: I want to focus and get clear on what I need to do. I have a lot of decisions to make, and frankly, I am feeling overwhelmed.

NC: *I hear that you have many decisions to make...*

Gail: I am confused and so ambivalent about what my course of treatment should be following my lumpectomy recently. I have been reading a lot, getting a lot of advice from my dear friends and from the doctors...so some are very medical model focused approaches and others are steering me in the direction of only alternative treatments.

NC: *Sounds like you have had a lot of people who care about you and are offering suggestions. You also have done a lot of research for considering your options. I hear how that could be overwhelming. Have you explored the benefits and challenges of each?*

Gail: The more I read, the harder it is to make a decision.

NC: *And what is your biggest hope in making your decision?*

Gail: I want a treatment that will help me get through this and not make me sick (begins to get teary-eyed).

NC: *(Listening...pause...) Can you share what you are experiencing now?*

Gail: When I was young I had lymphoma and I had chemo. I was so sick from the treatment, and I do not want to feel like that again (facial grimace).

NC: *It sounds like it was a really difficult time for you. Do you remember what helped get you through it?*

Gail: I was feeling so helpless. And I did have a lot of friends and family support.

NC: *What else was going on at that time in your life?*

Gail: I was young and had life ahead of me...I guess I was more hopeful.

NC: *So, I hear you saying on one hand, that you felt helpless. But I also hear you saying that you were hopeful. It sounds like you had a lot of courage to get you through a very challenging time.*

Gail: Yes, I did have courage to get me through a very scary unknown place.

NC: *Can you take a moment to connect with other strengths that have gotten you through this time...and perhaps other challenges in your life?*

Gail: (Pause)...I have a strong will once I put my mind to it...and I trust my intuition. That is how I discovered my cancer.

NC: *Intuition can be a powerful inner resource. If your intuition could speak to you now, what would it say?*

Gail: Gail, stay open...

NC: *Stay open?*

Gail: I feel myself resistant to even saying the words chemotherapy or radiation...any medical interventions...although I did agree to the lumpectomy that may have saved my life.

NC: *I think I hear you saying that you are resistant to medical interventions and that the lumpectomy may have been lifesaving?*

Gail: Yes, that is true.

NC: *So, on one hand, I hear you saying that you are resistant to chemotherapy and radiation...I also hear you saying that it could help you?*

Gail: And that is my dilemma.

NC: *Earlier, you mentioned a quality you identified in the past...being hopeful. Take a moment and reflect on what being hopeful means to you?*

Gail: (Pause)...I am looking forward to the future.

NC: *Take a moment and imagine yourself feeling hopeful in your future...see yourself...perhaps get an image of yourself at a future time...*

Gail: I see myself healthy and on the other side of this.

NC: *Can you describe what you see in more detail? (Gail closes her eyes for a few moments.)*

Gail: I am older and feeling very alive. I am at our favorite summer vacation spot on the Cape with my family...we are having a picnic on a steamy summer afternoon. I am healthy and in good shape.

NC: *What helped you along on this journey to being healthy as you have gotten older?*

Gail: Everything!

NC: Can you say more about what "everything" means for you?

Gail: Hmmm...I am just thinking that maybe it is not "either/or"?

NC: Either/or?

Gail: Maybe I can combine the best of both worlds: medical and alternative.

NC: I am noticing your energy really shifting when you connected with this possibility, a combination as a treatment option. What are you experiencing in this moment?

Gail: Intuitively, I believe...I know that this is the right direction for me.

NC: I hear you saying that you believe this is the direction for you and you are trusting your intuition?

Gail: Yes...and it gives me some clarity of doing what I believe...and it gives me hope that I can get through this on my terms. It is that the doctor I saw after my surgery was so medical and rigid and he frightened me.

NC: Take a moment to recognize your inner wisdom and your strengths and your opening to these new possibilities.

Gail: I am remembering being given the name of an integrative oncologist, and I have kept her card on my desk. She is in the area. I could make an appointment to meet with her and discuss my options. That is what I need to do...find a doctor and a team that I can work with.

NC: How does knowing what you need make you feel?

Gail: Hopeful. Thank you for assisting me in getting clear on my direction.

NC: Thank you for allowing me to be on this journey with you. What is one step you can take to assist you further in your becoming clear in your decision?

Gail: I am going to call the integrative oncologist...and again trust my intuition.

NC: That sounds like an important next step for you. Is there anything else you would like to explore today?

Gail: For today, I know that I made an important decision. I know that there are many areas that I would like to address in my life to become healthier. I would like to schedule a follow-up session.

NC: Wonderful. As you continue to see yourself healthy and to connect to your feelings of hopefulness, you may want to also connect to your strengths during this time. I wonder if you have ever kept a writing journal?

Gail: A long time ago. Actually, when I was going through my chemotherapy 30 years ago. Maybe it would be a good time for me to write down my thoughts...my last one was very negative.

NC: As you write down your thoughts can you imagine what your most positive and successful plan looks like for you? And what are your steps to have the best outcome possible. We can explore this together at our next session. Also, it is helpful for me to know more about you. Would you be willing to fill out the Integrative Health and Wellness Assessment so we can begin to explore your health and lifestyle as you mentioned earlier in our session?

Gail: Definitely.

NC: Let's review your next steps...

Gail: I am going to call the integrative oncologist for an appointment today. I will fill out the Integrative Health and Wellness Assessment. I will begin to journal, focusing on my strengths. Saying this out loud is very affirming and hopeful.

At end of session, Gail is given the IHWA long form (Chapter 6 and Appendix C-2) and a follow-up appointment is made for three weeks.

Gail's Action Plan

- Focus on a sense of hopefulness.
- Identify strengths and clarified choices.
- Dream about what can be and create a new future.
- Increase awareness over decision-making process.
- Explore through journaling her willingness and openness to reflect on the meaning of her cancer journey.
- Explore healthy lifestyle behaviors.

Nurse Coach Summary Notes

As an Integrative Nurse Coach, with knowledge of holistic modalities and strategies for treatment, the Nurse Coach explores and listens to where the client/patient is within her readiness for change. The session began with ambivalence about decision-making about cancer treatment. The client expressed her desire to be well and her commitment to herself to explore and discover a plan that could work for her. As the Nurse Coach deeply listened, the client discovered her inner knowing and tapped into her beliefs and her intuition to guide her and was supported in her process by the Nurse Coach.

Session 2 (three weeks later)

NC: *Good to see you, Gail. I look forward to listening to what has happened over the past three weeks since we last met.*

Gail: Well...I saw the integrative oncologist, who is wonderful. Her integrative oncology center offers acupuncture and herbs for any possible side effects to the treatments... my biggest fear. I can be an outpatient and do not need to go to the hospital, which I am thrilled about. Also, I learned that treatment is totally different now than when I had it 30 years ago. Today, you can get lower targeted doses of both chemotherapy and radiation and they encourage you to exercise so that the chemotherapy circulates throughout the body with minimum side effects.

NC: *It sounds like a lot of what you remembered has changed in a good way...*

Gail: I still remember lying in bed at the hospital and they told me that I had to rest. That was really hard at 21 years of age. My intuition always thought that I would feel better going out with my friends...and I was right! I have been carrying these memories for a long time and fearing them...

NC: *Sounds like you will have a totally different experience now. Perhaps you can continue to replace these new images for the old ones?*

Gail: I love this idea of seeing my treatment in a positive way and finally letting go of the old...Also, I will make plans to be with my friends who are my wonderful support network. One of my friends is a yoga teacher and has been encouraging me to take classes with her. I decided this after filling out the IHWA you gave me.

NC: *Tell me more about what you noticed filling out the IHWA.*

Gail: When I got to the Nutrition, Exercise, and Movement sections, it really caught my attention.

NC: *What caught your attention?*

Gail: I really do not like to exercise. Never did.

NC: *Any thoughts as to why?*

Gail: I was overweight growing up and couldn't move fast when playing sports.

NC: *Have you ever been engaged in any type of movement?*

Gail: I used to love to dance...(remembering)

NC: *What do you love about dancing?*

Gail: I love music. I grew up with music in my house as a child...jazz and rock and roll...

NC: *Can you recall the last time you danced and how it made you feel?*

Gail: At a family wedding a few months ago. It was fun. Music makes me smile (smiles) and makes me happy.

NC: *I hear you saying that dancing and music makes you smile and feel happy. Can you see bringing more music and dancing into your life?*

Gail: My yoga friend takes Zumba classes, and she always invites me to go with her. I also want to lose weight, and this might help me.

NC: *So I hear you saying that music and dancing makes you smile, and can also help you lose weight. You also mentioned earlier that it can help you in supporting your response to your treatment.*

Gail: Wow...I never thought that something I had forgotten and that was really important to me when I was younger could be good for me in many ways...

NC: *Do you have a favorite song to dance to?*

Gail: When I was young, I danced around the house to the Rolling Stones: Happy (starts singing, "a little love...will make you happy...").

NC: *Can you see bringing more music and dance into your life?*

Gail: I have music that I love and just haven't listened to in years...

NC: *It sounds like reconnecting to music and dance is a good next step.*

Gail: Definitely.

NC: *What else would like to discuss today?*

Gail: I am going to begin my first treatment next week.

NC: *So tell me about your plan.*

Gail: I will begin with low-dose radiation and possibly follow with chemotherapy since I had a few positive lymph nodes. I will take it one day at a time. I will also be scheduling my appointments with the acupuncturist to deal with any side effects. And I am going to dance! I also will begin yoga classes on Saturday mornings with my friend.

NC: *That sounds like a wonderful plan. Is there anything else you would like to reflect on before we finish our session today?*

Gail: When I was filling out the IHWA, I started to think about how I eat and I really know that it is important to my health.

NC: *Great. Would you be willing to keep a food diary until we meet next and note what you eat and any comments about how the food makes you feel? Bring it with you, and we can review it. You may also want to spend some quiet time before your upcoming treatments and imagine the best results possible. I would like to remind you that you have all of the tools within you to make this treatment work for you...and you have the external support, both friends and practitioners. I am here for you as you continue on your healing journey. (The session ended with a big mutual hug, and a follow-up session was scheduled in three weeks.)*

Nurse Coach Summary Notes

- The client connected with her joyful, playful self through music and dance.
- The client challenged her own beliefs.
- The client connected with her inner strengths to guide her treatment options.
- The client deepened awareness that a healthy lifestyle is associated with breast cancer survival and a reduction in recurrence.
- The client was able to accept treatment in an integrated manner using both medical interventions and alternative strategies to ensure success and diminish side effects.
- The client continued to explore her beliefs around health and illness.
- The client explored her challenges and strengths.

- The client explored her life balance and lifestyle, including nutrition, body weight, and movement and exercise (see Appendix E-13).

Session 3 (three weeks later)

NC: Good to see you again, Gail. How are you since our last visit three weeks ago?

Gail: I feel I am really doing well. I have had three radiation treatments at the office. I follow up with acupuncture the next day. I am taking some herbs including ginger tea for nausea and have really had no side effects and so far I still have my full head of hair (smiles). I also started yoga last week, and I pulled out some of my favorite oldies and I am dancing around my house. I am able to sleep at night with some herbal teas and relaxation tapes that a friend gave to me. I have been journaling, and that has been a wonderful way to reconnect to myself.

NC: It sounds like you have created a positive healing experience.

Gail: Surprisingly so...I realize that I carried so much fear and anxiety in anticipation of treatment and of my need to make this decision...I knew what I needed to do and once I got clarity, I now feel focused and feel like a warrior.

NC: Wonderful to listen to how you transformed your challenges and are connecting with your inner strengths and outer resources. I am curious. What are the qualities of a warrior?

Gail: A warrior is strong and courageous and confronts obstacles head on...sort of like walking through fire...and coming through to the other side safe.

NC: How does that make you feel?

Gail: I feel I have released something and I now have moments of feeling gratitude and I am connecting with hope and this really pulls me through in the moments of fear that can still come sometimes.

NC: It sounds like you are aware of when your vulnerability surfaces...and that you have chosen meaningful ways to connect with your inner strengths to work with this part of you.

Gail: Journaling has been helpful in learning more about myself at this time in my life. Also, I'm learning new ways to relax through yoga...and the relaxation tape to quiet my mind, especially at night...I put it on my iPhone as an app. I can even listen to it while I am waiting at the oncology center for my treatment.

NC: How wonderful that you have created your healing toolkit that you are bringing into your life.

Gail: I am feeling strong. I now am beginning to see a long life ahead of me. I am still young. I still have many hopes, including a new relationship in my future and even going back to college now that my kids are on their own. I want to improve how I eat since I only need to prepare meals for myself (laughs).

NC: It sounds like you envision a new life moving forward. How can you stay with this vision?

Gail: I am journaling about it and getting clarity within myself. I believe that I can create a new reality for myself.

NC: You mentioned food and meal preparation a moment ago. What did you notice when you filled out the tool?

Gail: My main problem is my sweet tooth...and eating late in the evening.

NC: Tell me more about your eating pattern.

Gail: Well, I often do not eat during the day...except for breakfast.

NC: What do you have for breakfast?

Gail: A bagel with cream cheese and two cups of coffee with sugar or Equal.

NC: Do you feel this breakfast nourishes and sustains you?

Gail: I get hungry by midmorning.

NC: *And what do you notice?*

Gail: I need coffee to keep my energy up…and usually a pastry with it.

NC: *Anything else you notice?*

Gail: It sustains me for a while but then my energy sinks again. When I do eat lunch, I grab something fast like a deli sandwich.

NC: *If you were to imagine eating differently, what would that look like?*

Gail: Everyone says that I should start my day with a good breakfast.

NC: *What do you believe about this approach?*

Gail: Years ago, I was on Weight Watchers, and ate often and always ate breakfast.

NC: *What was that experience like for you?*

Gail: I actually lost weight eating more. Also, I think my energy was better…and I didn't crave as much sugar.

NC: *So I hear you saying that when you ate regularly you had more energy and you lost weight?*

Gail: I heard Mehmet Oz speak on his show recently about eating in the morning to jump start metabolism, and somehow it helps the blood sugar.

NC: *It sounds like you know what would be best for you.*

Gail: My problem is that I really am not hungry in the morning. Some of my friends have protein smoothies in the morning.

NC: *Would you be willing to consider a protein shake in the morning?*

Gail: I would be willing to try. I have looked at them in the supermarket. Can you recommend one?

NC: *Many people use whey protein powder, and you can find that at your local market or health food store. You may want to read ingredients to avoid added sugars.*

Gail: Sounds like I could manage this. I will put it on my shopping list.

NC: *Based on what you have said about your sugar cravings and low energy, would you like information on what is called a "hypoglycemic food plan"? This involves eating several smaller meals daily, perhaps similar to Weight Watchers. Each meal consists of protein that can stabilize your blood sugar and cravings and give you fuel for energy. You can include healthy carbohydrates such as whole grains like quinoa and beans in measured amounts as you did on Weight Watchers.*

Gail: Great. This is just what I have been looking for.

NC: *Before we close today's session, can you review your food plan?*

Gail: I will purchase protein powder and begin my day with a protein shake. I will continue to keep my food journal and explore what foods I like within the hypoglycemic plan. I also will cut back on coffee.

NC: *This sounds great. Is this realistic for you at this time?*

Gail: I think so. I am motivated to get healthy.

NC: *Wonderful. How about giving yourself some time to integrate all of your wonderful new lifestyle tools and complete your course of treatment. You can implement them slowly over the next few months or as you feel will be best for you. Perhaps you can look at your action steps and set short- and long-term goals.*

Gail: I think that I will make major changes in my life over the next three months.

NC: *Sounds good. I am always here if you want to check in and to let me know how things are going.*

Gail: I feel really ready for changing my life. (At the end of the session the NC gave the forms, and this was followed by a hug.)

Nurse Coach Summary Notes

- The client guided her treatment plan.

- The client became aware of her innate resilience, tapping into her capacity for renewed health.
- The client sought the guidance and skills from her Integrative Nurse Coach and the interprofessional team.
- The client continued to explore her beliefs about her diagnosis.
- The client shifted from ambivalence to acceptance and action.
- The client discovered her strengths and innate capacity to heal the past and heal her present.
- The client chose the Western cancer treatment protocol of surgery, radiation, and the possibility of chemotherapy along with an integrative approach that resonated with her beliefs.
- The client chose to integrate journaling and self-reflection, acupuncture, nutrition, yoga, dancing, relaxation, and herbs into her treatment plan. She explored her beliefs and possibilities for optimizing her healing potential.
- The client will explore a new hypoglycemic food plan (Appendix E-10), including a protein shake in the morning.
- The client will continue to collaborate with her Integrative Nurse Coach on developing her next steps in the Lifestyle Health and Wellbeing plan.

Post Three-Month Summary

As sessions continued, Gail asked her Integrative Nurse Coach to speak with both her acupuncturist and oncologist and coordinate her interprofessional team and care plan. The Nurse Coach was able to assume this leadership role that supported her client. This gave Gail the added comfort knowing her team was communicating and enhanced her participation as she developed short- and long-term healthy lifestyle goals. Gail continued to explore awareness and mindfulness practices that assisted her in changing eating patterns, making new lifestyle choices, creating a healing environment in her home, and becoming aware of how stress impacted her wellbeing. After her treatment was over, she reflected back on her journey and that she achieved not only renewed health but a deeper sense of wellbeing for the first time. Increasing awareness using a food journal, mindful eating practices, and integrating imagery of her evolving self, all served to reinforce and strengthen her commitment to her health and wellbeing.

CASE STUDY 3: ANN—COACHING THE PATIENT WITH METABOLIC SYNDROME

Client's Presentation

Setting: Interprofessional medical practice

Ann's narrative: Ann is a 56-year-old business woman who travels to different cities three days/week to cover her work territory. She is divorced, supports herself, and has a good relationship with her two adult children. She has gained 10 pounds in the past two years following menopause, mostly around her abdomen and hips. She describes her work as a high-pressure job that consumes all of her time and energy. Ann scheduled a visit for guidance in changing her lifestyle and eating habits following her annual physical and her doctor's concerns. She shares the comfort of a few glasses of wine with associates several times a week, her only source of social contact. She craves carbohydrates and loves sweets. She described her main physical activity as "running through the airport to catch a flight," and often she is "short of breath." At her last physical, she had elevated lipids and high blood pressure along with an elevated C reactive protein (CRP), an inflammatory marker that her doctor appeared to be concerned about. She complained of generalized aches and pains and of feeling "old." She reported that her doctor told her that she had a classic case of metabolic syndrome that left her fearful and did not really understand what that meant although she had started reading about heart attacks as a leading cause of death in women her age.

Triggers: Diagnosis of metabolic syndrome.

Antecedents: Financial need to support family, family history, life stress.

Mediators: Aging process and diminishing stamina and energy.

Nurse Coach narrative: Ann was given a "diagnosis" that she did not understand as medical language can be intimidating and leave one anxious and fearful. Nurse Coaches speak both the language of medicine and healing and can deconstruct the language and ask the client for their understandings, reframing the conversation so they can understand and participate in the coaching process. Nurse Coaches can interpret medical jargon and be a nurse expert when needed. This also offers an opportunity to draw upon the client's inner strengths and offers shifting the client from feeling powerless and hopeless to empowered and hopeful. Once the Nurse Coach has listened to the client's narrative, the client has the opportunity to explore her/his current reality and begin to imagine what is possible. Inquiries to increase awareness and choice in lifestyle change include: What are my unique challenges? What factors will I use to weigh my options? What does success look like for me?

Session 1 with Nurse Coach (NC)

NC: Happy to meet you. Please share what brings you here today.

Ann: My nurse practitioner advised me that it is important that I make some changes in my lifestyle and referred me to you. I want to change but I do not know where or how to begin. I feel like my life is "out of control."

NC: How would you like to feel?

Ann: Healthier...especially as I get older...

NC: Can you describe what being healthy as you get older means to you?

Ann: I would be able to run to catch a plane and not be out of breath.

NC: Take a moment and reflect on why this is so important to you?

Ann: (after a moment's quiet pause and tears welling up) Many reasons. I want to feel healthy and have energy again.

NC: What is the first thought or image that comes up for you?

Ann: My daughter just got married, and I would love to be around to know my grandchildren. I come from an extended family where three generations of women cared for each other. I dreamed for many years of retiring and being a grandmother and helping my daughter. I do not want to be a burden on her.

NC: I hear you saying that you want to feel healthy and have energy. What do you believe are your challenges to feeling healthy and having more energy?

Ann: My work schedule and always being on the go.

NC: Can you say more about what that means for you?

Ann: It is hard to believe that I can change the downward spiral I am in. Now, I am often running to the airport, running to catch a plane, running to meetings and appointments. And you know, I am not a kid anymore.

NC: You just used an image of a spiral. Can you imagine your spiral going upward?

Ann: Right now it is difficult. I do not have a routine for myself, especially my meals, and I know that is a major problem. Living alone, I am out the door in the morning, grab a donut and coffee en route, and then some fast food at the airport food court at lunchtime. Then I have a drink with peanuts and pretzels on the plane. By the time I get to the hotel, I go to the bar and have a few glasses of wine to unwind. I eat whatever I can find, usually a burger and fries or pizza.

NC: *So when you describe your routine, what do you notice?*

Ann: I have no structure. I probably get little nutrition. And probably it is why I have gained weight and why I am having many other health issues.

NC: *It must be challenging traveling so much.*

Ann: This is my life but it doesn't work for me anymore but I need to support myself.

NC: *Can you imagine a way that it could work for you?*

Ann: I sound like I do not have control...but that is how I have been feeling and I don't like it!

NC: *I hear you say that you are wanting structure and to feel more in control. What would that look like for you?*

Ann: I guess I would plan more around my schedule when traveling...especially around food and my meals.

NC: *You have mentioned planning a few times? Can you say more about that?*

Ann: I know that I function best when I have a structure and a goal. That is how I am in my work in sales management and why I am so successful.

NC: *It sounds like you are successful because you have a system that works well for you. I wonder if there are skills you have in your work that you can apply to your personal life?*

Ann: I never thought of it that way. I always plan my work for the next day the evening before, especially since I am traveling to different cities half of my week. I keep a schedule of my meetings and appointments in Outlook on my iPhone. That provides a structure for me.

NC: *You describe that you are good at what you do. Tell me more about your qualities for being successful.*

Ann: I am organized. I meet my goals. I feel confident in my skills.

NC: *I hear you saying that you have wonderful skills that you use in your work. Can you think of how you can use your skills for success in your personal life to provide the structure I hear you say you need to be successful in attaining your health goals?*

Ann: I never thought about it like that.

NC: *Take a moment and see what that might look like? Where you might begin? (pause)*

Ann: I would begin by creating structure to start my day...eating a healthier breakfast before I leave the house. My daughter bought me some protein powder when she was visiting recently. I guess I could try that. I can bring food on the plane or buy a salad at the airport. I could make healthier choices at the hotel in the evening.

NC: *Does this feel like a realistic plan for you?*

Ann: Yes. I can also go to the market and make sure I have what I need. I can keep it on my iPhone in my notes and refer back to it every day.

NC: *I can feel your enthusiasm. I hear you saying that you will begin with breakfast and making better food choices when traveling and that this sounds like a good plan for you. Is there anything else that might assist you in your desire for feeling well?*

Ann: I was just remembering that when I was younger, I used to go to a gym when the kids were small. I would take an aerobics class while they were in day care.

NC: *In recalling that experience, what comes up for you?*

Ann: I loved feeling my body move. I am thinking that there are gyms at the hotels, and I never use them. I could go to the gym instead of the bar...(pause)

NC: *Take a moment, close your eyes if you choose, and focus on your breath...(pause) Now see yourself in your ideal state of health. Where are you? What are you doing? Stay* *with this image for as long as you like. When you are ready, open your eyes...(two minutes later)*

Ann: I was running after my (future) grandson on the beach by the shoreline. I was in my bathing suit...must have been at least 10 pounds thinner. (Ann smiles for the first time in the session.)

NC: *Did you notice anything else?*

Ann: I was not out of breath. I felt alive again...and I looked damn good!

NC: *What would it be like for you to feel like that again?*

Ann: I wish I could...

NC: *You may want to begin by recalling this image...and how you felt...and the feeling of going to the gym when you are at the hotel. Perhaps it can inspire you. Is there anything else you may want to consider to support your success?*

Ann: I do want to move more...not just at the airport running...I need to build up my stamina. I just had an idea: when I unpack, I can leave my sneakers at the door as a reminder to go to the gym...instead of the bar. I feel like that would give me structure and a goal.

NC: *I hear that you have a strong intention to change your routine and replace going to have a few drinks to unwind to going to the gym. Is that a realistic option for you?*

Ann: I am willing to try.

NC: *It sounds like a good plan. Let's review your next steps...*

Ann: I am going to make a protein shake every morning and bring food with me when I travel. And, I am going to remember to pack my sneakers and unpack them and leave them at the door when I check in to my hotel room to remember to work out.

NC: *How does that feel?*

Ann: I can do this!

NC: *Would it be helpful to record your activities in structuring your activities as you develop your routine? If you think it would be helpful, I can give you a Movement and Exercise Calendar.*

Ann: That would be great. (Ann was given the Movement and Exercise Calendar (Appendix E-12), and a follow-up appointment was made for two weeks.)

Nurse Coach Summary Notes

- The client reflected on meaning and purpose in her life.
- The client reflected on her strengths in her work life and on how to apply them in her personal life.
- The client deepened awareness of lifestyle factors that impact her quality of life.
- The client increased awareness of her relationship to food, eating patterns, and behaviors.
- The client agreed to keep a food journal and note all that she eats and drinks for one week.
- The client was given a Food Awareness Journal worksheet (Appendix E-5) and an Exercise and Movement Calendar (Appendix E-12).
- The client was given the Integrative Lifestyle Health and Assessment (IHWA) to complete and bring to her next session (see Chapter 6 and Appendix C-2 long form).
- The client will begin an exercise routine to replace her current routine of drinking at the hotel bar in the evening.
- The client will continue to focus on her strengths.

Session 2 (two weeks later)

NC: *Good to see you again, Ann. Tell me what has happened since we last met two weeks ago.*

Ann: Since I saw you last I have been keeping a food journal.

NC: *In keeping a food journal, what have you noticed?*

Ann: After writing everything down, I know that I want to eat healthier.

NC: *What does eating healthier mean to you?*

Ann: Making better choices. I notice how much coffee I drink throughout the day at meetings, airports, and in between...and how much sugar I use, and it is two packets in each cup. And that doesn't include the soda or sweetened iced tea. I think it keeps my energy going.

NC: *I hear you say that you need to keep your energy going? Tell me more about your energy.*

Ann: I guess I am used to being described by my colleagues as a powerhouse...have been all of my life. Now it seems that with my hormones, I don't sleep as well so I am always fatigued. I would like to feel like the old younger me again.

NC: *And what would that feel like?*

Ann: I would have energy.

NC: *How do you see yourself when you have more energy?*

Ann: I look vibrant and attractive.

NC: *What do you see contributing to your success in regaining your energy and feeling vibrant?*

Ann: Sleeping well. I am invigorated when I am outdoors and remember what it like when I used to jog down a country road. I felt strong in my body, mind, and spirit.

NC: *What are your qualities or strengths that can assist you feeling like this again?*

Ann: I am strong-willed and persistent. I can focus on the prize at work...although obviously it can be to my detriment.

NC: *Can you see using your strengths to guide your success personally?*

Ann: Sometimes I can. I think about friends my age who still run the New York Marathon every year.

NC: *I hear you saying that it is possible for you to feel this way again and move toward your vision for health and wellbeing.*

Ann: I am beginning to think it is.

NC: *So what is one change you believe you could make to move you closer to your image of health?*

Ann: I know that I need to cut back to one cup of coffee daily in the morning from my current four plus cups daily, each with three packets of sugar. I realize that means I need to give up at least four cups of coffee and eight teaspoons of sugar.

NC: *How does saying that feel?*

Ann: It would be difficult.

NC: *It sounds like on one hand, that you want to give up coffee and sugar while on the other hand, you need it to maintain your energy?*

Ann: I am afraid that I would crash and have no energy to do my work, and that happened when I tried to go "cold turkey" a few years ago.

NC: *You have tried this before. In order to be successful, it needs to work for you. As you know, both caffeine and sugar are stimulants. Can you think of how this can work for you?*

Ann: Yes. I could consider weaning off. That would definitely be less stressful.

NC: *Tell me about how you might begin.*

Ann: I think I can have a cup in the morning and one in the afternoon.

NC: This feels like a good plan for you?

Ann: Yes I can bring herbal teas with me on the road to drink in-between.

NC: Did you notice anything else in your eating patterns and food choices over the past week?

Ann: Yes. I eat too late at night, and I think it causes digestive problems including feeling bloated.

NC: Before our session ends, can I give you a Mindful Eating Practice (Appendix E-6) to do for at least two meals during each week and we can review at your next session?

Ann: Sound good. I will be traveling a lot over the next month and may have some challenges. I will schedule an appointment for next month.

Nurse Coach Summary Notes

- The client has increased her awareness and observed her food patterns and behaviors and how her energy is impacted by a high intake of caffeine and sugar.
- The client has chosen where to begin her process of change.
- The client is motivated and aware that she needs to set realistic goals for sustainable behavioral change.

Session 3 (one month later)

NC: Good to see you. How have you been since we last met?

Ann: I am happy to report that I have turned a corner.

NC: Tell me more.

Ann: Well...where to begin...over the past month I have cut back on caffeine and sugar as we had discussed. It was really difficult but I did it slowly. Actually am down to three cups a day of coffee but only one sugar in each, which is major for me.

NC: That is a big change. How do you feel?

Ann: At first, it was hard breaking the habit and I was irritable. Then after about two weeks, I started to notice that I had more energy. Also, I have started working out and I do leave my sneakers at the door at the hotel as soon as I arrive. It is an amazing reminder, and I smile each time I leave the room with them on. I started to make some change in my food choices on the road but not sure I am substituting with better choices and need some help in this area.

NC: Were you able to use the food journal?

Ann: I did.

NC: And what did you notice?

Ann: I still crave carbs but have been limiting them and focusing more on salads and proteins.

NC: How does that make you feel?

Ann: I find that if I eat several smaller meals a day, it sustains me.

NC: It sounds that you have found a rhythm of eating that seems to work for you.

Ann: Yes it sustains my energy.

NC: This is often referred to as a hypoglycemic approach of eating that encourages several smaller meals a day consisting of some protein such as chicken, fish, seeds and nuts, and beans and whole grains.

Ann: That is what I have been trying to do, and I think it is working.

NC: Would you like me to provide you with some materials that might guide you?

Ann: That would be really helpful.

NC: It sounds like you have implemented many changes. Can you review them?

Ann: So I cut back on caffeine and sugar...a work in progress. I have started going to the gym when I travel and basically stopped drinking. And I am trying to eat better. Did I say that I lost five pounds?

NC: *I want to acknowledge your success and motivation.*

Ann: Thank you, as you have really been a support as my Nurse Coach.

NC: *This is a partnership, and I am happy to have been able to be here with you on your journey. Before you leave, here is both a copy of the Hypoglycemic Food Plan (Appendix E-10) you mentioned and a copy of the Mediterranean Food Plan (Appendix E-9) for you to explore. It is basically the foods you mentioned in your food journal.*

Ann: You have given me the guidance I need. I would like to see how I can build on our work together, and I will call you at a future time.

NC: *That sounds like a good plan. You have a lot of tools, and you have your inner resources. I am here if you want to call and check in to let me know how you are. Thank you for allowing me to be part of your journey.*

Nurse Coach Summary Notes

As an Integrative Nurse Coach, working with Ann allows the Nurse Coach to listen to Ann's story from multiple perspectives. Listening with HEART (Chapter 2 TINC, Component 5), reflect on the questions that you might ask your client/patient. These coaching questions are for you to consider and to shape based on the person you are coaching. The key is to allow yourself to be curious and trust the therapeutic effect of being deeply listened to by the Nurse Coach. The Nurse Coach model knows the benefits of being fully present in the energy field she or he is sharing with another.

- The client expressed willingness to explore the change process.
- The client explored lifestyle challenges and barriers to change.
- The client increased awareness of food choices and behaviors.
- The client focused on her life skills and strengths to create new patterns and behaviors around food and exercise.
- The client created a wellness vision.
- The Nurse Coach focused on small steps to support the client learning new lifestyle patterns.
- The Nurse Coach acknowledged the client's successes.

CASE STUDY 4: SALLY—COACHING THE CLIENT WITH ENVIRONMENTAL HEALTH CHALLENGES

Client's Presentation

Setting: Employee health services

Sally's narrative: Sally, a 31-year-old woman, is employed as a medical surgical nurse manager in a busy metropolitan hospital where she works the evening shift. She has been married eight years and has experienced two miscarriages in the past two years and has not been able to become pregnant. She has a high-stress job, reports erratic eating and sleeping patterns, and has recently experienced unexplained weight gain. Sally was referred to the Nurse Coach through the Employee Assistance Program (EAP) at the hospital where she works. She had been experiencing an array of symptoms over the past year, including headache, fatigue, depression, and weight gain. All of her lab tests and scans appeared normal. Her OB/GYN physician recommended that she begin an antidepressant medication, and she has refused. She is hoping to become pregnant and anxious to find some answers to her symptoms.

Triggers: Stress at work due to short staffing and patient work load. Client is beginning to examine possible chemical exposures in her workplace. Frequent headaches and fatigue. Poor sleep patterns.

Antecedents: Family history of mother with breast cancer. Unexplained weight gain.

Mediators: Supportive work colleagues. She hopes to have a family.

Nurse Coach narrative: As the Nurse Coach listened to Sally's story with curiosity, she explored all of the possible triggers through a series of questions that related to both her timeline and her reason for coming for the visit. The Nurse Coach explored the client's beliefs about her symptoms from an integrative and holistic perspective. As a Nurse Coach, she is aware that environmental stressors can trigger similar responses to that of emotional stressors, including mood, energy, sleep, and weight gain. The Nurse Coach is aware that emotional stress can also make one more vulnerable to the impact of other stressors in the environment. The Nurse Coach supports the client/patient as she or he both connects to the story, increasing awareness of possible influences, and together explore the possibilities guiding the change process.

Session 1 with Nurse Coach (NC)

NC: Welcome, Sally. Please share with me what brings you here today.

Sally: I have not been feeling like myself. I can't explain it...and neither can the doctors.

NC: What concerns do you have about your current health?

Sally: Well, my main concern is that I have not been able to get pregnant.

NC: What do you believe are your challenges to becoming pregnant?

Sally: I honestly do not know. My husband and I love each other, and we have a good sexual relationship...although ever since I started my job a few years ago, I have been stressed and I have also gained weight...so I am not feeling as sexual. Also, I work evenings and when I come home, I am exhausted.

NC: Do I hear you saying that your current lifestyle including your schedule might be influencing your becoming pregnant?

Sally: I feel like I have a lot of stress and wonder how it can be affecting my sleep and my moods. I also wonder about chemicals in my workplace. We are constantly using cleaning products and chemicals for everything—wounds, floors, air, hands...I have done some reading about the association between chemicals and fertility...also chemicals and weight gain. I cannot explain my weight gain as my diet really hasn't changed.

NC: I hear you saying that you feel the environment at work might possibly be contributing to your health concerns?

Sally: Is it possible? I have read a lot about this and it makes me wonder.

NC: It sounds like you would like to begin by exploring possible influences in your environment. So let's explore this together and begin by you taking time now to fill out an Environmental Assessment that is part of a larger Health and Wellness Assessment as a place to begin exploring potential environmental links to your symptoms and concerns. (Sally is given this section of the IHWA long form and sits for about 10 minutes and completes this section.)

NC: What did you notice when answering these questions?

Sally: I think that both my home and workplace environment are toxic.

NC: What does that mean to you?

Sally: At home, I use disinfectants, and everything has a fragrance. A few years ago, we moved into a new home and renovated it in preparation for growing a family. We painted and put in new carpeting in the bedroom, and both gave off fumes. That is when I first started getting headaches and some of my symptoms of childhood asthma acted up. The smell is gone but I feel like I must be more sensitive to chemicals because now I can smell the chemicals used at work.

NC: Tell me more.

Sally: As soon as I walk onto the unit I can smell the chemicals in the air...probably a mix of cleaning products on the floor and sprays in the bathrooms and the perfume on some of the workers and visitors. A friend told me that some of these chemicals can contribute to my headaches, asthma, weight gain, and infertility. I wondered if that is true, and so I started doing my own research and found out that there are some strong associations.

NC: It sounds like you are becoming more aware of the chemicals in your workplace and at home as possibly contributing to your symptoms as well as difficulty in becoming pregnant. What do you feel might be helpful to minimize your exposures?

Sally: I started reading the ingredients in the products I am purchasing. I feel like an environmental detective. I want to go to some websites to get more evidence-based information to be able to make healthier choices. I need to get to the bottom of this and feel better. My husband and I are so ready to begin a family. Can you recommend some websites as there is so much out there on the Internet?

NC: I am happy to. There are two websites that come to mind, both were started by nurses. The Environmental Working Group is http://www.ewg.org. This can also link you to the safe cosmetics network to look at your personal care products that you use every day. The Health Care Without Harm website is http://www.hcwh.org and it explores the hospital environment.

Sally: This has really been important to me. I will do my homework. I would like to set up another appointment with you in a few weeks.

NC: I hear that you have a direction and a plan, and I would like to support you in your goals.

Nurse Coach Summary Notes

- The client is motivated to discover potential triggers impacting her health and wellbeing.
- The client is motivated to changing her personal environment.
- The client is an educated consumer seeking additional information.

Session 2 (two weeks later)

NC: How have you been since we saw each other last?

Sally: I have learned a lot, and I have a lot of environmental challenges to overcome, especially at work.

NC: Can you say more about your environmental challenges?

Sally: I looked at the products that I used in my home for cleaning and what I put on my skin and have changed them all.

NC: It sounds like you have been successful in making changes in your personal environment.

Sally: Well I went on the websites you suggested and started learning about endocrine disruptors and how they can interfere with normal hormones. They are everywhere! They are in fragrances and in skin lotions and plastics and pesticides.

NC: It sounds like you have discovered a lot. Tell me more about what you have changed.

Sally: I had already stopped using perfume and scented detergent. I also stopped microwaving in plastic containers: I am now reading labels and ingredients in my foods and stopped buying canned foods and drinking from plastic water bottles.

NC: It sounds like you have certainly made a lot of significant personal changes. What would you like us to address in our session today?

Sally: Here is my dilemma. I am able to change my personal environment as I feel I have some control over it even though it can be overwhelming...but how do I deal with all of the toxic chemicals in the workplace that I am sure affect me and everyone else?

NC: I hear you saying that you know your work environment is not safe for you and you would like to change it and make it safer but you do not know how?

Sally: Exactly. How would I begin?

NC: What is one environmental concern that affects you at work?

Sally: The strong-smelling cleaners that are used on the floors on my evening shift.

NC: How do they make you feel?

Sally: Respiratory and almost feel like a burning in my throat and coughing. Sometimes I get a headache.

NC: Have you noticed if others might be affected as well?

Sally: Several of the staff do have allergies...hmmmm...I wonder if it is affecting them as well.

NC: How might you find out?

Sally: I could have a conversation and ask if they are aware if the chemicals used on the unit bother them?

NC: That sounds like a good first step.

Sally: But can we actually change the hospital policy?

NC: Take a moment and think about working in an environment that supports your health goals personally and for your patients and co-workers.

Sally: We all deserve to work in a safe workplace environment. I will explore this with the staff and find out who purchases our supplies and if there are options.

NC: Reflect on what is one step you can take at work toward this goal? May I share that many hospitals are going through this same process for the environmental safety of both workers and patients. If you go to the Healthier Hospitals website, you can find a lot of information that might be helpful, http//www.healthierhospitals.org.

Sally: Wow, I had no idea that this is happening in healthcare.

NC: As you continue to increase your awareness of how chemicals might be affecting your health, let's review the changes you will implement in your personal life to move closer to your vision of health.

Sally: I will continue to eliminate personal care products that have endocrine disruptors. I want to phase out my cleaning products for greener products and I will microwave in paper or glass. My next step after reading the "dirty dozen" heaviest sprayed fruits and vegetables on the environmental working group website is to check out the local farmers market on Sunday as they sell a lot of organic fruits and vegetables.

NC: That sounds like a lot of change. Is it realistic for you?

Sally: What is realistic is feeling good, getting pregnant, and having a healthy family.

NC: As a nurse, and a global citizen, I believe this is an important part of your health and for the health of your children. I am happy to support you here at the hospital in any way I can. If you would be interested in more information on endocrine disruptors, I have some information I can share with you.

Sally: I would really appreciate that. [Sally is given the Common Endocrine Disruptors, Health Risks, and Prevention Tips (Appendix E-15)].

NC: Let me know how I can support you as you move forward in changing your personal and professional workplace environment.

Nurse Coach Summary Notes

As Nurse Coaches, we are also educators and client/patient advocates. Sally presents a story that expands our role for the wellbeing of not only herself, but her co-workers and her future family. Sally is an informed and motivated woman and nurse who is aware of the public health implications of the impact of chemicals in our environment.

Session 3 (three weeks later)

NC: Good to see you, Sally. What has happened since we last met?

Sally: I met with my co-workers, and I found out that some of them, especially the younger nurses, had the same concerns. I shared the Healthier Hospitals website with them, and we decided to write a letter and form an environmental committee at the hospital and go to our hospital administrator with our ideas. I was asked to be the spokesperson and met with the administration team last week. They agreed to research the products that they are using on all of the units.

NC: This sounds like an important conversation. How does it make you feel?

Sally: I am happy to be part of bringing awareness to others about how our environment can affect the health and wellbeing of both the workers and the patients. I am hopeful and happy to get involved in creating a safer workplace for everyone. My husband and I have also decided that if things don't change here soon, I will find another job in a healthier environment.

NC: You are a courageous nurse leader.

Sally: I really feel that this is part of my being a nurse. And I want to tell you something else...I discovered in my research something else that really bothers me...Triclosan, the antibacterial and antifungal agent that I use to wash my hands between patient rooms at least 50 times a day. And I am really beginning to wonder if this could be contributing to my infertility. It is a potent endocrine disruptor, and even the FDA is researching its safety issues. It also can fuel weight gain! I have a lot to work on and a lot to be thankful for. Thank you for this time together.

Nurse Coach Summary Notes

As the allotted three sessions came to closure, the Nurse Coach acknowledged Sally for strength and courage in working toward changing not just for herself but how she is changing the environment at work and contributing to the health of many others.

- The client became aware of making choices in her lifestyle health and wellbeing.
- The client became an environmental health advocate for herself and others.
- The client connected to life goals and took action to achieve them.
- The client demonstrated strong motivation to continue to make personal changes.

CASE STUDY 5: MARY—COACHING THE ELDER CLIENT

Setting: Visiting nurse at client's home

Mary's narrative: Mary is 93 years old and lives alone and rarely leaves her house. She has three grown children, all of whom live in other parts of the country. She has felt alone since her husband died over a decade ago, and she sees her family infrequently for their holiday visits. She remains mobile but recently began using a walker for balance, and she reports experiencing spells of "forgetfulness." Local church members look in on Mary and provide a part-time companion five days a week to shop, clean, and take her to doctor appointments. A visiting nurse who is also a Nurse Coach in the community attends Mary's church and has known Mary over the years. She visits Mary at her home and assesses her ability to live independently while providing some coaching skills exploring her life and goals at this time. The family was consulted and agreed, and the Nurse Coach set up an appointment after a brief phone conversation with Mary, who welcomed the visit.

Triggers: Difficulty living independently.

Antecedents: Concerns from family and church members.

Mediators: Cognitive and physical decline.

Nurse Coach narrative: Working with the aging population presents new challenges as many people are choosing to live independently into their later years. Home health nurses have the opportunity to listen and explore the client/patient stories as they evaluate and assess daily living skills. Support for elders in this phase of their lives is so important as often new choices need to be considered, including independent living challenges and end-of-life care.

Session 1 with Nurse Coach (NC)

NC: Thank you for inviting me to your home. I notice you have many plants, and they appear to be so well cared for.

Mary: Yes. Plants are my only companions these days.

NC: I know that the church members come and visit you. I wonder if have been attending some of the same church events?

Mary: No, I am not going out much.

NC: You don't go out much?

Mary: Only for doctor appointments, and the van picks me up.

NC: You live in an active senior community. Tell me about the activities they offer.

Mary: There are many activities. I used to go to the shows and even take art classes but... (she drifts away)

NC: What has changed for you?

Mary: My husband. We went everywhere together...(long pause)...he died a few years ago, and my life just stopped. We went to the theatre downtown, and they have a beautiful clubhouse here where we would go to shows.

NC: (Listens and knows it was over a decade ago that her husband died.)

Mary: I lost interest in everything. I felt disconnected to the world...to myself...He was everything to me...a wonderful man.

NC: He sounds like a wonderful man.

Mary: Oh yes. We had a good life. I loved traveling and going out.

NC: Would you be willing to tell me about a favorite trip?

Mary: Oh yes. And I can show you some photos from when we were on a cruise to Alaska. We danced at night and went to shows. The natural environment was breathtaking. (Mary showed the Nurse Coach photos and describes in detail the trip with her husband. After a while, she became tired and needed to rest. She thanked Nurse Coach for visiting.)

NC: It was wonderful visiting with you today. Thank you for sharing your wonderful life. May I visit you again as I would love to hear more about your travels?

Mary: I would like that.

NC: I will come by next week.

Nurse Coach Summary Notes

Mary has lived a full life and wants to remain independent in her home and with her memorabilia and memories until the end.

- The client is evaluated for skills of daily life and ability to live alone.
- The client stories are what appear to be most important to her at this time in her life.
- The client was monitored for health issues. (On a recent visit to her primary care physician for progressive fatigue, she was found to have an HbA1c of 9.7%, a blood pressure of 190/106, and PHQ-9 score, suggesting major depression. Although she was taking medication for hypertension and an SSRI for her depression, her symptoms did not appear to improve.)
- The client's family has requested additional support services, which led to the Nurse Coach visits.

Session 2 (one week later)

NC: I am happy to see you. How has your week been for you since I was here?
Mary: The days are getting longer, and being alone is so hard.
NC: Can you imagine some new activities in your life?
Mary: Oh, I don't know.
NC: You have a lot of church friends who would love to see you. There are Sunday activities after church. Would you like to go?
Mary: How would I get there? I can't drive anymore. I can barely walk.
NC: The church has a van, and many of your friends go to church in the van.
Mary: Oh. I didn't know that.
NC: Can I arrange this for Sunday?
Mary: I think I would like that.
NC: Perhaps there are other programs you would like to attend here in the community center? You know, they also have a van to pick you up. I brought the program with me, and I can review the activities with you. (As I reviewed the activities, Mary's attention was aroused by the program on "Telling your Story.")
Mary: You know, I think I have a story to tell...I would love to leave it to my grandchildren and great-grandchildren who hardly know me anymore. They all lead such busy lives and live in so many far-away places, and I can no longer travel to visit them.
NC: That sounds like a wonderful idea. It looks like they provide a recorder that you can talk into and then a volunteer can transcribe your story onto paper. Would you like to try that?
Mary: I would like that. I do not have a lot of time left but I would like to share my life. When I was a little girl in Ireland I came over on a boat to Boston. I worked and went to school and had wonderful teachers. That is where I met my husband and married and traveled the world for his business and for pleasure and met so many wonderful people. We had a good life.
NC: It sounds like you have had a very fulfilling life that would be wonderful to share. I can call for you and see how this can be arranged. I will see you in church on Sunday.

Nurse Coach Summary Notes

- The client is seeking meaning and leaving a legacy for her family.
- The client is open to outreach efforts to stay engaged in her faith-based community.
- The client is evaluated for her health and monitored.

Session 3 (two weeks later)

NC: It was wonderful to see you at church last Sunday...and so many of your friends were happy to see you.

Mary: I was happy to see them. You never know if it will be the last time...

NC: Do you want to talk about what you mean by "maybe the last time"?

Mary: I am beginning to feel like I am not going to be around too much longer.

NC: Can you say more about what you are feeling?

Mary: It is just a feeling that my time is coming.

NC: What are you hoping for at this time?

Mary: A peaceful death.

NC: What do you see helping you to have a peaceful death?

Mary: I would like to see my children and my grandchildren and be with them again.

NC: That sounds like a wonderful idea. Have you spoken with them about this?

Mary: No, not yet.

NC: It sounds like it is time to have this conversation.

Mary: Yes, it is.

NC: Would you like to make a call now?

Mary: Yes, but I cannot remember my daughter's number. I think it is written on the note pad by my bed.

NC: (Goes and finds daughter's number, dials it, and hands phone to Mary who speaks with her daughter. Her daughter makes plans to make reservations and to call her siblings and other members of the family to organize a visit the next month.)

Mary: That was so wonderful to speak with my daughter. I am so happy that I will see everyone. It will be a special occasion.

Nurse Coach Summary Notes

Mary knew that her light was slowly dimming. She was clear that she wanted to control her life until her last breath. She signed up for the class and recorded her life story, which provided her with wonderful moments of joy and sadness. Her family arrived for a visit filled with love and memories. Mary died a month later.

CASE STUDY 6: MARIA—COACHING AROUND *SUSTO*: A CULTURAL ILLNESS

Client's Presentation

Setting: Community hospital

Maria's narrative: Maria, a migrant farm worker, relocated to South Florida from the highlands of Guatemala. She frequently experienced abdominal pain and nausea. One evening, her cousin brought her to the emergency room of the local hospital. After a work up, nothing was found and Maria was given a prescription for her stomach pain and was sent home. At her follow-up visit, her symptoms had progressed and she was to be admitted to the hospital for further tests and her cousin accompanied her. The nurse noted that her pulse was rapid and her breathing was shallow. When the nurse began to ask some questions about her condition, her cousin shared that Maria was extremely worried and felt helpless and isolated from her family. In listening to the story, the nurse discovered that Maria recently received tragic news that several members of her family had been in a terrible car accident back in her village in Guatemala. Maria's cousin diagnosed her as afflicted by *susto*, a "folk illness" triggered by severe fright (from the verb *asustar* in Spanish that means "to frighten"). This story had not been told to the busy ER doctor on intake. The nurse sat down with Maria in preparation for her discharge home and wanted to explore her treatment options through Maria's beliefs for what she needed to assist her in getting relief from her pain. The nurse spoke Spanish and was able to communicate with Maria without an interpreter. The Nurse Coach had connected with Maria earlier in the ER.

Triggers: Fear and loss.

Antecedents: Separation from family and feeling isolated from community and culture.

Mediators: Indigenous beliefs and hope in going to a local healer.

Nurse Care Coordinator (NCC) narrative: In preparation for planning Maria's discharge from the hospital and for providing continuity of care, Maria was assigned to the Nurse Care Coordinator who had been Maria's translator in the ER on two separate occasions. The Nurse Care Coordinator was aware of the cultural beliefs of the local indigenous farm worker community, knowing that the cultural dimensions of health extended beyond physical symptoms and that medical interventions had repeatedly demonstrated its limitations. Integrating cultural competencies and nurse coaching skills, the NCC was effective in exploring patient outcomes for healing on multiple levels.

Session with Nurse Care Coordinator (NCC) (using nurse coaching skills)

NCC: Hello (speaking in Spanish). You may not remember me but I was in the emergency room when you arrived and I translated for you. I am here to see you as you are being discharged today and if there is anything that you need that I can assist you with.

Maria: I remember you (nods and smiles and takes the nurse's hand, looking into her eyes).

NCC: The tests did not show anything but I know you are still having abdominal pain. Do you have an idea of what might be causing your symptoms?

Maria: She nods yes and says "susto."

NCC: You call your problem susto? Can you tell me more about it?

Maria: It is because I am very worried about my family and do not know if they are okay. They are so far away.

NCC: It must be very difficult for you. What do you think can help you at this time to relieve your pain?

Maria: The doctors cannot help me. There is a healer (curandero) in my neighborhood and I need to see him.

NCC: What are the most important results you hope to receive with the curandero?

Maria: He will call in the ancestral spirits to protect my family whether they are alive or dead. He will create a ritual for them to cross peacefully and not be alone.

NCC: That sounds like it is very important special ritual.

Maria: Yes.

NCC: Who do you know that can contact the healer for you?

Maria: My cousin who is here to take me home but she doesn't believe in this anymore. She says it is from the "old country."

NCC: Would you be willing to ask her to assist you in going to the healer?

Maria: It is the only way for me...and for them...(Maria and her cousin spoke, and they agreed to go to the healer together. They needed to go to a local market to purchase some offerings including incense, herbs, and an egg. As Maria was preparing to leave, she appeared visibly relieved as if something was lifted from her and she was no longer holding her hand on her abdomen. The healing had begun.)

Nurse Coach Summary Notes

Having established a prior relationship in a vulnerable moment, the Nurse Care Coordinator was able to explore with Maria the meaning and beliefs about her health and her explanatory model. Everything shifted in this profound yet brief therapeutic encounter as Maria experienced a feeling of genuine concern by the nurse, allowing for authentic communication. Maria experienced a feeling that her beliefs and her story's meaning of what was needed to get well was being acknowledged, respected, and listened to. Physiologically, this exchange may have lowered her stress response, slowed her pulse, softened her breath, shifted her energy, and lessened her pain (see Chapter 18).

SUMMARY

- Case studies demonstrate the interaction of the bio–psycho–social–spiritual–cultural–environmental factors that are present when a client/patient request a Nurse Coach or nurse coaching.
- Case studies explore the client/patient list of concerns and benefits to each aspect of their lifestyle behaviors.
- Case studies examine client/patient options for changing behaviors and focus on core values, strengths, motivators, and reasons for change.
- Case studies identify the client/patient and stages of change, challenges, obstacles, and beliefs that may interfere with behavioral change.
- Case studies demonstrate nurse coaching and how to co-design strategies for possible solutions for behavioral change leading to sustained change.

NURSE COACH REFLECTIONS

After reading this chapter, the Nurse Coach will be able to bring awareness and personal insight to the following questions:

- What concerns do I have about my current health?
- How might my current behaviors influence my health or future health concerns?
- Do I believe that my current lifestyle supports my health and wellbeing?
- What changes do I want to make in my current patterns or behaviors?
- What do I believe to be my challenges or obstacles (stand in the way) for moving forward?

REFERENCES

Note: See Chapters 7, 8, and 9 for additional references related to Integrative Lifestyle Health and Wellbeing (ILHWB).

Nightingale, F. (1860). *Notes on nursing: What it is and what it is not* (p. 1). London, UK: Harrison.

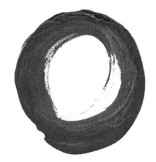

CHAPTER 11

Awareness and Choice

Bonney Gulino Schaub

> When I was a child, I remember reading that Sir Isaac Newton... said in his last hours: "I seem to myself like a child who has been playing with a few pebbles on the sea shore — leaving unsearched all the wonders of the great ocean beyond."
>
> *Florence Nightingale, 1872*

LOOKING AHEAD...

After reading this chapter, you will be able to:

- Explore the Vulnerability Model as a way of listening to the story.
- Identify forms of fight-or-flight patterns that can be obstacles to achieving desired coaching goals.
- Help clients/patients to recognize these fight-or-flight patterns.
- Empower clients/patients to learn awareness practices that make positive change possible.

DEFINITIONS

Psychosynthesis: An approach to working with people that includes the psychological and spiritual aspects of the person. It was developed by Roberto Assagioli, MD, of Florence, Italy in the early 20th century. He pioneered the integration of imagery and meditative practices into patient care.

Subpersonalities: Differing and sometimes conflicting patterns of thinking, feeling, and behaving that exist within our overall personality.

Vulnerability: The underlying feeling of uncertainty and threat to survival that all living beings experience.

Willfulness: A pattern of trying to exert power and/or control over difficult situations.

Will-lessness: A pattern of trying to escape difficult situations and challenges.

Willingness: Being open to learning and creative thinking when faced with challenges.

THE CHALLENGE

Patients or clients coming to meet with a Nurse Coach are motivated by the need to make changes in their life that they have been unable to make on their own. There are many reasons patients or clients show up. It may be from a desire to address their health and wellness challenges, or they may be coming at the recommendation of their healthcare provider, family member, or friend. They may be coming in response to a significant change in their life circumstances such as grief or loss. They may show up wanting to get in shape, be healthier, and have more energy. But whatever the variety of stated reasons, the common theme is the recognition that they need to change.

If change was easy, people would not need a Nurse Coach. They would just keep walking along directly to their goal. But, the client/patient has instead taken the action to find and meet with a Nurse Coach. Showing up is itself an important action step, reflecting that there is some aspect of this person that she or he is willing to change. As a Nurse Coach, this initial willingness is where you start. The first task at hand is to help the person identify what he or she is hoping for in his or her present life situation. This process can also identify deeper hopes and goals as a person moves toward meaningful and sustainable change.

The initial willingness for change will meet resistance from the person's habitual ways of being. Our habits are patterns of thinking and behaving that reflect the attitudes, ideas, outlooks, experiences, and beliefs that have shaped who we are. As a result, our habits may feel like "us" and generate a certain loyalty because they are familiar and safe. There is the possibility of "taking refuge in the habitual as a way of dealing with suffering by connecting to familiar ideas or conceptual models of how the world is/should be, and who is within it" (Bruce, Schreiber, Petrovskaya, & Boston, 2011).

Subpersonalities

One way of approaching a person's habitual patterns is to recognize that these patterns are not representing the totality of this individual's capacities. A particular pattern may be a dominant part—but not the whole person. Moore (2013) posits that coaches can invite "all of a client's capacities into a coaching process," helping clients to "engage their whole selves" and "reach beyond their dominant capacities and agendas" to "bring forth the quieter and less assertive capacities," thereby engaging their full potential. This insight emerges from the subpersonality aspect of psychosynthesis (Assagioli, 1965).

Assagioli wrote: "We are not unified; we often *feel* that we are, because we don't have many bodies and many limbs, and because one hand doesn't usually hit the other. But metaphorically, that is exactly what does happen within us. Several subpersonalities are continually scuffling: impulses, desires, principles, aspirations are engaged in an unceasing struggle" (Ferrucci, 2009).

We can observe this conflict in the way people bring forth different aspects of themselves in different situations and relationships. A very successful business person may come for nurse coaching because of repeated failures in quitting smoking. The person is well aware of the negative effects of smoking and has actually suffered embarrassment because he or she sees it as a failure or weakness on his or her part. Clearly, the successful business person has qualities and skills and is capable of multitasking, working well with other people, managing others, and conceptualizing at a high degree of competence. Why have all these qualities and skills not been successfully employed in the service of smoking cessation? The ability to step back, become aware of, and observe these contradictory aspects of self can begin to uncover obstacles to success at quitting smoking.

Assisting a person to step back and notice a habitual pattern is an important step in being able to make changes. Having one tool or pattern of reacting does not work in the complexity of our daily life. The comment attributed to Abraham Maslow, "If you only have a hammer, you tend to see every problem as a nail," reflects the importance of having a bigger toolkit. The variety of awareness practices in Appendix F is part of expanding the toolkit available to both clients/patients and Nurse Coaches.

THE VULNERABILITY MODEL

The Vulnerability Model (VM) is a model for understanding the underlying reason for patterns of protective behaviors and the way these set patterns can be obstacles to change (Schaub & Schaub, 1997). It presents these patterns as rooted in the habitual ways that each person's fight/flight survival instincts are expressed. The biochemistry of fight/flight is hard wired into us and is frequently stimulated throughout the day at any moment that we feel threatened. In the Vulnerability Model, we look at these fight/flight patterns as manifestations of the way we, as living beings, use our life energy to protect ourselves. We use the word *will* to describe the directing of our life energy into these patterns.

What is it about being alive that is so threatening? All of us, without exception, are subject to change and loss in any moment, and deep down we know this to be true. This is the truth of our basic vulnerability in the world, our human condition, our existential reality.

Bruce et al. (2011) have worked extensively in palliative care. They documented and described the experiences of people and their families when they are confronted with a newly diagnosed terminal illness. They described the emotional impact of this as one of "groundlessnsess." The patients they interviewed spoke of being shaken to their core, of words being inadequate, and of this information causing them to have a new experience of the nature of reality. The curtain that had separated them from full awareness of their vulnerability has been abruptly drawn back. Bruce et al. refer to this as existential suffering.

Clearly, in order to go about and function in the world, we find ways to avoid awareness of this truth—but our vulnerability reveals itself each time we go into fight or flight. Fight/flight reactions are the signals that we just felt threatened by someone or something.

An understanding of vulnerability and the variety of reactions it evokes has the potential to strengthen both the Nurse Coach's client/patient relationship and the Nurse Coach's own self-development. Since we share this universal fact of our vulnerable human situation, the recognition of it gives us a deep common bond with everyone we meet and work with. Recognizing and being open to the potential value of vulnerability as a source of connection enhances the Nurse Coach's ability to be fully present with a client. The energy that has been absorbed in protecting and avoiding this truth becomes available to be applied in new, creative ways. Each part of the Vulnerability Model, as depicted in **Figures 11-1, 11-2,** and **11-3**, will now be discussed.

Our Will

In the Vulnerability Model, *will* is the part of our nature that directs the use of our life energy. We do this directing of energy all day long, every day, without any conscious awareness that we are doing so. For example, you think one thought, rather than another thought, because you have directed energy into the first thought. This process of energizing one thought, rather than another, in the Vulnerability Model outlook, is an act of *will*. One of the goals of the model is to make these acts of *will* conscious so that you can choose where you are directing energy in your daily life and in the path of your life. Each breath, thought, and action we have is composed and activated by our life energy, our *will*.

In itself, this is not a new idea. Every healing system makes reference to this life energy and its implications for health. Some examples of this include *ki* (reiki), *chi* (*chi gong, tai chi,* and acupuncture), *prana* (yoga and aryuvedic medicine), subtle energy (biofeedback), libido (psychoanalysis), and Holy Spirit (Christianity).

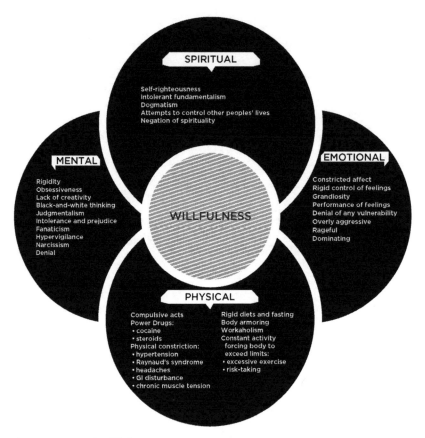

Figure 11-1 The Spectrum of Willfulness.
Source: Used with permission. Schaub, B. R., & Schaub, R. (1997). *Healing addictions: The vulnerability model of recovery.* Albany, NY: Delmar Publishers.

Health is the ability to maintain and live in a state of balance and equilibrium. Our biological systems maintain innumerable homeostatic processes to enable this to occur at the physiological level. But the concept of balance does not demand a steady state. It requires adaptability and the ability to restore balance in response to different circumstances and terrains. The way we direct our *will*, the way we harness and use our life energy, contributes to this desirable state of homeostasis and balance.

The uses of our life energy, our acts of *will*, are present in every aspect of who we are. They affect us across the spectrum of our bio/psycho/social/spiritual self. The Vulnerability Model highlights the balanced and unbalanced uses of our life energy.

The forceful, instinctive, fight use of this energy is referred to as willfulness, as seen in Figure 11-1. The flight expression of this energy is referred to as will-lessness, as presented in Figure 11-2. The point of balance and flow is willingness, as presented in Figure 11-3.

Despite your wishes, you were conceived.
Despite your wishes, you were born.
Despite your wishes, you live.
Despite your wishes, you die.

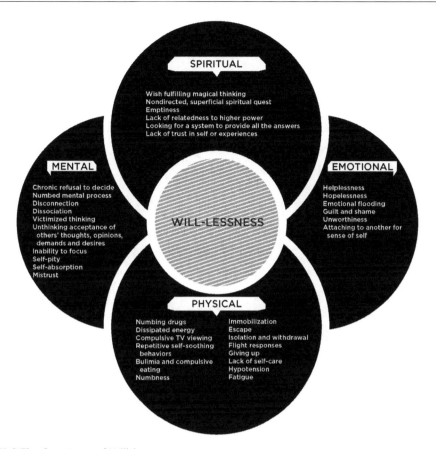

Figure 11-2 The Spectrum of Will-lessness.
Source: Used with permission. Schaub, B. R., & Schaub, R. (1997). *Healing addictions: The vulnerability model of recovery.* Albany, NY: Delmar Publishers.

> Despite your wishes, you are destined
> to deal with the consequences of your actions.
> So get on with it.
> *Rabbi Eliezar ha Kappar*

THE CHOICES: WILLFULNESS

Willfulness can pervade inner and outer behaviors in every aspect of life. There are circumstances when this is the most essential and appropriate response, times when certainty and action are required, but this approach is clearly not fitting in all circumstances. When coaching a person, examining what is or is not working is an important part of the coaching conversation.

We can operationalize the specific behaviors, attitudes, and responses that are associated with this willful way of being.

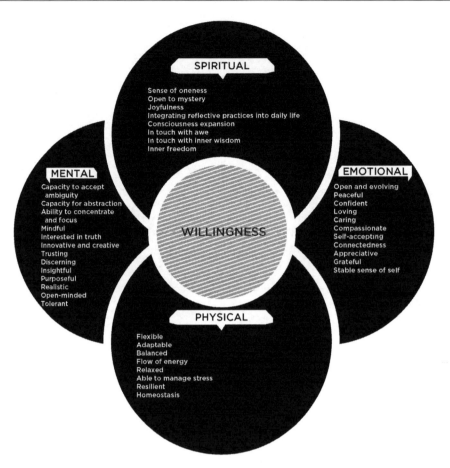

Figure 11-3 The Spectrum of Willingness.
Source: Used with permission. Schaub, B. R., & Schaub, R. (1997). *Healing addictions: The vulnerability model of recovery.* Albany, NY: Delmar Publishers.

Mental Willfulness

Mental willfulness is the forceful use of the mind to feel and assert power and control. This has the potential for misuse as seen in the following vignette.

Vignette: Marshall

Marshall was referred to coaching at his wife's insistence. He agreed to meet with the nurse coach to end his wife's nagging and also because he was going to a coach, not "a shrink." Marshall is a 45-year-old man who smoked marijuana daily. He was a college graduate who had been in the Peace Corps and at one time taught high school math. He lost his job as a teacher 15 years ago because he was found smoking marijuana in his car on his lunch break. He never accepted the fact that this was inappropriate behavior for a high school teacher, maintaining that the principal and other teachers were jealous of him. He pridefully insisted that he was the most popular teacher in the school because he could relate to the kids. He never returned to teaching because he said the system was filled with "losers and control freaks."

In the initial session, Marshall said he was coming to coaching to "get my wife off my back." She always complained about his marijuana use. Marshall worked intermittently in construction and his wife provided the primary family income working as a waitress. He told his Nurse Coach that he did not want his wife to complete college because she was only buying into the system. Marshall constantly found fault with any authority figures, and could recite a litany of circumstances to justify this opinion.

Observation

When the coach asked Marshall what had motivated him to set up an appointment, he said he only came to the session to placate his wife. Marshall displayed many characteristics of willfulness, as seen in Figure 11-1. Characteristically, a person with a very strong reliance on this pattern of thinking and feeling only shows up for coaching under duress. They do not judge their thinking or behavior as negative. They often see it as someone else's problem, for example, a spouse's, a supervisor's, or an authority figure's. There is no motivation to change.

Rigidity

Mental willfulness is characterized by rigidity of thinking. If we understand that the intention underlying willful thinking is to ward off vulnerability, then it makes sense that forming rigid, dogmatic attitudes would be one way to create an illusion of power and invulnerability. The person always has the answer. The refusal to tolerate ambiguity, confusion, or relativity results in a reliance on a black-and-white view of the world. Consequently, judgmental attitudes and intolerance of indecision are common characteristics. Extremes of this thinking result in prejudice, racism, and fanaticism.

Obsessing

Mental rigidity can also be seen in obsessive and hostile thought patterns. A person may ruminate about past injustices and embarrassments. Commonly, he or she relies on the defense mechanism of projection: accusing others of feelings, thoughts, and behaviors that he or she has. This pattern of willfulness will be very challenging in a coaching relationship. There is a refusal to take responsibility, or to even acknowledge that taking responsibility is an option. The logic in this thinking attributes all problems to the actions and attitudes of other people, places, and things, which then provides justification for all of his or her own failures in life.

Lack of Creativity

Absence of creativity, poor adaptability, and paucity of problem-solving skills all result from this constricted thought pattern. The mind is preoccupied with vigilance and anger. It is not given the ability to relax, imagine, or intuit. The person is cut off from some of the most resourceful and adaptive qualities of the mind.

Emotional Willfulness

Emotional willfulness is the misuse and manipulation of feelings to gain power and control. The following vignette describes a pattern of emotional willfulness. It also describes the origins of this behavior.

Vignette: Marco

Marco was referred to a Nurse Coach through the Human Relations (HR) department at his job. He was a project manager in the company's Information Technology department and had been referred because of complaints about his angry outbursts and insulting comments to his co-workers. He is an intelligent man who overcame a lot of obstacles to complete his education and get this job. He was surprised about the complaints about his behavior. He thought people were too sensitive. He told the Nurse Coach that he had always needed to fight for anything he got.

Marco told his Nurse Coach that as a teenager he had not done well in school. He had been socially awkward, always seeking approval and attention from other kids. What he had going for him was that he was big and strong. He was able to get by with his aggressiveness and fighting ability. After high school, he worked his way through college. He knew he was smart and didn't want to do menial work with losers. Marco acknowledged that he was provoked by his co-workers' whining and complaining. He recognized that they often felt intimidated by him but that was how he got things done.

Observation

Marco was highly motivated to work on changing his behaviors. His work was extremely important to him as both a source of income and self-esteem. His ability to have some awareness of the origins of his behavior suggested that he will be able to learn skills to manage his reactivity. Awareness of patterns allows the possibility of making choices to react differently.

Rage

Marco displayed classic characteristics of emotional willfulness. He had created a wall around his emotions, occasionally allowing for explosive verbal displays of rage that were then "resolved" by silence. In meeting with his Nurse Coach, Marco displayed some insight into his reactivity, but having insight does not necessarily lead to changes in behaviors. His coach introduced practices to increase Marco's ability to self-observe and take a breath before reacting. He was interested in learning these practices. He and the Nurse Coach established a plan for continuing these practices on his own.

Marco was also taught the Let Go practice when he noticed himself beginning to feel angry. See Appendix F-3 for the script of this practice. Marco's growing ability to self-observe made him want to explore how and why these patterns of reactivity occurred. This exploration went beyond the role of a Nurse Coach. Marco decided to pursue psychotherapy, and so he was given the names of two psychotherapists, colleagues of his Nurse Coach. He also chose to continue his work with the Nurse Coach for continued support in deepening the awareness practices.

Constricted Affect

Another expression of emotional willfulness is constricted affect. The person exerts control over expression of any feeling. This was Marco's "silent treatment" that he exhibited after his outbursts of rage.

Performance of Feelings

Performance of feelings is an insincere, false, contrived, and/or seductive emotional style used by a person to manipulate and control others. This inauthentic display of emotions can be very convincing. For the person who uses this, it can become so deeply habituated that he or she loses any awareness of genuine emotional reactions or experience.

Grandiosity

Grandiosity is a prime willful emotion. It heightens the person's mood through inner fantasies of self-worth and criticizing and demeaning the worth of others. Since grandiosity is not based on anything real, it eventually collapses, usually through a perceived slight or criticism. Then the person swings into the will-less emotion of humiliation. This is a classic emotional pattern. The root of the pattern is vulnerability, but the grandiosity (the defense) will be more obvious and on the surface. If you are dealing with a person who displays grandiosity, you can know, with absolute certainty, that this person is easily humiliated even though it is not overtly displayed.

Physical Willfulness

Physical willfulness is the misuse of the body's energy in a forceful, strained, constricted way to exert power and control. It is important to make the distinction between a person who chooses to push him/herself into doing something that is personally important and meaningful versus a person who feels compelled to do it. The following vignette offers a description of physical willfulness.

Vignette: Gloria

Gloria, a 35-year-old single woman, was referred to a Nurse Coach by her oncologist. She had been treated for breast cancer and had a mastectomy. Her doctor was concerned because Gloria's blood pressure was elevated and in addition, she was insisting she had to resume jogging and was pushing herself too much. She had gained 5 pounds since her surgery and was extremely upset about this. She timidly admitted that she had even tried to estimate how much her breast had weighed to add that amount to the 5 pounds she had gained.

In her high school years, Gloria had been preoccupied with her weight, frequently taking nonprescription weight loss products or laxatives. When she went to college, she started using cocaine on a daily basis. She liked it because it made her feel confident and it reduced her appetite. Gloria stopped taking cocaine after about a year of using it. After she stopped the cocaine, she started running. She wanted to be sure she would not gain weight. She also loved the high she felt when she ran.

In recent years, Gloria had to run at least eight miles a day, four miles in the morning and four after dinner. She was determined to not gain any weight and ran even when she had injuries. If she did not run this distance she feared she would get fat. This would then cause her to become anxious and irritable.

Gloria stated that she was coming for health coaching to learn some stress management skills to help her blood pressure. She was taking medication for her hypertension and was being monitored by her physician. She did not want to have to raise her dosage. She also took Valium occasionally if she could not sleep and she was worried because she was getting anxious about her weight gain.

Gloria did not understand why her doctor was worried about her running and her careful monitoring of her weight. She viewed this as her way of taking care of herself. She admitted that she had not told her doctor of her past use of cocaine and said she was able to stop using it when she became a serious runner. She took great pride in this accomplishment.

Observation

The Nurse Coach and Gloria agreed to focus on using stress management practices to help lower her blood pressure. They contracted to meet for three sessions. Gloria was given two awareness practice worksheets to use at home. See Appendices F-5 and F-7 for practice worksheets and Chapter 12 for a clinical description of the use of these practices.

Physically Willful Behaviors

Physical willfulness is expressed through activities that are attempts to use, control, or manipulate the body in ways that create feelings of power or invulnerability. Behaviors such as excessive exercising, as seen in Gloria's case, create the illusion that one can exert control over life. Gloria will force her body to bend to her will, which will not be stopped by illness, fatigue, injury, bad weather, or the pressure of other responsibilities.

In meeting with Gloria, the Nurse Coach is struck by the fact that her cancer diagnosis and treatment is never mentioned. She expresses great pride in the fact that prior to "this surgery" she maintained the same weight she had in college. Gloria's only concern is about her weight gain.

Physical behaviors that are characterized by willfulness include:

- rigid diets, excessive fasting, and anorexia
- use of substances to heighten feelings of power and/or push limits, such as methamphetamine, cocaine, steroids, excessive caffeine and power drinks, and so-called "smart drugs" such as Adderal
- risk-taking behaviors such as driving a car aggressively and recklessly
- participating in dangerous sports
- extremes of body-building

These behaviors are often treated with pride as indicators of mastery, victory, and superiority. Even though these behaviors may bear a resemblance to athleticism and health-promoting activities, they can in fact be damaging and destructive to the body. The body's signals are ignored and defied. At the most essential level, any awareness or feelings of vulnerability are overridden by the focus on physical power. Gloria has used exercise and focus on her weight as a distraction from and "powering over" her vulnerability.

Physical Symptoms of Willfulness

Physical willfulness is characterized by physical strain, exertion, force, and inflexibility. These ways of being in the body result in physical constriction. Some examples of medical problems that are aggravated by this constriction are:

- the constriction of blood vessels leading to hypertension
- Raynaud's phenomenon
- headaches
- muscle strains and spasms
- gastrointestinal disturbances such as irritable bowel syndrome

Body Armoring

Another form of physical willfulness is seen in body armoring. Body armoring is the conscious and unconscious control of the body as a major coping style, resulting in rejection of the body as a source of pleasure or contact. This is often present in people who have experienced physical or sexual abuse. Extreme control of the body is an attempt to ward off the profound vulnerability that the abuse has created.

Drivenness

Physical willfulness is seen in drivenness—the desperate need for constant activity and busy-ness, done with a sense of time urgency. This is sometimes referred to as hurry sickness. It is clearly seen in workaholism.

The dilemma with many of these physically willful behaviors is that they are admired and rewarded by the popular culture. Extreme examples include anorexic fashion models or waiflike ballerinas or gymnasts who sustain their appearance by starvation, diet sodas, nicotine addiction, and other drug use. Another example is seen in workaholic businesspeople who are so much "in demand" and so successful that they have no time for a personal life or meaningful intimate relationships.

Spiritual Willfulness

Spiritual willfulness is the misuse of spirituality to feel power and control. Such willfulness is the root cause of the abuses that can take place in religious and spiritual groups. In the following vignette, the client, Barbara is mistreated by Jason, a yoga teacher, and his rigid and judgmental spiritual outlook.

Vignette: Barbara and Jason

Barbara is a 42-year-old woman who was referred to a Nurse Coach because of great pain from the death of her newborn. The loss had occurred three months prior to the referral. Initially, she had gone for spiritual guidance for help in dealing with the turmoil of her feelings. Barbara remembered that when she was a child her spiritual life had been a source of comfort and reassurance for her. When her friend's sister was killed in an accident, she had successfully prayed every night for her nightmares about this event to stop. At this point in her life, she had moved away from the religion she had been raised in. She had been on a search for something that she could believe in.

Barbara met with Jason, a yoga teacher she had worked with in the past. She spoke to Jason about her most personal spiritual feelings. She described visiting a cathedral in Italy and being moved to tears by the beauty of the place. She also described walking along the beach early in the morning, watching the sun rise, and feeling incredibly joyful. She said she wished she could connect with this peacefulness now, but she is too angry and distraught.

Jason seemed to be listening thoughtfully and intently. Suddenly, he interrupted her and told her that she needed to let go of all those old experiences. She was clinging to an illusion. She needed a bigger picture. She needed to recognize that this life is about karma. What is she supposed to be learning from this experience? She is coming from a place of being too attached. She needs to meditate more and be in the moment.

Observation

Barbara's loss was very much in the moment, and she was in pain. She experienced Jason's comments as judging her and causing her to feel ashamed about what she had shared with him. She was not spiritual enough in his eyes. At first she was devastated by what he had said. The profound shame reaction she had just experienced resulted in her leaving the meeting feeling light-headed and ungrounded.

Barbara's mind did not really agree with what Jason said, but at an emotional level, she felt like a very young 42-year-old child ashamed of herself and walking down the street in a world of adults. She felt hurt, disappointed, and alone.

Jason's response to Barbara was a classic example of spiritual willfulness. If Jason had experienced any doubts that his worldview might not have the answer for Barbara, he did not express it in any way. He asserted his spiritual belief as the truth. He needed to do this to override any inner experience of his own doubts or vulnerability. Spiritual willfulness asserts itself in the same way as willfulness expressed mentally, emotionally, and physically. It moves into control, power, anger, and manipulation. People like Jason clearly cannot tolerate ambiguity. Everything must be one way—their way. They cannot tolerate doubts. Jason sounded as if he had all the answers, but in fact what he had was a fear of not knowing. If we could enter his mind, we would find swings from absolute knowing to absolute self-doubt. Jason's swings, from knowing everything to knowing nothing, are the spiritual equivalent of swinging from grandiosity to humiliation at the level of emotional vulnerability.

Spiritual willfulness can manifest itself in the following ways:

- self-righteousness
- fanaticism

- attempts to monitor other people's inner lives
- intolerant forms of fundamentalism and dogmatism

There can be tolerant forms of fundamentalism and choosing personal expressions of religious conservatism. A person can accept such spirituality for him- or herself but still be respectful of and not threatened by the beliefs and practices of others.

Negation of Spirituality

A very different manifestation of spiritual willfulness is observed in people who refuse to consider any concept of a higher power, universal reality, or larger sense of life's purpose, cycles, and processes. They display a prideful insistence that their logic and their rational thinking can understand everything. They demean and dismiss any consideration of spiritual reality as irrational or illogical. They aggressively reject anything that has not yet been "proven" by science. This pattern of thinking is demonstrated by Victor's therapist in the following vignette.

Vignette: Victor

Victor is a 35-year-old professional cabaret singer who had been diagnosed as HIV positive 10 years ago. He had started working with a Nurse Coach because he was feeling a decline in his energy, and it was frightening him. He felt a need to make some changes in his life, and he wanted some direction.

After assessing Victor's physical condition and referring him to an acupuncturist colleague, the Nurse Coach introduced meditation and imagery practices into the coaching. These were self-care skills she thought Victor could use for managing his fears. He had many interesting experiences with his meditations and eagerly discussed them in his coaching sessions. He felt supported by his Nurse Coach when discussing these new meditative explorations. He felt the meditation contained even more potential for deepening his sense of purpose. He began to understand that his love of music and his singing brought him into a profound sense of spiritual connectedness.

One of his most fascinating meditative experiences was a sense that his consciousness could travel and experience other dimensions of reality. This experience of an expansion of consciousness was very reassuring to him when contemplating his own death.

Victor had very limited financial resources and had lost his health insurance. He became aware of a research project at a major medical center that was exploring the relationship of stress reduction with long-term survival for HIV patients. In exchange for participating in this project, he would receive free medical care. He eagerly joined the program. The treatment modality was a cognitive behavioral psychology approach to stress management, and his therapist was a graduate student.

In his first session with the therapist, Victor enthusiastically told him about his meditation practice and all he had learned about an expanded sense of reality. The therapist listened with disdain to Victor's descriptions. The therapist could barely tolerate such ideas and felt completely certain that Victor was indulging in wishful thinking and escapism. He told Victor that he needed to begin to think about and make plans based on reality. This therapist had no doubts about his own opinion and was unable to give Victor's experiences any respect. The therapist himself had never experienced such meditative states of consciousness. In fact, he rejected the whole idea of meditating. He was sure, almost aggressively absolute, about his view of what Victor had experienced.

Summary

Willfulness is characterized by rigidity and the need to control self and others. At its core are fears of loss of control and the unknown. The control is an attempt to wall off conscious awareness of essential vulnerability. The resulting effect is the loss of creativity and openness to new possibilities. It can result in the loss of meaningful relationships, and spiritual isolation. This pattern is constrictive and confining and limits a person's capacity to be adaptive in his or her life, as seen in **Table 11-1**.

Table 11-1 Willful/Fight Reactions.

Willful/Fight Reactions
Fight in your mind
Hypervigilance
Silent, ongoing criticism of others
Inflexible thinking, black-and-white thinking
Frantic defense of opinions
Desperate need to be right
Inflated and arrogant self-image
Manipulative mind
Judgmental mind
Cynicism
Fight in your feelings
Easy to anger
Rage as a way of control
Aggressiveness
Grandiose mood
Constricted withholding of feelings
Fake performance of feelings
Denial of hurt and vulnerability
Restlessness, impatience
Desire to dominate
Fight in your body
Constricted vascular system
Tension headaches
Gastrointestinal distress
Rigid diets, anorexia
Body armoring and stiffness, e.g., neck pain and low back pain
Forcing your body to exceed limits (i.e., risk taking, extreme sports)
Fight in your spirit
Religious-based, self-righteous condemnation of others
Spiritual arrogance, having the answers
Dogmatic rigidity
Cynical negation of spirituality

Source: Used with permission. Schaub, R., & Schaub, B. G. (2013). *Transpersonal development: Cultivating the human resources of peace, wisdom, purpose and oneness.* Huntington, NY: Florence Press.

THE CHOICES: WILL-LESSNESS

Those who stay awake too late at night
neglect the body;
Those who walk alone
neglect the heart;
Those who allow the mind to be idle
neglect the soul.

All these forfeit life—
Even while they live, they are dead.
Rabbi Chanina ben Chachinai

Willfulness is about fight and power. In contrast, will-lessness is about flight, escape, and numbness. Vulnerability is avoided by behaviors that are diffuse, chaotic, ineffectual, and confused. Acts of will-lessness look, on the surface, to be without choice. As a Nurse Coach, you should be aware that choice is very much involved in will-lessness.

Mental Will-lessness

Mental will-lessness is the misuse of the mind to feel numb. The forms of mental will-lessness include:

* chronic refusal to decide
* numbing of mental processes through disconnection and disassociation
* unthinking acceptance of other's thoughts and desires
* victimized thinking

The following vignette reflects a person functioning from a place of mental will-lessness.

Vignette: Veronica

Veronica is a 43-year-old single woman who was referred to a Nurse Coach for help in decreasing her debilitating anxiety. She had significant financial stressors. Veronica was working at what she referred to as a "dead-end job" that barely met her financial needs. She was single and had a very limited support system. She had significant debt from unpaid medical bills for breast cancer treatment at the age of 39.

She hated her current clerical job but felt she had to stay at the job because it provided health insurance. Her acquaintances were involved in promoting and selling holistic health products and convinced Veronica to get involved in this business because they said it had amazing possibilities to bring her supplemental income. The business appealed to her because she had always been interested in holistic health and had specialized in vegan cooking at the catering business she had previously worked at. She was reluctant to make the financial commitment required to get started. These "friends" were insistent and kept pushing her to get involved. They belittled the work she was doing, saying she was not being true to who she was. They finally convinced her to go to one of the marketing seminars where she would learn how to market and promote herself.

When she was at the meeting, she felt embarrassed because everyone there was so upbeat and excited about what they were doing. The marketing leader, Frank, kept saying that only losers were afraid to take the steps to be successful in life and that this business was an amazing opportunity. He made joking remarks about people who had come to other meetings and left because they had been too afraid to be successful. The group had all these slogans and positive statements they would recite together to get them ready to go out and recruit other sales reps. There was so much energy in the room that Veronica began to feel that these people had something she wanted. She finally signed up and made a commitment to be involved in the complete training program that would prepare her to do the marketing.

Observations

Veronica got involved with the group and paid for the training with her credit card because she was reassured that this was a fantastic investment. Once she started to attend the meetings, she began to feel uncomfortable with what she had gotten involved with. Her fear of being wrong in her decision or looking foolish in front of the acquaintances stopped her from fully acknowledging what she was feeling disturbed about at the meetings. She felt upset by Frank's practice of manipulating and humiliating certain people in the group. It was definitely creepy, but she was just not "willing" to let these perceptions guide her in what to do. She was not "willing" to let her mind fully process what she was experiencing. Veronica's fear of looking foolish, of not being liked, or being a loser did not make this processing impossible, but it certainly did make it more difficult. She chose not to focus her mind on these perceptions. She distracted herself whenever she began to try to think the situation through and make a clear decision.

Disconnecting from the Mind

Mental activity includes the processing of our rational thinking, our images and imagination, our intuition, our memories, our emotions, and our physical sensations. We instinctively synthesize all of these complex experiences and, in time, try to derive learning from them.

We think of the mind as a way to understand things better. Sometimes, in fact, the mind is utilized as a way to know nothing, to avoid, to be numb, or to experience oblivion. Mental will-lessness is a way of refusing to use the mind. A person like Veronica is refusing to learn from experience. Mental will-lessness is the choice of disconnecting from what your thinking mind is telling you. This disconnect is often accompanied by surrendering to being distracted by meaningless, trivial thoughts and activities.

Refusal to Trust Instincts and Intuition

Veronica's instincts were warning her, but she did not allow her mind to make meaning of these reactions. She felt she could not back out because it would be too humiliating to be making a mess of things again. She felt vulnerable and feared she would be mocked when the group found out about her concerns. She felt so unsure of herself, but she was also worried that the "friends" who had brought her into this group would not like her. They might even be mad at her if she left.

Chronic Refusal to Decide

The chronic refusal to decide includes avoidance, denial, and procrastination. For example, distractibility is a method of self-protection used by many people. What does someone accomplish by procrastinating, by staying away from an action or a decision? One avoids setting in motion an unpredictable response to the action or decision. Procrastination can be influenced by a foreboding feeling that "something bad" will happen if the decision is made or the action is taken. "Something bad" includes rejection, failure, and incompetence. No one wants to experience such things. If such negative outcomes are expected, then they can only be avoided by not taking the action or making the decision.

Unthinking Acceptance of Another's Thoughts and Desires

This form of will-lessness is oriented around avoiding conflict at all costs. By agreeing with things that she does not agree with and by accepting things that are unacceptable, Veronica is seeking to keep others placated. The outer conflict is avoided. The inner conflict is not. The person using this form suffers greatly inside while at the same time feeling some relief that she has kept everyone else happy and, therefore, not angry at her.

Victimized Thinking

Victimized thinking is a mental pattern pervaded by self-reference, self-absorption, and self-pity. It often disguises anger at others and anger against the self for being so fearful.

It often leads to a decision to do nothing or to justify self-destructive or self-defeating behavior.

This pattern is evident in the following vignette.

Vignette: Jane

Jane is 27 years old and was referred to a Nurse Coach for smoking cessation. She worked at a copy center and graphic design studio. Her employer was putting pressure on all the employees who smoked to quit. The boss had recently quit and was complaining that it made it harder for him to have his workers standing around outside the shop smoking. Jane told her Nurse Coach that her boss had the classic "convert" mentality. He had quit so he wanted to convince everyone else that they should too.

Jane explained that quitting smoking was not that important to her, but she was doing it for the sake of keeping her job. She also mentioned that her doctor had done some breathing tests on her last visit and told her she needs to quit. Jane expressed anger at all the people telling her what to do. She said she would give it a try because cigarettes are too expensive now, but "I'll probably spend more money on food." She was very concerned about gaining weight since she gained weight the last time she quit smoking.

Another reason Jane gave for being ambivalent about quitting was that on 9/11 she had been downtown on her way to school when the World Trade Center was attacked. She saw the second plane hit. She breathed in all the toxic dust and smoke, and she thinks her lungs are probably already damaged from that experience.

Jane said she thought a great deal about the world since then. She said nothing ever changes, and that good people are always crushed by power-hungry leaders. She concluded that her relapse to smoking cigarettes was a minor matter compared to the sick world she has to live in. She also said her best friends all smoke, too. Within her vision of the world, this makes perfect sense: the world is a terrible place, it makes her upset, she needs something to soothe herself—give in, smoke, it doesn't matter anyway.

Observations

Jane views the world as something being done personally to her. She rationalizes that she cannot fight all the depressing realities of life. This kind of thinking can pervade a person, fostering a sense of powerlessness. It also serves as an excuse for not taking any healthy actions.

Emotional Will-lessness

Emotional will-lessness is a focus on hopeless and helpless feelings and moods in order to be too numb to make decisions and take actions. The following vignette describes how this pattern appears in behavior.

Vignette: Evelyn

Evelyn is a 31-year-old woman referred to a Nurse Coach for pain management. She had been dependent on pain medication following a car accident at the age of 28. She had recovered from her dependence on prescribed pain medications one year ago, but had suffered from anxiety and phobias ever since the accident. She was not able to drive after dark because her accident had taken place at night. She avoided certain roads that would bring her in the vicinity of where the accident had occurred.

She had recently begun a relationship with Piero, a much older man she had met at her food co-op. Evelyn experienced relief in dating someone who she felt totally understood her, accepted her, and could take care of her. He did not judge her for her anxieties and fears. She became dependent on him. At the same time, she panicked at any hint of problems in the relationship, believing she would fall apart without Piero's help.

Attaching to Another for Sense of Self

Evelyn's attachment to her pain medications had been intense. They had helped her cope with the trauma of her accident. Removing them from her life left her with a sense of emptiness, a void. She was preoccupied with anxiety and vulnerability. This made it impossible for her to feel any new sense of herself. Anxiety kept her busy just trying to survive. In Piero, she saw someone she could be—Piero's girlfriend. She judged herself harshly for still being anxious: after all, the accident was almost 3 years ago. She did not have any particular feelings for Piero. In actuality, she was emotionally numb as often as she could be in order to blunt her anxiety and memory of the accident.

Depression

Other emotions associated with will-lessness are feelings of hopelessness, helplessness, and unworthiness. These feeling states are classically associated with clinical depression. When working with a client in this state of mind, referral to a counselor for psychotherapy may be warranted.

Physical Will-lessness

While physical willfulness is characterized by strain, exertion, force, compression, constriction, and rigidity, physical will-lessness is characterized by:

- numbness
- collapse
- escape
- withdrawal
- immobilization
- giving up
- flight responses
- procrastination

These choices can lead to symptomatic levels of:

- loss of libido
- bulimia and compulsive eating
- lack of self-care and attention to personal hygiene
- repetitive self-soothing behaviors such as masturbation
- fatigue and listlessness
- compulsive use of TV or other on-line distraction

These symptoms are all related to withdrawal of energy. Hypotension can be thought of as insufficient energy being exerted within the circulatory system. Likewise, a lack of energy and engagement with the world is an aspect of loss of libido. This absence of passion can be reflected in every part of life. Mindless self-soothing such as compulsive masturbating is numbing and enervating. The self-soothing aspect of compulsive food binging and purging also brings on numbness. Again, energy is drained from the person. People often describe feeling light-headed or "stoned" after an episode of purging, while overeating results in feeling bloated and lethargic. Lack of attention to personal hygiene reflects withdrawal of energy from even the most basic physical activities.

A pattern of physical will-lessness is seen in the following vignette.

Vignette: Warren

Warren is a 58-year-old man referred to a Nurse Coach for life direction and help with career decisions. He had been unemployed for the past year. He lives with his wife and has three grown children who are living on their own. He had worked for a local tire manufacturing company for the last 25 years but was laid off. Initially, after the loss of his job, Warren spent time working on his favorite pastime: setting up model train layouts in his basement. He eventually became bored with this and also did not want to spend the money on materials. He began watching television during the day and often napping. At night, he put on the television to help him fall asleep. When Warren was awake, he kept the television on constantly, even if he was occupied with some other activity.

Numbing Behaviors

Warren displayed lethargy, excessive sleeping, and compulsive TV watching. These are all will-less physical acts performed to avoid any awareness of feelings. Warren was a person who never talked about his feelings, and he felt shame at the possibility of revealing anything about how betrayed he felt about losing his job. His layoff had come as a total shock because he had just received an excellent evaluation from his foreman.

Spiritual Will-lessness

In spiritual willfulness, a client's energy is caught up in knowing all the answers to life's questions. In spiritual will-lessness, the dissipated energy is not enough to even engage in struggling with spiritual questions and answers. The will-less client looks exclusively to others as sources of guidance. He or she looks to others to provide the energy for the quest. Will-lessness in spiritual life is characterized by nondirected, immature, magical, superficial, and, unfortunately, empty attempts to satisfy natural spiritual feelings and impulses.

From the perspective of the Vulnerability Model, spiritual development is crucial to health and well-being. It has great relevance for connecting people with a sense of meaning and purpose that motivates people to make life-affirming changes. Helping a client to connect with this aspect of self becomes an important step on the way to making positive choices and changes.

For many people, their religion is the way they relate to spirituality. "*Religion* refers to an organized system of beliefs shared by a group of people and the practices related to that system. Ritual, worship, prayer, meditation, style of dress, and dietary observances are examples of such practices." (Burkhardt & Nagai-Jacobson, 2013). For others, their religious affiliation is a social or cultural identity, or they may feel ambivalence toward their religion because aspects of it are hard to believe. There is also a growing population of people in the United States that identify themselves as "nones," meaning that they are not affiliated with any religion (Pew Research Center, 2012).

Spirituality refers to something more essential to human nature than a particular religion. It is not unusual to hear people say they are "spiritual" but not "religious." Spirituality is the innate impulse in each person to know about the universe they are born into. "Spirituality is at the core of the individual's existence, integrating and transcending the physical, emotional, intellectual and social dimensions... A person's spiritual dimension encompasses much more than a doctrine established by others. This dimension allows one to experience and understand the reality of existence in unique and direct ways that go beyond one's usual limits" (Landrum, Beck, Rawlins, Williams, & Culpan, 1993, p. 26).

The following vignette presents a client who is struggling with will-lessness in the domain of spirituality.

Vignette: Jessica

Jessica is a 47-year-old married woman referred to a Nurse Coach for help with deep grief over the death of her sister in a car accident. As a child, Jessica had been enriched by her church attendance. Soon after her marriage, however, she stopped going to church. Her husband had always been critical of the churches she attended, finding fault with the minister or the other parishioners. She finally gave up trying to attend because she did not want to go alone. At the same time, she did not want to deal with her husband's negativity.

During the past 18 years, Jessica had explored many different spiritual practices and philosophies. Each time she found a new spiritual book or group, she would wholeheartedly embrace this new perspective as the answer she had been searching for. She would use her latest spiritual insight as the answer to everything. However, she never followed through on any deeper exploration or practice. She said she could not because her husband would undermine her interests or get angry about them.

At the heart of these repeated capitulations was a belief that she could never achieve true insight and knowledge. What would happen if she really tried to develop spiritually and failed? Consequently, she settled for living with a profound sense of emptiness. When she experienced the sudden death of her older sister, she went in to an emotional crisis without any spiritual practice or perspective to help her.

Jessica's vignette demonstrates:

- magical thinking
- emptiness
- lack of relatedness to God or some concept of a higher power

Magical Thinking

Magical thinking is a child-like belief in having immediate, wish-fulfilling, and simplistic answers to the complex situations of life. For Jessica, magical thinking was based on expecting all the answers to come from outside of her. As a result, when she found a spiritual method or system of thought, she immediately, and without discernment, started applying that system's answers to all her personal problems and her spiritual questions. She wanted desperately to have a system to identify with so that her searching could be over, so that she could feel safe.

This approach is destined to be unsatisfying because the person never personalizes or integrates any system. In Jessica's case, she tried to memorize the ideas and vocabulary of the systems she read about. She quoted spiritual systems without truly knowing them. The heart of her magical thinking was hoping a system would have all the answers so she could avoid the issue of her poor relationship with her husband and her vulnerability.

Lack of Confidence

Jessica's magical thinking was partly the result of having no confidence in her intelligence. She was a good worker, had friends, and was interested in art and culture, but still lived with great doubt about her intellect. She found it difficult to defend her thinking in the face of any conflict. In other words, when she felt anxious and vulnerable, she became will-less. Behind her desire to have a system that had all the answers was her inability to feel confident in her own answers.

Emptiness

A second important factor contributed to her desire for a system that had all the answers: she was desperate to fill an emptiness. Emptiness is an emotional experience marked by absence, longing, varying degrees of numbness, and feeling that something essential is missing. She found it hard to describe this emptiness since it was characterized mostly by what was not there.

There is the possibility of moving from an essential sense of emptiness to a discovery of connection and oneness. There is evidence derived from current brain research showing that there is am innate capacity of our brain to experience states of oneness and union that have been called "absolute unitary being" (Newberg & D'Aquili, 2001). This oneness "...refers to the part of your nature that is capable of uniting with the energy of the universe beyond the limits of your mind and body" (Schaub & Schaub, 2013).

Even though mainstream western psychology has thus far shown minimal interest in spirituality, the entire area of spiritual development is a rich subject for the Nurse Coach working from an integrative perspective. Experiencing a state of oneness "helps to heal the fears related to your vulnerability as a separate self trying to survive in an uncertain world" (Schaub & Schaub, 2013). This will be elaborated on in exploring Willingness.

Lack of Relatedness to God or Higher Power

As a child, Jessica had strong feelings of contact with God. She stopped going to church to avoid conflict with her husband. As an adult, she had not experienced any of the relatedness to God that she enjoyed in childhood. Relatedness to God is a feeling of living with oneness and a deeper presence in the self and in the world. The lack of this feeling was a loss of major proportions for her.

Jessica presents an example of someone who is blocked from spiritual development by emotional, psychological issues. Most directly, she is cut off from worship because she fears her husband's anger. These fears are the result of her childhood fears of her father. She cannot assert her spiritual needs with her husband. She never commits herself to regaining or renewing her spiritual life.

Obstacles to Spiritual Development

Jessica needs the Nurse Coach's assistance in recognizing how her spiritual will-lessness keeps her from deeper healing. Spiritual will-lessness is an example of an obstacle to spiritual development. Obstacles to spiritual development are emotional attitudes and fears that block the opening of the personality to spiritual consciousness.

Addressing blocks to spiritual development may sound like territory beyond the Nurse Coach's role, but, in fact, just the opposite is true. In *Mental Health Psychiatric Nursing* (1984), Shannon, Wahl, Reha, and Dyehouse state:

> "...the nurse needs to be able to assess the individual's spiritual needs... The term spiritual refers to the search for a meaning in life and a belief in powers greater than oneself. In assessing the spiritual dimension, the nurse uses all of her interpersonal skills: listening, communication, observation, and interviewing. Because spiritual needs are often expressed subtly instead of overtly, the nurse needs to be sensitive to detect the expression of spiritual needs" (p. 215).

Many people suffer from blocks to this development and cannot reach this degree of emotional healing. As Landrum et al. (1993) advise:

> "The spiritual dimension is the most elusive for many people because of the individual nature of spirituality for each person and because of the tendency, particularly in Western culture, to emphasize what is tangible. Our spiritual dimension deals with a reality that is not tangible and that is more than what we are able to perceive through our senses" (p. 26).

A Nurse Coach has the opportunity to follow and encourage the client in his/her journey from living in vulnerability to living with wisdom and compassion through his or her spiritual development. The goals of spiritual development are therefore not abstract or esoteric. They are emotional and practical. Spiritual development is the deeper part of health and wellness: feeling at one with the world. Nurse coaching has the potential to help a client identify his or her best path toward experiencing feeling at ease, centered, and at one in harmony with life. Flaherty, in describing components of satisfaction and effectiveness, includes the soul as an essential area of competency to consider. He includes compassion and kindness as qualities to notice in the coaching client as well as the "experience of connectedness to the rest of humanity/life-forms on earth" (Flaherty, 2010, p. 74).

Summary

Will-lessness is a choice. Made repeatedly, it does not work. Nevertheless, it must be understood as an attempt to manage vulnerability. In this regard, it needs to be honored. Of course, there are always exceptions. There are times when will-lessness is exactly the best choice, the most intelligent survival technique. The Nurse Coach, in understanding the process of will-lessness and its manifestations on the mental, emotional, physical, and spiritual levels, can help the client to make the healthiest choices possible. Examples of will-less reactions that can be obstacles to change are listed in **Table 11-2**.

Table 11-2 Will-less Reactions.

Will-less Reactions
Flight *in your mind*
Worrying and ruminating
Chronic refusal to decide, maintenance of confusion
Inability to think clearly
Numbed mind, dissociation
Mindlessness
Ongoing search for distraction
Self-pitying, victimized thinking
Automatic people-pleasing
Indifference
Flight *in your feelings*
Anxiety, nervousness
Helplessness
Hopelessness
Escape into feelings, overwhelmed
Feelings of numbness, frozen
Shame, desire to hide
Guilt without having done anything wrong
Co-dependence
Flight *in your body*
Wired, anxious sensations
Compulsive TV watching
Repetitive self-soothing such as excessive masturbation
Eating too much, stuffing
Avoidance of situations
Lack of basic self-care

(continues on next page)

Table 11-2 (*Continued*).

Will-less Reactions
Flight in your spirit
Religious wishful thinking
Nondirected spiritual dabbling
Emptiness
Lack of relatedness to a higher power or larger vision of life
Lack of meaning

Source: Used with permission. Schaub, R., & Schaub, B. G. (2013). *Transpersonal development: Cultivating the human resources of peace, wisdom, purpose and oneness.* Huntington, NY: Florence Press.

THE CHOICES: WILLINGNESS

A person's inner wisdom is more available when in a state of balance and centeredness. It brings the ability to recognize old patterns and be willing and open to new ideas and ways of being. This quality of willingness is what allows the client to consider new possibilities, create new strategies, and make sustainable, life-affirming choices. The quality of willingness is reflected in the vignette below. Note that Bill is aware of a pattern that is creating difficulties at work. He is willing to examine it and decide to practice new ways of reacting.

Vignette: Bill

Bill was returning to work with a Nurse Coach he had worked with in the past. He was experiencing great anxiety and needing to make decisions about his life. He was having trouble with his small business. He daydreamed about doing violent things to his competitor. He also daydreamed about letting his business fail and of going off to a foreign country and starting his life over. What should he do—should he actually carry out his illegal daydreams or should he get out of his business altogether? His fantasies and feelings went back and forth.

In working with his Nurse Coach, he began to realize that he had to tolerate the uncertainty and ambiguity of his situation. He had to be willing to stay with the discomfort of not knowing. For Bill, this was an emotional challenge. His daydreams of violence and of going off to a foreign country were both fantasies of ways to get rid of the uncertainty of his situation.

Through his coaching conversations and awareness practice experiences he was developing a capacity to notice his own thoughts and feelings. The growing capacity for awareness broadened his ability to recognize more and more clearly a larger perspective on what he was dealing with both personally and with his business. He was able to acknowledge the wise choices he had made in the past. He was recognizing that there is a middle way in most circumstances, and he was acknowledging that he had to be willing to tolerate ambiguity, one day at a time.

Observation

The impulse to get rid of negative feelings was part of an old pattern for Bill. His reactive choices—violence or move away—were ways of thinking left over from his adolescence that had gotten him in trouble in the past. Through previous work with his Nurse Coach, Bill had been able to develop a greater ability to watch the process of these thoughts. This coaching relationship had helped him to become a successful business owner. He had not acted out on these thoughts in many years. His current feelings of vulnerability, generated by the potential downturn in his business, had resulted in his recognizing that he needed to return to coaching for a "tune-up." Bill saw this as an opportunity to re-examine what he had learned and explore additional strategies for working through his business troubles.

Self-awareness, Choice, and Self-responsibility

It bears repeating that willfulness and will-lessness are attempts to maintain health in the face of vulnerability. The fact that you can observe people swinging back and forth between these two ways of being can be recognized as attempts to achieve homeostasis. The desire is to experience a balanced sense of self—not too anxious or too depressed, not too angry or too afraid.

A balanced sense of self has the quality of feeling centered, grounded, at ease, and stable. In this state, you feel you have all your resources fully available to you. You trust yourself. You feel you can act effectively in the world.

In the face of this desire for a balanced sense of self, the willful and will-less responses need to be honored, not judged as pathological. They simply turn out to be poor choices because, over time, they do not work. Bill swings from impulses toward violence (willfulness) to impulses toward "escaping" to a foreign country (will-lessness) to resolve his business anxieties. Made repeatedly, these swings increase vulnerability and instability. In the Vulnerability Model, willingness is seen as the better choice.

THE EXPERIENCE OF "WILLING"

The transpersonal psychiatrist Roberto Assagioli said that the inner experience of willing takes place:

> "...During periods of silence and meditation, in the careful examination of our motives, in moments of thoughtful deliberation and decision, a 'voice', small but distinct, will sometimes make itself heard, urging us to a specific course of action, a prompting which is different from that of our ordinary motives and impulses...it comes from the central core of our being" (Assagioli, 1965, p. 9).

Dynamic Balance

Willingness is not a static state. It is an active balancing between the extremes of willfulness and will-lessness. This ideal of dynamic balance is spoken of in various spiritual and philosophical teachings. It is a concept known by many names, as seen in **Table 11-3**.

Table 11-3 Cross-cultural Concepts of Dynamic Balance.

- the balance of yin and yang energies in Taoism
- the Soto Zen way of effortless effort
- the concept of passive volition in biofeedback training
- the Greek ideal of the golden mean
- the Buddhist path of the middle way
- the AA advice of finding a place of wisdom from which to know when to change something and when to accept something
- Roberto Assagioli's concept of the balance and synthesis of opposing impulses in the personality
- the profound common sense of moderation in all things

Source: Used with permission. Schaub, B. R., & Schaub, R. (1997). *Healing addictions: The vulnerability model of recovery.* Albany, NY: Delmar Publishers.

THE ACTIONS OF WILLINGNESS

Willfulness and will-lessness are extremes. That is why both of those choices in time exhaust the person. Willingness is a balanced, easier, more adaptive response to life. This place of balance and ease is often the experience that coaching clients express as a goal they would like to work toward. The three actions of willingness are seen in **Table 11-4**.

TABLE 11-4 A.A.A.: The Three Actions of Willingness.

A. A. A.: THE THREE ACTIONS OF WILLINGNESS
A. A. A. refers to the three actions that lead to living with willingness: attention, noticing what is actually happening, and choosing a life-affirming response.
Action Step 1: Attention. This refers to bringing awareness to our inner experience. The inner experience might be a thought, an image, an urge, an impulse, a sensation, or a mood. This step stresses the point of not turning away from our experience, trying to ignore or avoid it. The spirit of this step is to be open to noticing our experience.
Action Step 2: Actually. This refers to the action of keeping our attention on the experience long enough to discern what is actually happening.
Action Step 3: Affirming. Having taken the above two actions, the person now has enough information to be able to choose a positive, affirming thought or behavior in response. It is important to note here that a person cannot choose how to feel. He or she can choose how to think and act, and these thoughts and actions will produce new feelings.

Source: Used with permission. Schaub, B. R., & Schaub, R. (1997). *Healing addictions: The vulnerability model of recovery.* Albany, NY: Delmar Publishers.

The First Action: Turning Our *Attention* Toward Ourselves

In nurse coaching, the first action of willingness is to turn attention toward vulnerability. If everything was going fine for a person, they would not need a Nurse Coach. The first action is getting clarity on exactly what the challenge is that has brought a person to the coaching relationship. For example, is it the recent medical diagnosis itself—or some life-defeating reaction that it has triggered inside the client?

The Second Action: Discerning What Is *Actually* Happening

The second action is to keep attention on the thought or feeling long enough to truly know what it means. There is not one uniform reaction that people have to a medical challenge. The Nurse Coach helps the client get to the essence of what this challenge means to the person.

This action counteracts the tendency to immediately get away from the vulnerability. Instead, with attention kept on it long enough, the need to get rid of it is replaced by insight into the vulnerability.

The key insight, which is experienced and learned over and over again, is that the vulnerability is tolerable, normal, and passes without anything bad happening. This is the key emotional fact for a person facing a challenge. This awareness opens up innumerable possibilities for making new choices. As Whitmore (2009, p. 70) puts it, "We have a measure of choice and control over what we are aware of, but what we are unaware of controls us."

The Third Action: Choosing an *Affirming* Response

Tolerating vulnerability could be seen as a goal. A healthier goal is to develop new, life-affirming responses to vulnerability. The third action of willingness is exactly this: a new response. We define the new response as choosing a life-affirming thought or behavior in the face of a vulnerable moment.

The inner conversation can then be one that notes the internal, fearful thoughts and feelings and is able to pause and choose the best response, not the reactive one. This is a basic self-care skill.

Practice: Willingness

The following imagery practice explores the experience of willingness. Whenever you are guiding a client through any imagery practice, be sure to take a few breaths and pause between each suggestion. This gives your client time to connect with his or her process. See Appendix F-8 for a willingness practice worksheet. See Chapter 12 for further discussion of imagery and awareness practices.

1. Take a few moments to reflect on a goal you have for yourself. It can be any kind of goal as long as it is a real possibility and not just a fantasy.
2. Close your eyes and bring attention to your breathing.
3. In your imagination, experience a path extending from where you are to the top of a tall hill...Now, imagine your goal and place it on the top of the hill.
4. Now, starting from where you are, experience yourself willing to travel along the path...As you move along, become aware of the obstacles that try to pull you off the path...Notice these obstacles...Now reconnect with your sense of purpose and your willingness to reach your goal.
5. Experience yourself on the top of the hill and fully identify with the goal...Allow yourself to feel what it is like having achieved the goal.
6. When you feel ready, bring your awareness back to the room and make some notes on what you have experienced.

Discussion of Willingness Practice

This practice can clarify the following issues:

- the goal
- the inner obstacles to the goal
- the inner strengths needed for achieving the goal
- the potential for staying on the path despite the obstacles
- the possibility of achieving the goal
- the experience of succeeding
- the rewards for achieving the goal

These clarifications enhance willingness. They give the person specific information about the challenge being confronted. Without specifics, the person is often blocked by vague doubts and moods, and the goal can seem hopelessly remote. The person experiences a nondirected struggle, a generalized frustration. The Nurse Coach helps the client see the real possibility of success.

This willingness practice can bring a nondirected struggle into focus and give it direction. Obstacles can be identified as specific problems to be addressed on the way to the goal. Vague feelings of incompetence can be replaced by directed actions to solve specific problems. This exercise can be repeated many times. The information is always new and relevant in the present moment.

Taking Actions

By taking actions, feelings change. A common mistake people make is to think they should wait until they feel better before taking an action. This is an attempt to keep feelings in a comfortable zone. The person feels too vulnerable to take any risks. Implicit in this thinking is the belief that the action will be difficult and painful. Often, the belief is that the action will not succeed and even worse, will lead to rejection, failure, and shame. To keep from being rejected, the person does not take the action. This thinking is based in the belief that "I'm going to fail." As a result of failure, he or she will experience shame. This basic, negative belief can be the obstacle to envisioning success.

In the face of this belief, taking an action is almost an act of faith. In the terms of the Vulnerability Model, it is an act of willingness. It is a willingness to test the vulnerability and to find out that it is tolerable. Often, when the action is taken, it turns out to be not as bad as anticipated and may actually be experienced as a relief. As a result, the negative belief is proven untrue.

Taking actions and experiencing the results becomes an important learning process for the client in a coaching relationship. To make this process more effective, certain self-care skills are extremely helpful. Awareness practices that support skills in acting from an attitude of willingness will be described in Chapter 12. As you will see, the practices and attitudes of willingness open clients to their internal wisdom and their natural drive to have meaning and purpose available to them in their life.

SUMMARY

- The Vulnerability Model describes patterns of willfulness and will-lessness that clients/patients struggle with in making positive changes in their lives.
- By appreciating these patterns and struggles, Nurse Coaches can bring awareness and compassion to the clients/patients sitting in front of them.
- Resistance to change will emerge in the habitual patterns of willfullness and will-lessness. From the perspective of the Vulnerability Model, these resistant patterns are normal and understandable and can be skillfully worked with once self-awareness is established.
- The Vulnerability Model does not propose, unrealistically, that we get rid of these resistant patterns. Rather, it says we can notice them but choose not to engage with them.
- The way through these struggles, and the direction of energy toward the achievement of sustainable coaching goals, is the process of willingness.

NURSE COACH REFLECTIONS

After reading this chapter, the Nurse Coach will be able to bring awareness and personal insight to the following questions:

- What have I identified as my patterns of response to vulnerability?
- What are the changes that I would like to make in my life?
- How have I managed challenges in the past?
- When have I been successful in making positive changes?
- What part of me was most active and supportive of success?
- What do I understand about the personal obstacles and blocks that came up for me?

REFERENCES

Assagioli, R. (1965). *Psychosynthesis: A manual of principles and techniques.* New York, NY: Viking Press.

Bruce, A., Schreiber, R., Petrovskaya, O., & Boston, P. (2011). Longing for ground in a ground(less) world: A qualitative inquiry of existential suffering. *BMC Nursing, 10*(2). Retrieved 08/15/2013 from http://www.ncbi.nlm.nih.gov/pubmed/21272349

Burkhardt, M. A., & Nagai-Jacobson, M. G. (2013). Spirituality and health. In B. M. Dossey & L. Keegan (Eds.). *Holistic nursing: A handbook for practice* (pp. 721–749). Burlington, MA: Jones & Bartlett Learning.

Ferrucci, P. (2009). *What we may be: Techniques for psychological and spiritual growth through psychosynthesis.* New York, NY: Tarcher/Penguin.

Flaherty, J. (2010). *Coaching: Evoking excellence in others* (3rd ed). New York, NY: Elsevier.

Landrum, P., Beck, C., Rawlins, R., Williams, S., & Culpan, F. (1984). The person as a client. In C. Beck, R. Rawlins, & S. Williams (Eds.), *Mental health psychiatric nursing: A holistic life-cycle approach* (pp. 17–39). St. Louis, MO: C. V. Mosby.

Moore, M. (2013). Coaching the multiplicity of mind: A strength-based model. *Global Advances in Health and Medicine, 2*(4), 78–84.

Newberg, A., & D'Aquili, E. (2001). *Why God won't go away: Brain science & the biology of belief.* New York, NY: Ballantine.

Nightingale, F. (1872). Address from Miss Nightingale to the probationer-nurses in the 'Nightingale Fund' at St. Thomas's Hospital, and the nurses who were formerly trained there (p. 1). London, UK: Spottiswoode.

Pew Research Center (2012). *Religion & public life project.* Retrieved 07/11/2013 from http://www.pewforum.org/Unaffiliated/nones-on-the-rise-demographics.aspx

Schaub, B., & Schaub, R. (1997). *Healing addictions: The vulnerability model of recovery.* Albany, NY: Delmar Publishers.

Schaub, R., & Schaub, B. G. (2013). *Transpersonal development: Cultivating the human resources of peace, wisdom, purpose and oneness.* Huntington, NY: Florence Press.

Shannon, C., Wahl, P., Reha, M., & Dyehouse, J. (1984). The nursing process. In C. Beck, R. Rawlins, & S. Williams (Eds.), *Mental health psychiatric nursing: A holistic life-cycle approach* (pp. 198–236). St. Louis, MO: C. V. Mosby.

Whitmore, J. W. (2009). *Coaching for performance: GROWing human potential and purpose* (4th ed.). London, UK: Nicholas Brealey Publishing.

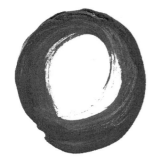

CHAPTER 12

Awareness Practices

Bonney Gulino Schaub

The world, more especially the Hospital, is in such a hurry, is moving so fast, this it is too easy to slide into bad habits before we are aware...

Florence Nightingale, 1873

LOOKING AHEAD...

After reading this chapter, you will be able to:

- Help clients/patients to connect with their inner wisdom as an on-going resource for sustaining positive changes.
- Identify the mind–body–spirit effects of awareness practices such as meditation and imagery.
- Learn awareness practices that promote the ability to make healthy choices.
- Recognize thoughts and patterns of behavior that reflect willingness to change.
- Guide your client/patient through awareness practices that enhance the capacity to sustain changes.

DEFINITIONS

Absolute unitary being: A natural state in which you temporarily suspend all self-centered fears and enter into a feeling of oneness with the primal energy of life.

Mental imagery: The conscious use of the power of the imagination for therapeutic purposes.

Relaxation response: A coordinated mind–body shift from an agitated, aroused sympathetic nervous system to a calm, balanced, parasympathetic response as a result of a meditative practice.

Transpersonal experience: The experience of connection with inner peace, wisdom, purpose, and oneness that exists when one is liberated from the habits and patterns of personality.

CONNECTING WITH INNER RESOURCES OF WISDOM

Although the clear light of reality shines inside their own minds, most people look for it outside.

—*Padmasambhava*

The goal of coaching is "building awareness, responsibility, and self-belief" (Whitmore, 2009, p. 18). An important objective of deepening awareness of inner knowing is to enable an individual to assume responsibility for choices and actions. The process of connecting with this inner resource leads to the strengthening of self-belief.

The variety of awareness practices presented in this chapter are mind–body–spirit techniques that are derived and modified from diverse cultures and spiritual traditions: prayer, imagery, meditation, contemplation, breath awareness, mantra, and *qi gong*.

These practices help to quiet the mental chatter of worry and fear, allowing a subtler "voice," a subtler source of knowing, to be available. When listening to the client/patient's story, be curious to learn about past experiences where he or she had a sense of knowing that resulted in deep satisfaction, resilience, or success. What inner resource did he or she feel connected to that was trusted and provided guidance?

A person may be surprised when asked about her or his inner wisdom or guidance. It is very likely that she or he has not been asked about this before. Their response might be "I just had an intuition," or "I just knew what to do," or "I think it must have been luck." It can be quite exciting for a person to learn that connection with an inner source of wisdom, and knowing it can be nurtured. This human potential can become more available to her or him when she or he learns to use imagery and other awareness practices for self-care and self-development (Schaub & Schaub, 2013).

It is essential for the Nurse Coach to trust that each client/patient has the potential to connect with his or her own resources of life-affirming inner wisdom. This reinforces the energy of willingness and reduces the negative influence of habitual willful and will-less patterns that are presented in Chapter 11.

Willingness is the client/patient's act of directing energies toward healthy, life-affirming choices and actions.

SKILLS AND PRACTICES THAT OPEN AWARENESS AND FREEDOM TO CHOOSE

When confronting challenges and experiencing obstacles to change, a person needs to be willing and ready to learn and utilize new inner skills. The safest, most successful changes come when people listen deeply to what is essential and meaningful for them and create plans of action from this place of self-knowledge.

The Origin of Awareness Practices in Nurse Coaching

Awareness practices have their origins in Eastern and Western spiritual traditions. As a professional working in a multicultural society, however, it is not appropriate for you to introduce awareness practices in the context of a spiritual tradition. The working context for the Nurse Coach is secular and science-based. Awareness practices need to be offered within this context.

Assagioli and Jung

The origins of the secular and science-based use of awareness practices in healthcare began in the early 20th-century work of Roberto Assagioli (1965) in Florence, Italy and Carl Jung (1933) in Zurich, Switzerland. They had served as physicians through two World Wars in Europe. As psychiatrists, they saw the urgent need for traumatized clients to discover, in their own nature, the paths to resiliency and inner strength. Assagioli emphasized meditative awareness practices and imagery for positive growth, and Jung stressed the discovery of guiding inner wisdom through symbol study, visualization, and dream work (Schaub & Schaub, 2013).

They were both knowledgeable about the spiritual roots of their awareness practices. Assagioli taught himself Sanskrit in order to read the Indian spiritual texts in their original language and personally meditated in an adaptive form of Buddhist mindfulness. Jung studied Eastern and Western alchemy and spiritual philosophy and traveled to indigenous tribes to study with their shamans. They both chose the word *transpersonal* (meaning *beyond the personality*) as a more accurate term than *spiritual* in describing their integration of science and spirituality.

Their pioneering work is the origin of the integration of a diversity of approaches to awareness practices introduced into healthcare in America beginning in the 1970s. Herbert Benson's (1975) clinical application of mantra meditation to evoke the relaxation response, Elmer and Alyce Green's (1977) pioneering research on biofeedback and higher states of consciousness, Ken Wilber's (1977) expansive integral psychology model that contributed to the conceptualization of the Theory of Integral Nursing (Dossey, B., 2013), John Welwood's (1983) work on the introduction of mindfulness into psychotherapy, Lawrence LeShan's (1989) groundbreaking work in mind–body medicine, Jon Kabat-Zinn and T.N. Hahn's (1990) important work of introducing mindfulness and yoga into a hospital-based program for pain management and stress reduction, Larry Dossey's (1994) exploration of the influence of prayer and the nonlocal mind in healing, and many others have expanded upon the original contributions of Assagioli and Jung.

National Institutes of Health

Meditation, imagery, prayer, yoga, *t'ai chi*, and other spiritually based awareness practices are now recognized and accepted as components of the practice of mind–body medicine. They offer adjunctive and supportive additions to standard medical care. The National Center for Complementary and Alternative Medicine of the National Institutes of Health advocates that health professionals should become "catalysts and guides" in teaching these awareness practices (NCCAM, 2011).

THE SCIENTIFIC BASIS OF AWARENESS PRACTICES

Meditation-Based Practices

Applied forms of meditation are the most commonly researched awareness practices. Meditation in general is a beneficial practice for focusing the mind and calming the body. The following lists are summaries of some of the benefits of this calm meditative state. There is a rapidly expanding body of research on meditation. Through searching the NIH website at www.ncbi.nlm.nih.gov/pubmed, you can keep current on the most up-to-date studies.

Physical Benefits

The ability of Western science to quantify specific physiological changes due to meditation resulted in greater acceptance of the introduction of these practices into mainstream healthcare. As you read through this list of beneficial changes resulting from meditation, think about the implications for their application in your nurse coaching work:

- strengthens integrative fibers in the executive center of the brain
- grows new neurons and gray matter in the executive center of the brain
- calms down the amygdala (the fear center of the brain)
- helps a person to manage pain better
- lowers respiration to a degree ordinarily reached only after seven hours of sleep
- increases alpha and theta brainwaves associated with deep rest in the body

- reduces heart rate
- reduces concentrations of blood lactate, which is associated with anxiety
- improves breathing patterns of patients with bronchial asthma
- reduces blood pressure in hypertensive patients
- reduces premature ventricular contractions in patients with heart disease
- reduces symptoms of angina pectoris
- reduces sleep-onset insomnia
- reduces stuttering
- reduces blood sugar levels in diabetic patients
- reduces psoriasis
- reduces salivary bacteria

Mental and Emotional Changes

As you read through this list of self-reported mental and emotional changes due to meditation, think about how these changes have useful implications for nurse coach practice:

- reduces distracted attention
- reduces the negative mental states of inner criticism and worry
- increases the experience of a calm, focused mind
- increases concentration
- increases short-term memory
- increases objective thinking
- increases access to intuitive and creative thought
- reduces fight/flight reactivity
- improves performance through imagery rehearsal
- reduces death anxiety
- increases your ability to notice your emotions
- empowers you to self-regulate difficult thoughts
- increases the emotion of tranquility

Spiritual Benefits

Of all changes due to meditation, those most difficult to measure are the spiritual changes. Nevertheless, these changes warrant special consideration. Research supports spirituality as a factor in healing, adjustment, recovery, and health promotion (Carmody, Reed, Kristeller, & Merriam, 2008). Self-reported spiritual changes from meditation and imagery include:

- experiencing pure, endless, and boundless awareness
- feeling solid and grounded like a rock
- feeling a lightness of being
- feeling serenity and contentment
- feeling a quiet joy pervading all things
- feeling unity with all beings

The Relaxation Response

How can meditation produce such an array of changes? The variable that is involved in many of these changes is the "relaxation response." The relaxation response was a term coined by Harvard cardiologist Herbert Benson (1975) to describe a coordinated mind–body shift from an agitated, aroused sympathetic nervous system to a calm, balanced, parasympathetic response achieved through meditative practice. Additionally, the meditative state extends the "relaxation response" beyond its normal cycle, bringing deep rest and restoration to the body. Physical manifestations of stress, such as increased heart rate, pulse rate, blood pressure, and muscle pain and stomach acidity are all lowered by the relaxation response.

Many of the mental/emotional changes produced by meditation can also be attributed to the stress-reducing effect of the relaxation response. As one example, nervousness makes it difficult for you to concentrate and remember, but meditation's relaxing feature will increase your concentration and memory (Jha, Stanley, Kiyonaga, Wong, & Gelfand, 2010).

Brain Research and the Essence of Meditation

A research picture is emerging that may show us the essential action of meditation. It involves the brain's neuroplasticity. To develop the picture and see its possible benefits, we need to start with a perspective on one of our inner resources—awareness.

Your awareness is different than your thinking mind. It notices what you are thinking, but it does not think. It notices feelings in the body, but it is not those feelings. Right now, as you read this, you are aware of yourself reading, but your awareness is not reading. Instead, your awareness is concurrently noticing what you are reading, noticing what you think of it, noticing how you feel about it, noticing the room you are in, and so on. Awareness notices what is going on, but it is not any of those things that are going on.

You cannot see your awareness. You cannot touch it, you cannot feel it. To date, researchers have not been able to find it in the brain. Awareness remains a physiological mystery. Yet it is not a mystery in our daily experience. Quite the contrary: It is always with you, always working for you, always noticing. And if you did not have awareness, you would have no experience at all. Awareness does not seem to be a thing that we can see or get our hands on, and yet it makes everything exist for us.

The brain research offers a startling new fact about awareness: As soon as your awareness notices something, another part of your brain starts a narrative about what you have noticed (Farb et al., 2007). This noticing/narrating interaction has many clinical implications. The narrating function is speculated to be the brain's way of comparing what you just noticed to what you know about yourself. This self-referencing comparison is a way of determining if the new thing you just noticed is a threat or not. In other words, noticing followed by narrating is a self-preservation process. The coaching process seeks to introduce new narratives into the brain/mind so that new behaviors can result.

Awareness practices aid this new process in two ways. First, they quiet down the habitual narrating region of the brain. This is demonstrated in the fact that meditators can focus more fully on an object, are less distracted, and can remember more about what they have noticed: more focus, less distraction, more memory (Jha et al., 2010).

Clinical Uses

This research points to many practical applications of awareness practices in working with coaching clients/patients. The following list indicates health and wellness issues that can be ameliorated by awareness practices:

- reduce stress symptoms: e.g., high blood pressure, stomach distress
- reduce anxiety in the face of an upcoming medical procedure
- reduce insomnia without medications
- train students to relax and focus during tests
- teach company employees to prevent stress-related illnesses
- train a performer or athlete to enter a state of calm concentration

- expand serenity and spirituality for clients facing major life challenges
- reduce anxieties and worries without medication
- reduce social fears and self-conscious shyness
- reduce the fear of dying
- release the tension of grief
- help clients identify their values and life direction

A source for current research on meditation is the Mindfulness Resource Guide website. It includes the *Mindfulness Research Monthly (MRM)* that, in addition to providing the most recent research, also has an archive of previous MRMs (http://www.mindfulexperience.org).

The Importance of Personal Practice for Nurse Coaches

When you introduce any awareness practice to a client/patient, you will be more confident and most effective if you have had personal experience with the practice. You will then have a deeper understanding of what the process is and will be better able to teach and guide someone through her or his own experience. Your comfort level will help your clients/patients to gradually let go of their apprehension and be open to the dormant resources awaiting them in their own nature.

Healthcare providers are vulnerable to stress and burnout from processing all the suffering that they bear witness to on a daily basis (Goodman & Schorling, 2012). The added value for the Nurse Coach in having personal experience with awareness practices is in building his or her own self-care toolkit. Included in this toolkit is the wellbeing that comes from spiritual development via the practices (Sahebalzamani, Farahani, Abasi, & Talebi, 2013). Appendix F has practice sheets for all the practices presented.

Imagery and Awareness Practices

Imagery awareness practices engage the use of the imagination for creating and implementing action plans that work. Imagery has the ability to be a proactive awareness practice that can focus on choices, actions, and intentions and how to carry through on them. Clients often feel a strong sense of hopefulness and validation when they learn to experience and appreciate this inherent resource.

The reference to imagery practice can be misleading because it suggests inner pictures. Visual imagery is not the way everyone experiences their imagination. In a suggestion to "Close your eyes and imagine a lemon," imagining a lemon may be experienced with any of our senses. An individual may have a stronger sense of the smell of a lemon, or the taste or tactile sense of it. There may also be an emotional response for a person who has a strong like or dislike of lemons or associations of lemons with a memory. People tend to have sensory preferences in the way they connect to imagining, and it is important for them to know this at the outset of working with imagery practices.

When introducing imagery and other forms of awareness practices to clients, it is important to tell them that you will be working together to explore the practices that are most comfortable and effective for them. They can be reassured that there is no one "right way" to use these tools, and learning what is personally effective will be part of your collaboration. The client can also be assured that they have the choice to continue or stop a practice at any point.

In introducing imagery and awareness practices, there are classic performance anxiety concerns that can arise for both client and coach:

- What if nothing happens?
- What if something upsetting happens?
- What if I do it wrong?

Your client may be concerned that she or he will not be able to imagine anything. You may be concerned that your client/patient did not succeed at getting the suggested images. Your client/patient may be concerned that "too much" information or emotion will come up and you may have this concern as well. Your client/patient may want your approval and want to be be liked by you. You as the Nurse Coach may be concerned about having your client/patient's approval and want to be liked as well.

Understanding that these personal reactions are normal will help you to be aware of these feelings when they arise. This awareness then allows you to not respond from a reactive place. You will be able to choose the responses that are best for your patient/cient.

As with the meditative awareness practices, it is important for you to experience these imagery practices personally. This experience will engender self-confidence as well as trust in the effectiveness of these techniques. This will also help you to get a sense of pacing when guiding a person through her or his individual experience. A common mistake that is made by new practitioners is to move too quickly through the process. Becoming comfortable with pauses and silence are part of learning to work in this way. Whenever you are coaching someone through imagery or another awareness process, be sure to take a few breaths and pause between each suggestion. This helps you to be fully present and allows the client time to connect with inner experiences. It also provides role modeling when you reflect your own comfort level and trust in what is being experienced.

Mind–Body Effects of Imagery and Awareness Practices

There has been a significant amount of research on the mind–body effects of imagery awareness practices just as there has been on the mind–body effects of meditation. A comprehensive survey of the research on the physiologic effects of imagery awareness practices cites their impact on a wide range of systems and symptoms as follows:

- increasing internal blood flow, demonstrated by increased temperature in specific skin areas
- increases in heart rate resulting from imaging sexually or emotionally arousing situations
- alterations in body chemistry such as gastric secretions and salivary pH
- muscle stimulation as shown in electromyography
- immune system responses
- wound healing
- systolic and diastolic blood pressure changes in response to images of fear and anger

The Creative Possibilities Emerging from Imagery and Awareness Practices

All new ideas and creations originate in the imagination. Imagery practices open the person up to considering new possibilities and solutions. These mind–body skills, with their ability to calm anxiety and promote well-being and resilience because of their physiological effects, can also bring unexpected and creative and spiritual insights and possibilities (Braud, 2003; Ferrucci, 1990; Schaub & Schaub, 2014; Sheikh & Sheikh, 2003).

Metaphors and Images of Transpersonal Experiences

There are dormant resources of peace, wisdom, purpose, and oneness in each person without exception (Dossey, L., 2013; Schaub & Schaub, 2013). These resources are referred to as "transpersonal" because they objectively exist beyond the habits and patterns of personality.

We can experience these healing resources through mind–body practices or spontaneously, in an unexpected moment of time. Throughout human history, in all cultures and traditions, people have told fables and myths; crafted art and symbols; acted out dramas and dances; created music, rhythms, and songs; and established sacred spaces and sacred rites, all to induce contact with these resources. We need to step out beyond our ordinary, ordered way of thinking and expression to access the often ineffable quality of these resources. In our time, we have neuroscientists measuring and mapping the brain to locate the places within our brains that are activated when transpersonal resources are awakened (Hanson, 2009).

The subtlest factor to measure, but one now being explored in brain research, is how meditation awakens dormant resources in the brain. Among these inner resources, there is the state of "absolute unitary being" in which, through awareness practices, you can temporarily suspend all self-centered fears and enter into a feeling of oneness with the primal energy of life (Newberg, D'Aquili, & Rause, 2001). This is the territory that the spiritual traditions point us toward as our desired state of being.

When clients/patients are experiencing profound vulnerability, they often seek the reassurance that this contact provides. Nurse Coaches can learn to listen to and open clients/patients to their powerful inner healing resources.

Clients/patients often find it difficult to find words that fully describe or express the qualities and impact of their transpersonal experiences. Language is inadequate. The person may rely on metaphors and images to express the nature of what has transpired.

As one example, Rachel had come to meet with a Nurse Coach following reconstructive surgery after her second mastectomy. She spoke about a spontaneous experience of expansion and light she had on her way home from a doctor's visit.

Vignette: Rachel

I was driving home...the doctor had said my surgery went well and she was pleased with the way the incision was healing. I was hurrying to get home in time for my kids, and feeling bad that I might be late...They have been through so much...and I was thinking about how much I love them...Suddenly I was filled with an incredible feeling of opening wide up...I was filled with light and felt connected with everything...the sun was glorious and it filled me...I don't know how long it lasted...but then I was aware that I was in my car and still driving home, but now I knew everything was going to be all right. I felt in a state of bliss...That experience changed everything for me. I can truly say I no longer feel afraid...It's hard to explain...

Rachel said it had been a startling event. She did not identify with the religion she had been raised in, but the experience "felt like a spiritual thing." She felt great reassurance in having had the experience. Rachel also said it reminded her of how much she loves being in nature, especially at the ocean.

Rachel's experience released her from feeling immobilized by her fear and vulnerability. It sparked her interest in coming for nurse coaching to learn practices that would help her explore ways she could stay connected to the deep joy that had been present in that event.

The transpersonal opening that Rachel described has been studied in research on posttraumatic growth (Calhoun & Tedeschi, 2004). The seemingly paradoxical fact is that, for some people, stark confrontation with their vulnerability can lead to feeling liberated from fear and an enhanced state of wellbeing. This awakened state has also been described by Fanslow-Brunjes (2008) in her pioneering work with hospice patients and Firman (2012) in her work with cancer patients.

Whitmore (2009) writes about introducing awareness and imagery practices in coaching that will open someone up to a wider perspective. He describes guiding the coaching client/patient to "the reservoir of potential, of creativity, of innovation, of aspiration, of peak experience, the absolute of joy, love, and compassion." This exploration of human possibilities is studied in the field of transpersonal development (Schaub & Schaub, 2013).

The following quote addresses the nature of Rachel's experience:

The sense of wonder is based on the admission that our intellect is a limited and finite instrument of information and expression, reserved for specific practical uses, but not fit to represent the completeness of our being...It is here that we come in direct touch with a reality which may baffle our intellect but which fills us with the sense of wonder which opens the way to the inner sanctuary of the mind, to the heart of the great mystery of life and death... (Govinda, 1990)

Rachel referred to "opening" and being "filled with light" as a way to describe her experience. The list in **Table 12-1** offers some of the other symbols and metaphors associated with transpersonal experiences.

Table 12-1 Symbols and Metaphors of Transformation.

Symbol or Metaphor	Transformative Experience
Introversion	Exploration of the true self; self-knowledge; inner journey to the soul, to beingness
Deepening/descent	Journey to the underworld of the psyche; confronting the difficult aspects of the self, the shadow; entering a cave; the heroic journey of facing fears
Ascent/elevation	Climbing a mountain to reach a higher plane of awareness
Expansion/broadening	Enlarging perspective; taking in the wholeness and seeing beyond one's small, individual perspective
Awakening	Awakening from the dream or from illusions; opening to the truth or reality of what really matters
Illumination	Bringing in the light of the human soul; spiritual light to transform or "enlighten" a situation; moving from darkness to light; bringing in life energy
Fire	Purification; spiritual alchemy; candles, lanterns, bonfires, ceremonies of transformation
Development	Growth, blossoming; potentials waiting to become real
Love	Opening the heart; compassion and generosity, forgiveness
Path/pilgrimage	"Mystic way;" the journey of outward exploration; seeking to be changed by new experience or knowledge
Rebirth/regeneration	Birth of the new being; resurrection
Freedom/liberation	Liberation of psychic, physical, and spiritual energy to align with creation and creativity

Source: Copyright © 2014 by Bonney Gulino Schaub. Adapted from Assagioli, R. (1965). *Psychosynthesis: A manual of principles and techniques.* New York, NY: Viking Press.

Awareness Practices That Evoke and Support Positive Perspectives

When a Nurse Coach begins the coaching relationship with a client/patient, an important starting point will be listening for this person's potentials, strengths, and resourcefulness. The process of unlocking these potentials can be enhanced with the introduction of awareness practices that help the client to recognize what has been meaningful and rewarding in the past. Motivation and positive actions will be maximized if the client/patient establishes goals that are aligned with what is personally truly important. The following practice has the potential to facilitate this objective. The practice sheet for Connecting with Meaning and Purpose is in Appendix F-9.

Practice: Connecting with Meaning and Purpose

1. Close your eyes or just lower them if you prefer and begin by bringing your awareness to your breath...follow your breathing...just noticing it...the sensation of the inhalation and the exhalation...
2. As you do this, just allow your chair to hold you, allowing your shoulders to drop, letting your arms feel heavy...just letting go and staying connected to your breath...
3. And now let your awareness go into your imagination...and into your memory...and reconnect with a time when you experienced a sense of meaning and purpose in your life...a sense of wholeness...take your time with this and let the details come to you...
4. And now begin to realize what the essence of that time was...What was at the heart of it for you?...take your time...
5. Allow yourself to deeply connect with what you were experiencing...What allowed it to happen? What supported it?...take your time...
6. Now, let go of the practice and turn your attention to noticing how you are right now...
7. Take as much time as you need...and when you feel ready, at your own pace, bring your attention back to the room...

This practice was introduced to Philip, a 19 year old, home from college for the summer. He had been referred to a Nurse Coach by the gastroenterologist he had consulted because he was having stomach aches. The results of his medical work-up were all negative, and he was referred for coaching because he was "stressed out." Phillip stated that he wanted to get himself straightened out before returning to school in five weeks.

As a business major, Phillip was working hard at school and getting good grades, but was very anxious. The Nurse Coach had introduced Phillip to a breath awareness practice for his stress in his first meeting. (See Appendix F-5 for the Connecting with Breath: Exhaling for Twice as Long as Inhaling practice sheet.)

Phillip responded well to this in the sessions, but did not practice at home. He was very concerned about going back to school and was worried about his stomach aches returning. He also began to express doubts about his major, saying that his dad wanted him to major in business. His dad's view was that the only purpose in working was to make money: There was no sense in paying a fortune for college if it was not going to pay off.

In doing the awareness practice, Phillip remembered taking care of his injured dog when he was 12 years old. His golden retriever, Buddy, had been his pet since he was little. Buddy had been hit by a car and had two broken legs. Phillip was so surprised by this memory and was even a bit embarrassed at how emotional it was for him. He remembered that he felt so focused on helping his dog, comforting him, changing his dressings, helping him to eat, and eventually helping him to get up and walk again. Phillip also remembered that his father had teased him for being so emotional about his dog.

The Nurse Coach acknowledged how skilled and caring Phillip had been. She also noted his perseverance despite his father's teasing. She asked Phillip what meaning he gave to the fact that this was the memory that came to him. He quickly responded that he knew he wanted to do some work that would help people. He could not stand the idea of working in an office and just doing "business stuff." He commented that he had actually noticed his belly relaxing when he connected with the image. He said it was funny because now it was so obvious to him that this is what he did when he worried—he tightened up his belly and held his breath.

The awareness practice gave Phillip clarity about what why he was so stressed about school. He needed to tell his parents about wanting to change his major. He worked out a strategy and plan to do this.

The awareness practice went beyond just confirming for Phillip that he wanted to change his major. It connected him with the deeper meaning and purpose of why he wanted to do this. He was genuinely surprised about the clarity that emerged. This allowed him to overcome his obstacle to communicating with his parents.

Connecting with Wisdom Figure

We have the ability, with the use of imagery, to connect with an inner advisor. This process of inner dialogue "is so named due to an assumption that through the imagery experience, the individual dialogues with an inner advisor who is a symbolic emanation of inner wisdom, the inner physician, or higher Self" (Baer, Hoffman, & Sheikh, 2003).

People connect with personally meaningful images of wisdom figures when doing these practices. **Table 12-2** provides an overview of the nature of the types of figures that may arise in this practice.

Table 12-2 Wisdom Figures and Guides.

- Religious figures—Buddha, Jesus, Moses, Mary, Jah, Rumi, etc.
- Spiritual practitioners—monks, rabbis, priests, shamans, saints, etc.
- Figures of myth, literature, legend, folk tradition, etc.—Athena, Yoda (*Star Wars*), King Arthur's quest for the Holy Grail, goddesses, wizards, fairies, etc.
- Admired, loved people from one's personal life such as grandparent, teacher, mentor, etc.
- Historical figures—Martin Luther King, Florence Nightingale, etc.

Source: Copyright © 2014 by Bonney Gulino Schaub.

Wisdom Figure Practice

1. Lower or close your eyes, relax your shoulders, and begin to follow your breath...
2. Begin to reflect on something you are wondering about at this point in your life...perhaps something about a decision you are trying to make...or something about yourself you are trying to understand better...or something about which you need guidance...
3. Try to identify the question you are asking yourself. What's the question that gets to the heart of the matter? It's okay if you don't get it exactly.
4. And now for a moment return to your breath...
5. And now begin to move from your breath to your imagination, and begin to imagine a road or path stretching out in front of you...one you know or one you create...
6. Get a sense of walking on this road or path...What's around you?
7. And now begin to imagine, in the distance, a wise being or a wisdom figure of any kind...any kind at all...coming toward you...

8. Ask your question...and be open to whatever happens...take as much time as you want...

    Go to Chapter 13, Case Study #4 – Marianna, for a clinical example of the use of this practice. The Wisdom Figure practice sheet is in Appendix F-10.

Stress Management

Stress management and self-care techniques can include meditation, prayer, imagery, and movement-based quieting and grounding practices such *t'ai chi* and *qi gong*. The Nurse Coach can introduce these tools at any point in the coaching process.

Focusing on Breath

Breath is literally a potential source of inspiration. Each of these stress reduction practices starts with focusing on breath. Two of the practices work exclusively with the breath. All of these have the potential to enhance awareness as well as provide relaxation.

Meditation teacher Lama Govinda (1990) writes:

> ...Breathing is the only vital function which, in spite of its independence from our normal consciousness and its self-regulating and self-perpetuating subconscious character, can be raised into a conscious function, accessible to the mind. Due to this double nature, breathing can be made the mediator between mind and body, or the means of our conscious participation in the most vital and universal functions of our psychosomatic organism. (p. 115)

Practice: Centering with Breath for Stress Reduction Simple Breath Awareness

One simple technique you can use to practice for yourself, and teach others, is counting breaths. Counting breaths is a first step in many forms of meditation. (The Centering for Stress Reduction practice sheet is found in Appendix F-7.)

1. Ask your client/patient to notice his or her breathing.
2. Instruct your client/patient to count his or her next out-breath as 1.
3. Instruct your client/patient to continue to count the out-breaths until he or she reaches 10 and then start from 1 again.
4. Let your client/patient continue with this practice for about 5 minutes.
5. Suggest that your client/patient slowly bring his or her awareness back to the room and open his or her eyes.
6. Ask your client/patient to discuss with you what he or she experienced.

Discussion of Practice

One of the first physiological responses to stress is alteration of breathing patterns. Typically, the breath becomes more shallow and rapid. The simple act of centering by bringing attention to breathing tends to bring the breath back into a more relaxed rhythm. The relaxation is enhanced by the fact that the mind is being given a simple focus. For many people, this centering can be a dramatic revelation of their ability to shift out of a stress state and into a relaxed state.

As with all stress management techniques, they work best for the people who actually use them on a regular basis. The challenge for the Nurse Coach is to motivate people to develop regular stress management practices.

It is always easier to "sell" something that you truly believe in. The importance of the Nurse Coach personally working with these techniques cannot be emphasized enough.

Your own success with using these practices will increase your effectiveness in motivating your client/patient.

Practice: Imagery for Stress Reduction: Connecting with a Safe Place

The imagination is a powerful force in human nature. It can re-experience the past, picture the future, and bring creativity into the present. It can dream up magically ideal wishes as well as the worst catastrophes. In this practice, the power of the imagination is directed toward communicating calm to the body. (The Safe Place Imagery practice sheet is found in Appendix F-11.)

1. Ask your client/patient to notice her or his breathing.
2. Allow your client/patient to do this for a few minutes.
3. Ask your client/patient to begin to imagine a safe place.
4. Ask your client/patient to imagine being in this place in as much detail as possible.
5. Ask what it feels like to be there.
6. Ask your client/patient to notice what it is about this place that evokes this sense of safety.
7. Have your client/patient bring her or his awareness back to the room whenever she or he feels ready.

When your client brings her or his attention back to the room, ask her or him to discuss the experience with you. Help your client/patient to recognize that this safe place is available to her or him in the imagination whenever it is needed.

Discussion of Practice

When introducing practices that engage the client/patient's imagination, it is important to recognize that people do not have to "see" the imagined scene in order to gain the benefits of imagery. Some people may experience this safe place with a visual image. Others may think about it, connecting with auditory information, or feel it as a kinesthetic experience. Our imagination can be experienced by all of our senses as well as in our emotions. This is an important point to explain to your coaching client/patient.

Practice: Exhaling for Twice as Long as Inhaling

This practice is very effective because, in addition to its physical effects, it requires some concentration and often takes a number of tries before it can be achieved. This focused attention, in and of itself, is of value to the client/patient because it distracts from the inner chatter and worry. Eventually, the client/patient can get a real kinesthetic sense of this and practice it without needing to do the counting. At this point, the client/patient can use it as needed—at a meeting, on the bus, while stuck in traffic, etc. The mental focus can remain on the task at hand, while the body drops into a relaxed state. (The Connecting with Breath: Exhaling for Twice as Long as Inhaling practice sheet is in Appendix F-5.)

1. Do all the breathing, both inhalation and exhalation, through your nose.
2. Notice the sensation of the passage of breath in and out through your nostrils.
3. Now begin to allow your exhalation to be twice as long as your inhalation.
4. The key element to this practice is the ratio—the shorter inhalation time and the longer exhalation. You can inhale for a count of 3 and exhale for a count of 6, or 4 and 8, or whatever is comfortable for you.
5. Give yourself time. It will take a little while to get comfortable with this.
6. After a while, when you get a good feel for this rhythm, you can stop the counting and continue with the long exhalations.

Discussion of Practice

When breathing through the nose, the inhalation activates the sympathetic nervous system. The exhalation through the nose activates the parasympathetic nervous system. This balancing, homeostatic effect is present in all the systems of the body. It may be helpful to explain to your client/patient that the sympathetic system is the one that is activated with stress: it is the activation of your fight/flight response. The parasympathetic system is the counterbalancing, or quieting, of this activation. Therefore, in doing this one-two breath rhythm, you are providing twice as much activation to the quieting, parasympathetic nervous system. For some people, this scientific explanation engenders confidence in utilizing this technique.

Stress Management and Fear of Loss of Control

Stress management techniques such as the practices listed above are clearly designed to reduce stress. The Nurse Coach should be aware, however, that some people can experience an increase in stress from such practices. Some people are in a constant state of vigilance as described in the discussion on willfulness. The reduction of stress, and the increase in relaxation, can be the first time the person has lowered her/his defenses. The result can be:

- a flooding of traumatic memories
- an episode of vulnerability
- a feeling of having no defenses available

These reactions tell us how much control the person needs to feel safe. One person described it as being "naked" in front of the nurse. The Nurse Coach should proceed slowly when this type of reaction is encountered. Communicating calm and acceptance of this response can, in and of itself, be an important message to the client/patient. Such feelings should be respected.

The first step in dealing with such a reaction is to help the client/patient to talk through the experience. Examine the fears together. Often, once the mind has acknowledged the fears, the technique can be modified and tried again with less fear. It is also an opportunity to discuss the availability of other resources. A referral to a counselor may be suggested if the client/patient feels he or she wants to more deeply explore and understand these responses.

SUMMARY

- An important goal of nurse coaching is to assist the client/patient to be empowered by building a self-awareness that opens up new possibilities and choices.
- An important component in this process is to guide the client/patient to connect with his or her inner wisdom by learning awareness practices.
- These practices have a wide variety of bio/psycho/spiritual effects.
- It is important to explore with each client/patient which of the practices is most acceptable and effective for that individual.
- It is important for the Nurse Coach to experience the awareness practices personally to be able to introduce them with confidence and skill.
- Nurse Coaches will themselves benefit from finding practices that support their health and wellbeing.

NURSE COACH REFLECTIONS

After reading this chapter, the Nurse Coach will be able to bring awareness and personal insight to the following questions:

- When am I aware of my inner wisdom?
- What awareness practices do I find most helpful for my self-care?
- When have I had transpersonal or spiritual experiences?
- How did I understand these experiences at that time?
- How do I express my creativity?

REFERENCES

Assagioli, R., (1965). *Psychosynthesis: A manual of principles and techniques.* New York, NY: Viking Press.

Baer, S. M., Hoffman, A. C., & Sheikh, A. A. (2003). Healing images: Connecting with inner wisdom. In A. A. Sheikh (Ed.), *Healing images: The role of imagination in health* (pp. 141–176). Amityville, NY: Baywood Publishing.

Benson, H. (1975). *The relaxation response.* New York, NY: William Morris.

Black, D. S. (Ed.). *Mindfulness Research Monthly.* Retrieved from http://www.mindfulexperience.org

Braud, W. (2003). Transpersonal images: Implications for health. In A. A. Sheikh (Ed.), *Healing images: The role of imagination in health* (pp. 448–470). Amityville, NY: Baywood Publishing.

Calhoun, L. G., & Tedeschi, R. G. (2004). The foundations of posttraumatic growth: New considerations. *Psychological Inquiry 15*(1), 93–102.

Carmody, J., Reed, G., Kristeller, J., & Merriam, P. (2008). Mindfulness, spirituality, and health-related symptoms. *Journal of Psychosomatic Research 64*(4), 393–403.

Dossey, B. (2013). Nursing: Integral, integrative, and holistic–local to global. In B. M. Dossey & L. Keegan (Eds.), *Holistic nursing: A handbook for practice* (pp. 3–57). Burlington, MA: Jones & Bartlett.

Dossey, L. (1994). *Healing words: The power of prayer and the practice of medicine.* New York, NY: Harper Collins.

Dossey, L. (2013). *The one mind: How our individual mind is part of a greater consciousness and why it matters.* Carlsbad, CA: Hay House.

Fanslow-Brunjes, C. (2008). *Using the power of hope to cope with dying.* Fresno, CA: Quill Drive Books.

Farb, N., Segal, Z., Mayberg, H., Bean, J., McKeon, D., Fatima, Z., & Anderson, A. (2007). Attending to the present: Mindfulness meditation reveals distinct neural modes of self-reference. *Social Cognitive and Affective Neuroscience, 2*(4), 313–322. First published online August 13, 2007. doi:10.1093/scan/nsm030.

Firman, D. (2012). The call of the self in chronic illness. *The International Journal of Psychotherapy, 16*(2), 48–57.

Ferrucci, P. (1990). *Inevitable grace: Breakthroughs in the lives of great men and women: Guides to your self-realization*. Los Angeles, CA: Jeremy P. Tarcher, Inc.

Goodman, M. J., & Schorling, J. B. (2012). A mindfulness course decreased burnout and improves well-being among healthcare providers. *International Journal of Psychiatry in Medicine, 43*(2), 119–28.

Govinda, L. A. (1990). *Creative meditation and multi-dimensional consciousness*. Wheaton, IL: The Theosophical Publishing House.

Green, E., & Green, A. (1977). *Beyond biofeedback*. New York, NY: Delacorte Press/Seymour Lawrence.

Hanson, R. (2009). *Buddha's brain: The practical neuroscience of happiness, love and wisdom*. Oakland, CA: New Harbinger.

Jha, A. P., Stanley, E. A., Kiyonaga, A., Wong, L., & Gelfand, L. (2010). Examining the protective effects of mindfulness training on working memory and affective experience. *Emotion, 10*(1), 54–64.

Jung, C. G. (1933). *Modern man in search of a soul*. New York, NY: Harcourt Brace Jovanovich.

Kabat-Zinn, J., & Hahn, T. N. (1990). *Full catastrophe living: Using the wisdom of your body and mind to face stress, pain, and illness*. New York, NY: Bantam Dell.

LeShan, L. (1989). *Cancer as a turning point: A handbook for people with cancer, their families and health practitioners*. New York, NY: Plume-Penguin.

National Center for Complementary and Alternative Medicine (NCCAM). (2011). *Meditation for health purposes – executive summary*. Retrieved 09/18/13 from nccam.nih.gov/news/events/meditation08/summary.htm

Newberg, A., D'Aquili, E., & Rause, V. (2001). *Why God won't go away: Brain science & the biology of belief*. New York, NY: Ballantine.

Nightingale, F. (1873). *Letter from Miss Nightingale to the probationer- nurses in the 'Nightingale Fund' at St. Thomas's Hospital, and the nurses who were formerly trained there* (p. 2). London, UK: Spottiswoode.

Sahebalzamani, M., Farahani, H., Abasi, R., & Talebi, M. (2013). The relationship between spiritual intelligence with psychological well-being and purpose in life of nurses. *Iranian Journal of Nursing and Midwifery Research, 18*(1), 38–41.

Schaub, R., & Schaub, B. G. (2013). *Transpersonal development: Cultivating the human resources of peace, wisdom, purpose and oneness*. Huntington, NY: Florence Press.

Schaub, R., & Schaub, B. G. (2014). *The Florentine promise: A seekers guide,* Huntington, NY: Florence Press.

Sheikh, A. A., & Sheikh, K. S. (2003). Death imagery: Confronting death brings us to the threshold of life. In A. A. Sheikh (Ed.), *Healing images: The role of imagination in health* (pp. 471–488). Amityville, NY: Baywood Publishing.

Welwood, J. (1983). *Awakening the heart: East/west approaches to psychotherapy and the healing relationship*. Boulder, CO: Shambhala Press.

Whitmore, J. W. (2009). *Coaching for performance: GROWing human potential and purpose* (4th ed.). London, UK: Nicholas Brealey Publishing.

Wilber, K. (1977). *The spectrum of consciousness.* Wheaton, IL: The Theosophical Publishing House.

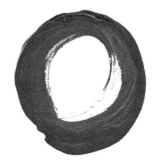

CHAPTER 13

Case Studies:
Awareness and Choice

Bonney Gulino Schaub

Nursing should not be a sacrifice, but one of the highest delights of life.

Florence Nightingale, 1897

LOOKING AHEAD...

After reading this chapter, you will be able to:

- Listen to the client/patient's story considering the mind–body–spirit aspects of what has brought this person to work with a Nurse Coach.
- Have a greater awareness of the diversity of life challenges that coaching clients/patients are confronted with.
- Listen to the client/patient's story with the intention of identifying the strengths and capacities this person possesses.
- Guide the client/patient to cultivate self-awareness and an enhanced ability to make choices.
- Guide the client/patient to learn skills in self-care and stress reduction.

DEFINITIONS

See Chapters 11 and 12 definitions that are related to the following case studies.

COACHING CLIENTS: EXPLORING AWARENESS AND CHOICE

A Nurse Coach brings a broad clinical model and framework to the coaching conversation. She or he listens to the client/patient narrative from multiple perspectives. See Chapter 2, Theory of Integrative Nurse Coaching (TINC) and Component #5 Listening with HEART to explore these areas in a coaching session.

CASE STUDY 1: ELIZABETH—COACHING THE GRIEVING CLIENT

Client's Presentation

Setting: Nurse Coach's office

Elizabeth's narrative: Elizabeth is a 58-year-old nurse seeking help following the unexpected death of her mother. On her initial visit, Elizabeth recounted the circumstances of her mother's death. She had visited her widowed mother who lived alone and had gone out to do some errands for her. Upon her return, Elizabeth found her mother slumped over in a chair at the kitchen table. Elizabeth called 911 and immediately began CPR, but it was obvious that her mom had died.

Triggers: Client had been grieving for several months, and had set up an appointment to meet with a Nurse Coach at the suggestion of a work colleague who was concerned about her.

Antecedents: Client's father had died of lung cancer the previous year after a long illness. Client's mother became dependent on her for driving, shopping, and other errands.

Mediators: Client lives alone; client has no significant other; client enjoys journaling and creating poetry.

Session 1 with Nurse Coach (NC)

(Client has just related story about finding her mother and administering CPR.)

NC: I hear how traumatic this experience has been. Such a profound shock...

Elizabeth: (sobbing, wiping her eyes with tissues and taking a deep breath and sighing)

NC: What are you hoping for in coming to meet with me today? Pause...

Elizabeth: I need to be able to talk about what I'm feeling. My doctor gave me Valium to calm me down but I don't like taking it. I get embarrassed because I become teary whenever anyone asks me how I'm doing. That's why I was given the Valium.

NC: Tell me more about your feeling embarrassed, what's that about? Pause...

Elizabeth: I think I should be handling things better...

NC: What would that look like?

Elizabeth: Oh you know, I would be able to answer without crying. I feel my friends think I was too dependent on my mom. We enjoyed so many of the same things. We'd go to the theater or the beach...she was an interesting and joyful person...

NC: How do you feel about the relationship you had with her?

Elizabeth: Well, I don't have any sisters or brothers and I haven't had a serious relationship in many years, so I think we were very dependent on each other. I judge myself too...

NC: How does this relate to your concerns about your friends' reactions?

Elizabeth: That's hard to describe...(pause)...I guess I feel defensive.

NC: What do you tell yourself when you feel defensive?

Elizabeth: I know about the stages of grief, the Kubler Ross stuff...I know there isn't a set time table...pause...It felt strange to not buy a Mother's Day card last week...(tearful)

NC: What are you experiencing right now?

Elizabeth: I'm remembering placing her on the floor and doing CPR...(shudders)...I knew it was too late, but I kept trying...I can feel the sensation of trying to blow into her mouth...(pauses and touches her mouth)...I can't believe I'm saying this, but I was so angry at her in that moment...We had argued just before I left, about all these errands she was asking me to do. It's not fair that that's my last memory of her...(long pause)

NC: What are you experiencing right now?

Elizabeth: There's so much I want to say to her...(client looking upward...tearful)...

NC: I'm hearing how painful this is for you. Can we take a moment to pause here and reflect on what you have just said? It would be helpful to take a moment to center yourself. Would that be OK?

Elizabeth: Yes...

NC: Okay, Elizabeth, get yourself comfortable in your chair, uncross your legs and place your feet flat on the floor, allow your shoulders to drop and rest your hands on your belly, just below your navel...Okay...and now, bring your awareness to the sensation of your hands in contact with your belly, noticing the sensation of touching the fabric of your shirt...any other tactile sensations...skin touching skin...skin in contact with the air in the room...(pause)...now notice the sensation of the weight of your hands resting on your belly...(pause)...notice the temperature of your hands...(pause)...Now that you've noticed so many sensations of your hands, notice that you can become aware of even subtler sensations...inside the skin sensations such as tingling...or pulsing...just allow yourself to be absorbed in noticing...Now lift your hands, and hold them with palms facing, at about waist height, as if you were holding an inflated balloon and bring all your awareness to noticing that space between your palms...just noticing, being curious...and if you notice any sensations as you do this play with this a bit , slowly moving your hands a little closer or farther apart...and whenever you feel ready, gently place your hands back on your belly, reconnect with your breath and notice the rise and fall of your belly with each breath...whenever you feel ready, bring your awareness back to the room and open your eyes...(Elizabeth kept her eyes closed for a few moments, then opened them and paused before she spoke)

Elizabeth: Hmmm...That felt so calming. It felt like we were doing it for a long time.

NC: What was most helpful in this experience?

Elizabeth: I felt myself really focusing on my hands. They felt warm...I liked the sensation of resting them on my belly. It felt soothing. Then they were so tingly and bouncy...it really got me out of my head.

NC: We only spent about seven minutes doing that practice. It's striking how we can have such a different experience of time when we focus our attention in this way. You went to a very deep place of centering.

Elizabeth: That felt good. It feels cleansing...

NC: Just before we did this practice you had been talking about the fact that you had so many things you wanted to say to your mom. What are your thoughts about that now?

Elizabeth: I realize that I am not really mad at her. I felt so guilty about feeling angry...That was me feeling panicked and helpless.

NC: That is such an important awareness.

Elizabeth: Yeah. I hope she didn't suffer. I'm sorry she was alone...In the work I've done I've seen so many people suffer so much...maybe it was a mercy for her...my dad suffered.

NC: Perhaps you could journal about what you experienced and the thoughts that came up for you.

Elizabeth: I think I will do that. I used to journal when I was in nursing school. It helped me to deal with all the new experiences I was having. Some of those feelings seem related to what I'm experiencing now. I also used to write haiku...I always loved that poetry...

NC: Okay. That sounds like a good plan. Can you also imagine doing the awareness practice on your own if you need to quiet and center yourself?

Elizabeth: Yes, I want to try that too.

NC: We have to stop now and we can make another appointment if you like.

Elizabeth: Yes, I think this is a good plan for now. I'd like to work with you for a while.

NC: Okay. It could be helpful for you to bring in your journaling or poetry if you are comfortable doing that.

Elizabeth: That's an interesting idea. I'll think about it.

Elizabeth's Action Plan

- Elizabeth will work with Nurse Coach weekly for unspecified period of time.
- Given practice sheet, Appendix F-2: Hands on Belly with Energy Ball.
- Elizabeth will journal about her experiences with this practice.

Nurse Coach Summary Notes

- The client described the reason she was coming for coaching.
- The client identified what she was hoping for in coming for coaching.

- The Nurse Coach focused on staying in the present moment in terms of what the client was experiencing.
- The client experienced clarity on what she was troubled by.
- The Nurse Coach introduced a self-care practice that allowed the client to gain deeper self-awareness as to what she needed. This skill provided the client with a tool she could use outside of the session.
- A plan was created for further action the client could take after the session—journaling and writing poetry about her experiences.
- A follow-up appointment was agreed upon.

CASE STUDY 2: GISELLA—COACHING THE CLIENT WITH TEST ANXIETY

Client's Presentation

Setting: Nurse Coach's office

Gisella's narrative: Gisella is a 25-year-old woman referred for coaching by her cousin who is a nurse. Gisella had worked as an LPN while attending nursing school. She had gotten excellent grades and, following graduation, had been hired as an RN at the same hospital. One year prior to coming to coaching Gisella had failed the nursing boards. The day before the exam, her sister, who lives in New Mexico, had been hospitalized after being injured in a car accident. Gisella, who lived in New York, was very upset that she was unable to visit her because she needed to take the exam. She thought this distress caused her to lose focus, and she believes this is why she failed.

Gisella had been avoiding applying to retake the exam because she was terribly anxious and sure she would fail again. She was living with her aunt because after failing the boards, she lost her nursing job and had to give up her apartment. She had been asked to stay on as an LPN but was too embarrassed to go back to that role since she had been working as an RN. She felt it would have made it obvious to "everyone" that she had failed.

Triggers: Increased emotional and financial distress as a result of failing nursing boards exam.

Antecedents: In terms of degree of shame that Gisella experienced, she was aware that it was related to her history. She grew up in New Mexico, a place where her family had lived for generations, "even before it was part of the U.S." She remembered walking in town with her mother and sister and being called "filthy Mexicans." Her mom was always scrubbing and cleaning their home, and Gisella knew it was because of the prejudice they had experienced.

Mediators: Gisella has been living with her cousin and aunt since losing her nursing job. She needs to be able to work as a nurse so she can live on her own. Her cousin and aunt are getting impatient with her since it was supposed to be a temporary arrangement.

Session 1 with Nurse Coach (NC)

Gisella: I'm avoiding registering to retake the exam and I keep telling myself I should do it.

NC: What's preventing you?

Gisella: I can't imagine studying again. I don't even know if I want to be a nurse anymore. Maybe it was a mistake to think I could do it.

NC: You worked as a nurse for a while before you took the exam, what was that like for you?

Gisella: My supervisor liked me and was so supportive, that's probably why I was able to do it. She was always encouraging me...I was so humiliated when I failed the boards.

NC: What did you do when you found out about it?

Gisella: You mean after I got hysterical and crawled into my bed? I called in sick to work and didn't tell anyone.

NC: I hear how painful it was for you.

Gisella: I couldn't face Anna [her supervisor] but knew I had to go in and tell her in person. She tried to console me, but I just kept crying. I was so pathetic, it was embarrassing and I just wanted to leave.

NC: Then what did you do?

Gisella: I went home. Anna called me in the evening to say I should reapply to return to my LPN position and take the licensing exam again. She was sure I would pass, I had just been in too much stress because of my sister's accident. She was very sweet.

NC: It sounds like she has a lot of confidence in you. That means a lot. She was working with you and supervising you every day for a number of months. What do you think it is about you and your work that gives her that confidence?

Gisella: She thinks I'm smart and sometimes I'm overly careful and slow because I don't want to make a mistake. She says she trusts me because of that.

NC: So it sounds like there's a part of you that's a perfectionist. That can be a big asset at certain times, like when you're caring for patients.

Gisella: Yeah...I guess so. It does make me very hard on myself.

NC: So what are you hoping for in coming here today?

Gisella: I need to get over myself and retake the exam. I need to work, I need to be able to support myself. What's my alternative, working in McDonalds? That would probably be easier, but I couldn't live on that.

NC: What went in to your decision to become a nurse?

Gisella: My mom had been a nurse's aide and she always wanted me to become a nurse. She died when I was in the 11th grade. She had a heart attack.

NC: Had your mom been ill for a while?

Gisella: She had high blood pressure and was always very tired from working. I didn't know she was so sick. It was a shock. I ended up living with my aunt, her sister. My dad was never in the picture.

NC: What about your sister?

Gisella: She's five years older than me, and she joined the Navy when she got out of high school. She wanted to get away.

NC: So, you had a lot to deal with. It's quite impressive that you got yourself through school and finished your degree. There's definitely a part of you that can be very determined and focused. It sounds like that perfectionist part of you can really drive you to succeed.

Gisella: I guess so, but I really screwed up now. I feel so stupid.

NC: Listen to how you put yourself down. It will be important for you to notice that and challenge that negative voice.

Gisella: I guess I do that a lot.

NC: Well, you started out our meeting saying you think you should retake the boards, but you've avoided doing that. Is that what you want to focus on?

Gisella: Well, there is an on-line review course I want to take that will help me study for the boards and it goes for six weeks. It's expensive, but I need to do it. My cousin told me you could help me to focus and be able to study again. That's why I came here today. I need to accomplish something quickly.

NC: *Okay. So you're saying you have six weeks to accomplish this. We can work together to create a plan for accomplishing that. How do you feel about that?*

Gisella: You make it sound like it's easy to do.

NC: *I can teach you some practices that you can work with to help you reach your goal.*

Gisella: Yeah...That's what Bella [her cousin] said. Will it be meditation?

NC: *There are many ways we can work with our mind for focus and relaxation, so we will see what works the best for you. Have you ever tried any meditation or imagery or breathing practices?*

Gisella: Not really. We did have to do some reading about some kinds of meditation in nursing school, but I could never do it. I'd always fall asleep when I tried.

NC: *Well I will guide you into a practice that involves noticing your breath. Noticing your breath is a way to practice focusing attention.*

Gisella: Okay, I'll try.

NC: *Okay, so will you be comfortable closing your eyes, I'll close mine too?*

Gisella: Okay.

NC: *Let's begin by noticing the breath, noticing the sensation of breath passing through your nostrils, notice the in breath...and then the out breath...the inhalation...and now the exhalation...Every time you become aware of a distracting thought, or noise or sensation, just notice it and return to noticing your breath...Every time you exhale, let go of any tightness or tension you notice and allow yourself to be more deeply held by the chair...notice all the places your body is in contact with the chair...and really allow the chair to hold you...Now I'm going to ask you to repeat, silently to yourself, a simple three-word phrase over and over again in your mind...as you inhale say your name...and as you exhale say let go...just continue to slowly repeat this for several minutes...as you become distracted, just bring your awareness back to this phrase...Pause...Okay, now let go of the words and keeping your eyes closed, just notice how you are...take your time and when you are ready, open your eyes...(Gisella opened her eyes and sighed.)*

NC: *So what did you experience?*

Gisella: At first I didn't think I could do it. I even thought I might sneeze from focusing on my nose...but then when you said about noticing other thoughts, that helped because I knew it was okay...

NC: *What else did you experience?*

Gisella: It was funny when you said to let the chair hold me. I noticed I could shift a little and relax some more. Then you said to say "let go" and I don't remember anything after that until you said "open your eyes."

NC: *Okay, interesting that you could notice so many different things going on in such a short time.*

Gisella: How long were we doing that?

NC: *Less than five minutes.*

Gisella: Really. It felt much longer.

NC: *Well, there was a lot competing for your attention. That's what awareness practices can help you to recognize so you can focus when you need to.*

Gisella: Do you really think this could help me to study?

NC: *Well, if you practice, it will help you to build focus. What do you think?*

Gisella: Well, I have to sign up for the review course on-line and take the boards.

NC: *So what are the steps you want to take to make that happen?*

Gisella: I need to find out when the next course starts and sign up. I need to get the practice exam books that go with it and I need to find out when I can retake the exam.

NC: *You could have done that two weeks ago. What's different now?*

Gisella: I got myself here so something changed. It's not like I just heard about you. I don't know.

NC: Are you ready to make a commitment to find out about the course and register?

Gisella: Yes. And I will learn how to focus. I need to do that.

NC: Okay. I'll give you a work sheet with the awareness practice we did so you can practice on your own. Is there anything else?

Gisella: I think I need to work with you up until I retake the exam. I could come every other week.

NC: Great, I'd be happy to work with you on preparing for the exam. May I make a suggestion?

Gisella: Sure.

NC: Tell yourself you are "taking the exam." You won't be retaking it. You've never taken it before, it's a different exam. Let's look forward.

Gisella: Okay. I get it.

Gisella's Action Plan

- Gisella and Nurse Coach made an appointment to meet in two weeks.
- Given practice sheet, Appendix F-3: Let Go, to continue working with on a daily basis.
- Gisella will register for review class and exam.

Nurse Coach Summary Notes

- Client needed support in taking actions to study for nursing boards.
- Client focused on her failure, and the Nurse Coach supported the client when she expressed her distress.
- Nurse Coach focused on client's achievements and success in school and in her work.
- Client learned to work with breath awareness and "let go" when she was focusing on "failure."
- Client returned for three more sessions and practiced breath awareness and "Let go" technique in each session.
- In taking practice exams at home, client found it helpful to pause in between questions and connect with her breath before going to the next one.
- Client became aware that she overthought her responses when she came to challenging questions rather than trusting her first response, which was usually the correct one, so she practiced telling herself "Gisella, let go" when she noticed she was doing this.
- Client used these skills when taking the board exam and passed.

CASE STUDY 3: LARRY—COACHING THE CLIENT FOR PAIN MANAGEMENT

Client's Presentation

Setting: Nurse Coach's office

Larry's narrative: Larry is a 67-year-old retired accountant who was addicted to pain killers for 15 years. It began when he had back surgery and knee replacement surgery within a year of each other. He got the pills "legally" from three different doctors.

    Recently Larry decided to stop taking his pain medications after going into a rage with one of his doctors. He had asked the doctor about some plan to wean and then stop medication. The doctor asked if the pills were "working." The client said yes, and the doctor responded by saying that he saw no reason to "fix what isn't broken." Larry left the doctor's office and went home and flushed all his pills down the toilet.

Larry sought out working with a Nurse Coach at the suggestion of a friend he had confided to about his situation. He explained to his friend that he had already stopped "cold turkey" two months earlier, but he felt his resolve was weakening. He said he needed support and tools to have alternatives to "popping pills anytime I feel any bad sensation." He was concerned about his willpower giving out.

Triggers: Angry at himself for becoming dependent on pills; feeling vulnerable to resuming his dependence on pain medications.

Antecedents: Recently retired; feeling bored and wanting to do some meaningful volunteer work; needing healthy skills for managing pain.

Mediators: Strong desire to improve health; has stopped drug use for two months; has a brother in Alcoholics Anonymous.

Session 1 with Nurse Coach (NC)

After relating history of dependence and current concerns:

NC: What's worked so far?

Larry: Mostly rage. I was furious with the doctor, and I said to myself "F—- you, I'm not taking that crap anymore."

NC: What's different now?

Larry: I guess the rage is gone. Now it's just me with me. I hear my mind telling me I can take some without getting back into the habit. It makes sense, but I know myself. If I do something I do something all the way. If I get back into the pills, I'll just use them anytime I feel like it. No holds barred.

NC: Hmm...isn't that also how you stopped?

Larry: I'm not getting what you mean.

NC: I mean that you totally went for it when you stopped. All at once, cold turkey.

Larry: That's how I do things. Sheer willpower.

NC: So we're together today because you want something else or something more to keep this good thing going?

Larry: I need someone else to think this through with me.

NC: Who else have you been able to talk to about your situation? Where else have you gotten support?

Larry: I really haven't had anyone. My wife doesn't really know the full extent to which I was using. It didn't interfere with me functioning for the most part. I had my own business and was very successful and I'm retired now. I have a lot of time on my hands. I talked to a friend who has been in AA for many years. He didn't know what to say, but he offered to take me to a meeting. But I didn't relate to that. Don't get me wrong, I know it works for him. My brother's in AA too and it was a life saver, but his life had been in shambles. No, I wouldn't feel like I belonged there.

NC: What does your wife know about you coming to see me?

Larry: She thinks I'm coming for stress management because I've been very irritable and angry a lot for the past couple of months. She doesn't understand why I seem so stressed out. She's a teacher and she's still working so she doesn't see me most of the day. It frustrates me that I can't be honest. I'm sick of hiding things but I'm embarrassed by this.

NC: I hear your vulnerability. You've achieved a great success with your willpower, but you're feeling a need for something more. That's a very important level of self-awareness. It's the first step to learning more ways to handle your challenge, more than pure willpower.

Larry: But I don't feel strong enough now, that's why I came here today.

(Larry is shifting in his seat and fussing with his shirtsleeves, rolling them up and then unrolling them.)

NC: What are you experiencing right now?

Larry: It's what I go through. My back is beginning to stiffen up, and I'm beginning to get worried that it's going to get worse. It's always the fear that it's going to get worse that sets me off.

NC: Let's try something. Close your eyes...(Client seems surprised at this suggestion, but does close his eyes)...Now bring your attention to your breathing in your nostrils...Don't do anything to your breathing...Just notice it...(Client waits about 20 seconds)...And now say inside your mind, about six times, "My right hand feels warm and heavy...my right hand feels warm and heavy" (Client waits about 20 seconds)...And now, slowly, at your own pace, begin to turn your attention toward noticing how you are...(Client waits about 10 seconds)...And now, slowly, begin to come back this way and, when you're ready, open your eyes...(Client opens his eyes and looks around the room)...How are you?

Larry: Very relaxed...wow...what was that?

NC: How's your back?

Larry: Better. Still a little stiff but no big deal. Doable. How did you do that?

NC: How did you do that, right? You did it.

Larry: When I was doing that I stopped thinking it might get worse.

NC: Interesting...What do you make of that?

Larry: I don't know, what do you make of that?

NC: Well, let's review what just took place. You were shifting in your chair and I asked what you were experiencing and you told me that your back was stiffening up. Then what did you tell me?

Larry: Yeah, I said I always get scared it's going to get worse.

NC: Then I suggested that you close your eyes and bring your attention to your breath and then tell yourself that your right hand is feeling warm...

Larry: Right, I did that over and over for a few minutes

NC: And then what happened?

Larry: I was thinking about something else and then my back felt better. Wow, it's about the fear, isn't it?

NC: It certainly seems that fear was a big factor.

Larry: Wow. That's intense. Fear has gotten a hold of me lots of times in my life.

NC: Well, notice how quickly you were able to get free of it with this practice. You can practice that skill, it would just require a commitment to actually do it.

Larry: Oh, my good old willpower.

NC: I'll give you a practice sheet so you can do this at home. We can work together on this if you like. There are a number of practices you can try.

Larry: I don't want to get back to taking pills. This is definitely worth a try.

Notes on technique:

This relaxation technique functions in two ways:

1. The mental suggestion that "my right hand feels warm and heavy" is a distraction technique. It is understood in pain management that a major part of the pain is very real physiologically but a contributing part of the pain is the mind becoming aggravated and afraid of the physical sensations. The mental suggestion distracted Larry away from his growing worry that his back will get worse.

2. The mental suggestion is also a mind–body technique. The "warm and heavy" state is accomplished by a generalized state of relaxation resulting in an increase in blood volume and blood flow to the extremities. The increase in warmth is objectively real. A person can feel the increased warmth of her or his hands by simply placing then on his or her cheeks. Noticing this change can empower a client to realize how he or she can affect her or his own body state.

Larry's Action Plan

- Larry and his Nurse Coach agreed to meet weekly for four weeks.
- Larry was given practice sheet, Appendix F-1: Breath Awareness and Auto-Suggestion.
- Larry set up a schedule to practice in the morning after his wife leaves for work.

Nurse Coach Summary Notes

- Client is sincerely motivated.
- Client became aware of fear as a component of his medication dependence.
- Client is intelligent and capable of insight and self-exploration.
- Nurse Coach focused on client's positive experience in overriding fear with use of mind–body technique.
- On-going assessment will need to be made to determine if client will need referral to counselor to further address his fear.
- Nurse Coach will consider referring client for acupuncture in the future.
- Nurse Coach helped client to explore and imagine what would be a meaningful and gratifying way for him to channel his energy now that he is retired.

CASE STUDY 4: MARIANNA—COACHING THE PATIENT AROUND TREATMENT DECISIONS

Client's Presentation

Setting: Nurse Coach's office

Marianna's narrative: Marianna was a highly sought-after public relations professional with many prominent clients. She regularly attended elegant events in New York City and often had to travel internationally with her clients. She was a beautiful woman who appeared healthy and vibrant. She had been successfully treated for thyroid cancer at 16 years old. Marianna was currently being treated for metastatic lung cancer. She believed that her current cancer was most likely caused by all the radiation treatment she received as an adolescent.

Marianna had grown up in Colorado. She moved to New York after attending college. She was now 42 years old. She had been referred for nurse coaching by a friend because she was struggling with what to do about her treatment. She had gone through a number of different experimental protocols over the past two years. She had experienced brief periods of remission, but now was needing to make more decisions on how to proceed with her care.

Triggers: Diagnosis of metastatic lung cancer; starting to feel symptomatic—breathless and fatigued at times.

Antecedents: Initially rejected by family when she came out as lesbian; recently renewed contact with parents by telephone; mother came to New York to visit her after this new diagnosis.

Mediators: Strong community of friends willing to help her; strong sense of purpose in working politically to protect LGBT rights; fully enjoys social and cultural events available through her network of colleagues and friends; determined to continue working " 'til the end."

Prior Contact with Nurse Coach

Marianna had been in psychotherapy for several years with a therapist she felt strongly connected to. She had discussed with her therapist a friend's suggestion that she consult with a Nurse Coach for additional support. Marianna was needing to make decisions about treatment and wanted to talk through her fears and confusion. The therapist agreed that this was a good plan.

The Nurse Coach worked with Marianna over a period of six months. During this period of time she had received two courses of chemotherapy as well as extensive radiation therapy. The in-person coaching sessions were scheduled for every two weeks. There were also phone meetings for regular check-ins, especially when Marianna was feeling weak and fatigued. She continued to work during this time, going for treatment early in the morning and then to her nearby office.

Initially the coaching work focused on breathing techniques which Marianna could practice whenever she needed to ground and focus herself. See Appendices F-1, F-5. Marianna chose to use the focusing on breath practice even though her lungs were the site of her cancer because it had been a helpful technique in the past. She found this improved her ability to focus and was helpful when it came to making treatment and self-care decisions. She also wanted to feel connected to her lungs and breath in a positive way.

For six months Marianna did quite well, successfully finishing up planning for and attending a major work event. She enjoyed experimenting with various wigs when she lost her hair, even getting a blond one for variety. Marianna had decided to stop working with her therapist for a while because of all her healthcare appointments. The therapist agreed to be available on an as-needed basis.

One day Marianna contacted her Nurse Coach asking to be seen as soon as possible. She arrived for her coaching session looking ashen and exhausted. She needed to meet because she had been told that lesions were appearing on her brain. Her radiologist wanted to start treating these brain lesions as well as start her on a new chemotherapy protocol. The thought of losing her mental capacity terrified Marianna more than any other loss. She wanted to meet with her Nurse Coach for help in deciding if she wanted to consent to this treatment.

This news changed the direction of her coaching sessions. Marianna had not spoken seriously about her mortality in her previous sessions. She preferred to make joking allusions to it. Now she was clearly shaken. Medical challenges were not new to her but this news opened her up to allowing deeper transpersonal work to be part of the coaching conversation.

Session 1 with Nurse Coach (NC)

NC: You sounded very worried on the phone, what's going on, Marianna?

Marianna: I'm terrified…You remember the last time we met…I said I was feeling weird? My head was foggy and I was getting dizzy? I thought it was probably because of the radiation being more frequent. Also, sometimes I get sinusy and that does it too…(getting tearful, which was very unusual for her)

NC: Okay, Marianna, just take your time…Whenever you feel ready let me know what's going on…(long pause).

Marianna: My worst nightmare has come true—my brain is affected, my brain!!

NC: *How can I help you now?*

Marianna: I haven't been able to sleep for two days. I haven't been able to tell anyone...Do you believe it, I'm embarrassed by this, how stupid is that?...you see, I'm already sounding stupid...

NC: *What does stupid mean to you?*

Marianna: It means I can't trust myself. I have to make a decision about whether I want to do this or not.

NC: *So you want to be able to trust yourself. What has helped you to trust yourself in the past?*

Marianna: I don't know, I just trusted myself, after all I just trusted that getting on a plane and leaving Colorado Springs was the right thing to do...I guess that was a no-brainer... Oh my God, do you believe what I just said?...okay, okay, take a breath, take a breath (she pauses and focuses on her breath for a few seconds).

NC: *Well that was a very important decision and the wisest part of you knew it was right, even if it may have been a bit scary...That wise part of you is still present, you have been guided by it many times without even thinking about it...*

Marianna: Well, where is it now? I need it now.

NC: *Well, what question would you ask it if you felt in touch with it?*

Marianna: I'd just ask what should I do?

NC: *Okay, we can work together and I can guide you to get in touch with that part of you. How would that be for you right now?*

Marianna: It's hard to believe that it's there...(sniffling)...okay, I think it's okay.

NC: *Place your hands on your belly, Marianna, and bring your awareness to noticing the rise and fall of your belly with each breath...*

Marianna: Yeah, this is what I do on the plane...

NC: *Okay, so just take a moment to practice that, noticing the rise and the fall, the rise as you inhale and the slight dropping down as you exhale...the rise...the fall...the in...the out...(Marianna is beginning to look more peaceful, face relaxing, breathing more slowly) Now bring your awareness up to your nose, notice the sensation of breath passing through your nostrils...the in...the out...notice the slight cool sensation of the breath as it enters your nose...now bring your awareness to the center of your forehead...notice the sensations here...now bring your awareness inside to your imagination and experience yourself in a beautiful, peaceful setting in nature...experience this place with all your senses...the smells...the sensation of the air in contact with your skin...the colors around you...the sounds...Now notice in the distance a very wise being, and experience yourself approaching this being...feel yourself moving toward this being and when you are close enough begin to communicate with this being, bringing your question and be open to whatever answer or information you experience. I'm going to be silent now... allow yourself to stay in this space for as long as you want and whenever you're ready, slowly open your eyes and bring your awareness back to this room...take as much time as you need...(Marianna was deeply relaxed, breathing slowly, her eyelids closed and fluttering slightly and after a couple of minutes she opened her eyes.)*

Marianna: Hmmm, that felt like a very long time...(pause)

NC: *What did you experience, Marianna?*

Marianna: It was quite a surprise...I was in the mountains near where I grew up. I saw a cave in the distance and I knew it, it's where I used to go with my friends as a child. I went into it and there was an old Indian man sitting in there with a fire in front of him... I really loved him, he was very kind and wise, I trusted him and he blew some of the smoke towards me...he was gesturing and saying "Come home...come home." I started to cry, and he smiled, saying "Don't be afraid, you've been here before"…It was very reassuring…(long pause)…It's so amazing that I had that memory. I loved those caves and we would look for pictures in them. We played cowboys and Indians and I was always the Indian. I always wanted to be the Indian.

NC: *How are you feeling right now?*

Marianna: I feel so peaceful and calm. I can't really describe it, it's more than that…I don't know, it just feels good.

NC: *What do you need right now?*

Marianna: I need to stay with this feeling and think about it. He was so strong and reassuring.

NC: *Let's close our eyes and take a moment to center and just check whether there is anything else you need to say or do.*

Marianna: Okay…(closed her eyes for a few moments). That felt good.

NC: *We have to stop now, so I'd like to suggest that you give me a call later today to let me know how you are doing.*

Marianna: Okay, that sounds good. I'll do that.

See practice sheet, Appendix F-10: Connecting with Inner Guide.

Continuation of Marianna's Narrative after Coaching Session

Marianna called that evening and said she was still working on her experience. A week later she called and said she had decided to go back to Colorado. She had called her mother, and her mother asked her to come home and stay with her. She was starting to make arrangements to do so. The Nurse Coach agreed that she would be available for phone contact with Marianna if needed. Marianna said this plan felt right to her.

Six weeks later the Nurse Coach received a note from Marianna's friend Helen telling her that Marianna had died. The friend had accompanied Marianna back to Colorado and met her parents. Helen said that her dear friend was so happy to be back in the mountains, and they had visited the cave that had been in the imagery. It had been a very moving and blessed experience for both of them. Marianna was exhausted the next day and died peacefully a few days later.

Nurse Coach Summary Notes

- Working with Marianna was truly a process of accompanying her on a profound journey of transition and transformation.
- The Nurse Coach did not make any assumptions about what Marianna needed or wanted.
- The Nurse Coach communicated her comfort level and ability to be present with a state of "not knowing."
- This allowed the client to be open and present to her self-determination and inner wisdom.
- The Nurse Coach fully trusted the therapeutic value to the client of experiencing being deeply listened to.
- The Nurse Coach did awareness practices with the client, role modeling staying present with breath, knowing the value of being fully present in the energy field being created, and shared with client.
- The Nurse Coach is bearing witness to a person's most intimate contact with the mystery each of us will have an opportunity to explore in the future.
- The Nurse Coach respected and supported the client's informed decisions.

CASE STUDY 5: PETER—COACHING THE CLIENT WITH HYPERTENSION AND JOB STRESS

Client's Presentation

Setting: Nurse Coach's office

Peter's narrative: Peter is a 50-year-old married father of two sons. His relationship with his wife and sons is very rewarding and important to him, and he is highly motivated to be as healthy as possible. He had come for coaching because of job stress and his poorly managed hypertension. His cardiologist suggested medication for managing stress and anxiety, but Peter didn't want to take more medication.

Peter had been overlooked for a job promotion he had expected to get. He was told the management was hiring someone from outside the company for a "fresh perspective."

Peter had previously worked with his Nurse Coach 10 years ago. At that time he had just been diagnosed with a congenital heart defect. The diagnosis was a shock to him. He was reassured that it could be corrected with surgery. He received coaching prior to surgery to help him manage his fears about the process, and he continued after surgery. Peter had always enjoyed running and had looked to that activity both to manage his weight and his work stress. Nurse Coaching had helped him in the process of slowly regaining trust in his body and confidence in resuming physical activity.

Triggers: Following a routine physical, client was told his blood pressure had gotten higher and his doctor was recommending an increase in his medication. Peter had been "overlooked" for a promotion at work.

Antecedents: Peter received nurse coaching 10 years ago and had found it helpful. Both of his sons were away at college so more time was available to address his health challenges.

Mediators: Highly motivated to be as healthy as possible; loving relationship with wife and kids; looking forward to being more active and loves running.

Session 1 with Nurse Coach (NC)

NC: Hi, Peter. It's been a long time since we've seen each other.

Peter: Yeah. I need a tune-up. Really, I've been doing great over the past 10, wow…10 years. My boys are both in college now. Sheila (his wife) and I are great. She's still teaching at the college. It's my job that's a mess and my blood pressure is up.

NC: So what are you hoping for in having us working together again?

Peter: Well, I really need to regain some structure in my life. When we worked together before, I really took to using that "let go" (Appendix F-3) practice and it helped me so much. I also got back into the running and did it for years. I've completely dropped all that, and the doctor says my blood pressure is up. He raised my medication, and I don't like that he had to do that.

NC: So what do you think has contributed to this change?

Peter: Oh I have a good idea about that. My job has gotten really bad. I have more and more work because when people leave, they don't get replaced and last year, they increased the work day by an hour and didn't give us a raise. I didn't even know that was legal, but we don't have a union. Obviously the vibe at work is pretty bad, and yet people say "at least we have a job." The final straw was when I didn't get the promotion. I had been taking on more and more responsibility, and I was the logical one to get the job, but hey, surprise, it's not me. It's someone we've never seen before.

NC: *Wow, you've really been dealing with a lot. What has helped you the most in dealing with all this?*

Peter: Well, all my buddies at work are on the same page, so you know, misery loves company. But it doesn't really help or make things better. And every time the new boss sends me a memo or wants to speak with me I feel myself getting angry.

NC: *Yes, I hear that. Let's take a moment and just pause. You know what I'm going to suggest...*

Peter: Oh, I know, we're going to practice breathing...

NC: *Brilliant! Okay, close your eyes...rest your hands on your belly...and bring your awareness to noticing the sensation of the rise and fall of your belly with each breath...as soon as you are aware of being distracted, just come back to your hands...(Focusing on hands and breath for at least a minute and occasionally reminding the client to be aware of distraction and then choose to bring awareness back to the hands on belly— see practice sheet, Appendix F-4.) Okay, now Peter, just reflect back on the last few days and reconnect with an experience, it could be any time at all, when you felt a sense of inner calm or contentment...just take your time and when you feel ready, open your eyes. (Long pause...observing Peter's breath slowing down, rapid eye movements, his shoulders dropping, his facial muscles relaxing.)*

Peter: Yeah, I remember doing this...wow, it is amazing how quickly you can chill out. I immediately thought about the other night when my wife and I were eating out in our garden. We were eating cheese with tomatoes and basil that we had grown, we were having a glass of wine, and it was so delicious. Sheila's off in the summer and she really loves to garden. It was perfect.

NC: *What was perfect about it?*

Peter: Well, it all made sense. We were enjoying each other. We were surrounded by flowers. There was a sweet breeze. We saw two rabbits run across the lawn chasing each other. We were eating what the earth had given us. Work and all its nonsense was far away...I guess it was like what you taught me last time...it was "Peter...let go."

NC: *So what allowed that experience to take place?*

Peter: Hmm...That's an interesting question. I'm not sure...

NC: *Well, take your time, close your eyes again and reconnect...what understanding comes to you?...(pause)...*

Peter: You know, I was just there...I wasn't thinking about anything, just being there. That's what I often experienced when I was running. Sometimes I'd get back and I could hardly remember where I had been. It's also like that when I'm sailing on my little boat. It was as if I had been away a long, long time.

NC: *So you were fully present in the moment...*

Peter: Yeah, that's what it was...

NC: *Our entire physiology shifts when we go into that state. It's a healing shift, letting go of alarm and vigilence...letting go of tightening your muscles...this allows your blood to flow freely.*

Peter: Boy, do I need more of that.

NC: *Well, you were very successful in making changes when we worked together in the past...you really were skillful and that was quite a challenging time...*

Peter: Oh boy, that was a scary time. The boys were little. I didn't know what would happen to them if I didn't make it. I had never been seriously sick before and even though the doctors were saying it was almost a "routine" procedure, it wasn't routine for me. It was the first time I had really thought I might die...I remember how you helped me to not be obsessed with scary thoughts and scenarios...

NC: *What was most helpful in slowing that process down?*

Peter: It was good working with the "let go" because I could do that anywhere. I did it at work, and when I was driving. I really learned to notice when my mind was going to that scary place. I was really disciplined because I had really gotten scared. I was going for PT and follow-up visits, I was seeing you regularly. Sheila was really great with changes in what we ate and she always supported me in getting out and walking and then back to jogging...Eventually I was feeling normal, almost forgetting all that.

NC: *So what changed?*

Peter: I think what happened was all the business and changes at work. That's been going on for about five years, I think that began to absorb me. At first it was even good to be distracted.

NC: *I can see that. You weren't just focusing on your health concerns?*

Peter: Yeah. It was back to normal. I could go out with my friends and have a drink and watch a ball game without worrying about driving home afterwards, I was never much of a drinker so it wasn't about too much booze, it was about being alone. For a few years I would never leave the house without my phone, even to go down the street to a store, in case I needed to call for help. I don't want that to happen again. I guess that's why I was so freaked out by the doctor raising my meds. It felt like I was going backwards.

NC: *Okay, so given what you've just said, what feels like a doable first step in taking care of yourself?*

Peter: Well, when we did the breathing before it really reminded me that I can go to that place. It reminded me that I can step back from the *mischegas* at work. I remember the last time you saying to focus on what I do have some control over, the choices I can make.

NC: *Okay, we can reconnect with that practice. Is there anything else?*

Peter: Well, I belong to a gym, but I never go. I leave too early, and I'm out of work too late. That extra hour is a killer, especially since it's not like the place closes at 6 PM.

NC: *So, you would like to have more exercise but you don't feel you have the time? Is there any other way you can bring some movement into your day?*

Peter: Well, at lunchtime I usually escape to my car where I listen to the radio or read a book and eat my sandwich. I just don't feel like talking to anyone because there are always so many gripes. There are some who walk at lunch, but I don't want to walk with them because I need some time alone. I guess I could fit in a 20-minute walk by myself and then eat. I had thought about doing that in the past, but I was afraid it would seem unfriendly to not join the group.

NC: *So does that feel like a doable plan?*

Peter: Yes, as long as the weather is good.

NC: *Okay. So we can end this session with taking a few moments to practice the Let Go exercise. How does that sound?*

Peter: Yes, that will be good.

Peter's Action Plan

- Follow-up appointment for next week, with five more sessions.
- Resume practice of the "Peter Let Go" exercise—given practice sheet, Appendix F-3: Let Go.
- Begin practicing Safe Place Stress Reduction—given practice sheet, Appendix F-11: Imagery for Stress Reduction—Connecting with a Safe Place.
- Have quick lunch at work and then walk for 20 minutes by himself.

Nurse Coach Summary Notes

- Client was motivated to take action to improve his health.
- Client had successfully worked with the Nurse Coach and used awareness practices in the past.
- Client recognized that he needed support and guidance in learning ways to quiet down his stress response to current challenges.
- Client needed help in stepping back from fear-based reactivity and letting go of the inner negative dialogue.
- Client was able to identify what gave him feelings of peace and gratitude and to remember this when he felt himself getting caught up in fear.
- Client felt empowered to make choices that supported his self-care and wellbeing.

CASE STUDY 6: VERONICA—COACHING THE PREGNANT CLIENT

Client's Presentation

Setting: Client's apartment

Veronica's narrative: Veronica was a 30-year-old married, third-year law student when she first contacted the Nurse Coach. She had just discovered that she was pregnant and was in a panic because she was about to start her final semester of law school, and pregnancy had not been in her plans. She had been referred for coaching by her nurse practitioner because she was considering terminating her pregnancy, but was in great conflict about it.

Veronica considered herself a very disciplined and focused person, and she had a clear vision of what she wanted to accomplish before she started a family. Her husband was ambivalent about what to do and said he would support her decision. After two coaching sessions, Veronica realized that she wanted to go forward with her pregnancy and arranged to take a leave from law school. At this point she stopped working with the Nurse Coach but was advised that the coach would be available in the future if needed.

Eight months later, Veronica contacted her Nurse Coach because she was on bed rest and had been told she was going to need a c-section because her baby was in a full breach position. She was in a panic at the prospect of the surgery and distraught because she had planned on natural childbirth. She was working with a midwife, was very engaged in her prepared childbirth classes, and taking pregnancy yoga classes. The C-section was not part of her plan. The Nurse Coach arranged to make a home visit.

Triggers: Client has been told she will need to have her baby delivered by C-section. Client is worried about the safety of her child because of the drugs they will be exposed to in the surgery.

Antecedents: Client prided herself on being organized and able to manage her life. This was an unplanned pregnancy that disrupted the client's sense of being able to control and plan her life.

Mediators: Client has a supportive and loving husband. Also has support from a sister. Client has maintained a healthy lifestyle and positive outlook once she decided to embrace her pregnancy.

Session 1 with Nurse Coach (NC)

NC: Hello, Veronica, how are you?

Veronica: Thank you so much for coming to my apartment. I really needed to speak with you. I'm a wreck.

NC: So sorry to hear that. Please tell me what's going on.

Veronica: Well, as I said on the phone, I was told I'm going to need a C-section. My midwife sent me to consult with the OB she partners with, and the doctor also said I will probably need a section. My baby is quite big, and they don't think there is enough room and time for it to turn. My due date is in two days.

NC: So what's causing you to be a wreck?

Veronica: Well, first of all I'm so scared about the baby having all those drugs because of the surgery. This isn't what I had planned. I was so focused on doing everything right for this pregnancy. I haven't had a sip of wine, no caffeine at all, I've taken all my vitamins and eaten only organic food, I'm taking yoga, and now the baby is going to be getting all those drugs.

NC: Veronica, I hear how nurturing and careful you've been. Your baby has really been given a good start. What do you think would help you right now in regard to the section? What do you need?

Veronica: I've asked my midwife so many questions. I've called her so many times. She reassures me, but I still get caught up in worrying.

NC: What has been most helpful for you these past months? I know you had a challenging start to this pregnancy.

Veronica: I was really able to make the transition. I surprised myself and I focused on making this a great experience. Tom (Veronica's husband) was always fussing over me and bringing me flowers.

NC: So it sounds like you have resources for the information you need, but your challenge is to work with your mind to help it stop worrying.

Veronica: Yes, I have to do that. I've really had a very good pregnancy. I was very lucky because I had very little morning sickness—it was only for about a week. Lately I've been getting leg cramps when I'm walking, but that's tolerable, no big deal. It's what I think about that's the problem.

NC: How has Tom reacted to this situation?

Veronica: He was only concerned about me being so disappointed. He was reassured that he can still be in the delivery room.

NC: That's great.

Veronica: Yes, but I'm still hoping I won't need it. My midwife tried to turn the baby, and my friend told me about a massage therapist who is very good at doing that, but Tom doesn't want that. He doesn't think it's safe. My sister doesn't like the idea either. She calls me every day and we talk. She thinks I'm silly in being so upset. She's had two kids and she keeps trying to downplay it, telling me about all her friends who've had sections.

NC: I wonder how your baby feels about it.

Veronica: Well, I'll never know that.

NC: Well you can use your imagination to find out. Would you be willing to try something?

Veronica: Yes, I guess so.

NC: Okay. I'd like to start with guiding you into a more relaxed state. Remember how we worked with focusing on breath when we first worked together?

Veronica: Yes, I practiced that for a while.

NC: Okay, great. So close your eyes and bring your awareness to your breath. Breathing through your nose, notice the length of your inhalations and exhalations...allow yourself to exhale for twice as long as you inhale...the length of the breath doesn't matter, it's the long exhalation that is important so you can inhale for a count of 3 and exhale for

6 or inhale for 4 and exhale for 8, whatever feels comfortable to you...be patient with yourself...it may take a few tries to do this...allow that long exhalation to be like a sigh... a letting go...allow the bed to hold you...take your time...Now, place your hands on your belly, keeping your attention on the sensations of your hands in contact with your belly...noticing all the sensations...the slight rise and fall with each breath...bringing your awareness to the shape of your belly and any shifts or other sensation you notice... (long pause)...use the power of your imagination to connect with your baby...(pause)... take as much time as you like and whenever you feel ready open your eyes...(Veronica closed her eyes for a long time. I even wondered if she had fallen asleep, but her hands didn't slip down from her belly so I knew she hadn't. I just stayed present connecting with my own breath so I was focused and calm. Eventually she opened her eyes which were teary and looked at me. "What are you experiencing?" I asked.)

Veronica: That was amazing...I really connected with her...She was so cozy and comfortable in there, I could feel her heartbeat...I felt sorry that I was trying to make her shift...I told her she was perfect just the way she is. I told her I loved her. I'm sure it's a girl. I'm so sorry I was trying to control her. Oh boy, that's me isn't it? I need to trust that she will be fine. I can't be feeding her my worries and fears.

NC: You made a very deep connection. That's what counts.

Veronica: I really saw her in my imagination. Do you think that it's possible it was really her?

NC: Well, I guess you'll know soon enough. How are you feeling right now?

Veronica: I'm feeling much more secure.

NC: Good. I'd like to take this one more step...How do you feel about that?

Veronica: Okay.

NC: Let's take another moment to connect with breath. Breath in whatever way feels best for you right now. As soon as you notice your mind wandering, bring your awareness back to your breath...(I take a long pause and notice Veronica breathing slowly, her eyelids fluttering...) Now, allow yourself to get an image of being here in your home, holding your baby...take your time and really experience it...whenever you're ready, open your eyes...

Veronica: I feel a lot safer. I know we'll be alright. Tom was here with me. He was so relieved that we are both peaceful. I could really feel her in my arms and Tom holding both of us...I will definitely have him do this breathing and imagery with me. He can put his hands on my belly too. He does that all the time anyway.

Veronica's Action Plan

- Practice Connecting with Breath: Exhaling for Twice as Long as Inhaling (Appendix F-5).
- Given practice sheet, Appendix F-6: Breath Awareness with Inner Dialogue.
- Practice imagery with husband—connecting with baby.
- Phone coach prior to going to the hospital.

   Two days later, Veronica called early in the morning.

Veronica: Hi, I'm packed and ready to go. Tom and I did the imagery together twice yesterday.

NC: Okay.

Veronica: I didn't sleep well but I kept going back to noticing my breath. It helped me to calm down. Tom can sleep through anything, so I was glad I could do that...

NC: Wonderful. You've become so good at using this, I'd love to hear from you when you're ready.

Veronica and Tom had a beautiful 9 lb. 2 oz. girl and named her Hope.

Nurse Coach Summary

- Client was a person who relied on structure and planning in managing her life.
- Unexpected events provoked great fear and vulnerability.
- Client experienced anticipatory anxiety because the birthing process was not going as she had planned.
- Nurse Coach focused on positive steps the client had taken.
- Nurse Coach determined that client needed to learn new skills to manage her anxiety.
- Client was able to change her feelings about the C-section.
- Client was able to focus on what was best for her baby.
- Client learned breathing practice to bring her back to the present moment.
- Client and husband learned to work with an image of a positive outcome.

CASE STUDY 7: CLARA—COACHING THE CLIENT WITH CAREGIVER STRESS

Client's Presentation

Setting: Nurse Coach's private practice office

Clara's narrative: Clara is a 54-year-old school nurse working full-time in a high school. She is married with two adult children, both of them living out of state. She has one sibling, a sister, with whom she has had a long-standing strained relationship. Clara is the Power of Attorney and the Healthcare Proxy for her mother. She also takes care of all her mother's finances and bills. Clara was referred for nurse coaching by her husband and a nurse colleague.

Triggers: Tension with husband. Taking too many personal days from work to handle "emergencies." Increasing fatigue.

Antecedents: Father's death in the past year with no time to process loss. Carrying full burden of responsibility for mother in regard to care decisions, POA, and Healthcare Proxy. Taking on full management of mother's finances.

Mediators: Supportive work colleagues. Trusts the current home care team to give good care—they are far superior to previous aides.

Session 1 with Nurse Coach (NC)

NC: What's brought you here today, Clara?

Clara: My husband is having a hard time with my mother's illness, and he and my friend have both told me I need to speak to someone about my situation with her.

NC: How did you feel about that suggestion?

Clara: Well, I know I'm dealing with a lot. My mom has Alzheimer's and I go to her house every day to check up on her. I am always exhausted. I work full-time and I visit her every day after work and on the weekend too. My husband is stressed out.

NC: How long has your mom been ill?

Clara: She's had a slow deterioration over the past five years. When my dad was alive he would cover up for her, so I'm not really sure when it started.

NC: Your Dad cared for her?

Clara: Yes he was a doctor so he wanted her at home—he hated nursing homes and found them depressing to visit. He hired full-time help in the daytime so he could still work part-time. I would go over a couple of days a week. A year ago he had a heart attack. He only survived a few days, but he made me promise I wouldn't put mom in a nursing home. He told me he had money for a live-in caretaker. It was so overwhelming. I didn't have time to deal with his death because I had to move in with my mom to go about finding a live-in caretaker. It was good that it happened in the summer because I was off.

NC: *This has been a very challenging year for you. What brings you here now, today as opposed to last month or last week?*

Clara: My husband thinks I need to cut back on visiting. He says I'm overdoing it. My friend says the same thing.

NC: *So what are you hoping for in coming?*

Clara: I need to figure out how to make my husband understand so he won't be angry at me. He says, "Get your sister up here to help you, she's retired." But that isn't an option. They haven't gotten along in years.

NC: *So one of your goals in coming to work together is to find a way to get your husband to understand your need to visit your mom every day? What do you think his understanding is right now?*

Clara: He keeps saying we're paying all this money for home care. Let them do the work.

NC: *Tell me about your visits with your mom—what is it like for you?*

Clara: I want her to know that she hasn't been abandoned—I usually help her with her dinner. She needs to be coaxed to eat healthy food. All she wants is ice cream. And I always tell her I love her...sometimes she asks where Dad is. I always say he loves her too. I want her to know she is loved. (tearful...rubbing her eyes)...I feel guilty that strangers are caring for her. They are wonderful women, but she often doesn't know who they are.

NC: *Help me to understand what you mean when you say you don't want her to feel abandoned.*

Clara: I feel I need to see her every day because most of the time now she doesn't even know who I am. She often thinks I'm her sister or her mother. I think she needs to see me every day so she feels at home.

NC: *Let's pause here for a moment. I hear all that you are processing in this situation. It could be helpful to take a pause, connect with breath, and get clarity on what you are experiencing...Have you ever practiced any form of relaxation or mind-body technique?*

Clara: I did some yoga in the past, but not in ages.

NC: *Did you do any breathing techniques at that time?*

Clara: No, we just lay down on the floor at the end of class, I think she called it the dead man's pose...I didn't like that name.

NC: *How would it be if we took a few moments to focus on breath and get more in touch with what's going on? I will do it too, I won't be watching you...I find it helpful for me as well...*

Clara: (Long sigh) Okay.

NC: *Take a moment to notice your breath...Inhaling and exhaling through your nose...allow yourself to put all your attention here...notice the sensation of breath passing through your nostrils...if you notice any distractions, just acknowledge them and then return to noticing your breath...distractions are normal...you can notice and choose to come back to breath...notice that there is a slight cool sensation as the inhaled air passes through your nose...take a moment to explore that sensation...just take your time and notice... Now become aware of the sensation of your exhaled air...it's warmer. Sometimes it's actually difficult to feel because your breath has traveled into your lungs and become warmed by your body...Now allow yourself to just focus on your breath in any way that you like...(I can hear Clara's breath slowing down and deepening.) If it feels ok, I'd like you to keep your eyes closed and I have a few questions.*

Clara: Okay.

NC: *What are you experiencing right now?*

Clara: I feel like I am far away from here...it's calm...

NC: *Okay, now from this calmer place, allow yourself to reconnect with your mom... (pause)...how are you doing?...*

Clara: I'm okay...I see her...

NC: *What are you feeling right now?*

Clara: I feel so close to her, I feel like I can touch her...

NC: *Okay. Take a moment and do whatever feels right in this moment and whenever you feel ready open your eyes...(Clara paused for a couple of minutes and opened her teary eyes.) What did you experience?*

Clara: I felt close to her...I told her that I loved her...she smiled at me...she didn't say anything, she just smiled...

NC: *What was that like?*

Clara: It felt good. It was reassuring...(pause)...I felt she knew I was there...It felt real.

NC: *What do you make of this experience?*

Clara: It did feel very real. It was so interesting that it felt like I was actually speaking with her and she heard me. She was more responsive than if I was actually there...

NC: *Hmmm...Interesting...how do you feel about this?*

Clara: I certainly didn't expect that to happen...

NC: *You and your mom have a deep connection even when you are not physically present with her...she is aware of your presence even when she is non-communicative with you. She feels your energy presence and it sounds like you had an experience of her energy right here in this room...*

Clara: Yes, I did. That felt good and reassuring. I wonder if I could do this at home. It felt freeing.

NC: *What do you mean by freeing?*

Clara: I wonder if I could do that on my own, when I am at home. It might help me to believe that we are not really separated just because I'm not next to her.

NC: *That's an interesting idea. What do you think you might do?*

Clara: I want to try this at home and maybe one day, rather than needing to go to mom's house at dinner, I could try to do this...I could tell my husband I'm trying this...(pause)... He really has been supportive...(pause)...it's just that he is always eating dinner alone and he worries about me.

NC: *How could you bring this practice into your day?*

Clara: I'll need to experiment with it. I'm not even sure I could do it on my own, but I want to try. Even if I can skip one day of going over there it would feel like progress. I'd love to cook my husband a special meal.

NC: *That sounds like a good start. We could set up a time for a phone check-in in a few days to see how the awareness practice is going. What would you like to do?*

Clara: That would be good. Then I could see you again next week to see how the week went.

Clara's Action Plan

- Follow-up appointment made to see each other in two weeks.
- Given practice sheet, Appendix F-6: Breath Awareness with Inner Dialogue.
- Clara will have a brief phone session to assess how the awareness practice is going.
- Clara will consider skipping a day of visiting mother.

Session 2

Clara spoke about how she didn't know what she believed in regard to god but she definitely didn't believe in the afterlife. She spoke about the sudden loss of her father and recognized that part of her strong commitment to her mother was because of her father's concerns about providing quality care. An awareness practice, just like the one that was conducted in the first meeting was offered in session 2. This time it was suggested that she connect with her father. Again she felt a deep connection through the imagery experience. She also sensed that her father would have wanted her to take care of herself. This was a profound experience, and Clara made a commitment to herself. She acknowledged that all the attention on her mother was causing her to neglect herself. In the past, she and her husband often took a walk together after dinner. She hoped she could begin doing that again on the days she didn't visit her mother.

Session 3

Clara reported that she and her husband briefly stopped in and visited her mother one evening and then went out to dinner. He told her he was relieved that she was working on making changes. He said he felt he was losing her. They also acknowledged how painful it is to see her mother in this state of deterioration. On a second night she stayed home and they cooked a meal together.

Clara acknowledged that she had come to realize that there was a part of her that is present for her mother even when she isn't physically there. She experienced this in her meditation and imagery. She self-consciously said "it's kind of a spiritual thing." Clara decided she wanted to write a letter to her mother expressing why she couldn't visit every day. She would spray the letter with lavender oil, a fragrance her mother loved. She would leave it in her mother's room. She said she felt that at some level her mother would feel the connection. Clara anticipated that there would be new challenges and decisions in regard to her mother and wanted to have the option to contact the Nurse Coach on an as-needed basis.

Clara's Action Plan

- Continue working with breath awareness and imagery practice.
- Make commitment to husband to stay home at least two days a week.
- Write letter to her mother.

Nurse Coach Summary Notes

- Client established a more realistic goal in regard to visiting mother.
- Client recognized the impact of her father's death on decisions in regard to her caregiver role with mother.
- Client opened to a more expansive, non-local, "kind of spiritual" sense of connection with her parents.
- Client improved relationship with husband by spending more time together.
- Client opened up to communicating with husband about the vulnerability felt in regard to mother's illness.
- Client recognized her neglect of self-care and planned to resume taking after-dinner walks with husband.

SUMMARY

- Case studies demonstrate the interaction of bio/psycho/social/spiritual factors that are present when a client/patient requests nurse coaching.
- Case studies demonstrate the process of Nurse Coach presence and deep listening to the client/patient's story.
- Case studies reflect the importance of the Nurse Coach's relationship-based care in effective coaching.
- Case studies show the interweaving of the variety of Nurse Coach communication and caring principles such as appreciative inquiry, motivational interviewing, awareness practices, focusing on the solution, directing the client/patient to their inner wisdom to make their choices, cultural considerations, and creation of personal rituals and plans for solutions.

NURSE COACH REFLECTIONS

After reading this chapter, the Nurse Coach will be able to bring awareness and personal insight to the following questions:

- How am I affected by the process of bearing witness to the depth of my client/patient's challenges?
- How do I manage my thoughts and feelings when my client/patient makes choices that are not what I would have chosen?
- How do I step back from the feeling that I need to "fix" things and have answers when I am asked a question by my client/patient?
- How do I bring awareness practices and self-care skills into my moment-to-moment experience when I am working with a client/patient?

Source: Copyright © 2014 by Bonney Schaub. Adapted from Schaub, B. G., & Schaub, R. (1997). *Healing addictions: The vulnerability model of recovery*. Albany, NY: Delmar Publishers.

REFERENCES

Note: See Chapters 11 and 12 for additional references related to Awareness and Choice.

Nightingale, F. (1897). *To the nurses and probationers trained under the 'Nightingale Fund'* (p. 2). London, UK: Spottiswoode.

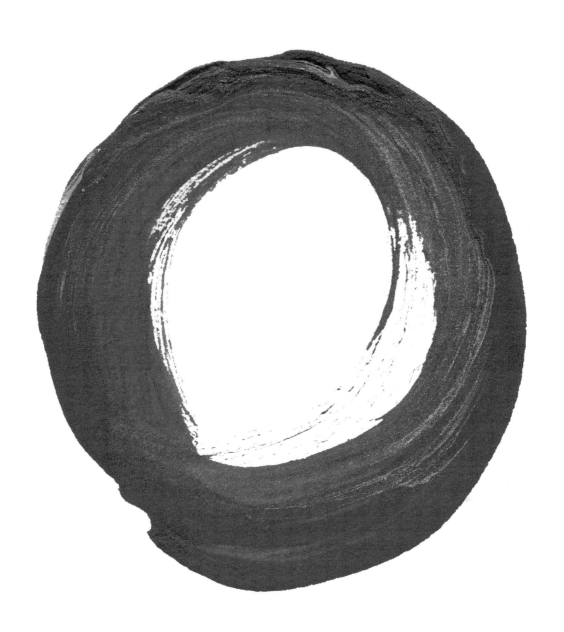

CORE VALUE 3

Nurse Coach Communication,
Coaching Environment

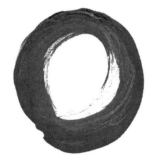

CHAPTER 14

Integral Perspectives and Change

Barbara Montgomery Dossey

> Does it not seem to you that the greater freedom of secular Nursing Institutions as it requires (or ought to require) greater individual responsibility, greater self command in each, greater nobleness in each, greater self possession in patience; — so, that very need of self possession, of greater nobleness in each requires (or ought to require) greater thought in each, more discretion, & higher not less obedience.
>
> *Florence Nightingale, 1872*

LOOKING AHEAD...

After reading this chapter, you will be able to:

- Discuss the change process from an integral perspective.
- Analyze the integral process and the four quadrants and its application in nurse coaching.
- Describe the four Nurse Coach Integral Principles.
- Examine the six lines of development for its application for Nurse Coach and client self-development.

DEFINITIONS

Integral dialogues: Transformative and visionary exploration of ideas and possibilities across disciplines where these four perspectives are considered as equally important to all exchanges, endeavors, and outcomes.

Integral healing process: Contains both the Nurse Coach processes and client/patient, family/significant others, and healthcare workers processes from four perspectives (see above). This leads to a deeper understanding of the unitary whole person interacting in mutual process with the environment.

Integral process: Comprehensive way to organize multiple phenomenon of human experience related to four perspectives of reality: (1) the individual interior (personal/intentional); (2) individual exterior (physiology/behavioral); (3) collective interior (shared/cultural); and (4) collective exterior (systems/structures).

Integral worldview: Examines values, beliefs, assumptions, meaning, purpose, and judgments of an individual's perceived reality and relationships from four perspectives.

NURSE COACHING AND AN INTEGRAL PERSPECTIVE FOR CHANGE

Nurse Coaches see clients as whole beings with each holding the capacity to connect deeply with her/his own inner wisdom and truth. These interactions assist clients to increase their sense of human flourishing—the individual's subjective experience about an optimal state of wellbeing where one's human capacities (growth, strengths, happiness, creativity, resilience, and life purpose, etc.) are recognized and defined (Dossey, 2013). Nurse Coaches accompany clients through the change and discovery process during coaching sessions. The shared field of the Nurse Coach and client come together where there is a sense of being in a safe relationship and a sacred space/environment that allows the coaching journey to move towards the client's desired goals.

Integral Process and the Four Quadrants

Nurse Coaches who analyze and translate an integral perspective in their coaching process increase their awareness of how the client is orienting in the world. This integral process represents a large map that helps to touch and link many aspects and resources for any situation. This integral process assists Nurse Coaches to more fully appreciate a client's worldview and process of discovery, as well as appreciate more deeply their own world-view and engage in new aspects of their own self-development (see Chapter 22) (Integrative Nurse Coach Certificate Program, n.d.; International Nurse Coach Association, n.d.).

An integral process is a comprehensive way to organize multiple phenomenon of the human experience related to four perspectives of reality: (1) *individual interior* (personal/intentional); (2) *individual exterior* (physiology/behavioral); (3) *collective interior* (shared/cultural); and (4) *collective exterior* (systems/structures) as seen in **Figure 14-1** (Wilber, 2000; 2005a; 2005b). On the outside of Figure 14-1, the left-hand quadrants (UL, LL) describe aspects of reality as subjective/intersubjective, interpretive, and qualitative. In contrast, the right-hand quadrants (UR, LR) describe aspects of reality as objective/interobjective, observable, and quantitative. When we fail to consider the subjective, intersubjective, objective, and interobjective aspects of a person's reality (always including our own), our endeavors are often fragmented and narrow. Many recognized theories and models do acknowledge the importance of various forms of reality, but the integral model recognizes all types of theories, data, phenomena, beliefs, experiences, and paradigms that can be placed in the most appropriate quadrant. The basic concept in an integral approach is that we must consider all points of view and possibilities. In addition to the four quadrants, the integral model explores the important elements of any comprehensive map of reality. Remember that we already have an awareness of these areas. The integral model simply assists us in further articulating and connecting all areas with more awareness in any situation.

This awareness extends to recognizing personal preferences and biases within each quadrant as seen in **Figure 14-2**. (See Theory of Integral Nursing [Dossey, 2013] for an in-depth discussion.) The Nurse Coach can offer the client a practice sheet (Appendix D-2) to create a personal chart of her/his personal statements in each quadrant. Each quadrant represents an *equal* one-fourth of reality, of the totality of our being and existence, and explains what you have observed or experienced within yourself and in others. The dotted lines between the quadrants represent that a change in one quadrant creates a change in all the other quadrants. A circle of healing in the center represents our integral coaching framework from the four perspectives described next.

Virtually all human languages use first-person ("I"), second-person ("we" or "you" and "me"), and third-person pronouns ("it" for exterior individual, or the plural "its" for exterior collective) to indicate three basic dimensions of reality. These four quadrants show

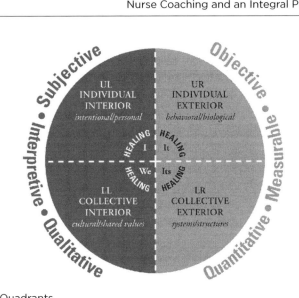

Figure 14-1 Integral Quadrants.
Source: Copyright © 2007 by Barbara M. Dossey. Adapted with permission from Wilber, K. (2000). *Integral Psychology*. Boston, MA: Shambhala.

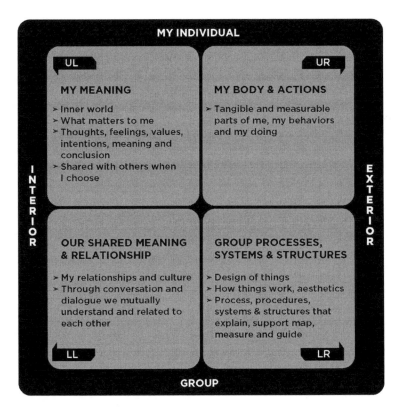

Figure 14-2 Personal Statements and the Four Quadrants.
Source: Copyright © 2014 by Barbara M. Dossey.

the four primary dimensions or perspectives of how we experience the world; these are represented graphically as the upper-left (UL), lower-left (LL), upper-right (UR), and lower-right (LR) quadrants. Each quadrant, which is intricately linked and bound to each other, carries its own truths and language (Wilber, 2000). These quadrants are as follows and seen in **Table 14-1**:

Table 14-1 Integral Model.

UPPER LEFT		UPPER RIGHT
INDIVIDUAL INTERIOR (intentional/personal)		**INDIVIDUAL EXTERIOR** (behavioral/biological)
"I" space includes self and consciousness (self-care, fears, feelings, beliefs, values, esteem, cognitive capacity, emotional maturity, moral development, spiritual maturity, personal communication skills, etc.)		"It" space that includes brain and organisms (physiology, pathophysiology [cells, molecules, limbic system, neurotransmitters, physical sensations], biochemistry, chemistry, physics, behaviors [skill development in health, nutrition, exercise, etc.])
• Subjective • Interpretive • Qualitative	I IT WE ITS	• Objective • Observable • Quantitative
COLLECTIVE INTERIOR (cultural/shared)		**COLLECTIVE EXTERIOR** (systems/structures)
"We" space includes the relationship to each other and the culture and worldview (shared understanding, shared vision, shared meaning, shared leadership and other values, integral dialogues and communication/morale, etc.).		"Its" space includes the relation to social systems and environment, organizational structures and systems [in healthcare-financial and billing systems], educational systems, information technology, mechanical structures and transportation, regulatory structures [environmental & governmental policies, etc.]
LOWER LEFT		LOWER RIGHT

Source: Copyright © 2007 by Barbara M. Dossey.

Upper-Left (UL). In this quadrant (subjective), we find the world of the individual's interior experiences: thoughts, emotions, memories, perceptions, immediate sensations, and states of mind (imagination, fears, feelings, beliefs, values, esteem, cognitive capacity, emotional maturity, moral development, and spiritual maturity). This is referred to as our "I" space.

Lower-Left (LL). In this quadrant (intersubjective), we find the world of our collective, interior experiences: shared values, meanings, vision, language, relationships, and cultural background. This is referred to as the "we" space.

Upper-Right (UR). In this quadrant (objective), we find the world of the individual's exterior things: our material body (physiology [cells, molecules, neurotransmitters, limbic system], biochemistry, chemistry, physics), skill development (health, fitness, exercise, nutrition, etc.), behaviors, practices, and anything that we can touch or observe scientifically in time and space. This is referred to as the "it" space.

Lower-Right (LR). In this quadrant (interobjective), we find the world of the collective, exterior things: social systems/structures, networks, organizational structures, and systems (including financial and billing systems in healthcare); information technology; regulatory structures (environmental and governmental policies, etc.); and the natural environment. This is referred to as the "its" space.

An integral understanding provides a powerful framework for nurse coaching and a way for the Nurse Coach to explore change. Coaching clients from an integral perspective is more likely to help them sustain change by increasing awareness about the current way of being and envisioning a desired new way of being (Hunt, 2009). This process includes a creative process of both embracing self and opening to a capacity to transcend and going beyond old patterns as discussed in Chapters 2 and 5.

Using a four-quadrant approach, the Nurse Coach is more likely to coach in a way that helps the client approach change and new behaviors and insights that can be embodied and sustained. Embodying a new capacity means that one starts with a new idea and then comes to understand its full meaning and implications. For example, a person becomes aware of using a focused breathing practice to become more present and to feel connected in the present moment. This self-awareness practice starts as an idea that then becomes an action, and ends as a capacity that is integrated throughout the day. In the next section, four Nurse Coach integral principles are discussed to assist in the translation of these concepts.

Nurse Coach Integral Principles

There are four Nurse Coach Integral Principles adapted from the Theory of Integral Nursing (Dossey, 2013) as follows:

Nurse Coach Integral Principle #1: Nursing coaching requires development of the "I." This first principle recognizes the interior individual "I" (subjective) space where each Nurse Coach values the importance of exploring one's own health and wellbeing—starting with personal discovery and development to become more integrally conscious of one's knowing, doing, and being in all aspects of personal and professional endeavors. This also includes addressing one's own shadow, referred to as the wounded healer—a composite of personal characteristics and potentials—of which one is unaware and that has been denied life expression (see Chapter 22). Through awareness practices (Chapter 12) and taking time for self-reflection, Nurse Coaches more easily understand how the ego can deny these characteristics because they may well be in conflict and incompatible with one's chosen conscious attitude.

Nurse Coach Integral Principle #2: Nurse coaching is built upon "We." This second principle recognizes the importance of the "We" (intersubjective) space where Nurse Coaches come together and are conscious of sharing their worldviews, beliefs, priorities, and values related to enhancing self-development. It includes being fully present and focused with intention to understand what another person (client/patient, family, significant other/s, or colleagues) is expressing, or not expressing, where deep listening is valued.

This focus begins an energy flow—by setting an intention for the healing process of the recipient—that moves from gross body (physical), to subtle body (light, energy, emotional feelings), to the causal body (infinity) where realization of not being separate from others is experienced. This energy healing is used to describe the subtle flow of energy within and around a person/s—creating a field that is experienced by the individual/s. This is the ability to be with empathy and open one's heart, to be present for all levels of the client's story (see Chapter 5).

Nurse Coach Integral Principle #3: Nurse coaching recognizes the "It" as behavior and skill development. This third principle recognizes the importance of the individual exterior "It" (objective) space where each person develops and integrates her/his action plan. This includes skills, behaviors, and action steps to achieve human flourishing and wellbeing. With some clients it may include exploration of conscious dying and end-of-life care as a normal process.

The Nurse Coach combines her/his nursing presence to assist clients to access personal strengths and capacities, and to release fear and anxiety that may surround change. Within this principle, Nurse Coaches move easily between the nurse expert role of educating, and the Nurse Coach role when listening to the client's concerns related to lifestyle, which may include disease management, assisting the client to identify goals and desired outcomes (see Chapter 7).

Nurse Coach Integral Principle #4: Nurse coaching recognizes the "Its" as systems and structures. This fourth principle recognizes the importance of the exterior collective "Its" (inter-objective) space where Nurse Coaches advocate for healthier communities, such as engaging group coaching on various topics (nutrition, stress management, exercise, etc.) at community facilities. Other group coaching may demonstrate how to create exterior healing environments and incorporate nature and the natural world whenever possible, including with outdoor and indoor healing gardens, use of green materials with soothing colors, and sounds of music and nature. Nurse Coaches are coming together with other interdisciplinary teams to examine their work, their priorities, use of technologies, and aspects of the technological environment, so that they deliver more effective client/patient care, coordination of care, and advocacy for care, wherever it is non-existent—local to global. This is the "collaboratory" in action (see Chapter 1).

These four Nurse Coach Integral Principles are necessary for the translation and implementation for the national initiatives such as Healthy People 2020 (U.S. Department of Health and Human Services, Office of Disease Prevention and Health Promotion, n.d.), the Patient Protection and Affordable Care Act (PPACA) (The Patient Protection and Affordable Care Act, 2010), and the National Prevention Strategy (U.S. Department of Health and Human Services, 2011). In the next section, six lines of development within the integral framework are explored.

Six Lines of Development

Wilber (2000; 2005a; 2005b) suggests six lines of development as follows: cognitive, emotional, somatic, interpersonal, spiritual, and moral. Nurse Coaches already focus on wholeness—body–mind–spirit–culture–environment—and they consciously touch these six lines and do so in relation to self, to others, and the natural world. This is part of being-in-the-world and is not imposed from the outside. It is already a part of our inherent makeup. Our nurse coaching challenge is to expand our consciousness and find new ways to deepen our integral understanding so that we coach from a depth that encourages exploration of new insights and possibilities for greater health and wellbeing. These six lines of development are illustrated in **Figure 14-3** in the upper left quadrant; they also apply to all quadrants. Each line appears differently to represent the dynamic developmental process where one line of development may be stronger than other lines depending on life's circumstances, which are always changing and evolving. The Nurse Coach can offer the client a practice sheet (Appendix D-1) to create a personal chart of her/his lines of development in each quadrant. This practice may shift the client to explore life challenges and raise one's consciousness to a higher level of awareness. Appendix D-2 is another client practice sheet with the self-development circle and the four quadrants. This discovery process often leads to finding more life satisfaction and balance as explored in Chapter 6.

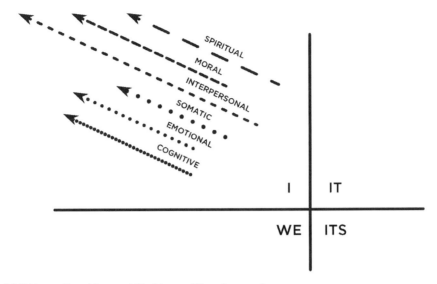

Figure 14-3 Nurse Coaching and Six Lines of Development.
Legend: Each line appears differently to represent the dynamic developmental process where one line of development may be stronger than other lines at different times depending on life's circumstances, which are always changing and evolving.
Source: Copyright © 2014 by Barbara M. Dossey. Adapted with permission from Wilber, K. (2005). *Integral operating system*. Louisville, CO: Sounds True.

1. **Cognitive: Awareness of What Is.** This is the capacity to make observations from different perspectives in a coherent manner. It is an awareness of what leads to new understanding related to possibilities, insights, action steps, breakdowns, and resistance to change.

2. **Emotional: Awareness of Spectrum of Emotions.** This is the capacity to skillfully recognize one's own emotional state in the present moment and what life conditions (present, past, future) are related; recognizing what situations evoke various emotions (challenges, difficulties, disappointments, joy, fears, anger, etc.). It is the ability to enter into the present moment and energy field with another person to listen deeply, noticing your own intuition to any emotional state/s that the person does not recognize.

3. **Somatic: Awareness of Body–Mind.** This is the capacity to feel, notice, and respond to one's body sensations (tired, tight, open, energized) and to connect these sensations with the present moment. It is the ability to skillfully access one's personal innate wisdom and make subtle shifts.

4. **Interpersonal: Awareness of How I Relate to Others.** This is the capacity to be engaged socially with others from different perspectives (I/We/It); to listen deeply to others' intentions, goals, and desires; and to offer appropriate support.

5. **Spiritual: Awareness of Ultimate Issues.** This is the capacity to explore feelings, thoughts, experiences, and behaviors that arise from a search for meaning around ultimate issues, questions, and concerns: "Who am I?" "What is my soul's purpose?" "How am I part of the interconnected web of life?" This includes from "me" to "us" to "all of us."

6. **Moral: Awareness of What to Do.** This is the capacity for choosing and caring about what is moral and ethical in personal behavior/s and action/s (includes from "me" to "us" to "all of us").

COACHING AND THE FOUR QUADRANTS

An integral approach to coaching is very useful to assist clients with change and to sustain changes. Joanne Hunt (2009), Founder and Master Certified Coach, Integral Coaching Canada, Inc. (Integral Coaching Canada, n.d.) has mapped the four quadrants and the role of the coach in each quadrant. This information on coaching from an integral and quadrants perspective and coaching conversations are foundational components of the Theory of Integrative Nurse Coaching as discussed in Chapter 2. **Figure 14-4** illustrates the common belief structures for change. **Figure 14-5** illustrates an integral and integrative Nurse Coach approach to change. **Figure 14-6** illustrates the Nurse Coach's understanding of the middle of coaching conversations with possible questions. The reader is referred to Chapter 5 for a further discussion of Nurse Coach presence and listening to the client's story. From this mapping, Hunt (2009) explores how different coaching schools believe change occurs and how these views shape the role of the coach. This integral process and the four quadrants are described next.

Upper-Left Quadrant (UL)

A UL coaching approach to change indicates that change occurs through bringing what is unconscious (what resides in the client's inner experience) into conscious awareness. The coach learns to hear it, recognize it, understand it, and give it voice. This inherent knowledge and wisdom comes from within the client.

Coach's Role with Upper-Left Quadrant (UL)

The coach's role is to hold the space and ask questions to more fully open the client to her/his inner world. This opening brings awareness of beliefs, fears, and obstacles as well as wisdom, inner truth, and intelligence. The coach listens attentively to be able to learn the client's perspective and underlying beliefs at both their personal and existential level. This coaching approach emphasizes the client's interiority—inner awareness, reflection, and wisdom, and the connections with possibilities beyond the self. With this approach, clients build cognitive capacities, increase their ability to choose, and make changes and broaden their emotional perspective and understanding. This alone will not always lead to translation and integration in daily life. It will be necessary to address the elements of all four quadrants to have a full perspective on the coaching process.

Upper-Right Quadrant (UR)

A UR coaching approach to change finds that change occurs through deliberate action and goal setting, breakthroughs, and completing projects.

Coach's Role with Upper-Right Quadrant (UR)

The coach's role is to help the client set her/his behavior goals and design an action plan. The coach works with clients as they begin to implement their plan. As clients accomplish goals, demonstrate new skills, and achieve new results, they build self-confidence and self-esteem. Clients may rely on a coach's skills and encouragement to sustain change.

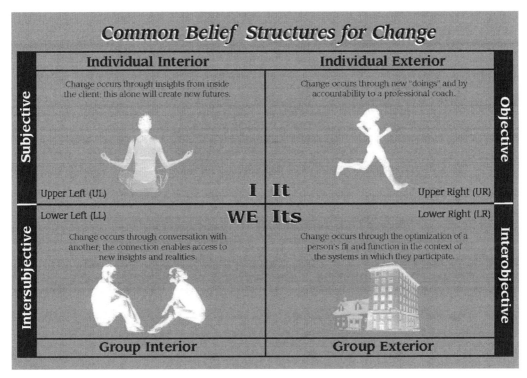

Figure 14-4 Common Belief Structures for Change.
Source: Copyright © 2010 by Barbara M. Dossey. Adapted with permission from Hunt, J. (2009). Transcending and including our current way of being. *Journal of Integral Theory and Practice*, 4(1), 1–20; and Integral Coaching Institute Canada, Inc. www.integralcoachingcanada.com

Lower-Left Quadrant (LL)

The LL coaching approach to change is sparked through interaction and shared meaning between individuals. This intersubjective sharing gives rise to new ideas and perspectives that would not be fully available in isolation.

Coach's Role with Lower-Left Quadrant (LL)

The coach's role is as a conversational partner, with the client being the "thinking partner." It is the voice of coach as "other" that helps expand and shift the client's perspective. This process occurs as the coach remains fully present, staying attuned to the story line and following threads that may spontaneously arise. This allows the possibility for deeper intimacy and insight and the client being witnessed and understood. Although the client accesses much information and new insights, there is a risk of the client being unable to sustain the change if other quadrants are not addressed as coaching will be insufficient and partial.

Lower-Right Quadrant (LR)

A LR coaching approach to change involves optimizing the function and fit of the client within the overall system (family, work, community). For example, within a work setting, the client may explore ways to improve skills, evaluate roles, and recognize expectations

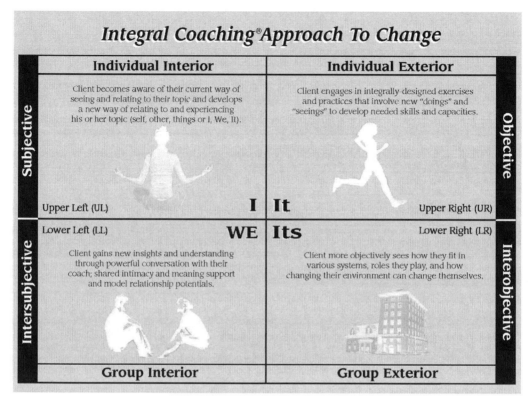

Figure 14-5 Integral Coaching Approaches to Change.
Source: Copyright © 2010 by Barbara M. Dossey. Adapted with permission from Hunt, J. (2009). Transcending and including our current way of being. *Journal of Integral Theory and Practice, 4*(1), 1–20; and Integral Coaching Institute Canada, Inc. www.integralcoachingcanada.com

or other issues relevant to the work environment. The question then may come up as to how to align with, or adapt to, contribute to, or influence the system, or move to another position or job where there is a better fit. If the system being explored is the family, then it becomes imperative to examine how the new behaviors impact the family.

Coach's Role with Lower-Right Quadrant (LR)

The coach's role requires a systems view and understanding around work or group interactions. The elements at play may include team structure, operating principles, organizational procedures, personal and professional relationships, and many other factors that come into play when working within a system. The coach works with the client to determine the dynamics and how to interact at the desired level within the system. The coach will help the client to determine the extent to which she/he can influence the system, or to discover if another system is a better fit. This also applies to coaching around family structure as in the above example. A focus on only this quadrant without connecting to the other quadrants is incomplete and partial.

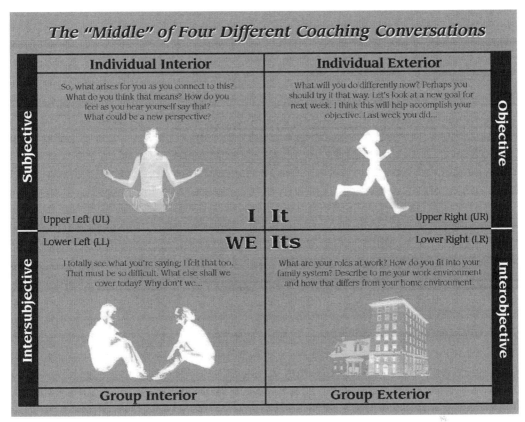

The "Middle" of Four Different Coaching Conversations

Individual Interior	Individual Exterior
Subjective	**Objective**
So, what arises for you as you connect to this? What do you think that means? How do you feel as you hear yourself say that? What could be a new perspective?	What will you do differently now? Perhaps you should try it that way. Let's look at a new goal for next week. I think this will help accomplish your objective. Last week you did...
Upper Left (UL) **I**	**It** Upper Right (UR)
Lower Left (LL) **WE**	**Its** Lower Right (LR)
Intersubjective	**Interobjective**
I totally see what you're saying; I felt that too. That must be so difficult. What else shall we cover today? Why don't we...	What are your roles at work? How do you fit into your family system? Describe to me your work environment and how that differs from your home environment.
Group Interior	Group Exterior

Figure 14-6 Middle of Four Different Coaching Conversations.
Source: Copyright © 2010 by Barbara M. Dossey. Adapted with permission from Hunt, J. (2009). Transcending and including our current way of being. *Journal of Integral Theory and Practice, 4*(1), 1–20; and Integral Coaching Institute Canada, Inc. www.integralcoachingcanada.com

Coaching Conversations

Coaching conversations have a beginning (reasons for seeking coaching and, if coaching sessions have started, a greeting, how are you, quick update), middle (where the majority of time is spent), and an end (agreeing on next session date, reviewing action plan, and other possibilities; or the completion of coaching sessions). (See Chapter 4 Nurse Coaching Process and Competencies and Standard 5: Implementation and Before the Coaching Interaction, Throughout the Coaching Interaction, and At the End of the Coaching Interaction.) After the client determines the topic for the coaching session, the Nurse Coach will use presence, intention, intuition, and deep listening to determine the most powerful questions to ask the client as discussed in Chapter 5.

Following the intake process in the initial coaching session, and during all coaching sessions, the Nurse Coach becomes aware of how the client orients in the world. Does the person come from a place of reflection (UL)? Is the client focused on actions and accomplishing a project or assignment (UR)? Does the client need to engage with another to explore meaning and understanding (LL)? Does the client seek to know the big picture within a system/structure (LR)?

Using silence, often referred to as the "power of the pause," throughout a coaching session allows time for both the client and the Nurse Coach to reflect on the process of discovery and insight. Further possibilities also emerge in the conversation, and the Nurse Coach may rephrase what the client shared, leading to an opportunity to go deeper into the client's story, as discussed in Chapter 2, Theory of Integrative Nurse Coaching, Component 5 and Chapter 5.

As the Nurse Coach listens to the client's responses to questions or insights, it is important to remember that moments of insight and "Ah-ha" are often examples of the mind grasping something new. This insight is often just transitory and not yet embodied as a lived experience. This is where the Nurse Coach and Client Guiding Principles (Appendix A-1) and the Integral Self-Development Circle (Appendix D-2) and Six Lines of Development (Appendix D-1) and coaching sessions evolve to guide the client to desired skill building and commitments to specific changes and goals.

Not all coaching leads to actions. Insights can be very useful in understanding barriers to change. They may result in identifying thoughts that get in the way of one's goals. In this way they are extremely beneficial. Assisting a person in the recognition of the need for an adjustment in attitude or in their challenging of a belief may, in and of itself, be the catalyst for change (see Chapter 15).

The Nurse Coach is aware that when clients are very expressive and make many connections this does not indicate embodiment of insights, goals, and actions. For a change to become embodied requires that a practice be repeated over and over again. This leads to the creation of new capacities and competencies. Clients learning how to use self-awareness and self-observation throughout the day become able to understand and recognize thoughts, actions, behaviors, body sensations, and postures in the moment when they occur and how they relate to the desired changes.

Nurse coaching from an integral perspective is more likely to create the conditions for sustainable change. To neglect any quadrant leaves a client with many insights and actions without a way to fully understand her/his challenges and succeed in integrating and sustaining the desired changes.

SUMMARY

- An integral process is a comprehensive way to organize multiple phenomenon of human experience related to four perspectives of reality: (1) the individual interior (personal/intentional); (2) individual exterior (physiology/behavioral); (3) collective interior (shared/cultural); and (4) collective exterior (systems/structures).
- Nurse Coaches recognize four integral principles—the individual interior "I"; the individual exterior "It"; the collective interior "We"; and the collective exterior "Its" in nurse coaching.
- An integral healing process leads to a deeper understanding of the unitary whole person interacting in mutual process with the environment.
- Nurse Coaches (and clients) explore six lines of development (cognitive, emotional, somatic, interpersonal, spiritual, and moral) to increase their capacities and competencies. They also explore these lines of development with clients/patients and others.
- Nurse Coaches are aware that using an integral perspective in coaching sessions allows for more flow within a session and assists clients to embody new behaviors for sustained change.

NURSE COACH REFLECTIONS

After reading this chapter, the Nurse Coach will be able to bring awareness and personal insight to the following questions:

- What ways do I integrate the integral principles in my life and nurse coaching?
- What new understanding and insights do I have about my own capacity to change a behavior(s) using an integral perspective and the four quadrants?
- What do I discover when I explore the six lines of development?
- What awareness practices help me become more aware of the interior and exterior qualities of my life?

REFERENCES

Dossey, B. M. (2013). Integral and holistic nursing: Local to global. In B. M. Dossey & L. Keegan (Eds.), *Holistic nursing: A handbook for practice* (6th ed., pp. 3–57). Burlington, MA: Jones & Bartlett Learning.

Hunt, J. (2009). Transcending and including our current way of being. *Journal of Integral Theory and Practice, 4*(1), 1–20.

Integral Coaching Canada, Inc. (n.d.). Retrieved from http://www.integralcoachingcanada.com/

Integrative Nurse Coach Certificate Program (n.d.). Retrieved from http://inursecoach.com/programs/overview/

International Nurse Coach Association (n.d.). www.inursecoach.com

Nightingale, F. (1872). *Address from Miss Nightingale to the probationer-nurses in the 'Nightingale Fund' at St. Thomas's Hospital, and the nurses who were formerly trained there* (p. 4). London, UK: Spottiswoode. (Privately printed.)

Patient Protection and Affordable Care Act (PPACA) 42 U.S.C. § 18001 et seq. (2010). Retrieved from http://democrats.senate.gov/pdfs/reform/patient-protection-affordable-care-act-as-passed.pdf

U.S. Department of Health and Human Services, Office of Disease Prevention and Health Promotion (n.d.). *Introducing healthy people 2020.* Retrieved from http://www.healthypeople.gov/2020/about/default.aspx

U.S. Department of Health and Human Services (2011). *National prevention strategy: American's plan for better health and wellness.* Retrieved from http://www.surgeon-general.gov/initiatives/prevention/strategy/report.pdf

Wilber, K. (2000). *Integral psychology.* Boston, MA: Shambhala.

Wilber, K. (2005a). *Integral operating system.* Louisville, CO: Sounds True.

Wilber, K. (2005b). *Integral life practices.* Denver, CO: Integral Institute.

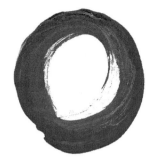

CHAPTER 15

Change and Two Theoretical Perspectives Towards Achieving Goals

Lisa A. Davis

> Rules may become a dead letter. It is the spirit of them that "giveth life." So is the individual, inside, that counts—the level she is upon which tells. The next is only the outward shell or envelope. She must become a "rule of thought"—to herself thru' the Rules. Every Nurse must grow. No Nurse can stand still, she must go forward, or she will go backward, every year.
>
> *Florence Nightingale, 1888*

LOOKING AHEAD...

After reading this chapter, you will be able to:

- Analyze the Transtheoretical Model (TTM) of Behavioral Change and the five stages of change.
- Explore the pros and cons for change.
- Conceptualize Barrett's Power as Knowing theory.
- Identify applications of Barrett's Power as Knowing theory in nurse coaching.
- Reflect on SMART goals and their relevance for coaching.
- Examine the GROW Model and the 4-step process.

DEFINITIONS

Affirmational resolution: An intentional declaration of a decision or goal.

Ambivalence: Contradictory attitudes are feelings toward an action or uncertainty about which approach to follow.

Decisional balance: Weighing the pros and cons that are associated with a change behavior.

Deep listening: Presence in the moment to understand what another person is expressing or not expressing; communication between two or more individuals in which the conventional division of self and ego is transcended by a sense of indivisible unity between all involved.

Motivator: A reason for action.

Positive psychology: Focus on the positive, adaptive, creative, and emotionally fulfilling aspects of human behavior.

Power profile: Awareness, choices, freedom to act intentionally, and involvement in creating change. These elements are seen only as a whole rather than separate.

Unitary: Indivisible, unpredictable, and ever-changing nature of human beings (Parse, 2003).

Values clarification: A nursing intervention in which a client can discover her/his own values by assessing, exploring, and evaluating the effect of personal values on decision-making. The role of the nurse is to facilitate this process.

TRANSTHEORETICAL MODEL (TTM) OF BEHAVORIAL CHANGE

The Transtheoretical Model (TTM) of Behavioral Change offers an explanation of how people change their health behaviors over time. The motivation to change may or may not be addressed depending on if the person sees change as a perceived threat, perceived benefit, and/or perceived capacity for change. TTM addresses both the intention to change and the process of change. Change is a staged process, and understanding the stages of change is essential if new behaviors are to be sustained and maintained. Beginning in 1995, James O. Prochaska and colleagues (1995) based their TTM on research; it is the most recognized model in the field of coaching, addictions, and wellness. The five stages of change (**Figure 15-1**) in the TTM are precontemplation, contemplation, preparation, action, and maintenance (Moore & Tschannen-Moran, 2010). This sequence is important.

Before a discussion of the process of change according to TTM, it is important to understand some of the underlying assumptions (**Table 15-1**). Behavioral change can appear at first glance to be simple, but it is very complex, requiring an understanding of underlying reasons for behaviors, barriers to change, and internal and external motivation to either promote or resist change. It is common for change to take a long time, even with years of coaching and/or counseling. Within each stage of change are elements that may remain the same, but can also vary widely (Norcross, Krebs, & Prochaska, 2011). For example, suppose a client developed a running program to enhance health and has been running two miles, five times a week for two years. This client would be considered to be in the maintenance stage. However, what if this same client begins a new job that requires a lot of travel, or sustains an injury, or moves to a much colder climate? All these new conditions affect how and when the client may run, and the client can either adapt to the new conditions of maintenance, or fall back to any of the previous stages.

Table 15-1 Assumptions Related to TTM.

1. No single theory can explain all the aspects of behavioral change.
2. Change takes time and occurs in stages.
3. The stages of change are both static and dynamic.
4. Without intervention, change may never progress past the early stages.
5. Most people cannot change all at once (e.g., "cold turkey"), but are more successful if change is incremental, in stages.
6. Specific process needs to be in place to effect progress through the stages of change.
7. Behaviors can be changed.
8. It is common for the individual to have several attempts at changes before successfully making it through all the stages.

Source: Adapted by Lisa A. Davis. From Prochaska, J., Reddig, C., & Evers, K. (2008). The transtheoretical model and stages of change. In B. Glanz, B. K. Rimer, & K. Viswanath (Eds.). *Health behaviors and health education: Theory, research and practice* (4th ed.). San Francisco, CA: Jossey Bass.

1. **Precontemplation (not ready for change):** Clients in the precontemplation stage, the "I can't" or "I won't" stage, are usually not interested in change in the foreseeable future (usually defined as six months), that they don't have a problem (DiClemente, Salazar, & Crosby, 2013). Also, they may have tried to change a health behavior over and over

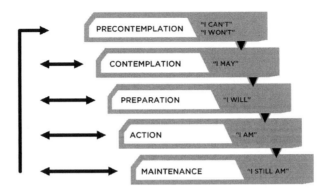

Figure 15-1 Stages of Change.
Source: Copyright © 2014 by the International Nurse Coach Association. www.inursecoach.com

again and are too discouraged to think of trying again. Change may not be contemplated because the client is uninformed or under-informed. Often, friends and family may perceive a need to change and begin nagging. If a client comes to a Nurse Coach in this stage, it is usually to satisfy a family member or friend. If a client does seek out a Nurse Coach in this stage, the Nurse Coach can help her/him sort out barriers that allow for a good feeling about the discussion. When clients are ready for change, they will return.

2. **Contemplation (thinking about change):** In the contemplation stage, the "I may" stage, a client can identify an unhealthy behavior, begins thinking about it, and considers taking action within the next six months. She or he has an awareness of the benefits of changing and is less satisfied with the status quo. In this "I may" stage, the client often feels that change will be difficult and ambivalence about change is to be expected. In this stage an affirmational resolution, an intentional declaration of a decision or goal, becomes the stimulus for change (DiClemente et al., 2013). The affirmational resolution results from decisional balance, in which pros and cons of change are contemplated and discussed. It is to be expected that the client will be ambivalent. In fact, in early discussion, the list of cons may be longer and more compelling than the list of pros (**Figure 15-2**). As the client moves through the stages of change, the benefits outweigh the cons, and become a motivator for change, but in the contemplation stage, the client needs to maximize the benefits of change and minimize the barriers to change in order to achieve decisional balance.

The Nurse Coach role in the contemplation stage is that of deep listening. The Nurse Coach assists clients to connect the dots between the change they seek and the shifts that will occur. Small steps at this stage are essential for the client to see a new possibility and achieve decisional balance. In this stage, the client is discovering new information by reading, talking, listening, and exploring some changes to determine if the small steps can be achieved. Other nurse coaching actions in this stage might include values clarification (**Table 15-2**) or guided imagery, in which the client imagines her-/himself in the contemplated mode of behavior. Supportive relationships help to keep a person motivated.

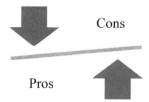

Figure 15-2 Decisional Imbalance.
Source: Copyright © 2014 by Lisa A. Davis.

Table 15-2 Values Clarification Strategies.

• Encourage consideration of values underlying choices.
• Ask open-ended questions to assist the client in reflecting on what is personally important.
• Assist client to prioritize values.
• Pose reflective, clarifying questions that give the client something to think about.
• Reinforce actions or statements that support the client's values.
• Support the client in communicating her or his values to others.
• Avoid use of this intervention with persons with serious emotional problems.

Source: Adapted by Lisa A. Davis. From Bulechek, G., Burcher, H., Dochterman, J., & Wagner, C. (2013). *Nursing interventions classification (NIC)* (6th ed.). St. Louis, MO: Mosby.

3. **Preparation (preparing for action):** In the preparation stage, the "I will" stage, clients have overcome their ambivalent feelings and know the barriers as well as identify some solutions. They intend to adopt the new behavior, usually within a month. They may have taken some action already, such as retaining services of a Nurse Coach or joining a health club. The client is developing a sense of self-efficacy or belief that they can commit to the change. It is important to remember that change will result in new skills and resources, and those take time to achieve. The Nurse Coach's role is to help clients in the preparation stage with a plan of action. The coach explores the difficulties of change and new behaviors, as resistance and ambivalence often arise as clients begin to change.

4. **Action (taking action):** Clients in action, referred to as the "I am" stage, are modifying their behavior, experience, and environment to facilitate the desired change (Norcross et al., 2011). Clients in this stage have identified new behavior/s and are integrating their new actions consistently. This stage lasts around six months. During this period, a lapse may occur, which is a single slip in a desired behavior. This can be reframed as a temporary setback and a learning opportunity, not a failure. New behaviors can be further compromised, causing the client to recycle. If this happens, it is important for the Nurse Coach to support the client, encouraging positive self-talk instead of shame and blame. This may happen numerous times during the action phase.

   Remember, this stage requires significant time and energy on the part of the client. Most coaching takes place in this stage when new habits, behaviors, and relationships occur. The Nurse Coach's role is to encourage the client to connect with her/his new behaviors and personal strengths and values. With support from a community, long-term change is more likely.

5. **Maintenance (maintaining a new behavior):** Clients in this "I still am" stage have new behaviors that have become a habit and are done automatically. It is usually six months to an indeterminate time from the beginning of a new behavior before maintenance is achieved. Both self-efficacy and self-reinforcing feelings are high in this stage as the

client is confident that a new behavior can be maintained and sustained. The aim of this stage is to consolidate gains and avoid relapse (Norcross & Prochaska, 2002). The Nurse Coach's role in maintenance is to assist a client to reconnect and appreciate her/his accomplishment and to continue to identify motivators for making these behavior changes. Lapses may occur as the client becomes bored and may slip into old patterns. This is when new goals need to be made and reinforced. If a complete relapse happens, integrate strategies that were also used in the preparation and action stages. The overall goal of nurse coaching is to facilitate movement through the stages until the client has achieved maintenance and remains in maintenance, as seen in **Table 15-3**.

Table 15-3 Examples of Client Behaviors That Affect Progress in TTM.

TTM Stage	Client Behavioral Cues	Nurse Coach Action
Precontemplation	"I can't." "I won't." "My (family member, physician, etc.) thought I should see you."	• Identify barriers • Be available when client is ready for change.
Contemplation	"I may." "It might help."	• Assist clients to connect the dots between the change they seek and the shifts that will occur. • Support client in imagining possibilities.
Preparation	"I will." "I can." "I plan to."	• Assess for and facilitate working through ambivalence and resistance. • Support positive self-talk.
Action	"I am."	• Encourage congruence with strengths and values. • Assess for balance.
Maintenance	"I still am."	• Reinforce self-efficacy. • Assist client to appreciate work. • Explore potential new goals.

Source: Copyright © 2014 by Lisa A. Davis.

Prochaska, Reddig, and Evers (2008) believe that most of us require some sort of intervention to progress past the early stages of change. Facilitating change can include several strategies by healthcare professionals, but the interventions of the Nurse Coach is one on which this chapter focuses. The Nurse Coach can guide the individual through the stages of change, being cognizant of the complexity of change and the importance of the stages to maintaining change. It is important to be aware of all the life events which can become barriers to change, and can result in a reversal of that change, or lead to reverting to a previous stage. Prochaska, Norcross, and DiClemente (1995) call this recycling. Figure 15-1 depicts this as arrows moving back up at each stage of change.

Norcross (2012) uses different terminology (**P**sych, **P**lan, **P**erspire, **P**ersevere, and **P**ersist), and these stages directly correlate to the stages in TTM. Norcross helps clarify the nonlinearity of the process as an upward spiral. If the person has a small slip, she/he will begin again with getting psyched about the desired change, planning the steps, etc. In fact, he identifies that relapse is more the rule than the exception. Prochaska et al. (1995) also caution that the probability of recycling must be considered. This is a crucial insight the Nurse Coach can use in guiding the client. Because the process is really nonlinear, the Nurse Coach should be cognizant of expressions of shame on the part of the client related to recycling. Use of positive psychology principles and nonviolent communication is helpful in coaching through an experience of recycling. In addition, the Nurse Coach should be aware of feeling guilt that the client experienced recycling and blamed her-/himself. For this reason, it is important to use positive psychology principles and self-care measures when a client is experiencing a period of recycling. In short, the Nurse Coach should have no attachment to the outcomes.

Predictors of Success in TTM

Blissmer et al. (2010) have identified several predictors that the client will be successful in change. First, clients with tailored interventions for change have more success than those who do not (Noar, Benac, & Harris, 2007). Second, those who express a greater intention to change are more successful in maintaining change. Also, the discrepancy between risk of not changing and the desired change is predictive, in that those who need to make the greatest change are less likely to be successful.

As could be expected, those who exert the greatest effort in achieving change are generally more successful. Finally, demographic variables such as age, gender, marital status, ethnicity income, and education can be predictive in changing health-related behaviors. Generally, females are more disposed to change, as are those who are younger. Those aged 65 and older are least likely to change. With regard to race, Caucasians are more likely to change. Those who are married (both men and women), those with higher income, and those with more education are more predisposed to change (Harper & Lynch, 2007; Pleis & Lethbridge-Cejku, 2007). Keep in mind these are just predictors and are based on counseling outcomes, not nurse coaching. It will be interesting to see, as data become more available, if nurse coaching will have similar, or better, results.

Pros and Cons of Change

Understanding these five stages of change assists integrative Nurse Coaches with how and when clients' behaviors can be altered and why clients struggle, recycle, fail, or quit with desired change. Remembering that self-change is a staged process, clients are usually thinking about the "pros" and "cons" of change and are asking themselves reflective questions such as the following (Moore & Tschannen-Moran, 2010):

- Why do I want to try and change my behavior? (pros)
- Why shouldn't I try to change my behavior? (cons)
- What would it take for me to change my behavior? (my strategy to overcome the cons)
- Do my "pros" outweigh my "cons?"
- What would it take for me to change the behavior and overcome the "cons?"
- Can I really do this?

The pros have to outweigh the cons for a person to actually sustain a change in behavior/s. People want to change fast and often set unrealistic goals with a new practice. Listen for client statements such as: "I won't do it;" "I can't do it;" "I may do it;" "I am doing it;" and "I am still doing it." As a Nurse Coach you can help the client uncover blocks and resistance that increase her/his sense of self-efficacy. When a person has a belief that she/he can change and a successful action takes place, this is more likely to be followed by other positive changes or a positive circular process (one good thing leads to another).

The opposite is also true when a client fails at a new behavior because the goal was unrealistic.

Helping people find strong motivators to change behavior, to understand their challenges, and to identify possible choices and solutions is key in coaching. When a client can find and understand an internal motivation to change, she/he can understand a current way of being. When a client's focus is on external motivators such as when a spouse or friend wants to see the change, it may lead to frustration, guilt, anger, and no readiness to change a behavior. Assisting the client with readiness to change in small steps is more likely to lead to the first steps of success. Success in one small area leads to increased confidence and a shift in one's self-dialogue about the pros of change. In the next section, the leading nursing theory on change is explored.

KNOWING PARTICIPATION IN CHANGE THEORY

Elisabeth Barrett (1983, 1989, 2003) developed the Knowing Participation in Change Theory. Her power theory elaborates on Martha Rogers' (1970) axiom that humans can participate knowingly in change. Barrett proposed that power is the capacity to participate knowingly in the nature of change characterizing the continuous mutual process of people and their world. Power as knowing participation in change is being aware of what one is choosing to do, feeling free to do it, and doing it intentionally.

According to this theory, power is inherently value free. The observable, measurable dimensions of power are awareness, choices, freedom to act intentionally, and involvement in creating change (**Figure 15-3**). The inseparable association of the four power dimensions is termed a person's or group's Power Profile. The Power Profile is not static; it varies based on the changing nature of the human-environment mutual process of various individuals and/or groups. These changes indicate: (1) the nature of the awareness of experiences; (2) the type of choices made; (3) the degree to which freedom to act intentionally is operating; and (4) the manner of involvement in creating specific changes that create an upward spiral towards change.

Barrett's theory is congruent with the TTM in that it deals with terms of change, but not causality. It is applicable to both individuals and groups. She sees power as knowing participation in change based on four inseparable dimensions: (1) awareness, (2) choices, (3) freedom to act intentionally, and (4) involvement in creating change (Figure 15-3). These, together and inseparable, are what Barrett calls her Power Profile. As you can see, the power profile is nonlinear, and neither is it static. The human and environmental factors involved in patterning vary constantly and are (Barrett, 1986; 2010, p. 49):

- *Nature* of the awareness of experience;
- *Type* of choices that are made;
- *Degree* to which freedom to act intentionally is operating; and
- *Manner* of involvement in creating specific changes.

The more effortless or rhythmic the person/group's life flow, the greater is the person's/group's capacity for knowingly participating in change. Barrett uses the term "life flow" to denote physical, emotional, social, and intellectual harmony. See Chapter 2 on Flow Theory. It is important to remember Rogers' (1970) unitary principle in this conceptualization because Barrett does not see physical, emotional, social, and intellectual as separate parts of human being, but as a whole, the whole being more than the sum of the parts.

Barrett (2010) differentiates what she states are the "two worlds we live in" without claiming one is better or worse than the other, but that the two worlds exist. In the

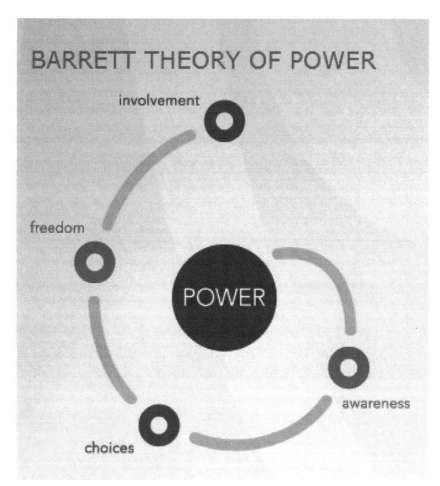

Figure 15-3 Barrett's Theory of Power as Knowing Participation in Change.
Source: Copyright © 2003 by E. A. M. Barrett. Used with permission.

material worldview, power is seen as control and as causal. In this thought mode, the client may state: "If I do this, that will happen." In the worldview of the unitary, what Barrett calls the spiritual, power is seen as freedom. In this worldview, the client may state: "If I do this, anything might happen." The elements of the power profile are the same for each worldview, but how individuals use it is different. As Barrett says, "power is power." We can use it for control or for freedom (**Figure 15-4**). For the Nurse Coach, understanding the worldview of the client, how they see their experiences, is a starting place for understanding their change possibilities. Irrespective of the worldview, Barrett believes living their power is in the best interest of the individual and that all people can knowingly participate in change. Also, power as freedom can be taught. She offers the following power prescription, "I am free to choose with awareness how I participate in changes I intend to create" (Barrett, 2010, p. 52). Look at the powerful words of this prescription—free, choose with awareness, participate in change, intend, create. What an impact these words of power

Barrett's Theory of Power as Knowing Participation in Change: Spiritual and Material Worldviews

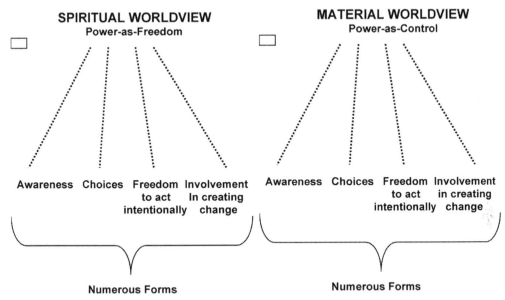

Figure 15-4 Barrett's Theory of Power as Knowing Participation in Change: Spiritual and Material Worldviews.
Source: Copyright © 2003 by E. A. M. Barrett. Used with permission.

can have in eliciting change talk and change behavior! She expands on the power prescription in **Table 15-4**.

Regardless of whether using TTM or Barrett's Theory of Power (or some combination thererof) as a theoretical framework, not all coaching sessions lead to (observable) actions. Insights can be very useful in understanding barriers to change, or to identifying thoughts that get in the way of one's goals and in this way are extremely beneficial. If a client's goal is to feel better about something, an insight can take her or him there. Some types of coaching do focus on action steps. Next steps may involve contemplation or reflection. Reflection in itself may involve skill building for clients. Remember to look for the client's intrinsic (internal motivators such as more life balance, less stress, hypertension management, reducing risk factors) and extrinsic (family member wants client to change, peer pressure) motivators, which can provide additional information on why she or he seeks ways to increase healthy lifestyle behaviors. In the next section, steps for achieving goals are explored.

Table 15-4 Power Prescription Questions.

Ask yourself the following:
- What am I aware of?
- What choices am I making?
- Am I following through on the choices I'm making?
- What actions am I taking?

(continues on next page)

Table 15-4 (*Continued*).

Then consider power dimensions in the proposed change:
- Do the changes I intend to create interfere with anyone else's freedom?
- Do the changes I intend to create attempt to control, dominate, manipulate, or bring harm to anyone?
- Do the changes I intend to create harm my health or shorten my life?
- Do the changes I intend to create violate what I know to be my truth?

Source: Copyright © 2007 by E. A. M. Barrett. Used with permission. Published as Barrett, E. A. M. (2010). Power as knowing participation in change: What's new and what's next, *Nursing Science Quarterly, 23*(1), 52.

SMART GOALS

Assisting a client to identify areas for change and action steps towards increased self-esteem can create a new level of potential engagement with a client towards increased health. The Nurse Coach's role is to help clients in the preparation stage with a plan of action that may include SMART goals (**Table 15-5**).

Table 15-5 SMART Goals.

S	Specific: State exactly what you want to accomplish (Who, What, Where, Why).
M	Measureable: How will you demonstrate and evaluate the extent to which the goal/s have been accomplished?
A	Achievable: Be creative and stretch for challenging goals within your ability to achieve outcomes using an action-oriented verb.
R	Realistic: How does the goal tie into your life and responsibilities? Is it aligned with your goal/s and what you want to achieve?
T	Time-lined: Set one or more target dates, "by when" and "frequency" to guide your goal to a timely and successful completion.

Source: Copyright © 2014 by the International Nurse Coach Association. www.inursecoach.com

The SMART acronym can be helpful in creating lasting, positive change. Goals should be **specific** in that they are easily described. They should answer the questions: "What?", "Why?", and "How?" Goals should be **measurable**. When will you know you have achieved the goal? The measurement should also be specific, such as "three times a week," rather than vague, such as "by the end of the year." Of course, the goal should be **achievable**. While it is important to be challenged, you don't want the client to be overwhelmed into stagnation. Along with that, the goal should be **realistic**. If the client has never run distance, it would be unrealistic to expect her or him to run a mile within a week. Lastly, goals should be **timely**. Goals should have a clear, but realistic time frame, such as "I will enroll in yoga class today," or "I will walk for at least one mile three days a week."

GROW MODEL

The GROW Model (**G**oal>**R**eality Check>**O**ptions>**W**ill) is one of the most frequently used conversational models in coaching (**Table 15-6**). This four-step progression model assists the client from defining an objective (**G**oal) through clearly defining the starting point (**R**eality Check), developing several potential possibilities for action (**O**ptions), and creating concrete actions steps with high buy-in commitments (**W**ill) that allow the person to actually achieve the desired goal with success. This works well to help a person with practice issues such as changing a habit (eating, exercise, workaholic, etc.) increasing performance with projects, and accomplishing practical things. The reader is referred to Chapters 10 and 13 for case studies that show the application and translation of the TTM and the Stages of Change, Knowing Participation in Change Theory, SMART goals, and the GROW Model in clinical practice. In the next section, the Patient Activation Measure is briefly explored as a validated tool that assists Nurse Coaches in working with clients towards change and how to sustain new behaviors.

Table 15-6 GROW Model Sample Questions.

Goal	What do you want to achieve?
	What is important to you right now?
	Describe yourself after achieving this goal.
	How will you know you have reached your goal?
	What do you want to happen that is not happening now?
	What is of value to you?
Reality Check	On a scale of 0-10, where are you with relation to your goal?
	What has helped you be successful so far?
	What are you working on right now?
	Describe your progress.
	What have you tried so far?
Options	What are your options?
	What could you do differently?
	Write down 5 options and then discuss which options are most appealing.
	What are some pros and cons to these actions?
	Have you done something similar in the past?
Will	What support do you need?
	What are the next steps?
	How will you start that?

Source: Modified by Lisa A. Davis. From Whitmore, J. (2009). *Coaching for performance: GROWing human potential and purpose* (4th ed.). Boston, MA: Nicholas Brealey Publishing.

PATIENT ACTIVATION MEASURE

The Patient Activation Measure® (PAM®) as seen in **Figure 15-5** indicates knowledge, skills, and confidence in management of one's own healthcare decisions. This tool not only gives insight into what drives activation of a new health behavior, but can also be predictive of perseverance with the change in behavior, and thereby outcomes. For the Nurse Coach, PAM can provide insights into learning opportunities with the client. Nurse Coaches meet the clients where they are and guide them to where they want to be with regard to health goals. This is achieved by encouraging small steps and tailoring educational/motivational coaching to each individual client. Research has shown this to be effective with regard to personal outcomes, quality of care, and cost of care (Hibbard & Green, 2013; Hibbard, Green, & Overton, 2013). **Figure 15-6** depicts specific actions for the client and for the Nurse Coach at each level of the activation of change.

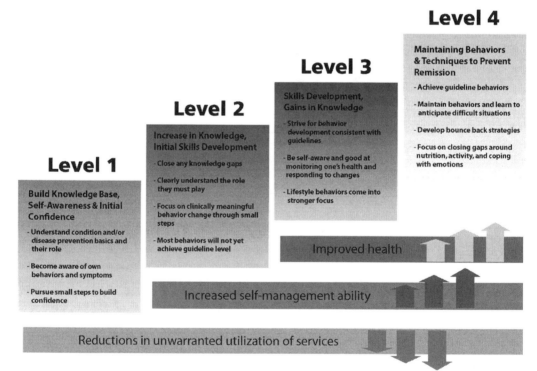 Level 1	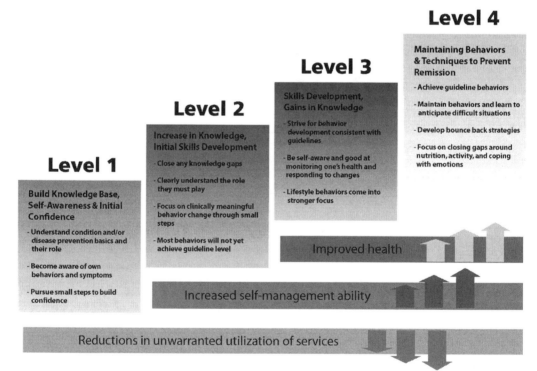 Level 2	Level 3	Level 4
Disengaged and overwhelmed	**Becoming aware, but still struggling**	**Taking action**	**Maintaining behaviors and pushing further**
Individuals are passive and lack confidence. Knowledge is low, goal-orientation is weak, and adherence is poor. Their perspective: "My doctor is in charge of my health."	Individuals have some knowledge, but large gaps remain. They believe health is largely out of their control, but can set simple goals. Their perspective: "I could be doing more."	Individuals have the key facts and are building self-management skills. They strive for best practice behaviors, and are goal-oriented. Their perspective: "I'm part of my health care team."	Individuals have adopted new behaviors, but may struggle in times of stress or change. Maintaining a healthy lifestyle is a key focus. Their perspective: "I'm my own advocate."

Increasing Level of Activation

Figure 15-5 Patient Activation Measure.
Source: Copyright © 2014 by Insignia Health Patient Activation Measure. Used with permission.

Figure 15-6 Patient Activation Measure and Specific Client Actions at Each Level of the Activation of Change.
Source: Copyright © 2014 by Insignia Health Patient Activation Measure. Used with permission.

SUMMARY

- The Transtheoretical Model (TTM) of Behavioral Change offers an explanation of how people change their health behaviors over time. The five stages of change are: pre-contemplation, contemplation, preparation, action, and maintenance.
- Behavioral change can appear at first glance to be simple, but it is very complex, requiring an understanding of underlying reasons for behaviors, barriers to change, and internal and external motivation to either promote or resist change.
- Most of us require some sort of intervention to progress past the early stages of change.
- In the TTM, relapse is more the rule than the exception. The Nurse Coach knows that the probability of recycling must be considered.
- According to Barrett's theory, power is inherently value free. The observable, measurable dimensions of power are awareness, choices, freedom to act intentionally, and involvement in creating change.
- Power as knowing participation in change is based on four inseparable dimensions: awareness, choices, freedom to act intentionally, and involvement in creating change. These, together and inseparable, are what Barrett calls her Power Profile.
- Barrett's theory is congruent with TTM in that it deals with terms of change, but not causality.
- Regardless of whether using TTM or Barrett's Theory of Power (or some combination thereof) as a theoretical framework, not all coaching sessions lead to (observable) actions.
- Remember to look for the client's intrinsic (internal motivators such as more life balance, less stress, hypertension management, reducing risk factors) and extrinsic (family member wants client to change, peer pressure) motivators that can additional information on why she or he seeks ways to increase healthy lifestyle behaviors.
- SMART goals are specific, measurable, achievable, realistic, and time-lined.
- The GROW Model (Goal>Reality Check>Options>Will) is one of the most frequently used conversational models in coaching.
- The Patient Activation Measure (PAM) indicates knowledge, skills, and confidence in management of one's own healthcare decisions.

NURSE COACH REFLECTIONS

After reading this chapter, the Nurse Coach will be able to bring awareness and personal insight to the following questions:

- After reviewing the TTM model, can I identify any other assumptions related to TTM? Do I agree with all those presented in this chapter?
- Reflecting on Barrett's Freedom as Power statement: "If I do this, anything might happen," how does this affect my perception of change?
- Can I write a SMART goal related to a change I would like to make in my own life? What was easy and what was difficult in the process?
- Using the SMART goal I have written, can I use some of the GROW questions related to that goal? How does this process compare with writing the SMART goal?
- Can I compare and contrast setting SMART goals and GROW questions with Barrett's Power Prescription questions?

REFERENCES

Barrett, E. A. M. (1983). *An empirical investigation of Martha E. Rogers' principle of helicy: The relationship of human field motion and power.* Unpublished doctoral dissertation, New York University, New York.

Barrett, E. A. M. (1986). Investigations of the principle of helicy: The relationship of human field motion and power. In V. Malinski (Ed.), *Exploration on Martha Rogers' science of unitary human beings.* Norwalk, CT: Appleton-Century-Crofts.

Barrett, E. A. M. (1989). A nursing theory of power for nursing practice: Derivation from Rogers' paradigm. In J. Riehl (Ed.), *Conceptual models for nursing practice* (3rd ed., pp. 207-217). Norwalk, CT: Appleton & Lange.

Barrett, E. A. M. (2003). Update on a measure of power as knowing participation in change. In O. L. Strickland & C. DiIorio (Eds.), *Measurement of nursing outcomes: Focus on patient/client outcomes* (Vol. 4, pp. 21-39). New York, NY: Springer.

Barrett, E. A. M. (2010). Power as knowing participation in change: What's new and what's next. *Nursing Science Quarterly, 23*(1), 47-54.

Blissmer, B., Prochaska, J., Velicer, W., Redding, C., Rossi, J., Green, G., Paiva, A., et al. (2010). Common factors predicting long-term changes in multiple health behaviors. *Journal of Health Psychology 15*(2), 205-214.

Bulechek, G., Burcher, H., Dochterman, J., & Wagner, C. (2013). *Nursing interventions classification (NIC)* (6th ed.). St. Louis, MO: C. V. Mosby.

DiClemente, R., Salazar, L., & Crosby, R. (2013). *Health behavior theory for public health: Principles, foundations, and applications.* Burlington, MA: Jones & Bartlett Learning.

Harper, S., & Lynch, J. (2007). Trends in socioeconomic inequalities in adult health behaviors among US states, 1990-2004. *Public Health Reports, 122*, 177-189.

Hibbard, J. H., & Greene, J. (2013). What the evidence shows about patient activation: Better health outcomes and care experiences; Fewer data on costs. Health Affairs *32*(2), 207-214.

Hibbard, J. H., Greene, J., & Overton, V. (2013). Patients with lower activation associated with higher costs; Delivery systems should know their patients' scores. *Health Affairs 32*(2), 216-222.

Insignia Health (2014). Patient activation measure. Retrieved from http://www.insignia-health.com

Moore, M., & Tschannen-Moran, B. (2010). *Coaching psychology manual.* Philadelphia, PA: Lippincott Williams & Wilkins.

Nightingale, F. (1888). *To the probationer-nurses in the Nightingale Fund School at St. Thomas' Hospital from Florence Nightingale 16th May 1888* (p. 2). (Privately printed.)

Noar, S., Benac, C., & Harris, M. (2007). Does tailoring matter: Meta-analytic review of tailored print health behavior change interventions. *Psychology Bulletin 133*, 673-693.

Norcross, J. (2012). *Changeology: 5 steps to realizing your goals and resolutions.* New York, NY: Simon & Schuster.

Norcross, J., & Prochaska, J. (2002). Using the stages of change. *Harvard Mental Health Letter, 18*(11), 5–7.

Norcross, J., Krebs, P., & Prochaska, J. (2011). Stages of change. *Journal of Clinical Psychology: In Session, 67*(2), 143–154.

Parse, R. (2003). *Community: A human becoming perspective.* Sudbury, MA: Jones & Bartlett Learning.

Pleis, J., & Lethbridge-Cejku, M. (2007). Summary health statistics for US adults: National Health Interview Survey, 2006. *Vital Health Statistics 10*, 1–153.

Prochaska, J., Norcross, J. C., & DiClemente, C. C. (1995). *Changing for good. A revolutionary six-stage program for overcoming bad habits and moving your life positively forward.* New York, NY: Harper Collins.

Prochaska, J., Norcross, J. C., & Hill, S. S. (Eds.) (2004). *Psychologists' desk reference* (2nd ed.). New York, NY: Oxford University Press.

Prochaska, J., Reddig, C., & Evers, K. (2008). The transtheoretical model and stages of change. In K. Glanz, B. K. Rimer, & K. Viswanath (Eds.), *Health behaviors and health education: Theory, research and practice* (4th ed.). San Francisco, CA: Jossey Bass.

Rogers, M. (1970). *An introduction to the theoretical basis of nursing.* Philadelphia, PA: F. A. Davis.

Whitmore, J. (2009). *Coaching for performance: GROWing human potential and purpose* (4th ed.). Boston, MA: Nicholas Brealey Publishing.

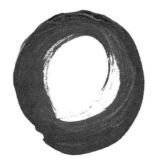

CHAPTER 16

Motivational Interviewing and Nonviolent Communication

Lisa A. Davis

...Let us value our training not as much as it makes us cleverer or superior to others, but inasmuch as it enables us to be more useful & helpful to our fellow creatures, the sick who most want our help. Let it be our ambition to be thorough good women — and never let us be ashamed of the name of "nurse." Let us each & all, realizing the importance of our influences on others — stand shoulder to shoulder & not alone, in the good cause.

Florence Nightingale, 1881

LOOKING AHEAD...

After reading this chapter, you will be able to:

- Explore motivational interviewing (MI) and its application in nurse coaching.
- Analyze the four MI general principles.
- Discuss the four elements of nonviolent communication (NVC).
- Incorporate NVC in coaching practice.

DEFINITIONS

Ambivalence: Having mixed feelings or contradictory ideas at the same time. Being indecisive. A state of feeling two or more ways about something, or when values are not aligned with change. A lack of commitment to change.

Change talk: Expressions by the client which indicate an intent to change, or how she or he will follow through with a desired goal; this change talk can be subtle and culturally specific.

Decisional balance: The process of evaluating the pros and cons of changing or not changing.

Discrepancy: Lack of agreement or inconsistency on steps with a decision or action steps towards a healthier behavior/s.

Empathy: Understanding the feelings of another. The capacity to vicariously experience the feelings or thoughts of another without having to have those thoughts or feelings expressed explicitly.

Motivation: What drives a person to make choices and take action.

Motivational interviewing (MI): Client-centered, semi-directive method for motivating change by exploring and resolving ambivalence within the client.

Nonviolent communication (NVC): Originates in compassion, in which violence is an anathema. It also assumes all humans have the same needs and our actions are a means of meeting those needs (Center for Nonviolent Communication, 2013).

Open-ended question (OEQ): Question in which there is no simple yes/no response. Open-ended questions encourage reflection and meaningful responses.

Pity: Expression of sorrow for suffering. Pity implies judgment and is often expressed with words or acts of comfort such as tears and a desire to spare the other from their discomfort.

Resistance: Pushing back with comments related to change, health behaviors, or other factors.

Self-efficacy: The belief that one has the capacity to begin and/or sustain change towards desired behavior/s.

Self-esteem: The belief that one has value and self-worth.

Sympathy: Feeling the sorrow or suffering of another. Sympathy is the sharing of, rather than understanding of, the feelings of another.

MOTIVATIONAL INTERVIEWING (MI)

The principles of motivational interviewing (MI) are very helpful in nurse coaching. Rollnick, Miller, and Butler (2008) describe MI as a "gentle" form of counseling to effect behavioral changes related to lifestyle. It is not directive, but taps into the individual's motivation to change. The process of the counselor/client relationship is collaborative and honors patient autonomy. The goal is to evoke not only the motivation to change, but also to recognize the resources the client already has to effect that change.

It is important to note that nurse coaching is not counseling and is only one methodology used in nurse coaching. MI offers the Nurse Coach a style of guiding clients to make their own decisions. It is an intervention strategy for helping the client make a desired change in behavior. Remember, there are two sources of motivation: *Intrinsic* sources are the internal motivators such as wanting to improve health, lose weight, or increase exercise; *extrinsic* sources are those external motivators such as a family member, watching a loved one suffer, or wanting a person to change. Sustained change comes from intrinsic motivators. This is the overarching aim of nurse coaching.

From the Nurse Coach perspective, the purpose of MI is to assist the client to explore possible changes in health behaviors by working with ambivalence and resistance. Ambivalence is when the client has mixed feelings or contradictory ideas at the same time and is indecisive. It is a state of feeling two or more ways about something, or when values are not aligned with change. This results in a lack of commitment to change. Resistance is seen when the client pushes back with comments made by the nurse related to change, health behaviors, or other factors. There are many causes of resistance to change such as anxiety, family or financial issues, or fear. Some signals to watch for in a coaching session are when the client does not contribute to a conversation, argues, changes the subject, interrupts, denies behaviors or words, or focuses on unimportant issues. Rolling with change behaviors is so essential; otherwise the client sees some progress and then may fall back to old behaviors and will feel like a failure by not being able to accomplish and sustain even small steps. Nurse coaching assists the client in moving beyond ambivalence and resistance to developing discrepancy (**Table 16-1**). Developing discrepancy is a guiding principle of MI and is discussed further in that section.

Motivational interviewing is guided by several theoretical frameworks. Prochaska, Norcross, and DiClemente (1995) offer the Transtheoretical Model (TTM) of Behavioral Change that can be applied to MI and involves five phases: (1) precontemplation, (2) contemplation, (3) preparation, (4) action, and (5) maintenance. See Chapter 15 for details. Elizabeth Barrett (1983, 2003), a nursing theorist, developed the Knowing Participation in

Change Theory which is based on power, or the capacity to knowingly participate in change (see Chapter 15).

Table 16-1 Examples of Ambivalence and Developing Discrepancy.

Ambivalence	Developing Discrepancy
I know I need to exercise, but I don't have time. I should eat better, but I don't like fresh vegetables.	I know I need to exercise, and I think I could for 20 minutes a day. I know I need to eat better and add more fresh food to my diet.
I am tired of hurting. I guess it is my cross to bear.	I want to feel better. I wonder what might help my pain.

GUIDING PRINCIPLES OF MI

The four MI guiding principles as seen in **Table 16-2** are (1) express empathy, (2) develop discrepancy, (3) roll with resistance, and (4) support self-efficacy, and are discussed next (Dart, 2011; Moore & Tschannen-Moran, 2010; Rollnick et al., 2008). Dart (2011) cautions that although these principles are simple, people are complex and caregivers must not lose sight of the individuality of all clients. Miller and Moyers (2006) identify four micro skills emphasized in MI, which can be remembered by using the acronym OARS (**O**–Open-ended questions, **A**–Affirming, **R**–Reflecting, and **S**–Summarizing) that elicit change talk. Another helpful acronym for motivational interviewing is GRACE. The components of GRACE are depicted in **Table 16-3**.

Table 16-2 Motivational Interviewing Basic Principles and Skills.

Motivational Interviewing Basic Principles	Basic Skills (OARS)
1. Express empathy 2. Develop discrepancy 3. Roll with resistance 4. Support self-efficacy	• Open-ended questions • Affirm • Reflective listening • Summarize (echo principle) to elicit change talk

Table 16-3 GRACE.

- **G**enerate a gap—*between current behaviors and stated values and interests*
- **R**oll with resistance—*seek to clarify, reinforce client's role as a problem-solver*
- **A**void argumentation—*promotes resistance*
- **C**an do—*increase client perception as capable, offer options, instill hope, affirm positive statements*
- **E**xpress empathy—*create sacred space to explore difficulty issues, reflective listening*

Principle One: Express Empathy

It is important to understand a person's story. Listening with the goal of holding the space expresses empathy and offers the client the opportunity to feel comfortable in sharing her or his experiences, needs, goals, and desires. The Nurse Coach's skillful listening and acceptance helps to facilitate change. Health issues can be overwhelming, and the client may express what seem to be conflicting goals, or have mixed feelings about health changes. This ambivalence is normal. For example, the client may state a need or desire to be more active, but then confess to hating to exercise. There may be a desire to make a health change, but also a comfort with the status quo. The client may state a reason to change, but then add a reason not to change. This takes the form of resistance talk. For example, the client may state the need to eat more fresh vegetables, then talk about how prohibitive the cost of fresh vegetables is.

Resist pushing for change, trying to "fix" or imposing personal beliefs on the client, even if they ask for an opinion. Expressions of pity or feelings of sympathy interfere with empathy and deep listening, thus it is important to avoid confusing pity and sympathy with empathy. Pity is grieving someone's experience. Sympathy is identifying with a person's experience from an emotional level.

To facilitate remaining empathic, use appreciative inquiry (AI) and the 4-D Cycle (Discover, Dream, Design, Destiny) to help the client move towards that change that becomes an inner tug that calls for change (see Chapter 17). MI works well with AI. Using AI, clients are called to use their creativity and to tap into their inner resources. As they dream big, they can see what is possible and also what they are being called to do.

Principle Two: Develop Discrepancy

Change is motivated by a perceived discrepancy between present behaviors and desired goals and values. In other words, it is the recognition of their ambivalence. Developing discrepancy is recognized when the client begins to talk about change. Again, an acronym is helpful in resolving ambivalence and developing discrepancy. This acronym is DARN (**Table 16-4**). The client presents the discrepancy and the reasons for change. According to Dart (2011), the goals of the Nurse Coach in developing discrepancy are:

- to assist the client in identifying their current status and her or his health goals, and
- to explore with the client how she or he can reach these goals.

To best meet these goals, the Nurse Coach uses open-ended questions and reflective listening. At least 50% of the coaching session is made up of open-ended questions (**Table 16-5**).

Table 16-4 DARN.

D — Desire is expressed and congruent with values and emotions to change
A — Ability with the confidence and self-efficacy to initiate and follow through with change
R — Reasons for change (both pros and cons)
N — Needs to include the importance of the desired changed and how this change fits into the client's needs

Table 16-5 Examples of Open-Ended Questions.

What are your reasons for considering this change?
What is the best experience you have had towards your desired future behavior?
What changes would you like to make in your current behavior/s?
What concerns do you have about your current health status? Behavior?
How might your current behavior lead to health challenges in the future?

Four Types of Reflective Listening

There are basically four types of reflective listening: Simple Reflection, Amplified Reflection, Double-Sided Reflection, Shifted-Focus Reflection (**Table 16-6**). To further understand these concepts, the analogy of a mirror is used and adapted from Moore and Tschannen-Moran (2010, pp. 68–72).

- **Simple Reflection.** Use a simple paraphrase and restate what client says. Following is a sample dialogue of simple reflection:

  Client: I don't have time to eat fresh vegetables. My family or friends don't either.

  Simple Reflection: I hear you say that you don't have time to eat fresh vegetables and that your family and friends don't either.

  Client: That's true, except for one friend that is so busy like me and she finds time for fresh vegetables and very healthy eating.

  Empathetic Simple Reflection: When you say you have a friend that integrates healthy eating, it sounds like you may be interested in how she does find time for healthy eating because you are so busy with your work and life.

- **Amplified Reflection.** These reflections maximize or minimize what the client says he or she can't do to change talk. By increasing or decreasing both the affect and the outcome, the Nurse Coach can facilitate new insights and reasons for change. It is important to be careful to deliver amplified reflections in change-neutral terms to avoid being manipulative, patronizing, or mocking. For example:

  Client: I don't have time to buy or fix fresh vegetables. My family and friends don't either.

  Amplified Reflection: I hear you saying that you don't know anyone who has time to buy or fix fresh vegetables and that it's impossible for you to fit eating fresh vegetables into your schedule.

  Client: It's not impossible for me to eat fresh vegetables. It's just that I don't find the time to stop by the store and buy vegetables that are already prepared or do it myself. Sometimes I actually do eat fresh vegetables, and I do have one friend that finds time every day, so maybe I could figure this out.

  Empathetic Amplified Reflection: When you say that you eat fresh vegetables on occasion, and that maybe you could figure out a way to eat them regularly, it sounds like you are *feeling stimulated* because your need for the benefits of more consistent healthy eating would be met.

- **Double-Sided Reflection.** These reflections reveal multiple perspectives at the same time and encourage clients to look at different angles/facets of their health needs. This is accomplished by comparing a current resistant statement with a prior readiness-to-change statement. This reflection allows the client to see another perspective for forward movement and action. For example:

  Client: I don't have time to eat healthy. My family and friends don't either.

  Double-Sided Reflection: I hear you say that you don't have time to eat healthy and that you family and friends don't either. But I've also heard you say that eating healthy makes you feel better and that eating healthy on a regular basis would be good for your health.

  Client: That's the problem. I want to eat healthy, and it does make me feel better, but it cuts into my busy schedule and time with my family. I wish I could figure out how to do both.

  Empathetic Double-Sided Reflection: When you say that you could make eating healthy stick if it didn't cut into time with your family and friends, it sounds like you are feeling discouraged because your needs for both eating healthy and connection are not being met.

- **Shifted-Focus Reflection.** In the shifted-focus reflection, the Nurse Coach assists the client to shift resistant-provoking topic to focus on another topic and possibility. For example:

  Client: I don't have time to eat healthy. My friends and my spouse don't either.

  Shift Focus: Because you don't have time to eat healthy, let's talk about your new walking routine you started with your partner. You said you liked this new routine.

  Client: Yes, it really makes me unwind, get out in nature, and not go back to surfing the Internet and the endless e-mails. I just hadn't thought about following the walk with chopping vegetables.

  Empathetic Shifted-Focus Reflection: It sounds like you are feeling happy with the walking routine and out in nature with your partner because it's helping you unwind. Would you be willing to tell me what you heard me say?

Table 16-6 Four Types of Reflection.

Simple Reflection (Analogy: flat mirror). Use a simple paraphrase and restate what client says.

Amplified Reflection (Analogy: convex or concave mirror). These reflections maximize or minimize what client says he or she can't do to change talk.

Double-Sided Reflection (Analogy: trifold mirrors). These reflections reveal multiple perspectives at the same time and encourage clients to look at different angles/facets of their health needs.

Shifted-Focus Reflection (Analogy: periscope). In the shifted-focus reflection, the Nurse Coach assists client to shift resistance-provoking topic to focus on another topic and possibility.

Source: Adapted by Lisa A. Davis. From Moore, M., & Tschannen-Moran, B. (2010). *Coaching psychology manual* (pp. 68–72). Philadelphia, PA: Lippincott, Williams & Wilkins.

Principle Three: Roll with Resistance

It is said that people do not resist change, but resist being changed. Resistance can be seen as a call to respond differently. To challenge the client's resistance or negative thoughts can reinforce negativity, and conversely, allowing the client to explore resistance can evoke feelings of acceptance (Dart, 2011). In rolling with resistance, the Nurse Coach facilitates client exploration of perceived barriers to achieve a desired health change. The client should be encouraged to examine new ideas about change. It is important for the Nurse Coach to remember the client is the primary resource for answers and solutions. The Nurse Coach avoids advising, educating, consoling, correcting, explaining, interrogating, etc. To facilitate acceptance rather than reinforce resistance, the Nurse Coach can use the following precepts (Moore & Tschannen-Moran, 2010, p. 71):

- From *correction* to *connection*. Correcting others makes them resist change.
- From *competence* to *confidence*. Claiming to know provokes more resistance.
- From *causes* to *capacities*. Moving from problems to new capacities is exciting.
- From *counter-force* to *counter-balance*. Arguing for change generates pushback; one must move to new awareness to generate positive self-talk.

Principle Four: Support Self-Efficacy

Self-efficacy is the client's capability to initiate and sustains change, which in turn leads to self-confidence. It promotes self-awareness. In supporting self-efficacy, the Nurse Coach acknowledges and praises positive plans and encourages the client to make choices.

Combining these for principles moves clients to action. When the client entertains that change is possible and change talk starts, motivation is tapped into, and this can lead to developing action steps for change. These small wins towards change create an upward spiral towards sustaining goals that can lead to new goals, new relationships, and new insights about what is possible (see Chapter 15).

Once readiness for change is ascertained, the Nurse Coach helps the client to set goals for change. Again, these are based on the client's needs. An acronym that may facilitate goal setting is SMART (Specific, Measurable, Achievable, Realistic, and Time-lined). This is discussed in detail in Chapter 15.

HELPFUL TOOLS IN MI

Decisional Balance

Decisional balance is the process of evaluating the pros and cons of changing or not changing. In decisional balance, the Nurse Coach facilitates the client's considering the pros and cons of changing or not changing. Open-ended questions help the client work her/his way through a decision for change. The client can develop a pros and cons or decisional balance worksheet (**Table 16-7**). The decisional balance worksheet should be approached in a clockwise manner, first addressing the advantages of staying the same, then, the downside of staying the same. Finally, the client would list the downside of changing, and finally, the advantages of changing. In the top two boxes, the client basically addresses his/her ambivalence. However, it is in the second box that possibilities open for change talk (Miller & Rollnick, 2009; Rollnick et al., 2008). In the third box, the client is addressing resistance to change, and even fear of loss. In the fourth box, along with listing the advantages of change, the client may voice some goals and initial plans to meet those goals. When the client deduces that the advantages of change outweigh the advantages of staying the same, she or he may express a readiness to change.

Table 16-7 Decisional Balance.

What is good about how things are now?	What is not good about how things are now?
Advantages of staying the same?	*Downside of staying the same?*
1	2
The benefits of change	The benefits of not changing
4	3
Advantages of changing?	*Downside of changing?*

Source: Copyright © 2014 by the International Nurse Coach Association. www.inursecoach.com

Rulers

Rulers are familiar in assessing a patient's pain and are very effective with exploring readiness to change and identifying the priority and confidence for change. First, ask the client about a readiness for change. The use of words or an actual printed readiness ruler that incorporates a Likert scale from 1 to 10 is very effective (**Figure 16-1**). A level of 0–3 usually reflects a lack of commitment. A level of 4-6 demonstrates ambivalence. A level of 7–10 indicates a person is ready to make a commitment. When using a scale, follow-up questions posed by the Nurse Coach can help the client to further think through a behavioral change. It is important to explore the exact meaning of these numbers to really understand the client's readiness, desire, and commitment using a straight question, a backward question, or a forward question (Dart, 2011):

- Straight question: Why a 5?
- Backward question: Why a 5 and not a 2?
- Forward question: What would need to be different to move you from a 5 to a 7?

Table 16-8 offers an example of a coaching session with a client after she/he completed the IHWA.

Table 16-8 Sample Conversation using a Readiness Ruler.

This client was referred to the Nurse Coach because she stated she wanted to take charge of her health and to try once again to stop smoking. She has a 40-year history of smoking.

Nurse: On a scale of 0–10 with 0 being not at all ready to quit smoking and a 10 being absolutely ready to quit smoking, how ready are you to quit smoking?

Client: Today I am at a 7.

Nurse: Can you tell me why you chose a 7 today?

Client: I can't enjoy my young grandchildren's activities. I also need to do this for my own health as I can't even do basic house cleaning or cooking without feeling short of breath. I've tried before and I know how hard it is to quit, but I have been successful before for over a year. Then I got stressed over some family issues, but I now want some help so I can see some progress.

Nurse: You really sound motivated to change, and I'm basing this on you didn't put yourself at a 2 or 3. What might it take to get you at an 8 or 9?

Client: There is no way I can answer that, but I will start with not smoking after meals so I think that is my plan right now.

Use of Hypotheticals

Allowing the client to speak in hypothetical terms is less threatening than speaking in real, personal terms (Rollnick et al., 2008). Using hypothetical situations may lead to more exploration of possibilities. Examples of hypotheticals are:

- Imagine how your life would be if...
- What do you most want in your life 10 years from now?
- If you make this change, what will be your greatest joy?
- What advice would you give a friend who was in this situation?

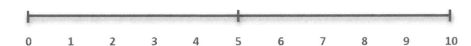

Figure 16-1 Readiness Ruler.

Remember the RULE and WAIT

The RULE acronym (**Table 16-9**) reinforces the purpose of MI for the Nurse Coach. It is tempting to try to "fix" the patient, which can paradoxically reinforce the status quo. It is important to resist this righting reflex in order for the client to fully explore her or his motivation to change (Hall, Gibbie, & Lubman, 2012). Keep in mind, the patient derives his or her own reasons for change. Listening with empathy is essential in understanding what motivates the patient and facilitating getting past ambivalence and resistance into developing discrepancy. Finally, positive outcomes depend on active input and participation from the client. The Nurse Coach empowers the client when drawing out her or his strengths and conveying belief and hope.

As has been emphasized throughout this discussion, the Nurse Coach is practicing empathetic listening. Part of resisting the righting reflex is resisting giving advice, or telling personal anecdotes, or even client teaching. Listening through silence and respecting that silence is of paramount importance to the Nurse Coach/client relationship. It is often in that silence that the client develops discrepancy. A helpful acronym to remember this is WAIT—**W**hy **A**m **I T**alking.

Table 16-9 RULE and WAIT Acronyms.

R — Resist the righting reflex	**W** — Why
U — Understand the clients motivations	**A** — Am
L — Listen with empathy	**I** — I
E — Empower the client	**T** — Talking

SUMMARIZING THE COACHING SESSION

In summarizing with the client, using MI, it is important to affirm positive behaviors, be respectful of decisions, offer information if appropriate, and express confidence in the client. Rollnick et al. (2008) identify that a summary of the client session allows the Nurse Coach to demonstrate how carefully she or he has listened, emphasize important points, and offer closure to the session. Reinforcing key points also refreshes the Nurse Coach's memory in order to make clear session notes. In addition, summarizing the session gives the Nurse Coach and client an opportunity to set goals for the next session.

NONVIOLENT COMMUNICATION (NVC)

An early model for nonviolent communication (NVC) is that of the Iroquois nation. In the 15th century, they developed a law of peace. This was more than just the absence of war, but a law. In fact, the word for "law" and "peace" was the same, and it was sacred. It was a way of life, gracious and wise. If a dispute arose, the disputing parties would enter the longhouse and speak their truth until a compromise was reached. The compromise was held sacred and inviolate. The precept of nonviolence was paramount, not only in their speech, but in their subsequent actions towards each other (Wallace, 1994).

NVC is used in MI as well as other nurse coaching activities. Nonviolence is a way of communicating which values and honors our common humanity in such a way that there is no need for language of blame, judgment, or domination (CNVC, 2013). It starts within ourselves (Sullivan, 2007) and includes not only our own communication with others, but also how we hear the needs of those who do not use NVC. Gaardner (Sullivan, 2007, p. 134) calls this "hearing with nonviolent communication ears." It is not only a way of communicating, but a path for healing. Nosec (2012, p. 833) adds that practicing NVC "both with self and others affords the opportunity to remain present with the intent to understand and maintain connection." In her qualitative study, Nosec (2012) noted three themes related to NVC. First, NVC fosters mutual respect. Second, it offers a way to reflect on needs and communicate nonviolently to self. Lastly, NVC offers a path for discovering each other's needs rather than emotions to get a sense of shared meaning and significance.

With NVC, there are four elements as seen in **Figure 16-2. First, make observations**, not evaluations or judgments. These observations are factual, based on objective information. Limiting descriptions of observations to the five senses (hearing, sight, smell, touch, taste) decreases the tendency to interrupt, criticize, judge, or exaggerate. Rosenberg (2003) observed, "nonviolent communication shows us a way of being very honest, but without any criticism, without any insults, without any putdowns, without any intellectual diagnosis implying wrongness" (www.cnvc.org). For example:

"I failed to do 20 minutes of exercise three times a week" (evaluation).
"I did 20 minutes of exercise three times this week" (observation).

Second, express feelings or emotions, not thoughts about what you have observed without assigning blame. For example:

"I feel tired."
"I was encouraged by...."

The following are thoughts; they do not express feelings and are referred to as "faux feelings." Faux feelings are usually followed by which such as "that", "like," and "as if," or a noun or pronoun (Rosenberg, 2003).

"My mother is controlling me."
"I feel like it won't work."

Third, **identify unmet needs that are the source of feelings**. Distinguishing between universal needs and strategies for meeting those needs is at the core of NVC. Universal needs include safety, connection, autonomy, trust, honesty, meaning, peace, physical wellbeing, play, self-worth, and understanding. For example:

"I need to feel I am valued."
"I need to be authentic."

The following are strategies and not universal needs:

"I need to get this project finished."
"I need to exercise every day."

Finally, **make requests for actions that can meet needs, not demands**. When the Nurse Coach is clear about the client's feelings and underlying needs, then she or he can move forward with confirming what is heard or on an agreed-upon action.

"Would you be willing to tell me what you heard me say?"
"What agreement would you like to make with regard to conscious eating?"

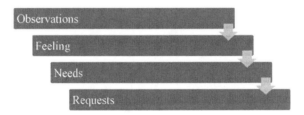

Figure 16-2 Nonviolent Communication: Four Elements.

Latini (2009) sees NVC as a spiritual practice, which involves mutual assisting, emphasizing the reciprocity, in expressing and receiving requests. Further, requests are not demands, and the other can say no without retributions; they are stated using positive language; and they must be specific enough to be doable. NVC is offered with gladness: "Behind every evaluation, there is an observation, behind every thought a feeling, behind every strategy a need, and behind every demand a request" (Moore & Tschannen-Moran, 2010, p. 67). It is important to note that NVC does not seek to diminish evil in life by putting a positive spin on everything. Flack (2006, p. 321) uses examples of the Jewish Holocaust in which "nonviolent" language became euphemisms for evil, citing "evacuation" for killing, and "change of residence" for deportation. NVC is not about creating euphemisms, but mutually respectful communication.

SUMMARY

- There are four guiding principles to MI (expressed empathy, develop discrepancy, roll with resistance, and support self-efficacy).
- With MI, listening with the goal of holding the space expresses empathy and offers the client the opportunity to feel comfortable in sharing her or his experiences, needs, goals, and desires.
- Change is motivated by a perceived discrepancy between present behaviors and desired goals and values. In other words, it is the recognition of their ambivalence. Developing discrepancy is recognized when the client begins to talk about change.
- In rolling with resistance, the Nurse Coach facilitates the client's exploration of perceived barriers to achieving a desired health change.
- Self-efficacy is the client's capability to initiate and sustain change, which in turn leads to self-confidence. It promotes self-awareness. In supporting self-efficacy, the Nurse Coach acknowledges and praises positive plans and encourages the client to make choices.
- Tools used in MI include decisional balance, rulers, and use of hypotheticals.
- In summarizing with the client, using MI, it is important to affirm positive behaviors, be respectful of decisions, offer information if appropriate, and express confidence in the client.
- NVC is used in MI as well as other nurse coaching activities.
- The four basic elements of NVC are observations, feelings, needs, and requests.
- In NVC, requests are not demands, and the other can say no without retributions; requests are stated using positive language and must be specific enough to be doable.

NURSE COACH REFLECTIONS

After reading this chapter, the Nurse Coach will be able to bring awareness and personal insight to the following questions:

*   By comparing and contrasting pity, sympathy, and empathy, can I identify a situation in which each would be appropriate?
*   What strategy could I employ for a client who cannot seem to get beyond ambivalence?
*   Which words could convey violence or judgment in common speech?
*   Was there a time when my needs were not met? How could I use NVC to change the outcome?

REFERENCES

Barrett, E. (1983). *An empirical investigation of Martha E. Rogers' principle of helicy: The relationship of human field motion and power.* Unpublished doctoral dissertation, New York University, New York.

Barrett, E. (2003). A measure of power as knowing participation in change. In O. Strickland & C. Dilorio (Eds.), *Measurement of nursing outcomes: Self care and coping* (2nd ed.). New York, NY: Springer.

Center for Nonviolent Communication (CNVC) (2013). *Center for nonviolent communication: An international organization.* Retrieved from www.cnvc.org

Dart, M. (2011). *Motivational interviewing in nursing practice: Empowering the patient.* Sudbury, MA: Jones & Bartlett Learning.

Flack, C. (2006). The subtle violence of nonviolent language. *Crosscurrents,* 312–327.

Hall, K., Gibbie, T., & Lubman, D. (2012). Motivational interviewing techniques: Facilitating behavior change in the general practice setting. *Australian Family Physician, 41*(9), 660–667.

Latini, T. (2009). Nonviolent communication: A humanizing ecclesial and educational practice. *Journal of Education & Christian Belief, 13*(1), 19–31.

Miller, W., & Moyers, T. (2006). Eight stages in learning motivational interviewing. *Journal of Teaching in the Addictions, 5*(1), 3–16.

Miller, W., & Rollnick, S. (2009). Ten things that motivational interviewing is not. *Behavioural and Cognitive Psychotherapy, 37,* 129–140.

Moore, M., & Tschannen-Moran, B. (2010). *Coaching psychology manual.* Philadelphia, PA: Lippincott Williams & Wilkins.

Nightingale, F. (1881). Letter from Florence Nightingale (pp. 2–3). London, UK: Spottiswoode.

Nosec, M. (2012). Nonviolent communication: A dialogical retrieval of the ethic of authenticity. *Nursing Ethics, 19*(6), 829–837.

Prochaska, J. O., Norcross, J. C., & DiClemente, C. C. (1995). *Changing for good: A revolutionary six-stage program for overcoming bad habits and moving your life positively forward.* New York, NY: Harper Collins.

Rollnick, S., Miller, W. R., & Butler, C. C. (2008). *Motivational interviewing in healthcare: Helping patients change behavior*. New York, NY: Guilford Press.

Rosenberg, M. (2003). *Nonviolent communication: A language of life* (2nd ed.). Encinitas, CA: PuddleDancer Press.

Sullivan, D. (2007). Nonviolence begins with speech: An interview with Emily Gaardner on the practice of nonviolent communication. *Contemporary Justice Review, 10*(1), 131–142.

Wallace, P. (1994). *The Iroquois book of life: White roots of peace.* Santa Fe, NM: Clear Light Publishers.

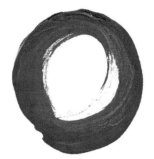

CHAPTER 17

Appreciative Inquiry

Lisa A. Davis

> Every Nurse must grow. No Nurse can stand still, she must go forward, or she will go backward, every year.
>
> *Florence Nightingale, 1888*

LOOKING AHEAD...

After reading this chapter, you will be able to:

- Evaluate assumptions about appreciative inquiry (AI).
- Examine the AI five principles.
- Describe the 4-D cycle methodology.

DEFINITIONS

Appreciate: To understand a situation fully and to recognize the full worth of a person and her/his life experiences; valuing.

Appreciative inquiry (AI): A relational construct based on affirmation, appreciation, and dialogue (Trajkovski, Schmied, Vickers, & Jackson, 2012).

Calling: A strong inner impulse, often described as "soul speak" or "heart speak."

Collaboration: To work jointly, as a Nurse Coach with a client, toward a common objective and together co-create goals and plans.

Core values: Beliefs or convictions that direct behavior and support purpose in life for the individual or group.

Energy: Life force; a sense of being stimulated to act.

Generative moments: Experiences in which clients are inspired towards change, growth, and a vision.

Organizational change: A structured approach in an organization for ensuring that changes are smoothly and successfully implemented to achieve lasting benefits.

Problem solving: Discovering, analyzing, and solving problems using a systematic approach based on perceived deficit.

Support: An environment in which assistance is perceived. This can include but is not limited to persons, equipment, faith, organization structure, weather, etc.

Transformational change: A marked or radical change for the better, whether personal, group, or organizational.

APPRECIATIVE INQUIRY (AI)

There are several affirmative rather than problem-based change models, to include motivational interviewing (Chapter 16), imagery (Chapter 12 and Appendix F), and asset assessment, where things of value to an entity or group are maintained and monitored.

Csikszentmihalyi (2003) has determined that the greatest rewards in life result in choices that lead to personal growth and social good (Chapter 14). In this chapter, appreciative inquiry (AI) is discussed as an affirmational approach to change.

AI is a relational construct based on affirmation, appreciation, and dialogue (Trajkovski et al., 2012). Developed as a management tool focusing on what works for groups and organization (Cooperrider, 1995; Cooperrider & Whitney, 2005; Sorensen & Yeager, 2002), AI focuses on positive and creative change rather than change based on a deficit or a problem to be solved. AI has been adopted by counseling psychology and coaching as a philosophy and approach for motivating change (Foster & Lloyd, 2007; Moore, 2008; Tschannen-Moran, 2007). Moore and Charvat (2007) identify that current behavioral models are derived from philosophies which focus on deficit, and that not following a prescribed behavioral pattern is the problem. Therefore, rather than focus on problems to be fixed or solved, AI focuses on exploring and amplifying strengths. This represents a tremendous paradigm shift for most people. Consider in your own life how much of your day is spent on problem solving. For most of us, problem solving is a day-long activity both at work and in our private life. Because the concept of solving problems or fixing is so ingrained, be aware that some people may not be ready to shift from problem solving to a focus on strengths. See Chapter 5 for discussion on strengths.

Moore (2008) offers six key characteristics of AI:

- Assumption of health and vitality
- Connection through empathy
- Personal excitement, commitment, and caring
- Intense focus through deep listening and attention
- Generative questioning, cueing, and guiding
- From monologue to dialogue

There are eight basic assumptions related to AI (Hammond, 1998; Southard, Bark, & Hess, 2013, p. 212):

- In every society, organization, or group, something works.
- What we focus on becomes our reality.
- Reality is created in the moment; there are no multiple realities.
- The act of asking questions of an individual or group has some influence on the individual or group.
- People are more confident and comfortable with moving forward (the unknown) when they carry forward parts of the past (the known).
- What we carry forward from the past should be what is best about the past.
- It is important to value differences.
- Language creates reality.

AI FIVE BASIC PRINCIPLES

With these assumptions in mind, there are five basic principles to AI (Tschannen-Moran, 2007; Tschannen-Moran, 2010) as seen in **Figure 17-1**:

1. **Positive Principle** (positive energy and emotions): Positive actions overcome an imbalance in energy and are stimulated by positive energy and emotion. Conversely, negative energy and emotion, which are part of finding fault or correcting weakness, lack the force needed to move in new, positive directions. While they may solve the problem at hand, they may also generate other problems, causing a downward spiral. Positive actions and outcome disrupt downward spirals and are the basis of transformational change. Pos-

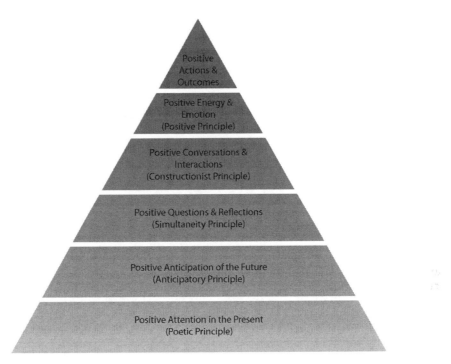

Figure 17-1 Appreciative Inquiry (AI) Pyramid.
Source: Adapted from Tschannen-Moran, B. (2007). Five-principle coaching. *AI Practitioner*, (May), 19–23.

itive energy expands awareness and thinking, increases abilities, and builds resilience. It offsets negative possibilities, thus it creates an upward spiral towards goals and outcomes.

2. Constructionist Principle (positive conversations and interactions): Positive energy and emotions generate positive conversations. They emphasize the present moment and changing future events. We invent stories and frameworks together in conversation with others. Inner work and "self-talk," while positive, are not enough. Shifting conversations and interactions with other people in a positive direction simultaneously creates a positive present. The social context is key to creating not only the present moment, but future moments. "Words do not create worlds unless they are shared with others" (Tschannen-Moran, 2007, p. 20).

3. Simultaneity Principle (positive conversations, questions, and reflections): Just as positive conversations create positive outcomes, positive conversations and interactions develop from positive questions and reflections. These questions and reflections are key to stimulating positive change. In fact, they are themselves a change. Every question or reflection has an effect, even if it is to reinforce what is already believed by the individual or group. Questions and reflections engender a sense of wonder, which is in itself transformational.

4. Anticipatory Principle (positive anticipation of the future): Positive questions and reflections result in positive anticipation of the future. When a positive anticipation is held, positive outcomes become possible. When positive outcomes are anticipated, individuals and groups become more resilient, hopeful, and creative about the future. In order for this to occur, more than just vague assertions that things will turn out is needed. Affirmational statements and holding a positive image are needed (Tschannen-Moran & Tschannen-Moran, 2011). Questions and reflections flow from the outlook we hold.

5. Poetic Principle (positive attention in the present): Positive anticipation of the future stems from positive attention in the present. This principle is based on mindfulness, intention, and attention. This principle inspires change. It is important to remember that problems do not go away, but other things become more important. When we focus on possibilities, we get more possibilities. When we focus on problems, we get more problems. The image of poetry in this principle evokes positive imagination.

Because it is foundational to AI, the poetic principle is depicted as the base of the AI pyramid. Positive attention to the present then leads to positive anticipation of the future (Anticipatory Principle), which in turn leads to positive questions and reflections (Simultaneity Principle), resulting in positive conversations and interactions (Constructionist Principle), which culminates in positive energy and emotion (Positive Principle). It is through these principles that the individual or group can achieve positive actions and outcomes as seen in Figure 17-1.

AI 4-D CYCLE: DISCOVER—DREAM—DESIGN—DESTINY

This philosophical framework of focus on the positive resulted in a methodology for AI known as the 4-D cycle. It is a way of coaching and a way of living that inspires an upward spiral of personal and professional development (Cooperrider & Whitney, 2005). The Nurse Coach can initiate the 4-D cycle by simply asking the client, "What would you like to talk about today?" Once that focus topic is identified, the Nurse Coach can facilitate the 4-D cycle of Discover, Dream, Design, and Destiny as seen in **Figure 17-2**.

Use expressed empathy in the AI process. Expressed empathy is the respectful understanding of another person's experience, to move conversations forward. Be alert to not confusing pity and sympathy. *Pity* means grieving someone's experience, usually due to circumstantial hardships. *Sympathy* is identifying with someone's experience primarily on an emotional level.

AI facilitates generative moments, those experiences where clients are aroused towards change and growth and a vision. Generative moments feel intense, deep, powerful, and moving—not difficult. The role of the Nurse Coach is to assist the client with agreement and commitment to goals, dreams, and vision. Generative moments often require that a client can allow her or his self to feel vulnerable with a Nurse Coach. This happens as the Nurse Coach listens deeply and has established the trusting relationship.

It is important to note that the 4-D cycle is not just facilitating by asking questions. It may be necessary to be creative in exploring the focus topics, which can involve asking the client to tell a story. Follow-up questioning may be used to help the client see the focus topic more clearly. Another strategy could be to use metaphor in the questioning (e.g., if the feeling you have after exercise is a color, what color would it be?).

It is also important to note that the 4-D cycle is not linear. As discussion progresses through the cycle, and the client gains more clarity, the focus topic might change (Trajkovski et al., 2012). That is normal. Health goals are broad and complex; as the client completes the cycle related to the focus topic, another aspect of the focus topic will most likely emerge. For example, if the focus topic is nutrition, the client may have developed a healthy dietary plan which works, but then she/he might decide to explore changing from a traditional diet which includes fish and chicken to an all-vegan dietary regimen. At that point, the cycle would start again.

The Nurse Coach should be aware of the tone of the dialogue. Remember, it should remain positive. If clients respond to questions or tell a story, they might revert to negative

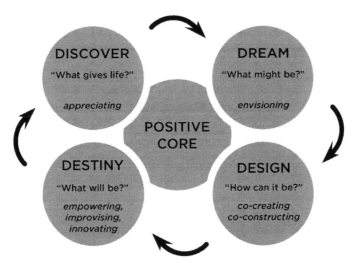

Figure 17-2 4-D Cycle of AI.
Source: Copyright © 2014 by the International Nurse Coach Association. www.inursecoach.com

speech, or what is problematic rather than what is positive. Remember, this is a paradigm shift for them. The Nurse Coach should use questions, responses, and affirmation to insure that the dialogue remains positive, desirable, and affirmational.

- **Discover:** AI makes the assumption that something is always working right in someone's life. Discovering a person's strengths increases her or his energy, self-efficacy, and belief in self. Questions in this phase address the client's core values about health (**Table 17-1**). These core values are those which give meaning to life, are a source of joy and contentment, and guide choices. As Palmer (2000, p. 3) states, "Before I can tell my life what I want to do with it, I must listen to my life telling me who I am." In the discovery part of the cycle, the Nurse Coach could ask about peak, or best, experiences regarding the focus topic. The Nurse Coach and client might also explore what drives success (Gaddis & Williams, 2008). This can lead to insight or stimulate thought for the client. Related to this, the Nurse Coach can ask questions about generative moments. These are "ah-ha" moments in which a change in energy may be noted as the client responds to the question or tells a story. It is in this phase that the seed is planted for what might be. Also, in this phase, in addition to asking questions, clarifying questions, or eliciting story, the Nurse Coach engages in appreciative statements. Once discovery is accomplished, the Nurse Coach and client move to the dream phase of the cycle.
- **Dream:** After the client has discovered the best of "what is," now help her/him to envision "what might be." The dream phase builds on the outcomes of the discovery phase. In this phase, the client challenges the status quo (Moore & Charvat, 2007). Dream-making uses left-brain and right-brain capacities. In this phase, in addition to questioning, the Nurse Coach might elicit personal stories, images, metaphors, and narratives. Questions might begin with: "What is the ideal...", "In a perfect world...", or, "If you had a magic wand... ." The hallmark of this phase is creativity. Questions can relate to calling, energy, or support. Once the dream is fully explored, the Nurse Coach will guide the client into the design phase, in which the dream becomes a target and the client senses anticipation.

- **Design:** In the design phase, the Nurse Coach and client collaborate to construct positive images of the client's future. Align the client's plan with the dream. Ask the client how her/his dream would manifest itself in terms of habits, practices, relationships, structures, systems, technology, resources, finances, etc. The goal is to create strong affirmative statements for the dream to become destiny or principles the client wants to preserve (Moore & Charvat, 2007). Create as many details as possible. Include commitments, offers, and requests in the design (**Table 17-2**). Have the client make commitments within one or two weeks, as this becomes relevant to the final phase—destiny.
- **Destiny:** This phase elevates energy and self-efficacy. This is an action process, and the goal is to make dreaming intrinsic to the client's way of being in the world. In this phase, the client aligns actions to her or his vision. As the plan comes to fruition, remember that strategies to accomplish this may need to be revised in this phase. It is also important for the Nurse Coach and client to review and celebrate accomplishments (Trajkovski et al., 2012). Remember that transformative change is a dynamic process (Carter et al., 2007). This phase may include one follow-up visit to review and celebrate change, a three-month follow-up visit, or even follow-up visits for five years (Trajkovski et al., 2012). The Nurse Coach and client need to negotiate follow-up based on the client's needs.

Table 17-1 Sample Questions Using the 4-D Cycle.

DISCOVER	DREAM
Peak/best experiences: Tell me about the best experience with this area of your wellness, and a time when you felt alive and engaged. What makes it exciting? Describe this experience in detail.	**Question of *calling***: "What is life calling you to be?"
	Question of *energy*: "What possibilities excite you?"
What drives success/core values: Tell me the things that you value most deeply, your family, your relationships, your work, and your hobbies?	**Question of *support***: "What's that positive core that supports you?"
	If you had a magic wand, what would you use it for?
Generative moments: Tell me about the key ingredients, both internal and external, that allows you to be your best and to have fun. Tell me about life-giving factors in your experience.	Imagine a perfectly healthy self. Tell me about what a typical day would be like. How do you feel?

DESTINY	DESIGN
What should be? What should you do first? Second? How will you...?	What can you do now which could give you what you imagined? What can you do in the next two weeks? Who would you go to for help in making this change?

Source: Copyright © 2014 by Lisa A. Davis.

Table 17-2 Design Phase Suggestions.

Commitments represent actions that the client will take.
Offers represent actions that the client volunteers to give.
Requests represent actions that the client seeks from others.

Source: Copyright © 2014 by Lisa A. Davis.

SUMMARY

- AI focuses on positive and creative change rather than change based on deficit or a problem to be solved.
- Positive actions overcome an imbalance in energy and are stimulated by positive energy and emotion. Conversely, negative energy and emotion, which are part of finding fault or correcting weakness, lack the force needed to move in new, positive directions. (Positive Principle)
- Shifting conversations and interactions with other people in a positive direction simultaneously creates a positive present. (Constructionist Principle)
- Just as positive conversations create positive outcomes, positive conversations and interactions develop from positive questions and reflections. (Simultaneity Principle)
- When positive outcomes are anticipated, individuals and groups become more resilient, hopeful, and creative about the future. (Anticipatory Principle)
- Positive anticipation of the future stems from positive attention in the present. This principle is based on mindfulness, intention, and attention. The poetic principle inspires change. (Poetic Principle)
- This philosophical framework of focus on the positive results in a methodology for AI known as the 4-D cycle: Discover, Dream, Design, Destiny.

NURSE COACH REFLECTIONS

After reading this chapter, the Nurse Coach will be able to bring awareness and personal insight to the following questions:

- In reflecting on the eight basic assumptions of AI, do I agree with all of them? Is there something I would add?
- Upon reviewing the five principles of AI, can I choose one to depict artistically? This can be a drawing or poem--anything that speaks to me about that principle.
- If I work with a client who wants to focus on having more energy during the day, can I develop at least three questions to ask during the discovery phase?

REFERENCES

Carter, C., Ruhe, M., Weyer, S., Litaker, D., Fry, R., & Stange, K. (2007). An appreciative inquiry approach to practice improvement and transformative change in health care settings. *Quality Management in Health Care, 16*(3), 194–204.

Cooperrider, D. (1995). Introduction to appreciative inquiry. In W. French & C. Bell (Eds.), *Organizational development* (5th ed.). New York City, NY: Prentice Hall.

Cooperrider, D., & Whitney, D. (2005). *Appreciative inquiry: A positive revolution in change.* San Francisco, CA: Berrett-Koehler Publishers.

Csikszentmihalyi, M. (2003). *Good business: Leadership, flow and the making of meaning.* London, UK: Hodder & Stoughton.

Foster, S., & Lloyd, P. (2007). Positive psychology principles applied to consulting psychology at the individual and group level. *American Psychological Association and the Society of Consulting Psychology, 59*(1), 30–40. doi:10.1037/1065-9293.59.1.30

Gaddis, S., & Williams, C. (2008). See yourself in 4-D: How to use Appreciative Inquiry to ignite positive change. *Prairie Rose, 76*(4), 17–19.

Hammond, S. (1998). *The thin book of appreciative inquiry* (2nd ed.). Plano, TX: Thin Book Pub.

Moore, M. (2008). Appreciative Inquiry: The why? The what? They how? *Practice Development in Health Care, 7*(4), 2014–220. doi:10.1002/pdh.

Moore, S., & Charvat, J. (2007). Promoting health behavior change using Appreciative Inquiry: Moving from deficit models to affirmation models of care. *Family Community Health, suppl. 30*(15), S64–S74.

Nightingale, F. (1888). *To the probationer-nurses in the Nightingale Fund School at St. Thomas' Hospital from Florence Nightingale 16th May 1888* (p. 3). (Privately printed).

Palmer, P. (2000). *Let your life speak: Listening for the voice of vocation.* San Francisco, CA: Jossey-Bass.

Sorenson, P., & Yeager, T. (2002). Appreciative Inquiry as an approach to organizational consulting. In R. Lowman (Ed.), *Handbood of organizational consulting psychology.* San Francisco, CA: Jossey-Bass.

Southard, M. E., Bark, L., & Hess, D. R. (2013). Facilitating change: Motivational interviewing and appreciative inquiry. In B. M. Dossey & L. Keegan (Eds.), *Holistic nursing: A handbook for practice* (6th ed., pp. 205–219). Burlington, MA: Jones & Bartlett Learning.

Trajkovski, S., Schmied, V., Vickers, M., & Jackson, D. (2012). Implementing the 4D cycle of Appreciative Inquiry in health care: A methodological review. *Journal of Advanced Nursing*, 1224–1234.

Tschannen-Moran, B. (2007). Five-principle coaching. *AI Practitioner*, (May), 19–23.

Tschannen-Moran, B. (2010). Appreciative inquiry. In M. Moore & B. Tschannen-Moran (Eds.), *Coaching psychology manual* (pp. 52–62). Philadelphia, PA: Lippincott Williams & Wilkins.

Tschannen-Moran, B., & Tschannen-Moran, M. (2011). The coach and the evaluator. *Educational Leadership*, (October), 10–16.

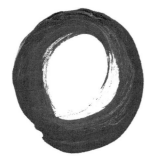

CHAPTER 18

Cultural Perspectives and Rituals of Healing

Susan Luck and Barbara Montgomery Dossey

...The effect in sickness of beautiful object, of variety of objects, and especially of brilliancy of colour is hardly at all appreciated... I shall never forget the rapture of fever patients over a bunch of bright-coloured flowers. I remember (in my own case) a nosegay of wild flowers being sent me, and from that moment recovery becoming more rapid...

Florence Nightingale, 1860

LOOKING AHEAD...

After reading this chapter, you will be able to:

- Explore how your cultural beliefs impact your health and lifestyle choices.
- Examine how your beliefs about health influence how you listen to your client's story.
- Identify the unique Nurse Coach role when working in diverse cultural communities.
- List your Nurse Coach cultural competences.
- Explore the process of rituals in health, lifestyle choices, and healing.

DEFINITIONS

Note: The term *patient* is intermittently used to connote within the cultural context of Western medicine where the person is assigned the "sick role" and thus surrenders as a passive participant in her/his treatment plan of care, while the healthcare provider is seen as the "all knowing" authority. In nurse coaching, the role of patient as client connotes shared participation in the decision-making process (see Chapter 1, Table 1-1).

Acculturation: The process by which an individual immigrant or group adapts or accommodates to a new culture.
Culture: The shared values, beliefs, attitudes, customs, rituals, symbols, and social structures that provide meaning and significance to a person's or a group's human behaviors around living in the world.
Cultural assessment: The recognition and honoring of a person's or group's cultural values, beliefs, customs, and practices that assist with implementation of cultural competent care.
Cultural awareness: Deliberate self-examination and in-depth exploration of one's biases, stereotypes, prejudices, assumptions, and "isms" one holds about individuals and groups who are different.

Cultural care: Healthcare delivered with knowledge of and sensitivity to cultural factors that influence health and illness behaviors of an individual client, family, or community.

Cultural competence: An ability to interact effectively with people of different cultures and socio-economic backgrounds, particularly in the context of human resources.

Cultural embeddedness: Process where the client is aligned with one's native culture, which influences her/his capacity to change and achieve desired lifestyle goals.

Ethnicity: Designation of a population subgroup sharing a common social and cultural heritage.

Ethnocentrism: Convictions of an individual's own cultural superiority that often blocks the capacity to be open to another person's worldview.

Rituals: Enactment of cultural beliefs and values; the repetition and patterns of behaviors and beliefs that have personal, healing worth.

CULTURAL PERSPECTIVES IN HEALTH AND HEALING

Nurse Coaches have a unique opportunity to explore the *soul* and *roots* of cultural meaning that binds people, families, and communities together. Culture is an integral, holistic, all-embracing concept that can be viewed as a social phenomenon that examines and weaves the past, present, and future (Engebretson, 2013). Culture is embedded in all individuals and groups and shapes experiences through a unique set of values, patterns of behaviors, traditions and rituals, and ways of seeing the world. Health beliefs are deeply held and embedded in one's earliest experiences. To cross the quality chasm and have a new health system for the 21st century we are challenged to deepen our understanding of cultural perspectives in health and healing (Institute of Medicine, 2001).

All societies develop strategies and systems to maintain health and treat illness. Health is viewed as balance in the inner and outer worlds—natural, familial, communal, and metaphysical. These shared dimensions of culture transcend all cultures and can describe beliefs and practices used to maintain health and wellbeing that include food, movement, social connections, rituals, healing practices, and traditions. In our current modern culture, we may refer to this approach as "lifestyle practices" as seen in **Figure 18-1**.

Explanatory Narratives

Everyone has their own explanatory narrative that encompasses the multidimensional layers of being human. Listening to our own story and the story of others reveals how values, beliefs, attitudes, customs, rituals, and symbols can open doors to exploring and expanding possibilities for growth and change. Our beliefs and customs can be a connector to our inner spirit and life force, and can also be self-limiting. As a client tells her/his story, it is a way of seeking wholeness and balance, while often in the midst of vulnerability, transformation, and/or transition. During this deep listening process, the Nurse Coach shifts into a new awareness and consciousness of co-participating with the client story in her/his healing process (see Chapter 5).

Nurse Coaches recognize that when listening to the client's story they become part of the client's environment as she or he centers and enters into an energy space or a field of shared consciousness. Throughout time, most cultural models have held a worldview that there is an interconnectedness of body, mind, and spirit. Disharmony or disruption in the external and/or internal environment is perceived as being out of balance and vulnerable. As living beings, we are a reflection of our world, and any environmental assault directly impacts our energetic patterns and wellbeing.

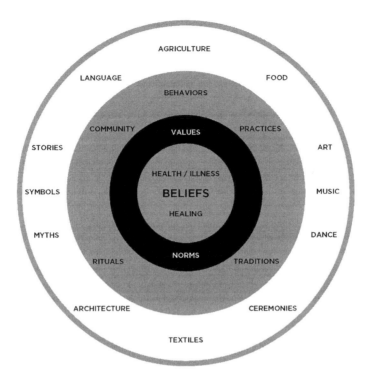

Figure 18-1 Dimensions of Culture.
Source. Copyright © 2014 by the International Nurse Coach Association. www.inursecoach.com

Health, illness, and healing all have explanatory models that reflect the traditions, rituals, and practices that represent dominant values and expectations and serve as a mirror reflecting the dimensions of a given culture. Maintaining and restoring health is important for the survival of all groups and communities. Healthcare systems, as in all other cultural systems, articulate prevailing philosophical concepts of social values and cultural norms. How one defines health and seeks solutions when ill will express how beliefs, attitudes, and images translate into biological messages to the world. Understanding the power and impact of one's beliefs and images around health, illness, healing, and dying has always been a provocative issue in cultural models and in medicine.

Exploring Personal and Cultural Meaning

As Nurse Coaches explore cultural diversity and listen to the client's narrative, we have the opportunity to reevaluate and redefine our personal and cultural meaning of health and healing. As the layers of culture intersect, the culture of our nursing profession may perform within the culture of a hospital, clinic, or community. In the Western allopathic health model, nursing and healthcare systems function within the cultural construct of medicine and biotechnology. Nurses can simultaneously work within several cultural frameworks, synthesizing and processing personal and professional expectations and roles.

Nurse Coaches are challenged to become aware of our unique set of cultural beliefs, biases, and expectations so that we can observe the influences and filters that we use in listening to the client's narrative. Nurse Coach behaviors are learned and reflect the values and norms of our profession and institutions and can accompany embedded meaning and patterns of behaviors that are also an expression of who we are.

Vignette: Jen

Jen, a pediatric nurse working in her local hospital, debated whether to get a flu vaccine this year, although hospital policy mandated it. Being just three months pregnant, Jen was being extremely cautious, and her belief was that the vaccine could be harmful to her baby. There were several cultural beliefs interfacing in her decision-making process. The dominant medical belief (and policy) is that flu vaccines are important for protection and prevention for both the nurse and the vulnerable patients she or he works with. Her doctor believed that as an expectant mother, if she transmitted the flu to her unborn child, there may be serious health consequences. The belief of Jen's friends and of the popular culture was that the vaccine might be detrimental to normal growth and development of her baby in utero.

In a nurse coaching model, how does a Nurse Coach work with a client in exploring the benefits and challenges of a given situation? How does the Nurse Coach explore her or his personal beliefs that might influence her or his Nurse Coach conversations? How can the Nurse Coach assist Jen in exploring her beliefs and inner wisdom to assist her in considering her choices and options?

Nurse Coach Reflection

Take a moment to reflect on your own beliefs about Jen's situation. Where do they come from? Are you able to listen to her story without bias or judgment? Does your worldview influence your coaching dynamic? Consider the coaching questions you might ask Jen that might assist her in making her decision?

As a nurse, have you been in a situation where your beliefs and attitudes are not congruent with the prevailing cultural norm? How can you deeply listen to your own voice and trust your intuition? Are you able to view the situation from all sides and contemplate the challenges and the possible benefits? How do you advocate for yourself? Do you recognize personal beliefs that may or may not serve you? Are you willing to be responsible for your actions in whatever choices you make?

CULTURAL HEALING SYSTEMS

All cultures use language to express meaning and communicate thoughts and ideas. There is a large set of concepts underlying language, and these concepts are embedded in interconnected networks of meaning individually and from the group. For example, reflect on the meaningfulness of your life. What culturally transmitted symbols and language do you access to evaluate life in relation to your purpose, values, and other meanings that also are mostly learned from the culture. Meaning is also linked to one's cultural identity. There are themes woven into patterns of meaning inherent across all cultural healing systems where health is viewed as a balance and harmony and where the individual is seen as a *hologram*—a microcosm of the grander macrocosm of nature and the universe. Nurse coaching can serve as a cultural bridge within our biomedical framework, in allowing the voice of the client/patient to be heard as we care for the whole person.

Allopathic Medicine and Its Explanatory Model

Allopathic medicine has its own explanatory model for health and illness as learned through a biomedical framework: physical assessment, diagnosis, and treatment options. The Western medical model conceives of illness as something entering the body from the outside, such as a virus, while someone from another culture may see illness as an intrusion of other entities, including ancestral spirits or demons. The treatment to exorcise the invader may be antibiotics in the case of infection, or it may also be a ritual and prayer in another cultural interpretation. Is there one model that includes all of the possibilities that might influence the healing process? When we listen to the story and engage the person in what she or he believes will ameliorate distress, can this influence outcome? Some persons believe their symptoms are the result of the "evil eye." This is said to be a look from a person that is believed by many cultures to be able to cause injury or bad luck to whom it is directed. How might this person who has received an "evil eye" integrate her/his own rituals to ease and relieve suffering? What meaning does the person give to her/his illness? (Luck, 1994).

In our current medical model, patients tend to not share their personal beliefs about their illness, the folk remedies they use, the traditional healers they have seen, or their use of nutrition and herbal supplements. They conform to a passive, compliant "patient" role expectation, accompanied by fear and vulnerability of the unknown. Patient "behaviors" conform to role expectations, usually in a setting that is unfamiliar and often perceived as insensitive and alienating.

Nurse Coaches seek insight into what a person believes caused the symptoms or illness and how her/his beliefs, attitudes, and values, as well as her/his family's response, and what she/he believes will assist in the health and healing process (see Chapter 10). Discovering one's personal interpretation of her/his illness experience can be a significant finding in analyzing what is needed. Nurse Coaches and healthcare providers can expect better outcomes when they position themselves as supportive partners and come from a mutual understanding and collaboration rather than trying to impose traditional Western medical practices that may offer only limited buy-in. The relationship between the provider and the client/patient can have the greatest impact on her/his health experience and potential outcome. The nurse coaching process may provides accessibility for lowering barriers to client/patient-centered care and diminish isolation and fear, opening communication for establishing trust and partnership.

Disease and Illness

Disease is a label from a medical perspective while *illness* is the lived experience that is culturally shaped and includes categorizing and explaining forms of distress. In a Nurse Coach encounter, the meaning of illness is explored within the context of the therapeutic relationship facilitating movement towards change.

Illness includes the individual's ability to determine how best to cope with distress and deal with practical problems of daily living. Perceived illness and resolution may include initiating changes such as food and nutrition, physical activities, sleep and rest, reaching out to family and friends, and seeking practitioners including allopathic, integrative, complementary, alternative, and cultural healers.

Common Symptoms Across Cultures

The most common symptoms in illness and in disease management across cultural systems include pain, depression, and loss of hope. The Harvard psychiatrist and anthropologist, Arthur Kleinman, in his *The Illness Narratives: Suffering, Healing, and the Human Condition,* describes the sick role as a passive one that ultimately, and in all traditions, must transition into becoming an active one where the participant shares in decision-making. In this model, chronic illness is viewed as a therapeutic ally, and the client/patient and the Nurse Coach each have reciprocal responsibilities and facilitate a caring partnership with positive outcomes (Kleinman, 1988).

Cultural Assessment and Embeddedness

Cultural assessment is used to determine how embedded the individual is in her or his traditional culture. Cultural embeddedness refers to how aligned one is with her or his native culture. The extent of the patient's cultural embeddedness has a major influence on coaching and the change process. Knowing the patient's degree of cultural embeddedness assists the Nurse Coach to know the patient and the family, which assists with exploring readiness to change, along with identifying opportunities, issues, and concerns towards achieving new desired health behaviors and goals. Patients who are highly embedded in their native culture tend to be more aligned with their traditions and are more committed to their original cultural values and beliefs. People who are less embedded and more acculturated tend to be more open to ideas from both cultures. Bicultural individuals can move easily between both cultures.

Nurse Coaches working in multicultural environments listen to and observe words, images, and symbols that have deep meaning to an individual, whether it be the proverbial chicken soup or a religious icon. The Nurse Coach remains curious in a caring and respectful way. The Nurse Coach begins asking questions that are curious, engaging, and nonthreatening, offering comfort and decreasing anxiety. Showing authentic interest and appreciation for food and celebration can become a healing dynamic and a bond between the Nurse Coach and the client/patient. Other questions can explore how embedded one is in her or his culture. Does the client/patient live exclusively within her/his own cultural neighborhood? Does she/he venture out into the larger dominant culture? People whose daily lives are spent within their own culturally defined neighborhoods are usually more culturally embedded than patients who leave the neighborhood. This is valuable information when exploring willingness to change and stages of change model (see Chapter 15).

Vignette: Maria

Maria, a migrant farm worker, relocated to South Florida from the highlands of Guatemala. She frequently experienced abdominal pain and nausea. One evening, her cousin brought her to the emergency room of the local hospital. After a work-up that included a CAT scan, nothing was found and Maria was given a prescription for her stomach pain and was sent home. At her follow-up visit, her symptoms had progressed and she was to be admitted to the hospital for further tests. Her cousin, again accompanying her, finally spoke with the nurse who appeared empathic, noticing the nurse holding Maria's hand as she took her pulse. The nurse noted that her pulse was rapid and her breathing was shallow. When the nurse began to ask some questions about her condition, her cousin shared that Maria was extremely worried and felt helpless and isolated from her family. In listening to the story, the nurse discovered that Maria recently received tragic news that several members of her family had been in a terrible car accident back in her village in the highlands of Guatemala. Maria's cousin diagnosed her as afflicted by Susto, a "folk illness" triggered by severe fright (from the verb *asustar* in Spanish that means "to frighten"). This story had not been told to the busy ER doctor on intake. The nurse sat down with Maria and asked her if she knew what might be causing her abdominal pain. Maria simply stated, "Susto."

An important element in a Nurse Coach model is to understand the cultural context within which the symptoms are being experienced. Further insight into what Susto means will support Maria to listen to her own story and devise her own rituals for healing. When the nurse, intuitively using a coaching process, asked Maria a question that had deep meaning for her explanatory model of why her health was declining, everything shifted in this profound yet brief therapeutic encounter: Maria experienced a feeling of genuine concern by the nurse and thus spontaneously offered an authentic and open response. Maria perceived feeling acknowledged, respected, listened to, and cared for. Physiologically, this exchange may have lowered her stress response, slowed her pulse, softened her breath, shifted her energy, and lessened her pain. In the next section, rituals of healing are explored to assist Nurse Coaches in their healing journey with clients/patients.

RITUALS OF HEALING

Whenever human beings are faced with challenges alone or come together in groups in societies, they develop rituals. Rituals give significance to life's passages. They provide form and guidance to our lives, prescribing behaviors during the perilous times when bodies, minds, and spirits are broken. Without rituals, we would have no map for how to act, and no occasion for people to share their common bonds of experience. Our nursing rituals easily blend with our nursing theories and evidence-based practice (Wolf, 2014) to show the sacred and profane of nursing through their performance. Within the complexity of everyday life and the fast-paced hospital/clinic environment, rituals create an intimacy to facilitate healing. In the next sections, we will further explore specifics related to rituals of healing and as a healing force (Achterberg, Dossey, & Kolkmeier, 1994).

Traditional and Self-Generated Rituals

Rituals are an enactment of cultural beliefs and values. Rituals have repetition and patterns of form and behaviors with personal and healing worth. They can be traditional or self-generated rituals. *Traditional* rituals are handed down through generations and have a history such as the way we celebrate births, deaths, holidays, and other special events with our families and friends. *Self-generated rituals* have no cultural history or tradition and are created in a very special way by each person or group.

Rituals have qualities that help us enter into the sacred space of the mind where we honor the core of our human experience and touch the power of the invisible force or whatever we name it. We create rites of separation from the old to new ways of thinking, behaving, and doing, where we integrate into new modes of living. Rituals work as a healing force because they contain steps for recovery, reduce anxiety and fear, and also reduce feelings of helplessness. They also evoke a higher power or healing source (**Table 18-1**).

Table 18-1 Rituals of Healing.

- Entering into a sacred space of mind
- Honoring the core of our own humanity
- Recognition of the power of the invisible forces that heal and connect and transcend
- Visible expressions of community bonding and support through biological, psychological passages of life
- Rites of separation from old ways of being and thinking and behaving, and integrative new modes of living
- Communication and celebration, solemnity, and occasions for deep inner silence
- The way all societies give meaning, richness, and structure to healing ceremonies

Source: Used with permission from Achterberg, J., Dossey, B. M., & Kolkmeier L. (1994). *Rituals of healing* (pp. 32–33). New York, NY: Bantam.

Structure of Rituals

Rituals contain a structure—a beginning, middle, and end. When we plan details in advance we avoid doing anything against our personal beliefs and values. Remember, there are no absolute rules. Healing rituals often call forth our community. In an illness or crisis, there is a disruption in life's harmony, and this disruption can touch many lives as it never occurs in a vacuum. Rituals help us with the restoration of harmony as we reweave the social fabric of our life and community. It is through community that a person can act and work on one's self or on another's behalf and are brought into harmonious relationship.

Characteristics of Rituals

Rituals have four major characteristics—intention, time, place, and people. *Intention* is when a person acknowledges the need to change, heal, or otherwise give attention to one's self. *Time* means to find moments to an extended period of time and to separate from your regular activities. *Place* means to locate a place or create a space that is conducive to inner work. *People* means that you find your team, be it a friend or a community, then hire a healing team if needed, and have family and friends to support you when needed. See the Ritual Guide to Getting Well (**Table 18-2**).

Table 18-2 Ritual Guide to Getting Well.

This *Ritual Guide to Getting Well* helps you decide what to do if you are diagnosed with the unknowable, the unthinkable, the awful, or the so-called incurable. By doing this, you can better determine how to survive treatment, yourself, your friends and family, and life in general.

1. Find a quiet place, a healing place, and go there. This might be a corner of your favorite room where you have placed gifts, pictures, a candle, or other symbols that signal peace and inner reflection to you. Or it might be in a park, under an old tree, or in a special place known for its spirit, such as high on a sacred mountain or on the cliffs overlooking a coastline or in the quiet magnificence of a forest.
2. Ask questions of your inner self about what your diagnosis or treatment means in your life. How will life change? What are your resources, your strengths, your reasons for staying alive? These deeply philosophical or spiritual issues often come to mind when problems are diagnosed. Listen with as quiet a mind as possible for any answers or messages that come from within, or from your higher source of guidance.
3. Take this time, knowing that very few problems advance so quickly that you must rush into making decisions about them immediately, without first gaining some perspective.
4. Find at least one friend or advocate who can be level-headed when you think you are going crazy; who can be positive for you when you are absolutely certain you are doomed; who can listen when your head is buzzing with uncertainty.
5. Love yourself. Ask yourself moment by moment whether what surrounds you is nurturing and life-giving. If the answer is no, back off from it. Kindly tell all negative-thinking people that you will not be seeing them while you are going through this. You may need never to see them again, and this is your right and obligation to yourself.
6. Assess your belief system. What do you believe? How did you get to believe it in the first place? What is really happening inside you and outside you? How serious is it? What will it take to get you well?
7. Gather information, keeping an open mind. Everyone who offers to treat you or give you advice has their lives invested in what they tell you. Stand back and listen thoughtfully.
8. Now go and hire your healing team. Remember, you hired them—you can fire them. They are in the business of performing a service for you, and you are paying their salaries. Sometimes this relationship gets confused. Make sure they all talk to each other. You are in command. You are the captain of the healing team.
9. Don't let anyone talk you into treatment you don't believe in or don't understand. Keep asking questions. Replace anyone who acts too busy to answer your questions. Chances are, they're also too busy to do their best work for you.

(continues on next page)

Table 18-2 (*Continued*).

10. Don't agree on any diagnostic or lab tests unless someone you trust can give you good reasons why they are being ordered. If the tests are not going to change your treatment, they are an expensive and dangerous waste of your time.

11. Sing your own song, write your own story, take your own spiritual journey through a journal or diary. A threat to health and wellbeing can be a trigger to becoming and doing all those things you've been putting off for the "right" time.

12. Consider these maxims in your journey:
    - Everything cures somebody, and nothing cures everybody.
    - There are no simple answers to complex issues of why people get sick in the first place.
    - Sometimes disease is inexplicable to mortal minds.

13. You will not be intimidated by the overbearing world of medicine or alternative health know-it-alls, but can thoughtfully take the best from several worlds.

14. You can teach gentleness and compassion to the most arrogant doctor and the crankiest nurse. Tell them that you need your mind and soul nurtured, as well as the best medical treatment possible in order to get well. If they are not up to it, you'll find someone who is.

Source: Used with permission from Achterberg, J., Dossey, B. M., & Kolkmeier L. (1994). *Rituals of healing* (pp. 32–33). Bantam: New York, NY.

Three Phases of Rituals

Rituals have three phases—separation, transition, and return. In the *separation phase*, the client/patient engages in a healing activity and enters into a healing state of consciousness. In the *transition phase*, the client/patient moves into an awareness of being changed in the healing process. In the *return phase*, the client/patient reenters life's activities, renewed and changed .

The separation phase has two distinct phases. The first is the *trigger*, which is often a trauma, illness, or crisis. The boundaries and routines have changed. The second phase requires *deliberate activities*, as normal activities have changed. It is moving from one form or place to another, and locating and creating a sacred healing place. This may be forming a circle with healing objects or being surrounded by a circle of friends. This is a symbolic act of breaking away.

The transition phase is the hero's journey, where we face the shadow of what we have repressed. We must determine what is real and worthy of this moment. When we find time alone to consider what is present, we can most often identify things that are in need of healing. The transition phase can be thought of as a symbolic death and rebirth. We enter into a heightened state of consciousness where we rehearse activities, gather information, and learn to reflect deeply.

The return phase is moving back to the activities of daily life and recognizing the challenges and connections of reentry. It is noticing any aspects of a healing state and being able to have a formal release of the old ways in order to embody and integrate new ways of being and living.

NURSE COACHING AND CULTURAL COMPETENCIES

Health and illness are not merely the end results of individual biology and behavior. What people believe and experience when they are ill is usually something far more complex and deeply interconnected with their daily lives. The way people think about health influences whether they are receptive to health information, willing to change health behaviors, and whether or not their health improves. How can Nurse Coaches and healthcare providers who spend less and less time with patients in the current system expand their clinical gaze to include the patient's health beliefs and perspectives?

The process of cultural competence consists of five inter-related constructs: (1) cultural desire, (2) cultural awareness, (3) cultural knowledge, (4) cultural skill, and (5) cultural encounters (Campinha-Bacote, 2002). Cultural competence is a process that continuously strives to achieve the ability to effectively work within the cultural context of the individual (client/patient), family, and community. This ongoing process involves the integration of cultural awareness, cultural knowledge, cultural skill, and cultural curiosity and openness. The foundational construct of cultural competence is the cultural encounter. Nurse Coaches can remember that all encounters are cultural encounters. Cultural competence involves the paradox of knowing—the more you think you know, the more you really do not know; the more you think you do not know, the more you really know.

Nursing has maintained its vitality in a dynamic process through a lens that includes honoring and respecting the uniqueness of each individual and embracing all of her/his dimensions and complexity. In a nursing paradigm, and within a client/patient-centered care model, cultural competency embraces the premise that all dimensions of the individual are connected. The empathetic witnessing of the existential experience of suffering can lead to practical coping strategies for the experience. The art of nurse coaching includes sensitive solicitation of the client's/patient's and family's/significant others' story around the illness. Integral to nurse coaching is being curious about culturally held beliefs and the causes one attributes to their symptoms.

Theory of Transcultural Nursing

Nurse theorist Madeleine Leininger's (2002) Theory of Transcultural Nursing is based on her ideas of care that contain a strong cultural anthropologic framework. Leininger encouraged nurses to conduct a holistic "culturalological" assessment in the major areas of worldview and social structure factors, including cultural values, beliefs, and practices; religious, philosophical, or spiritual beliefs; economic factors; and educational beliefs. She believed that care was the dominant focus of nursing, which needed a cultural environmental context to be understood and used to ultimately influence nursing care and patient centered care (Leininger, 2006). Leininger's Transcultural Theory is embedded in the Theory of Integrative Nurse Coaching where the client/patient is primary and the "disease" is secondary.

A major feature of Leininger's theory is the emphasis on the way individuals relate to health, wellbeing, illness, and death in different contexts and cultures. She defined a cultural assessment as a systematic appraisal of individuals, groups, and communities about their cultural beliefs, values, and practices, in order to determine explicit needs within the context of the people being served. The goal of a cultural assessment in nurse coaching is to listen to the client/patient narrative, which will allow the Nurse Coach to co-create a mutually acceptable and culturally relevant plan.

LEARN: Five-Step Cultural Assessment

Berlin and Fowkes (1982) recommend the five-step LEARN (**Table 18-3**) process in a cultural assessment. When introduced into the therapeutic encounter, it can improve communication and create a heightened awareness around cultural issues in medical and healthcare of the client/patient. The goal is to co-create with clients/patients where this is active engagement and commitment about the treatment plan. This assessment allows the Nurse Coach to enter into a coaching conversation with the client and family. Culturally knowledgeable and compassionate care supports and preserves valued traditions that give meaning to people's lives. Acknowledgment and maintenance of the client's cultural traditions show respect for the person, supporting the client's desire to engage in this practice.

Table 18-3 LEARN: Five-Step Process for Cultural Assessment.

LISTEN	*Listen* to the client's/patient's perception of the presenting problem.
EXPLAIN	*Explain* client's/patient's perception through a medical/nursing/integrative assessment that includes the physiological, psychological, spiritual, and cultural components.
ACKNOWLEDGE	*Acknowledge* the similarities and differences between the two perceptions. At times it is easier for the nurse to acknowledge cultural differences than to acknowledge and focus on similarities that the nurse and the patient have in common. Be sure to recognize differences and build on similarities to create a culturally relevant action and/or treatment plan.
RECOMMEND	*Recommend* and focus on client/patient active participation.
NEGOTIATE	*Negotiate* an action and/or treatment plan, recognizing that it will be beneficial to incorporate selected aspects of the patient's culture into the client/patient-centered plan.

Source: Adapted from Berlin, E., & Fowkes, W. (1982). A teaching framework for cross-cultural health care. *The Western Journal of Medicine, 139*(6), 934–938.

Theory of Explanatory Models (EMs)

Psychiatrist and anthropologist Arthur Kleinman's (1988) Theory of Explanatory Models (EMs) resonates with an integrative Nurse Coach approach of asking meaningful questions. He suggests that individuals and groups can have vastly different notions of health and disease than what the health providers tending to them address. He proposes that instead of simply asking patients, "Where does it hurt?" the provider needs to focus on eliciting the patient's answers to *"What," "When," "How,"* and *"What next."* In listening to the patient's narrative, there are five major categories of questions in order to explain the patient's perception of the illness. The questions are framed to elicit information on (1) etiology, (2) time and mode of onset of symptoms, (3) pathophysiology, (4) course of illness (including both severity and type of sick role), and (5) treatment for an illness episode as see in **Table 18-4**. Obtaining patients' explanations of their illness using their explanatory model are notions about illness, treatment, and possible amelioration of symptoms. When the client/patient, family, and significant others are supported to express their beliefs, concerns, barriers, and priorities in their care, a new dynamic emerges and engages the person in the mutual decision-making and setting of goals. As the Nurse Coach integrates explanatory models and supports meaningful cultural healing practices, this strengthens and facilitates client/patient partnerships, and develops dynamic approaches for care, and promotes the healing process.

Table 18-4 Nurse Coach Cultural Coaching Questions: Five Categories.

Etiology: "What"
> What do you call your problem (or illness)? What name does it have?
> What do you think has caused your problem (illness, symptoms)?

Time and Mode of Onset of Symptoms: "When"
> When do you think it started when it did?

Pathophysiology: "How"
> How does your sickness affect you now?
> How does it work?

Course of Illness Episode: "How" and "What"
> How severe is it?
> How short or long will it be?
> What do you fear the most about your sickness?
> What are the chief problems your sickness has caused for you?

Treatment for an Illness Episode: "What Next"
> What kind of treatment do you think you should receive?
> What are the most important results you hope to receive from this treatment?
> What is it you need to help you get well?

Source: Adapted from Kleinman, A. (1988). *The illness narratives: Suffering, healing, and the human condition*. New York, NY: Basic Books.

SUMMARY

- Nurse Coaches are uniquely positioned to be with a client/patient and explore meaning and beliefs she or he holds about her or his health and illness and what might help in the health and healing process.
- Nurse Coaches cultivate cultural competencies to assist individuals in their health and wellbeing and for achieving goals and improving health outcomes.
- Nurse Coaches view individuals within the context of their family, community, and culture, and honor the traditions embedded in their choices.

NURSE COACH REFLECTIONS

After reading this chapter, the Nurse Coach will be able to bring awareness and personal insight to the following questions:

- What are my personal beliefs and values about health and healing?
- What are the cultural influences that impact my own health choices?
- How do I feel when caring for a client/patient from a cultural background different from my own?
- How has my understanding of cultural competence influenced how I listen to a client/patient?
- As a Nurse Coach, how will I explore the client's/patient's narrative to understand her or his perceived meaning of her or his illness?
- What are the healing rituals that I create in my daily life?
- What new ritual can I bring into my life to enhance my wellbeing?

REFERENCES

Achterberg, J., Dossey, B. M., & Kolkmeier, L. (1994). *Rituals of healing.* New York, NY: Bantam.

Berlin, E., & Fowkes, W. (1982). A teaching framework for cross-cultural health care. *Western Journal of Medicine, 139*(6), 934–938.

Campinha-Bacote, J. (2002). The process of cultural competence in the delivery of healthcare services: A model of care. *Journal of Transcultural Nursing, 13*(3), 181–184.

Dobbie, A., Medrano, M., Tysinger, J., & Olney, C. (2003). The BELIEF instrument: A preclinical tool to elicit patient's health beliefs. *Family Medicine, 35*(5), 316–319.

Engebretson, J. C. (2013). Cultural diversity and care. In B. M. Dossey & L. Keegan (Eds.). *Holistic nursing: A handbook for practice* (6th ed., pp. 677–702). Burlington, MA: Jones & Bartlett Learning.

Institute of Medicine (2001). *Crossing the quality chasm: A new health system for the 21st century.* Washington, DC: National Academy Press.

Kleinman, A. (1988). *The illness narratives: Suffering, healing, and the human condition.* New York, NY: Basic Books.

Leininger, M. (2002). *Transcultural nursing: Theories, concepts and practices* (3rd ed.). New York, NY: McGraw Hill.

Leininger, M. (2006). Cultural care diversity and universality theory and evolution of the ethnonursing method. In M. M. Leininger & M. R. McFarland (Eds.). *Culture care diversity and universality: A worldwide nursing theory* (2nd ed., pp. 1–42). Sudbury, MA: Jones & Bartlett Learning.

Luck, S. (1994). Cross cultural healing. *Journal of Holistic Nursing, 12*(3), 237–238.

Nightingale, F. (1860). *Notes on nursing: What it is and what it is not.* London, UK: Harrison.

Wolf, Z. R. (2014). *Exploring rituals in nursing: Joining art and science.* New York, NY: Springer.

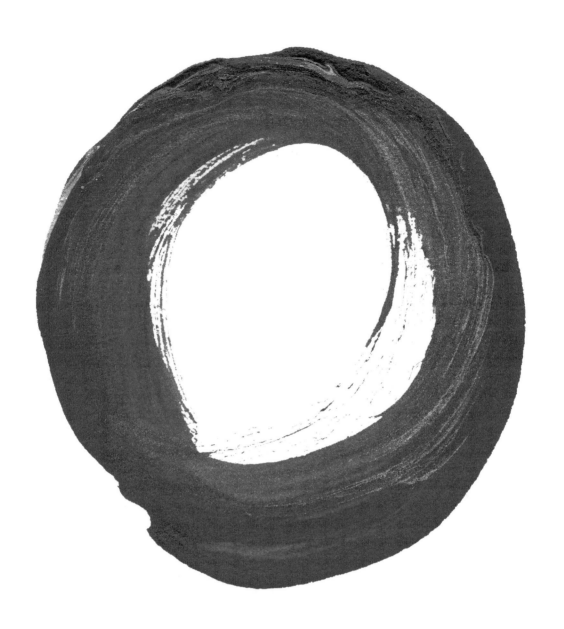

CORE VALUE 4

*Nurse Coach Education,
Research, Leadership*

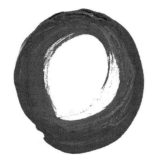

CHAPTER 19

Nurse Coaching and Education

Lisa A. Davis

So never lose an opportunity of urging a practical beginning, however small, for it is wonderful how often in such matters the mustard-seed germinates and roots itself.

Florence Nightingale, in Cook, E., 1913

LOOKING AHEAD...

After reading this chapter, you will be able to:

- Discuss the importance of holding space, ritual, invitation, pause, and teaching work as well as life in relation to teaching nurse coaching.
- Relate the role of facilitator to teaching nurse coaching.
- Develop nurse coaching course or workshop objectives.
- Design learning activities to enhance understanding of nurse coaching.

DEFINITIONS

Abstracting: Summarizing or converting concepts or ideas into models or metaphors.

Application/question cards: Index cards used in both teaching and evaluation that are given to students. At the end of the class, students are encouraged to write how they can use information or questions they have about information on the index card to be submitted to the teacher.

Checking in: Pausing during class or at the end of class to ask students how they are, what they are thinking, or what they need.

Discovery learning: An active teaching strategy based on natural curiosity, which builds on prior knowledge or experience in which the learner is encouraged to question. The goal of discovery learning is to promote deep understanding. Collaboration and discussion allow for that deeper understanding. It emphasizes the process rather than the end-product.

Facilitator: Teacher who addresses learning objectives in an indirect manner. The hierarchy of teacher/student is flattened, and teacher and student become co-learners.

Learning community: A group of students or workshop participants who take coursework together and share a common experience.

Learning environment: All the conditions present, both internal and external, that might affect learning. This can include, but is not limited to, room temperature, seating comfort, teaching tools, interruptions, course content, characteristics of the teacher, and characteristics of the learner(s).

Objective: Expected student/participant learning as a result of instructional activity.

Problem-based learning: Problem-based learning (PBL), also referred to as concept-based learning, is an instructional method that challenges students to "learn to learn", working in groups to seek solutions to real world problems or issues. The process replicates the commonly used systemic approach to resolving problems or meeting challenges that are encountered in life.

Service learning: A type of teaching that combines academic content with civic responsibility in some community project. The learning is structured and supervised and enables the student to reflect on what has taken place

Third things: Indirectly approaching a topic metaphorically by use of poetry, storytelling, art, etc. which allows for a "voice" other than that of the teacher or that of the student. The third thing can engage both teacher and student in such a way as to make all more aware of deeper meaning and deeper thought. The term "third thing" was coined by Parker Palmer (2004).

FACILITATING DISCOVERY

The goal of nurse coaching is to facilitate discovery. This chapter offers that practical beginning in teaching nurse coaching. First, discovery on the part of the Nurse Coach, and second, on the part of the individual being coached. Discovery learning as a framework for organizing workshops and classes is therefore quite helpful. In this framework, active involvement of the student is essential to the learning process, and what students take away from the learning opportunity is very individual. Therefore, learning objectives should be broad enough to allow for this individual discovery. Discovery learning is meant to stimulate curiosity and creativity, so activities that foster curiosity and creativity are optimal. Finally, with discovery learning, while some responses are better than others, there are no right or wrong answers. Students should feel free to explore, to fail, to excel, to ask questions, and to be held gently in the learning environment.

HOLDING THE SPACE

Part of providing a positive learning environment is engendering safety and trust. This requires very purposeful actions on the part of the teacher/facilitator. Parker Palmer (2004) speaks of providing an environment that is neither invasive nor evasive. The space should not discount or deny the innate wholeness of the individuals of the group, nor of the group itself. Conversely, the space should not refute the fact that there are individual struggles. Rather, in holding the space, the teacher and the learners are present to each other. Honoring the present helps us tune into who we are. Zorn (2010, p. 15) notes that honoring the present allows space for our "essential" self. "It is living and experiencing rather than controlling or solving." In holding the space, individuals need to trust that they will not be fixed nor judged. In fact, the teacher is really a facilitator of holding the space. Nurse coaching is not about solving problems, but providing a space in which people are allowed to arrive at their own solutions and set their own goals. This holding of space is just as important in a classroom or workshop as it is in the nurse/client interaction. This experience of holding space in the teaching/learning of nurse coaching reinforces the importance of this type of environment in a nurse/client session.

The role of the teacher is built upon the principles of warmth, indirectness, cognitive organization, and enthusiasm. Warmth conveys to someone that she or he is liked and accepted. Indirectness is the way of guiding the learner to find her or his own way rather than supplying pat answers to problems. Emily Dickinson (1830–1886) reinforces the notion of indirectness in her poem *Tell all the Truth but Tell it Slant:*

Tell all the Truth but tell it slant—
Success in Circuit lies
Too bright for our infirm Delight
The Truth's superb surprise As Lightning to the Children eased
With explanation kind
The Truth must dazzle gradually
Or every man be blind—

Cognitive organization involves developing a plan for teaching which includes not only the content of the lesson, but also incorporates sensitivity to the age, cultural background, motivation, and learning styles of the student. Enthusiasm for the subject matter is easily perceived by the student and enhances the learning environment (Loftin, Davis, & Hartin, 2010). Palmer (2007) reminds us that the most important thing the teacher brings to the classroom is her or his authentic self.

There are several things that enhance the facilitation of holding space. First, allow for community and collaboration. This is best done when people can make eye contact and not have barriers, such as desks between the members of the group. An open circle is the best seating choice for holding space. Members of the class can sit comfortably and see other members of the group. Lighting should be adequate for writing, but not harsh. Soft background music can be both inviting and soothing to the group prior to the session starting. It can promote a peaceful, welcoming environment.

The physical environment itself is just a part of holding space. The inner environment of all participants is equally important. Part of the role of the facilitator in holding space is to gently set some ground rules. Palmer (2007) provides some excellent "touchstones" for holding space as seen in **Table 19-1**. These tenets can be discussed at the beginning of class so all members know what to expect from each other, and from themselves.

Table 19-1 Touchstones.

The following ideas, based on the work of Parker Palmer (2004), increase the likelihood of working together productively.

1. **Be 100% present.** Set aside the usual distractions of things undone from yesterday, things to do tomorrow. Bring all of yourself to the work. Suspend multitasking.

2. **Listen deeply.** Listen intently to what is said; listen to the feelings beneath the words. As Quaker writer Douglas Steere puts it, "Holy listening—to 'listen' another's soul into life, into a condition of disclosure and discovery [which] may be almost the greatest service that any human being ever performs for another." Listen to yourself as well as to others. Strive to achieve a balance between listening and reflecting, speaking and acting.

3. **It is never "share or die."** You will be invited to share in pairs, small groups, and in the large group. The invitation is completely open. You determine the extent to which you want to participate in our discussions and activities.

4. **No fixing.** Each of us is here to discover our own truths, to listen to our own inner teacher, to take our own inner journey. We are not here to set someone else straight, or to help right another's wrong, to "fix" what we perceive as broken in another.

5. **Suspend judgment.** Set aside your judgments. By creating a space between judgments and reactions, we can listen to the other, and to ourselves, more fully.

6. **Identify assumptions.** Our assumptions are usually transparent to us, yet they undergird our worldview. By identifying our assumptions, we can then set them aside and open our viewpoints to greater possibilities.

(continues on next page)

Table 19-1 (*Continued*).

7. **Speak your truth.** You are invited to say what is in your heart, trusting that your voice will be heard and your contribution respected. Your truth may be different from, even the opposite of, what another person in the circle has said. Yet speaking your truth is simply that. It is not debating with, or correcting, or interpreting what another has said. Respond from your center, not to another's center. This behavior honors the previous speaker's comments without passing judgment. It also avoids introducing defensive feelings that distract from the listening.

8. **Respect silence.** Silence is a rare gift in our busy world. After someone has spoken, take time to reflect without immediately filling the space with words. This applies to the speaker as well. Be comfortable leaving your words to resound in the silence, without refining or elaborating on what you have just said. This process allows others time to fully listen before reflecting on their own reactions.

9. **Maintain confidentiality.** Create a safe space by respecting the confidential nature and content of discussions held in the formation circle. Allow what is said in the circle to remain there.

10. **When things get difficult, turn to wonder.** If you find yourself disagreeing with another, becoming judgmental, or shutting down in defense, try turning to wonder: "I wonder what brought her to this place?" "I wonder what my reaction teaches me?" "I wonder what he's feeling right now?"

Source: Copyright © 2014 by Lisa A. Davis. Adapted from Palmer, P. (2004). *A hidden wholeness: The journey toward an undivided life.* San Francisco, CA: Jossey Bass.

IMPORTANCE OF RITUAL

One thing that can serve to set the tone for honoring and respecting both the space and each other is to start each session with a ritual. Rituals not only reflect the values of the class, but can also function to create values for a class (Achterberg, Dossey, & Kolkmeier, 1994). Furthermore, rituals and symbols affirm knowledge and healing wisdom. They can "set the stage" for learning, so to speak. Think of your own rituals, often performed unknowingly, but if skipped can leave you off kilter for the entire day. Do you start your day with an affirmation, a special poem, certain music, exercise? Do you have a special "wake up" song for your child? These rituals reflect what is important to us and invite a meaningful start to the day. It is the same in the classroom—to celebrate and acknowledge everyone is there for the same reason. Examples of rituals are found in **Table 19-2** and further explored in Chapter 18.

Table 19-2 Examples of Rituals.

- Placing flowers or a live plant in the center of the learning circle
- Starting the session with a meditation or guided imagery
- Having each participant place a stone in the center of the circle
- Lighting a candle or a lamp
- Reading a passage from a book, or reading a poem
- Having students place a note with their deepest wish for the day in a bowl in the center of the circle and then burning them at the end (sending them to the universe)
- Drumming
- Singing/chanting
- Repeating an affirmational mantra
- Holding the space with silence

Source: Copyright © 2014 by Lisa A. Davis.

INVITING PARTICIPATION

Part of holding a space of trust is that all members are invited, rather than expected, to speak or act. Voluntary participation is a guiding principle of coaching, as is honoring silence. Silence can result in or be caused by profound reflection. The invitation, as well as honoring silence, precludes the pressure to conform with the group, however subtle. One way to physically demonstrate invitation to the group is to hold out the hand, palm up, as if reaching to connect with the group. If someone would like to respond, they may. Prolonged silence is a cue that no one wishes to respond. This act is invitational, as opposed to pointing to a participant, which can be more demanding. It connotes, "You, answer me." In the worst cases, the pointed finger is accusatory. Palmer (2004) offers an excellent example of the invitation. In structuring self-introductions at the beginning of a class, rather than say, "I'll introduce myself then everyone else introduce themselves, starting on my right," he begins with silence. He then invites the group to introduce themselves when they are ready. Everyone will have time to speak if they choose to. Prolonged silence indicates that everyone who wished to speak has done so. Inviting participation includes inviting questions. Nothing silences a group so much as a conscious or unconscious indication that a question is not welcome.

This is quickly perceived by all members of the group, not just the one posing the question. Conscious indications of unwelcomed questions include stating, "That's a stupid question," or, "Look it up in the book." Other, more subtle indicators are eye rolling, placing hand on hips, a deep sigh (Loftin et al., 2010). Inviting questions would be accomplished by stating, "There are no 'stupid' questions," or "I'm so glad you asked that."

THE POWER OF THE PAUSE

A common issue, particularly to the new educator, is focus on "content." There is so much information that needs to be covered. Information is overabundant. It is important to refrain from bombarding students with facts and figures. Research (Ayres & Paas, 2012) indicates that too much cognitive load compromises learning because there is a limited amount of working memory available to process all the information. It is overwhelming and disengaging. To maximize learning, limit facts and figures to manageable chunks of information interspersed with activities, breaks, or times of reflection, and trust this process. It is often hard as an educator to let go. It becomes an issue of control—control of the content, of the lecture, of the discussion—usually driven by fear that if we do not control the content, learning will not take place. Control makes you the expert to be listened to in a classroom setting. Letting go of this control allows you to listen more, and in so doing, experience those marvelous serendipitous insights that in education lead to the teachable moment. Thus, pauses keep the learning community in the present. A mind shift may be necessary to get away from the autocratic mindset of control to that of a shared learning experience facilitated by the teacher.

Zorn (2010, p. 5) beautifully describes the pause as fundamental, especially as we "pass over yet another threshold. Thresholds are sacred turning points—they mark the place where what is ending has not yet transformed into that which is about to be." The pause allows us to dwell with and reflect upon concepts and ideas, and it is in that time that deep learning takes place. At the edge of the subway platform in London is an admonition, "mind the gap." This can serve as a reminder to allow for the discovery that takes place in moments of mindful pause. As we know from life, pausing is not always easy, nor does it provide easy answers. It is too easy to fill time and space with tasks which keep us from introspection, compromise, intuition, and wonder.

TEACHING LIFE AS WELL AS WORK

As with so much of what we teach in nursing, both knowledge and skills, nurse educators are not just preparing future nurses, but also life skills for students to be productive men and women. This is certainly the case with Nurse Coach education. Self-care, deep listening, breath work, facilitation of goal setting, nonviolent communication, and all the other concepts used in coaching others also become personal life skills and insights for the Nurse Coach. Holding the space to allow this to happen is intrinsic to teaching nurse coaching.

DEVELOPING OBJECTIVES

Educational objectives are required by either college or university accrediting bodies, or organizations (AHNCC, 2012; AHNCC, n.d.; CCNE, 2013; SACS, 2012) that grant continuing education (CE) or university course credit. Knowledge, skills, and abilities expected of the Nurse Coach student and reflected in the objective statement should be consistent with pre-licensure and licensure expectations of registered nurses (Cronenwett et al., 2007; QSEN, 2014).

Bloom's Revised Taxonomy (Anderson & Krathwohl, 2001; Krathwohl, 2002) provides a framework for classification of objective statements (**Figure 19-1**). It is important to remember that objectives are written for the learner, not the teacher. A well-constructed objective provides students information about what they are to learn as a result of instruction. They also provide the teacher with some information about how to teach. For example, if the objective is to list the elements of the nurse coaching process, the teacher would not spend much time on this activity because the learning outcome is only to list the elements. There is no expectation of understanding the process or using the process. Changing the verb in the objective to "discuss" takes the objective to a higher level of the taxonomy and would require a lot more time to teach. The teacher would introduce the topic with the information the students needed to discuss, but the majority of the teaching plan would be aimed at developing questions to stimulate discussion. Lastly, the objective provides guidance on how to evaluate if the objective was met. In the first example above, if the students successfully listed the elements of the nurse coaching process, the objective was met. In the second example, if the students participated in discussion, the objective was met. The overarching guideline for teaching nurse coaching is to write objectives in which the outcome is deep learning and let those objectives guide the methodology you use to teach. What you do to maximize learning is the methodology, and we will address that later. What is it you want the learner to learn? Finally, what is the time-frame?

The well-constructed objective addresses the questions: who, what, and when. As stated earlier, the "who" is always the learner. The "what" always includes an action verb, which corresponds to the level on the taxonomy, which in turn indicates the desired learning outcome. The "when" is easy, and generally understood by the end of the lesson. **Table 19-3** provides some sample verbs which can be used in writing objectives in order to achieve learning at each level of the taxonomy.

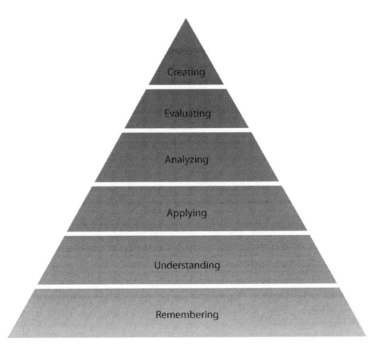

Figure 19-1 Bloom's Revised Taxonomy.

Bloom's Taxonomy is a classification system for levels of behaviors important to learning. The base of the pyramid is the most basic (easiest) learning requiring rote memorization with the top level, creating, being the most complex behaviors of learning. Keep in mind that the further you go up the pyramid, the more brain pathways are involved in learning, and the more likely the learning is retained long-term.

Source: Copyright © 2014 by Lisa A. Davis. Adapted from Krathwohl, D. (2002). A revision of Bloom's Taxonomy: An overview. *Theory into Practice*, *41*(4), 212–218.

Table 19-3 Sample Verbs for Each Level of the Revised Taxonomy.

Level	Defining Characteristic	Sample Verbs
Remembering	Retrieving information	Recognize Recall List Define Select
Understanding	Derive meaning from instruction.	Interpret Classify Summarize Compare Explain
Apply	Use what is learned in a specific situation.	Implement Demonstrate Construct Utilize Develop

(*continues on next page*)

Table 19-3 (*Continued*).

Level	Defining Characteristic	Sample Verbs
Analyze	Determine how parts fit together by induction or deduction.	Organize Differentiate Compare Contrast
Evaluate	Assess how standards or criteria are met.	Critique Deduce Interpret Appraise Support
Create	Put it all together in an original, novel way.	Generate Develop Produce Plan Adapt

Source: Copyright © 2014 by Lisa A. Davis.

LEARNING ACTIVITIES AND COURSE OUTLINES

Within the framework of discovery learning, learning activities are essential to curriculum development. Authentic learning activities (Lombardi, 2007) are designed specifically for discovery learning with the goal of not only building on what the student already knows, but also fostering confidence. Learning activities that are participative and challenge students to think deeply are optimal for nurse coaching. Another hallmark of learning activities within the framework of discovery learning is collaboration. Drawing knowledge from each other, listening deeply, willing to listen to other ideas and compromise, collaborating, and supporting each other in the learning process are valued. Teaching nurse coaches is enhanced by developing learning communities. This has been achieved by the International Nurse Coach Association (INCA, n.d.) and their Integrative Nurse Coach Certificate Program (INCCP, n.d.) developed by Barbara Dossey, Susan Luck, and Bonney Schaub. Learning communities share a common experience, and by doing so, develop a sense of community. **Table 19-4** offers some suggestions for activities to enhance learning of nurse coaching.

Table 19-4 Examples of Learning Activities.

Small group learning activities
- Breath-work
- Meditation
- Discussion
- Case studies
- Reflective journal writing
- Checking in*
- Service learning*
- Problem- or concept-based learning

Large group learning activities
- Breath-work
- Meditation
- Lecture

(*continues on next page*)

Table 19-4 (*Continued*).

- Abstracting
- Summarize
- Discussion
- Role play
- Case studies
- Application or question cards
- Social networking for learning community
  - Facebook™
  - Email
  - Linkedin™
- Third things*
  - Poetry
  - Storytelling
  - Art project
  - Art appreciation
  - Music
  - Movie clips
  - Humor

Dyad learning activities
- Role playing (Nurse Coach and client)
- Administer the IHWA tool
- Maintain client log and client file
- Reflective journal writing
- Debrief

Individual learning activities
- Reflective journal writing
- Contemplative walks
- Meditation
- Breath-work
- Field work (work with actual clients)
- Debrief

*See Definitions.
Source: Copyright © 2014 by Lisa A. Davis.

Developing objectives and topics that meet learning needs as well as accreditation/CE requirements is time-consuming. **Table 19-5** offers examples of course descriptions, objectives, topics, and activities/assignments for a 3 semester credit hour (SCH) graduate course and a 3 SCH undergraduate course. **Table 19-6** offers an example of a 1 SCH undergraduate course. **Table 19-7** offers the one-day INCA Introductory Nurse Coach workshop, and **Table 19-8** offers a one-day workshop for self-care.

Table 19-5 Nurse Coach Course Outlines.

Course Title	Nurse Coaching (Graduate level; 3 sem. cr. hr. [SCH])	Nurse Coaching (Undergraduate level; 3 SCH)
Course Description	This course is designed to develop students to nurse coaching competences, working with the whole person, using modalities that integrate body-mind-emotion-spirit-environment. The course is aligned with American Nurse Association (ANA) 6 standards of practice and 10 standards of professional performance for nurses.	This course is designed to introduce students to nurse coaching competences, working with the whole person, using modalities that integrate body-mind-emotion-spirit-environment. The course is aligned with American Nurse Association (ANA) 6 standards of practice and 10 standards of professional performance for nurses.
Required/Recommended Texts	*Required texts*: Dossey, B. M., Luck, S., & Schaub, B. G. (2014). *Nurse coaching: Integrative approaches for health and wellbeing.* North Miami, FL: International Nurse Coach Association.	*Required texts*: Dossey, B. M., Luck, S., & Schaub, B. G. (2015). *Nurse coaching: Integrative approaches for health and wellbeing.* North Miami, FL: International Nurse Coach Association.
	Other required materials (software, other readings, etc.): Personal journal Integrative Health and Wellness Assessment™ (IHWA) long and short form.	*Other required materials (software, other readings, etc.)*: Personal journal IHWA long and short form. *Website:* International Nurse Coach Association, www.inursecoach.com
	Recommended texts: Hess, D., Dossey, B., Southard, M., Luck, S., Schaub, B., & Bark, L. (2013). *The art and science of nurse coaching: The provider's guide to coaching scope and competencies.* Silver Spring, MD: Nursesbooks.org. Dart, M. (2011). *Motivational interviewing in nursing practice: Empowering the patient.* Sudbury, MA: Jones & Bartlett Learning. Deci, E. (1995). *Why we do what we do: Understanding self-motivation.* New York, NY: Penguin. *Website:* International Nurse Coach Association, www.inursecoach.com	

(continues on next page)

Table 19-5 (*Continued*).

Course Objectives	Objectives/Student Learning Outcomes –	Objectives/Student Learning Outcomes –
	1. Analyze nurse coaching and the nurse coaching process.	1. Overview nurse coaching and the nurse coaching process.
	2. Explore Integrative Health and Wellness Assessment (IHWA) tool and how it reflects integrative perspective of care.	2. Explore IHWA tool and how it reflects integrative perspective of care.
	3. Discuss deep listening and therapeutic presence.	3. Discuss deep listening and therapeutic presence.
	4. Discuss motivational interviewing (MI), nonviolent communication (NVC), appreciative inquiry (AI), and positive psychology.	4. Discuss MI, NVC, AI, and positive psychology.
	5. Conduct intake sessions with peer clients.	5. Conduct intake sessions with peer clients.
	6. Learn and practice breath awareness using various techniques.	6. Learn and practice breath awareness using various techniques.
	7. Analyze various theoretical models applied to nurse coaching.	7. Apply various theoretical models applied to nurse coaching.
	8. Incorporate clinical use of self-care.	8. Identify clinical use of self-care.
	9. Practice mindfulness and self-awareness.	9. Practice mindfulness and self-awareness.
	10. Discuss the relationship between food choices, environmental exposures, health, and disease.	10. Discuss the relationship between food choices, environmental exposures, health, and disease.
Course Topics	Introduction Identify faculty/student goals Overview of expectations Confidentiality Self-care activity IHWA tool (long and short form) Theoretical frameworks Deep listening and therapeutic presence Motivational interviewing Nonviolent communication Intake sessions Breath awareness Imagery Appreciative inquiry Mindfulness Food choices/nutrition Environment and health Nutritional self-care planning	Introduction Identify faculty/student goals Overview of expectations Confidentiality Self-care activity IHWA tool (long and short form) Theoretical frameworks Deep listening and therapeutic presence Motivational interviewing Nonviolent communication Intake sessions Breath awareness Imagery Appreciative inquiry Mindfulness Food choices/nutrition Environment and health Nutritional self-care planning

(*continues on next page*)

Table 19-5 (*Continued*).

	Coaching sessions Putting it all together	Coaching sessions Putting it all together

Activities/Course Requirements	Client coaching log (10 sessions)
	Peer coaching log (10 sessions)
	Food journal with insights
	  (personal and with one client)
	IHWA with insights (personal)
	Midterm exam
	Final exam
	Reflective paper
		Client coaching log (10 sessions)
		Peer coaching log (10 sessions)
		Food journal with insights
		  (personal)
		IHWA with insights (personal)
		Midterm
		Final exam
		Integrate nurse coaching into a
		  nursing care plan/care map

Source: Copyright © 2014 by the International Nurse Coach Association. www.inursecoach.com.
Copyright © 2014 by Lisa A. Davis.

Table 19-6 Nurse Coach Undergraduate Course (1 SCH) Outline.

Course Title	Introduction to Integrative Nurse Coaching
Course Description	Exploration of the role of the Nurse Coach in healthcare and nursing practice, and the importance of self-care as part of professional development. Focus is on the impact of lifestyle choices and behaviors that impact health and wellbeing. Includes nurse coaching skills of awareness practices and motivational interviewing, as well as how to implement these skills into patient care.
Required/Recommended Texts	*Required text*: Dossey, B. M., Luck, S., & Shaub, B. G. (2014). *Nurse coaching: Integrative approaches for health and wellbeing*. North Miami, FL: International Nurse Coach Association. *Recommended books*: Kabat-Zinn, J. (2103*). Full catastrophe living: Using the wisdom of your body and mind to face stress, pain, and illness* (revised ed.). New York, NY: Bantam. Brown, R. P., & Gerbarg, P. L. (2012). *The healing power of the breath: Simple techniques to reduce stress and anxiety, enhance concentration, and balance your emotions*. Boston, MA: Shambhala. *Other required materials (software, other readings, etc.)*: Integrative Health and Wellness Assessment (IHWA) short form. Downloading apps to mobile device for: awareness practices; wellness reminders; and health behavior tracking (e.g., nutrition, physical activity) for accountability with SMART goals.
Course Objectives	• Explore the Nurse Coach role in promoting healthier communities. • Analyze impact of lifestyle behaviors related to chronic diseases. • Explore coaching skills that nurses can bring to clinical settings. • Explore Nurse Coach self-development (self-reflection, self-assessments, self-evaluation, self-care). • Complete two assessments using the Integrative Health and Wellness Assessment (IHWA). • Experience conducting/receiving a coaching session with/from a nursing student peer.

(continues on next page)

Table 19-6 (*Continued*).

Course Topics	Nurse Coach competencies Nurse Coach process • Establishing a relationship • Identifying what stage of change client is in within the Transtheoretical Model • Identifying opportunities, issues, and concerns from IHWA • Establishing client-centered SMART goals • Empowering and motivating clients, focusing on strengths • Motivational interviewing Self-reflection Self-assessment Self-care
Activities/Course Requirements	Self-care activities Working with a student peer in dyads Experiencing various awareness practices (breath-work, imagery) Using IHWA tool

Source: Copyright © 2014 by the International Nurse Coach Association. www.inursecoach.com.
Copyright © 2014 by Christine Gilchrist.

Table 19-7 Introduction to the Art and Science of Nurse Coaching (6.5 Contact Hours).

Course Title	Introduction to the Art and Science of Nurse Coaching
Course Description	Integrative Nurse Coaching is a natural extension of nursing practice to address the healthcare needs of our nation and world. To model health and wellness, the Nurse Coach engages in four areas of self-development (self-reflection, self-assessments, self-evaluation, self-care) to enhance growth, overall health, and wellbeing.
Recommended Texts	Handouts provided in workshop Dossey, B. M., Luck, S., & Shaub, B. G. (2015). *Nurse coaching: Integrative approaches for health and wellbeing.* North Miami, FL: International Nurse Coach Association.
Course Objectives	• Define integrative nurse coaching. • Identify the difference in the nursing process and the Nurse Coach process. • Explore Nurse Coach self-development (self-reflection, self-assessments, self-evaluation, self-care). • Explore the Integrative Health and Wellness Assessment (IHWA). • Experience using the IHWA in a coaching session with a peer.
Course Topics	Define nurse coaching Nurse Coach practice areas Nurse Coach competencies Nurse Coach process • Establishing a relationship and identifying readiness for change • Identifying opportunities, issues, concerns • Establishing client-centered goals • Creating structure for interaction • Empowering and motivating clients to reach goals • Assisting client in evaluating goal achievement

(*continues on next page*)

Table 19-7 (*Continued*).

	Self-reflection Self-assessment Self-evaluation Self-care Use the Integrative Health and Wellness Assessment (IHWA)
Activities/Course Requirements	Self-care activities Using IHWA tool

Source: Copyright © 2014 by the International Nurse Coach Association. www.inursecoach.com

Table 19-8 Self-Care 1-Day Workshop (7.5 Contact Hours).

Course Title	Integrating Self-Care
Course Description	This course explores self-care activities to be used personally, but also taught to clients. Included are stress management pathophysiology, motivational theory and empowerment, and health and wellness theoretical frameworks.
Required/Recommended Texts	Personal journal
Course Objectives	• Explore motivational theory in relation to self-care activities. • Review stress response and introduce relaxation response. • Demonstrate self-care activities. • Reflect on incorporating self-care activities. • Evaluate effectiveness of self-care activities.
Course Topics	Stress Stress response Relaxation response Motivational theory Self-care activities • Deep breathing • Guided imagery activity • Journal writing
Activities/Course Requirements	Journal writing Participation in entire workshop for CE

Source: Copyright © 2014 by Lisa A. Davis.

SUMMARY

• Discovery learning is an appropriate framework for developing coursework related to nurse coaching.
• Part of providing a positive learning environment is providing trust and a safe environment. Establishing an environment in which the students and teacher(s) are present to each other. The teacher becomes the facilitator of holding the space.
• Rituals are important and can serve to set the tone for honoring and respecting both the space between, and the space within classroom or workshop participants.

- Teaching nurse coaching is accomplished much as coaching itself—by invitation. Participants are not forced to respond nor judged if they do not respond. Silence is honored.
- Too much cognitive load compromises learning. Allowing for pauses gives participants the opportunity to dwell with and reflect on concepts and ideas. It is in that time that deep learning takes place.
- Nurse educators are not just preparing future nurses with nursing knowledge and skills, but also teaching life skills for students to be productive men and women.
- Bloom's Revised Taxonomy provides a framework for developing course or unit objectives that give students information about what they are to learn as a result of instruction. They also provide the teacher with information about how to teach.
- Learning activities should be designed to not only build on what is known, but also to foster confidence. Learning activities foster active learning which is optimal for deep learning.
- Sample coursework to include course descriptions, objectives, topics, and activities/assignments are provided.

NURSE COACH REFLECTIONS

After reading this chapter, the Nurse Coach will be able to bring awareness and personal insight to the following questions:

- How are teaching about nurse coaching and providing nurse coaching similar and/or different?
- What do I value most about nurse coaching, and how can I convey that to others?
- How can I reconcile the need for concrete objectives required by accrediting bodies/continuing education to the more subjective experience of allowing the learner to derive what she or he needs from the course/workshop?

REFERENCES

Achterberg, J., Dossey, B., & Kolkmeier, L. (1994). *Rituals of healing: Using imagery for health and wellness.* New York, NY: Bantam Books.

American Holistic Nursing Credentialing Corporation (AHNCC) (2012). *AHNCC nurse coach certification program.* Retrieved from http://ahncc.org/images/AHNCC_WEBSITE_RELEASE_STATEMENT,_MAY_21,_2012-1.pdf

American Holistic Nursing Credentialing Corporation (AHNCC) (n.d.). *Certification in nurse coaching, NC-BC and HWNC-BC.* Retrieved from http://ahncc.org/certification/nursecoachnchwnc.html

Anderson, L., & Krathwohl, D. (2001). *A taxonomy for learning, teaching and assessing* (abridged ed.). Boston, MA: Allyn and Bacon.

Ayres, P., & Paas, F. (2012). Cognitive load theory: New directions and challenges. *Applied Cognitive Psychology, 26,* 827–832.

Commission on Collegegiate of Nursing Education (CCNE) (2013). *Standards for accreditation of baccalaureate and graduate nursing programs.* Retrieved from http://www.aacn.nche.edu/ccne-accreditation/Standards-Amended-2013.pdf

Cronenwett, L., Sherwood, G., Barnsteiner J., Disch, J., Johnson, J., Mitchell, P., Sullivan, D., & Warren, J. (2007). Quality and safety education for nurses. *Nursing Outlook*, *55*(3), 122–131.

Dossey, B. M., & Keegan, L. (2013). *Holistic nursing: A handbook for practice.* Burlington, MA: Jones & Bartlett Learning.

International Nurse Coach Association (INCA) (n.d.). Retrieved from http://inursecoach .com/

International Nurse Coach Certificate Program (INCCP) (n.d.). Retrieved from http://inursecoach.com/programs

Krathwohl, D. (2002). A revision of Bloom's taxonomy: An overview. *Theory into Practice*, *41*(4), 212–218.

Loftin, C., Davis, L., & Hartin, V. (2010). Classroom participation: A student perspective. *Teaching and Learning in Nursing*, 5, 119–124.

Lombardi, M. (2007). Approaches that work: How authentic learning is transforming higher education. *Educause Learning Initiative*, 1–16.

Nightingale, F. (n.d.). In Cook, E. (1913). *The life of Florence Nightingale* (Vol. II, p. 406). London, UK: Macmillan.

Palmer, P. (2004). *A hidden wholeness: The journey toward an undivided life.* San Francisco, CA: Jossey Bass.

Palmer, P. (2007). *The courage to teach: Exploring the inner landscape of a teacher's life.* San Francisco, CA: Jossey Bass.

QSEN (2014). Quality and safety education for nurses. Pre-licensure KSAs. Retrieved from http://qsen.org/competencies/pre-licensure-ksas/

Southern Association of Colleges and Schools (SACS) Commission on Colleges (2012). *The principles of accreditation: Foundations for quality enhancement.* Retrieved from http://www.sacscoc.org/pdf/2012PrinciplesOfAcreditation.pdf

Zorn, C. (2010). *Becoming a nurse educator: Dialogue for an engaging career.* Sudbury, MA: Jones & Bartlett Learning.

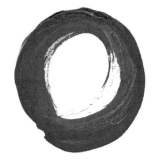

CHAPTER 20

Nurse Coaching and Research

Heidi Taylor and Deborah McElligott

In dwelling upon the vital importance of sound observation, it must never be lost sight of what observation is for. It is not for the sake of piling up miscellaneous information or curious facts, but for the sake of saving life and increasing health and comfort.

Florence Nightingale, 1860

LOOKING AHEAD...

After reading this chapter, you will be able to:

- Understand and apply research findings as part of an evidence-based nurse coaching practice.
- Participate with others in identifying research questions and activities.
- Use the Integrative Health and Wellness Assessment (IHWA) as a research tool.
- Identify future research opportunities in nurse coaching.

DEFINITIONS

Note: The terms "research report" and "research article" are used interchangeably in this chapter.

Aggregate: Gathering information from different sources together into one collective group.
Data: Information that is collected and analyzed. Plural form of the word datum.
Database: A collection of related information.
Decision tree: A diagram with logical steps that assists in decision-making.
Evidence-based practice: Integrating clinical knowledge, expertise, research findings, and other evidence, including patient perspectives for care decisions.
Generalizability: To infer what is learned from a small group of people to the larger population they represent.
Institutional review board (IRB): Group of people who represent various disciplines and interests and who review research projects before the study commences to ensure that the human subjects' rights will be protected.
Narrative data: Information in the form of words and stories; spoken or in text form.
Numeric data: Information in the form of numbers.
Phenomenon: A fact, occurrence, or circumstance that is observable or experienced.
Praxis: Practice informed by theory and research.
Primary source: The author as the person who generated the ideas that are published.

Qualitative research: Studies that involve collecting nonnumeric, often narrative, data to deeply understand phenomena.

Quantitative research: Studies that involve collecting numeric data and analyzing the data statistically.

Reliability: Of an instrument; the consistency with which an instrument measures what it is intended to measure.

Secondary source: The author as summarized or quoted from primary sources.

Statistical significance: The extent to which statistically analyzed findings were due to chance relative to a pre-determined level of probability.

Validity: Of a measurement instrument; the extent to which the instrument measures what it purports to measure.

THE SPIRIT OF INQUIRY

Nurse coaching is, among other things, a process of asking questions. Clients seek answers to important health and wellness questions when they receive services from a Nurse Coach. Likewise, Nurse Coaches engage in self-inquiry and self-care to ensure an authentic presence in coaching relationships. The ability to question one's self is necessary to the cultivation of a "spirit of inquiry where all health professionals are encouraged to question their current practices" (Melnyk & Fineout-Overholt, 2011, p. 11). This spirit of inquiry is considered foundational to evidence-based practice. Without such a culture, healing interventions might never be developed or improved through the collection and analysis of evidence that support their use.

Among the competencies identified for Nurse Coaches is the ability to use the "best available evidence, including theories and research findings, to guide and enhance professional Nurse Coaching practice" (Hess et al., 2013, p. 40). Consistent with all professional nurses, Nurse Coaches are compelled to utilize research findings in their coaching practices. This chapter provides a basic overview of research utilization for Nurse Coaches who are novices in reading and utilizing research reports. For more experienced research consumers and researchers, this chapter provides examples for using existing tools for collection of data in a nurse coaching practice for the purposes of research as well as suggestions for future research initiatives.

THE ROLE OF RESEARCH IN EVIDENCE-BASED NURSE COACHING PRACTICE

As nursing theory provides a strong base for patient-centered care, research is a vehicle to evaluate the way we translate that theory into an evidence-based practice, thus forming nursing praxis. The evidence-based practice process identified for nursing practice is applicable to nurse coaching (Melnyk & Fineout-Overholt, 2011). "Evidence-based practice" and "research utilization" are terms that are often used interchangeably. In this chapter, evidence-based practice is understood as being built upon and constantly informed by a broad body of informational resources, not just published reports of research studies. However, utilizing research findings effectively is a cornerstone of evidence-based practice and can contribute to a more meaningful experience for clients and Nurse Coaches. Furthermore, using basic research strategies in a private practice or collaborating with others in research studies can provide important insights into best practices and further develop the evidence in support of nurse coaching as an effective approach to improving health and wellness outcomes.

For Nurse Coaches practicing within a holistic framework, many of the phenomena expressed through interventions and holistic nursing practice cannot be easily observed or measured (Zahourek, 2013). However, nurses often practice in cultures where the scientific method of recording observable phenomena and analyzing for statistical objectivity or significance is considered the gold standard in research. In the scientific community, there is a growing understanding of the complex nature of human health and healing. As a result, broadened views about diverse research approaches are emerging as valid pathways to new knowledge. Nurse Coaches have a responsibility to understand the nature of the unseen and immeasurable phenomena and to ensure that interventions are safe and efficacious (Zahourek, 2013). Though the scientific method may seem limited in its ability to reveal the whole of human experience, Nurse Coaches working from a position of holism recognize the value of all sources of knowledge.

For these reasons, developing the necessary skills for reading, understanding, and utilizing research findings in the nurse coaching practice is essential for responsible partnerships with clients. Additionally, it is important for Nurse Coaches to recognize researchable questions and to participate in research activities that extend the knowledge base for nurse coaching.

RESEARCH STARTS WITH PROBLEMS AND QUESTIONS

All research begins with problems to be solved and questions to be answered. When a Nurse Coach has a question about how to best care for a client, many kinds of resources may be consulted such as textbooks, protocols, guidelines, and research reports. In this context, the Nurse Coach is a consumer of research and other available knowledge. Sometimes the answer cannot be found in the existing sources. In other words, there is a gap in our knowledge about how to solve the problem. In this case, the Nurse Coach may decide that a research study to answer a specific question about a problem needs to be conducted. The Nurse Coach may then move into the role of researcher or becomes part of a research team to design and conduct a research study that may help answer the question (**Figure 20-1**). When acting as either the consumer of research, a member of a research team, or the primary researcher, skill in navigating the broad range of resources is essential. Knowing how to find relevant research reports and make sense of them is fundamental to evidence-based practice.

FINDING THE RELEVANT RESEARCH

The information landscape is constantly changing, and it is not possible to provide a complete description of the many ways in which a Nurse Coach can locate relevant research reports and articles. For Nurse Coaches in private practice who are not affiliated with a healthcare or academic setting, the retrieval of high-quality research materials may be challenging. In such cases, developing collaborations with colleagues who work in academic and healthcare institutions can be very helpful. Many Nurse Coaches, regardless of their practice arrangements, have access to many information resources (**Table 20-1**).

The Internet has made accessing information easy for everyone, but it has also added a level of complexity to filtering out irrelevant or poor-quality information. This can add to frustration and ineffective use of time. Surfing the web is not the same as searching databases, and Nurse Coaches are advised to develop information literacy skills.

The idea of using a library at a time when information is so easy to access from a home or mobile computer seems outdated. However, it is important to remember that librarians are experts at information retrieval. Many libraries participate in consortia with a network of other libraries of varying types and offer interlibrary loan arrangements or can facilitate retrieval of hard-to-locate information.

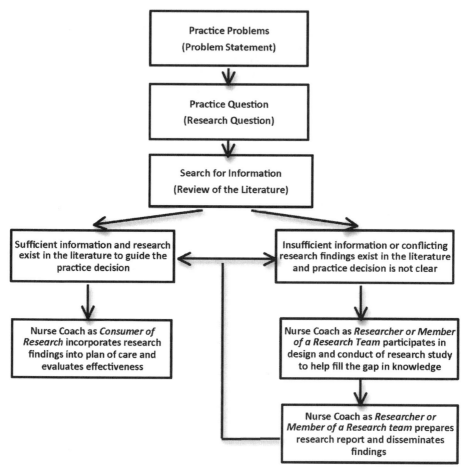

Figure 20-1 Nurse Coach as Consumer of Research and Nurse Coach as Research.
Source: Copyright © 2014 by Heidi Taylor.

READING AND UNDERSTANDING THE RESEARCH REPORT

A research report is a detailed description of a research study. When it is written by the researcher who conducted the study, it is known as a primary source. When it is summarized by someone other than the researcher who conducted the study, it is known as a secondary source. It is usually best to use the primary source whenever possible in making a decision about best practice.

It is helpful to think about the research article as the primary way in which scholars and practitioners in the field communicate with one another about the problems that need to be solved and the research activities designed to solve the problem. By necessity, research articles are rich with technical detail, highly ordered in their presentation, and, depending on the nature of the research that was conducted, potentially complex and difficult to understand if the reader is unfamiliar with terms and research processes.

The researcher's intention in writing the article is to anticipate the questions other professionals in the field might have about the research and to follow generally accepted writing styles in presenting the work. For these reasons, the research article can be intimidating. A basic understanding of the structure of a research report and research processes is necessary when utilizing research for an evidence-based Nurse Coaching practice. A good dose of patience may also be necessary; reading research reports can be like learning a new language.

Research articles follow a fairly consistent structure with minor modifications depending on the nature of the study and editorial standards of the publication. This is very helpful when comparing one study to another. **Table 20-2** illustrates and describes the key sections of a research article.

Table 20-1 Finding Relevant Research.

Web sites	• Many professional organizations and other groups maintain highly reliable information and research reports that are free to access using the Internet. • Scrutinize the quality and source of the information and look for possibility of bias in the report of findings. • Noteworthy resources for EBP include: the Cochrane Collaboration; the Agency for Healthcare Research and Quality (AHRQ); the Joanna Briggs Institute (JBI).
Online databases	• Useful in locating research articles and reports. • Provide information about published research. • Full-text versions of the articles may be available. • Examples: Cumulative Index of Nursing and Allied Health Literature (CINAHL®), MEDLINE®, and OVID® • Subscriptions are often expensive; best to obtain through an academic or health system library.
Online journals	• Journals are often available online as well as in print. • Some are available exclusively online. • Most require subscriptions, some are free.

Source: Copyright © 2014 by Heidi Taylor.

Table 20-2 Key Sections of a Research Article.

Abstract	• Often limited to a specific word count, the abstract • Concise summary of the way research was conducted and the findings • First element of the article that should be read • One way to determine if the research is relevant or valuable
Introduction/ background	• States the problem and the questions • Should convince the reader that the problem is worth studying • Should clarify understanding of the nature and scope of the problem
Review of the literature	• Purpose is to highlight existing evidence • Provides the state of the most current knowledge on the subject • Usually includes classic pieces and publications from the last 5–10 years
Sample	• Participants (sometimes referred to as subjects) • Represents a population that is the focus of the research

(*continues on next page*)

Table 20-2 (*Continued*).

	• Quantitative research designs 　○ Designed to include participants who accurately reflect the characteristics of the population of interest 　○ Facilitates the ability to make generalizations to the broader population based upon what was learned from the participants 　○ Random selection of participants (all members of a population have an equal chance of selection—considered the gold standard for sampling) 　○ Random sampling may not be possible; other options acceptable • Qualitative research designs 　○ The participants are specifically recruited because they have particular knowledge, experiences, or views related to the study. 　○ There is no random selection of participants. 　○ Sample sizes are usually smaller than in quantitative studies. 　○ Small sample size does not limit the usefulness of the information.
Methods	• Includes information about the research design, variables, data collection instruments and procedures, population and sample, intervention (if applicable), and the plan for analysis of the data
Variables	• Qualities, properties, or characteristics of persons, things, or situations that can change or vary 　○ *Dependent variables*: outcome or response to be explained or predicted 　○ *Independent variables*: stimulus or activity manipulated or applied to create an effect on the dependent variable 　○ *Extraneous variables*: interfere with the variables being studied 　○ *Demographic variables*: characteristics of participants that cannot be changed (e.g., as age, gender)
Data collection	• Quantitative studies 　○ Using any of many different measurement instruments to quantify variables and collect information 　　▪ Physiologic measures 　　▪ Observational measures 　　▪ Structured interviews following questionnaires 　　▪ Questionnaires 　　▪ Scales 　　　• Rating 　　　• Likert 　　　• Visual analog 　○ All data is collected before analysis begins • Qualitative studies 　○ Using spoken words, observations, and texts to collect information 　　▪ Interviews 　　　• Semi-structured interviews 　　　• Probes 　　　• Open-ended interviews 　　▪ Focus groups 　　▪ Observation 　　▪ Collecting stories 　○ Data is analyzed during and after data collection

(*continues on next page*)

Table 20-2 (*Continued*).

Results	A report of the key findings with respect to the research questions
Discussion	Discusses study findings in relation to other studies, implications for practice, and strengths and limitations of the study
Conclusion	A brief summarization with suggestions for future research
References	A list of resources that were cited in writing the article

Source: Copyright © 2014 by Heidi Taylor. Adapted from Burns, N., & Grove, S. (2011). *Understanding nursing research building an evidence-based practice* (5th ed.). Maryland Heights, MO: Elsevier Saunders.

RESEARCH METHODS

There are many ways to conduct research. However, most research methods can be categorized in one of the two major classifications of research methodology, quantitative or qualitative. Each of these methodological approaches has its own set of rules, procedures, and research designs (**Tables 20-3** and **20-4**).

Distinguishing between articles describing quantitative and qualitative methodologies is really quite simple on the surface. Quantitative research methods lead to the collection of numeric data that are analyzed using some form of statistics to answer the research question(s). Qualitative research methods lead to the collection of stories and narratives, and the words are analyzed to answer the research question(s). Both of these research approaches are based in quite different philosophical positions, and as a result, are often debated for their credibility among different camps.

The decision to collect numeric data or narrative data is directed by the research question. For example, the research question "Do clients with Type 1 diabetes who receive motivational therapy by a Nurse Coach in addition to the standard medical treatment have better regulation of Hemoglobin A1c (Hgb A1c) levels than clients who do not receive motivational interviewing from a Nurse Coach?" will require the collection of numeric data (Hgb A1c levels) to answer the question. This question will drive the researcher to quantitative research designs and statistical analysis.

The research question, "What is it like to experience guided imagery from a Nurse Coach as an intervention for chronic back pain?" will require the collection of richly descriptive narratives (that are not bounded by a questionnaire or survey) to answer the question. This question will drive the researcher to qualitative research designs and some appropriate form of narrative analysis.

One source of confusion for some people is the way in which the term "qualitative" is used when describing a research methodology. As previously mentioned, Nurse Coaches often work with qualitative phenomena (e.g., pain, suffering, compassion, anxiety, sadness, etc.). These are phenomena that are subjectively experienced in highly individualized ways. But if the researcher applies a numeric score to the qualitative phenomenon and analyzes the numbers, the method becomes quantitative (e.g., pain scales).

It is important to remember that the research question drives the design; the design should not drive the research question. In cultures where the scientific method is valued above all other ways of knowing, it may be argued that quantitative research is more credible than qualitative research. But neither research methodology is inherently "better than" the other. The most credible research method is the one that best answers the research question.

Table 20-3 Quantitative Research Methodologies and Selected Designs.

Research Designs	Purpose and Characteristics
Descriptive	• Acquire information about a variable in its natural state. • No intent to change or modify the situation or to determine cause-and-effect
Correlational • Descriptive correlational • Predictive correlational	• Describes variables and examines the relationships among the variables • Predicts the value of one variable based upon the value of another variable • No intent to determine cause-and-effect

Experimental
• Pretest-posttest
• Randomized clinical trial
	• Used to identify cause-and-effect
	• Offers the greatest amount of control possible to exclude influencing factors other than cause that is being studied
	• *Must* have three characteristics to be an experiment:
	  ○ Randomization
	  ○ Control
	  ○ Manipulation of the independent variable

Quasi-experimental	• Searches for cause-and-effect in situations where complete control is not possible or when randomization is not possible. • Manipulation of the independent variable must be present.

Source: Copyright © 2014 by Heidi Taylor. Adapted from Burns, N., & Grove, S. (2011). *Understanding nursing research building an evidence-based practice* (5th ed.). Maryland Heights, MO: Elsevier Saunders.

Table 20-4 Qualitative Research Methodologies and Selected Research Designs.

Research Designs	Purpose and Characteristics
Phenomenology	• Explores the person's experiences as uniquely lived by the person • Describes and interprets the meaning of the experience
Grounded theory	• Emerged from discipline of sociology • Based on symbolic interaction theory with the view that reality is created by attaching meaning to situations • Results in a theoretical framework grounded in the real experiences of the participants • Often accompanied by a diagram displaying the interactions of the social processes identified
Ethnography	• Developed by anthropologists to study cultures • Studies the behaviors from within the culture (emic) or outside the culture (etic)
Historical	• Examines the events of the past • Explores, describes, and analyzes a process or event during a specific period of time

Source: Copyright © 2014 by Heidi Taylor. Adapted from Burns, N., & Grove, S. (2011). *Understanding nursing research building an evidence-based practice* (5th ed.). Maryland Heights, MO: Elsevier Saunders.

More recently, researchers are valuing multidimensional approaches to research design known as triangulation and mixed methods (Zahourek, 2013). These designs combine the use of qualitative and quantitative approaches and may use two or more different sampling strategies, data collection procedures, and other research process elements (Nieswiadomy, 2010; Zahourek, 2013). Additional methods include synthesis, systematic (or integrative) reviews and meta-analysis. Synthesis of sources is a process used in the systematic or integrative review and involves compiling, analyzing, and interpreting findings from a selected group of studies (Burns & Grove, 2011). Meta-analysis focuses on the statistical findings in multiple studies, large and small, with the intent of finding meaningful estimates of measures on a larger scale (Burns & Grove, 2011).

MEASUREMENT AND DATA COLLECTION

In quantitative studies, the way in which data are collected and variables are measured is an important consideration for the research. When numbers are assigned to a variable, it is being measured and implies a quantification of the variable (Nieswiadomy, 2012). But not all numbers mean the same thing when they are applied to a variable.

In the research context, the numbers that are used to measure a variable can be categorized by their level of measurement, also referred to as a measurement scale. There are four levels of measurement: *nominal, ordinal, interval,* and *ratio.* These are described in **Tables 20-5** and **20-6**. The level of measurement necessary to adequately answer the research question is an important consideration when deciding on a data collection instrument and analysis procedures. Measurement error exists in all types of measures and must be considered in any research process. Data collection in qualitative research is not intended to lead to quantification of the variables (with the exception of demographic data that may be used to describe the sample characteristics). In qualitative studies, information is collected through the use of interviews with participants, focus groups, observation of participants, examining written texts, collecting stories, and other creative methods (Burns & Grove, 2011). Unlike quantitative studies in which the data are first collected and then analyzed after data collection is completed, qualitative data are analyzed during data collection and beyond. Often, what the researcher hears, sees, or reads while collecting the data determines who will be sampled next and what new questions, observations, or texts are needed to answer the research question. It is a very fluid and nonlinear process intended to elicit rich, true, and deep meaning.

Table 20-5 Levels of Measurement Described.

Level of Measurement	Description
Nominal	• Used when a number is assigned to name a category of the variable for labeling and categorizing only • No meaning to the number in terms of value of the variable • Gender, ethnicity, marital status, political affiliation, and religious preference are examples of variables assigned nominal level data • No mathematical meaning to this level of measurement • Cannot make meaningful comparisons between the categories based upon the number alone • This level of measurement is considered the lowest, or least meaningful.

(continues on next page)

Table 20-5 (*Continued*).

Level of Measurement	Description

Ordinal	• Illustration: Gender
	  ○ Would not be able to say that males (named with the number 2) have two times as much gender as females (named with the number 1).
	• Adds the dimension of rank ordering
	• Helps to determine who has more or less of the of property being measured
	• Can make comparisons between members of the sample
	• Limited in the mathematical operations that are meaningful
	• Illustration: Sadness
	  ○ Measured by a scale (e.g., 0 = none, 1 = mild, 2 = moderate, 3 = severe, 4 = disabling)
	  ○ Could conclude that the people with disabling sadness had more sadness than those with moderate sadness, but it would not be possible to determine individual differences in sadness among the participants

Interval	• Adds the dimension of an equal distance between the numbers
	• Can make more meaningful mathematical computations, such as a mean
	• Can make more precise comparisons between members of the sample
	• Illustration: Temperature
	  ○ Distance between each degree on the thermometer is numerically the same.
	  ○ Temperature reading of 97.7° is the same distance away from 98.7° as 99.0° is from 100°.
	  ○ 0° does not mean an absence of the property of temperature

Ratio	• Considered the highest level of measurement
	• Adds the attribute of having an absolute zero point, meaning an absence of the property being measured
	• Illustrations: weight, length, and volume
	  ○ Value of zero means there is an absence of the property.
	  ○ Statistically, interval and ratio level data can be used the same way.

Source: Copyright © 2014 by Heidi Taylor.

Table 20-6 Levels of Measurement Basic Characteristics.

Level of Measurement	Names	Rank Orders	Equal Interval	Absolute Zero
Nominal	✓			
Ordinal	✓	✓		
Interval	✓	✓	✓	
Ratio	✓	✓	✓	✓

Source: Copyright © 2014 by Heidi Taylor.

RESULTS IN A QUANTITATIVE STUDY

Understanding and interpreting the statistical results in quantitative studies can be a barrier to reading and using research articles for many nurses. Even if nurses have taken a course in statistics, the skills may be infrequently used and statistical terms and symbols long forgotten. Although a deep knowledge and skill level in statistics is not needed to make sense of the statistical information in most research articles, it can be helpful to understand why there are so many, sometimes exotic-sounding, statistical tests identified by the researchers. Simply stated, the type of statistical test used is determined by several factors including the level of measurement at which the variable is measured and the number of variables involved. Each statistical test was developed to manage certain conditions of the data. There are many decision trees available to help determine which statistical test is appropriate to use under certain circumstances.

Statistics are used to essentially answer three broad questions in quantitative research: how the variable can be described, how variables are related, and how groups are different from each other on a variable. In a nutshell, statistics help us describe things, see relationships, and compare differences. This is all done using mathematical formulae that can be simple or quite complex. Thankfully, mathematicians and statisticians have perfected these strategies, and for the Nurse Coach who desires a deeper understanding of statistics, a plethora of resources are available. A brief description of these three statistical approaches is useful (**Table 20-7**).

Table 20-7 Basic Statistical Approaches of Quantitative Research with Exemplar Tests.

Type	Purpose	Statistical Test	Minimum Level of Measurement
Descriptive	Examine characteristics, behaviors, and experiences	**Measures of central tendency** Mean • the arithmetic average of a set of data	Ordinal (with caution)
		Median • the middle-most score in the exact center of a set of data	Ordinal
		Mode • the numerical value that occurs most frequently in a set of data	Nominal
		Measures of dispersion Range • the difference between the highest and the lowest scores in a set of data	Ordinal
		Variance • indicates the spread or dispersion of the scores	Interval
		Standard deviation • on average, how the set of scores deviate from the mean	Interval
Relationships	Examines the extent to which values of one variable are related to, or associated with, the values of another variable	**Correlation coefficients** Pearson product-moment correlation (Pearson r)	Interval
		Spearman Rho	Ordinal

(*continues on next page*)

Table 20-7 (*Continued*).

Type	Purpose	Statistical Test	Minimum Level of Measurement

Differences	Comparing groups on a variable to determine if the difference between the means of the group is likely to have occurred by chance	• *t* Test
		  ○ comparing two groups
		• Analysis of variance (ANOVA)
		  ○ Comparing more than two groups
		• Chi-square
		  ○ Comparing sets of frequencies
			Interval
			
			Interval
			
			Nominal

Source: Copyright © 2014 by Heidi Taylor. Adapted from Nieswiadomy, R. (2012). *Foundations of nursing research* (6th ed). Upper Saddle River, NJ: Pearson.

Descriptive statistics are mathematical operations that describe and summarize data. They are categorized as measures of central tendency and measures of dispersion. Nurse Coaches and researchers are often interested in the relationships between and among variables. For example, the Nurse Coach may want to know if the client's anxiety score on a measure of anxiety decreases as the amount of time spent in meditation increases. Correlational statistical tests are a special case of descriptive statistics used to determine the nature of relationships, but because they go beyond pure description, are sometimes presented as a separate type of statistics.

A common correlational test is the Pearson *r*. This technique results in a correlation coefficient abbreviated as *r* (think "relationship"). The *r* value will be a number between –1.0 and +1.0. The closer the *r* value is to 1.0, either positive or negative, the stronger the relationship. The closer the *r* value is to 0, the weaker the relationship. If the value has a negative number, it means the relationship is negative; a higher score on one variable is associated with or related to a lower score on the other variable. As one score goes up, the other goes down. A positive number means the relationship is positive; whatever one score does, the other does the same thing. As one score goes up, the other score goes up. As one score goes down, the other score goes down. In both cases, these are positive correlations because the variable scores are moving in the same direction, not opposite one another.

So what constitutes a strong or weak relationship? An *r* value of less than +0.3 or –0.3 is considered a weak correlation; a value between +0.3 to + 0.5 or –0.3 and –0.5 is considered a moderate correlation; and an *r* value above +0.5 or –0.5 can be considered a strong correlation. Burns and Grove (2011) appropriately caution that weak relationships can sometimes be disregarded when they may, in fact, have meaning when considered in the context of other variables. For Nurse Coaches and researchers, a holistic view of this quantitative measure is necessary.

It might be tempting to infer that the correlation that was found in the sample that was studied can be generalized to the population it represents, but that would be incorrect. Before one can make that inference, another statistical test (discussed in the next section) must be conducted to determine whether or not the correlation coefficient is significantly different from zero (Burns & Grove, 2011). It may also be tempting to argue that a strong correlation coefficient indicates that one variable "causes another variable." Correlation does not signify cause and effect; it only signifies an association between the variables. If correlational statistics cannot help Nurse Coaches understand causality, what statistical tests can? How can a Nurse Coach determine if an intervention that was found to be effective in a research study will likely be effective in other clients? Researchers use a variety of statistical tests (again, sometimes with exotic names) that have been specifically designed to meet certain conditions of the data or design. As is true with correlational analysis, statistical tests of differences are selected based on the level of measurement used for the variable, the number of variables, the independence of one group from the other, and other factors. A commonly used analytical technique for analyzing differences between two groups, or samples, is the *t*-test. The *t*-test will be used to illustrate how to interpret findings when they are reported for differences between groups.

Let us assume that a Nurse Coach who is certified in aromatherapy is interested in determining if the use of essential oils will reduce the experiences of nausea and vomiting among cancer patients receiving chemotherapy. The research team would need to design a study in which two groups of patients are observed; one group will receive the treatments with essential oils while receiving chemotherapy, and the other group will receive chemotherapy in the standard way without essential oil treatments. Let us assume that the two groups were essentially the same for all characteristics that could affect their experience with nausea and vomiting. The only difference between the two groups was the use of the essential oils.

Let us further assume that at the end of the study, the research team noted that the mean (average) number of occurrences of nausea and vomiting in the group that received the essential oil treatments was less than the mean number of occurrences of nausea and vomiting in the group that received the standard of care. But how can the researchers know if this difference between the two groups' means happened purely by chance or because the essential oils really made a difference?

The only way to know is by subjecting the data to a statistical test of difference; in this case, the *t*-test. The *t*-test compares the mean scores on a variable (nausea and vomiting) between two groups (the group that received essential oils and the group that did not). It is not necessary to know the mathematical formula to understand the finding; one only needs to look for the *p*-value. The *p*-value indicates the probability that the difference between the two groups happened by chance and not because one group was treated differently than the other. During the planning phase of the research study, even before any data is collected, the researcher decides a decision point, or specific value of *p*, that will indicate whether the difference between the two groups is likely to be due to chance. That is known as the alpha level (α) or level of statistical significance. The alpha level can be one of three standard numbers; .05, .01, or .001. Simply interpreted, it means that the researcher is willing to accept that 5 times out of 100 (.05), or 1 time out of 100 (.01), or 1 time out of 1,000 (.001), any difference may be found between the groups on the mean occurrences of nausea and vomiting happened by chance.

The data from the study are then subjected to the mathematical and statistical tests. Let us assume that the researchers set an alpha level of 0.5 as the decision point for determining statistical significance. Let's further assume that the researchers find a *p*-value of 0.036 when they compared the actual means of occurrence of nausea and vomiting between the two groups. Since the actual *p*-value (.036) is less than the alpha level (.05), the researchers can say that there is a statistically significant difference between the two groups of patients. Because the mean number of occurrences of nausea and vomiting was lower in the group who received essential oil treatment than the number of occurrences in the group who received standard care, we can further say that the group who received essential oil therapy had a statistically significant lower incidence of nausea and vomiting. In this case, the likelihood, or probability, that the difference between the two groups happened by chance was only 3.6 times out of 100.

In all studies, it is important to consider not only the statistical significance of a finding, but also the clinical significance. Some findings may not be statistically significant, but because the intervention carries a low risk of harm and there appeared to be some benefit to some patients, the Nurse Coach may decide to incorporate the intervention in practice.

RESULTS IN A QUALITATIVE STUDY

The results of qualitative research are usually reported narratively, though in some cases diagrams may be used. Descriptive statistics may be included, but are only used to describe the characteristics of the sample. The results will be presented in the form appropriate to the specific research design. For example, in phenomenological studies, themes that emerged from the interviews will be presented. In grounded theory studies, a theory will be presented that may include a diagram of the theoretical relationships between the concepts.

USING RESEARCH TOOLS

The purpose of research may be to answer a question, support a new method of practice, or build on evidence reported in prior studies. As mentioned above, research studies may be either qualitative or quantitative. When conducting quantitative research in nurse coaching, as in other areas, we need to use valid and reliable tools.

CHOOSING A TOOL

Researchers may decide to create their own tool, or use an already published tool. It is important to note that publication of a tool does not ensure validity and reliability. To ensure that a tool is valid and reliable, it must be free from bias, able to measure what it is designed to measure, and able to produce consistent results. Reliability, the degree to which a tool produces consistent and stable results (Zahourek, 2013) may be determined by various methods including: test-retest reliability (the same test is given twice and scores are correlated or compared); parallel forms reliability (two forms of the same test are given and then results correlated); inter-rater reliability (different raters agree in the assessment); test for internal consistency (different test items probing the same area obtain the same results). This may be measured by tests such as Kuder-Richardson Formula 20 (KR20) or Cronbach's alpha. Reliability is reported in a range from 0 to 1.0 with 0 being no reliability and 1 being perfect. Usually, a report of .80 is considered good, and below .50 is considered poor (Colin & Wren, 2014; Cronbach, 1971).

Validity of a tool means the tool measures what it is supposed to measure; the data are meaningful and appropriate (Zahourek, 2013). Validity may be measured by tests such as the Kaiser-Meyer-Olkin (KMO), where the statistic predicts how well the data will factor (a score of .60 or higher is acceptable) and the Bartlett's Test of Sphericity, where the validity and suitability of the responses collected to the problem are reported (a score less than 0.05 is acceptable) (Garrett-Mayer, 2014). There are various types of validity including: face validity (the tool appears to be measuring what it is designed to measure), construct validity (ensures the tool is measuring what it is designed to measure, using a panel of experts), criterion-related validity (correlates test results with another criterion of interest), formative validity (applied to outcome assessment), and sampling validity (panel of experts ensures all areas of inquiry are included) (Garrett-Mayer, 2014).

INTEGRATIVE HEALTH AND WELLNESS ASSESSMENT (IHWA)

One example of a nursing theory with a designated tool that supports research in the field of nurse coaching is the Theory of Integrative Nurse Coaching (TINC) (Chapter 2). The designated tool is the Integrative Health and Wellness Assessment (IHWA) (Chapter 6). As described in Chapter 6, the IHWA examines eight components of health and wellness: (1) Life Balance & Satisfaction, (2) Relationships, (3) Spiritual, (4) Mental, (5) Emotional, (6) Physical (nutrition, exercise, weight), (7) Environmental, and (8) Health Responsibility. There is an IHWA short form (Appendix C-1) and an IHWA long form (Appendix C-2) described below.

The original IHWA (Appendix C-2 long form) was developed with 149 Likert scale questions to provide a formal assessment of the eight identified components. The scale had boxes to check: never, almost never, once in a while, almost always, and always. Each of the eight areas also had three questions on readiness to change, priority to change, and confidence in the ability to make the change. The rating scale had boxes to check: now, in two weeks, next month, within six months, and in one year. With those three additional questions in each of the eight categories, there were a total of 179 questions. Each of the eight components also had a space for a qualitative response for an action plan for each category, and to list three changes that could be implemented into one's current lifestyle over the next three months. With the construct validity completed, it was determined that the IHWA had some similar questions in sections and the tool was further refined to 132 Likert scale questions in the specific statements related to each category. This form requires about 15–30 minutes to carefully and reflectively complete.

The construct validity of the IHWA was first evaluated through a factor analysis in a study involving 211 participants from a community hospital in central Wyoming. The Kaiser-Meyer-Olkin (KMO) statistic score was acceptable at .772 (Nelson, 2012). The Bartlett's Test of Sphericity examined the suitability of the answers on the IHWA to health and wellness. The results of this analysis were statistically significant, indicating that the model fit was adequate. The IHWA long form included all the concepts of the Theory of Integrative Nurse Coaching that fully assess the eight components of health and wellness (Nelson, 2012).

The IHWA short form is 36 questions that were adapted from the 179 questions IHWA (long form) focusing on the same eight components of health and wellness. The IHWA short form was used in a quasi-experimental study examining the effect of an integrative wellness program on a control and study group (McElligott et al., 2014). In this study, the construct validity was determined by factor analysis. Factor analysis is one way to shorten a long questionnaire, keeping the important questions so valuable information would not be lost. The tool performed as proposed by the authors with the 36 questions loading as a single measure for integrative health; the sample size was not large enough to test each of the eight components as individual components. The KMO was .82 and Bartlett's Test of Sphericity was statistically significant. The 36 questions were examined for reliability using Cronbach's alpha for both the control and study group to ensure equal reliability. The IHWA had a good reliability using Cronbach's alpha with a score of .93 for the control group and .88 for the treatment group. (McElligott et al., 2014). Thus, the initial analysis of the IHWA short form supports the tool as valid and reliable.

USES OF THE IHWA

Further use of the IHWA with larger populations will enable factor analysis of each respective measure, as well as add to the support of the tool as a measure of integral health.

While the IHWA has been used in institutional review board (IRB)-approved research studies, it can also be used in both individual and group coaching session. The 36-question tool has been used in individual coaching sessions, when time, individual preferences, or literacy skills were issues. It provides an introduction to self-assessment and frequently generates discussion around clients' areas of concern. In addition, completion and discussion of the tool provides an indication of clients' readiness to change, the priority and the confidence level in making the desired change. The form can be comfortably read and discussed with individual clients and is not overwhelming for clients who are not familiar with self-assessment or long forms. Comments range from "I never thought of all of this before" or "How does this relate to my wellness?" or "No one ever asked me all of this before" to "I never have time to meditate" or "What does nontoxic mean?"

In addition to individual assessment, the short form is easy to distribute and complete in a group setting. It can be used as an educational tool in large groups, allowing participants to complete and then discuss themes, either as a whole or breaking up into small groups. It can also be used in a group coaching setting (usually limited to eight or fewer participants) where results are discussed and group wellness goals are set. It is important to note that in group coaching, the team, not the individual, is the client, and therefore, goals are driven by the group, not an individual or the coach (Donner & Wheeler, 2009). The tool works well with worksite groups where one goal may be peer support for wellness activities, or for disease management groups with specific goals in mind.

It is often refreshing to use this tool with cardiac or diabetes support groups when the prior focus has been based on a medical model and not a holistic approach to wellness. The shift is from education and recommendations to self-discovery and goal setting. Clients actually score their results and often marvel weeks later when they see an increase in readiness, priorities, and confidence level scores. As there are only three or four questions in each area of wellness, I have not seen a significant change in subscores of each area when working with groups, but this is a potential area for future research.

Another way to use the IHWA is to combine it with other valid and reliable tools in a research study. For example, in one study it was combined with the perceived stress scale and the mindfulness attention awareness scale with a control and study group. In that particular study, it was noted that as the IHWA scores increased, so did the mindfulness awareness and perceived stress. The discussion revolved around the group studied (during a stressful period in their lives) and that as wellness increased, they became more aware of their surroundings and identified stressors—the first step to stress management.

Finally, the IHWA may be used in qualitative research through the identification of various themes that arise after completing a holistic self-assessment. Coaching discussions, coaching dialogues, questions, or insight could all be reported, thus adding to our field of knowledge in the coaching area. Demographic tools (examining age, gender, race, culture occupation, income, etc.) can all be correlated to the IHWA to see if there is a specific response, either good or poor, to this type of assessment—further leading to our spirit of inquiry.

CONTRIBUTING TO RESEARCH ACTIVITIES

Nurse Coaches can contribute to research activities in a number of ways. Through careful observation of client experiences and outcomes in a Nurse Coaching relationship, questions about best practice will emerge. Ensuring that interactions, interventions, and client outcomes are well documented will assist in the collection of the necessary data for research. Collaborating with other Nurse Coaches and researchers to explore the nature of the Nurse Coach/client partnership can lead to improved data collection strategies and stronger evidence. Using similar or standardized data collection instruments for assessment (such as the IHWA), intervention, and outcomes across practices and settings could enhance collaborative research initiatives.

Asking relevant clinical questions that can be easily searched and researched contributes to evidence-based practice and the development of new knowledge. One strategy is to use a question template known as PICOT (Melnyk & Fineout-Overholt, 2011; Baldwin, Schultz, Melnyk, & Rycroft-Malone, 2013). PICOT stands for **P**atient population, **I**ntervention or issue of interest, **C**omparison intervention or issue of interest, **O**utcome, and **T**ime. Question templates can be used to frame questions focused on interventions, prognosis or prediction, diagnosis or diagnostic test, etiology, and meaning. The question template used for interventions is used here as an example.

In _____ (P), how does _____ (I) compared to _____ (C) affect _____ (O) within _____ (T)?

Templates assist in clarifying the purpose and variable of a research study and can assist the Nurse Coach in communicating with other colleagues about researchable problems.

FUTURE DIRECTIONS FOR NURSE COACHING RESEARCH

Research opportunities in nurse coaching are limited only by the imaginations of those in the practice. Zahourek (2013) appropriately argues that all holistic therapies are in need of investigation to ensure a comprehensive evidence base to support integrative healing practices. Additionally, Zahourek posits that many of the phenomena of interest to holistic nurses (and Nurse Coaches) are not easily measured in a reductionistic scientific study. These phenomena may not even be amenable to language that can describe them. Any work to advance our ability to communicate about intangible experiences will enhance the body of knowledge. New research methodologies are needed to support the study of these very complex phenomena.

Future research will require significant collaboration among and between all professionals interested in health and wellness outcomes. Such collaboration necessitates a culture of professional humility and openness that challenges the prevailing culture of hierarchies in knowledge, research, and professional practice. To that end, interdisciplinary teams collaborating across many settings studying aggregated data and experiences will contribute significantly to the advancement of art and science of health and wellness. Certain infrastructure developments around data collection, management, and analysis will be necessary. Regional hubs for research-related activities in which small private practices can link with large systems to aggregate findings and experiences could provide one form of such an infrastructure.

Research is needed to determine if self-care of the Nurse Coach or other providers contributes to improved outcomes in clients and patients. Some authors are beginning to note the importance of "positive side effects" (Weeks, 2014) and "unanticipated benefits" (Hsu, Bluespruce, Sherman, & Cherkin, 2010) in whole person, integrative care that are not necessarily captured when one is focused on a particular outcome. Sometimes, there may be no change in the outcome being researched, but many positive changes in other aspects of the client or patient's life that may be due to the intervention. These phenomena deserve more study, and current methodological constraints for allowing them to be revealed must be improved.

Finally, it is important to remember that skepticism about the effectiveness of coaching and other holistic approaches is a good thing. Pushing the boundaries of current methodologies and paradigms will not lead to better understanding of the mysteries of health and healing unless it is balanced by a healthy dose of skepticism.

SUMMARY

- A spirit of inquiry facilitates a culture of evidence-based practice and research.
- Research findings are one of many possible sources of information for an evidence-based nurse coaching practice, but they provide an important cornerstone to such a practice.
- Nurse Coaches are consumers of existing research and can serve as a researcher or member of a research team to develop research studies.
- Relevant research can be found in many locations, and the Nurse Coach needs information literacy skills to effectively locate and utilize high-quality resources.
- Reading and understanding research articles requires the development of some basic research and statistical knowledge and skills.
- The Integrative Health and Wellness Assessment (IHWA), long and short forms, provides a useful assessment tool as well as a valid and reliable data collection instrument for research.
- Nurse Coaches can contribute to research by asking researchable questions, partnering with other Nurse Coaches and researchers to design and implement research studies, contributing health and wellness outcomes data from practice experiences, and participating in analyzing data for future research initiatives.
- Future directions in nurse coaching research will push the boundaries of current methodologies that may be barriers to understanding complex and often immeasurable phenomena.

NURSE COACH REFLECTIONS

After reading this chapter, the Nurse Coach will be able to bring awareness and personal insight to the following questions:

- How do I know whether my nurse coaching practice is helping my clients/patients achieve their goals for health and wellness?
- How can I use the existing research findings about nurse coaching in the best way in my own practice?
- How can I contribute to the research efforts that inform an evidence-based nurse coaching practice?

REFERENCES

Baldwin, C., Schultz, A., Melnyk, B., & Rycroft-Malone, J. (2013). Evidence-based practice. In B. M. Dossey & L. Keegan (Eds.). *Holistic nursing: A handbook for practice* (6th ed., pp. 797–814). Burlington, MA: Jones & Bartlett Learning.

Burns, N., & Grove, S. (2011). *Understanding nursing research building an evidence-based practice* (5th ed.). Maryland Heights, MO: Elsevier Saunders.

Colin, C., & Wren, J. (2014). *Exploring reliability in academic assessment.* Retrieved from http://www.uni.edu/chfasoa/reliabilityandvalidity.htm

Cronbach, L. J. (1971). Test validation. In R. L. Thorndike (Ed.), *Educational measurement* (2nd ed.). Washington, DC: American Council on Education.

Donner, G., & Wheeler, M. (2009). *Coaching in nursing: An introduction*. Indianapolis, IN: International Council of Nurses and Sigma Theta Tau International. Printing Partners.

Garrett-Mayer, E. (2014). *Statistics in Psychosocial Research Lecture 8 Factor Analysis I*. John Hopkins Bloomberg School of Public Health. Retrieved from http://ocw.jhsph.edu/courses/statisticspsychosocialresearch/pdfs/lecture8.pdf

Hess, D. R., Dossey, B. M., Southard, M. E., Luck, S., Schaub, B. G., & Bark, L. (2013). *The art and science of nurse coaching: The provider's guide to coaching scope and competencies*. Silver Spring, MD: Nursesbooks.org.

Hsu, C., Bluespruce, J., Sherman, K., & Cherkin, D. (2010). Unanticipated benefits of CAM therapies for back pain: an exploration of patient experiences. *Journal of Alternative and Complementary Medicine, 16*(2), 157–163. doi: 10.1089/acm.2009.0188

McElligott, D., Mishanie, N., Okane, K., Friedman, I., & Nelson, J. (2014). The effect of an integrative wellness program. Unpublished study.

Melnyk, B., & Fineout-Overholt, E. (2011). *Evidenced-based practice in nursing and healthcare: A guide to best practice*. Philadelphia, PA: Lippincott Williams & Wilkins.

Nelson, J. (2012). Unpublished report. Healthcare Environment, St. Paul, Minnesota. 2/12/12 Schultz, Melnyk, Rycroft-Malone (p. 805).

Nieswiadomy, R. (2012). *Foundations of nursing research* (6th ed.). Upper Saddle River, NJ: Pearson.

Nightingale, F. (1860). *Notes on nursing: What it is and what it is not* (p. 70). London, UK: Harrison.

Weeks, J. (2014). Secret sauce and the positive side effects in whole person integrative medical care [online blog]. Retrieved from http://www.huffingtonpost.com/john-weeks/integrative-medicine_b_4755238.html

Zahourek, R. (2013). Holistic nursing research: Challenges and opportunities. In B. M. Dossey & L. Keegan (Eds.), *Holistic nursing: A handbook for practice* (6th ed., pp. 775–796). Burlington, MA: Jones & Bartlett Learning.

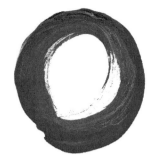

CHAPTER 21

Nurse Coaching and Leadership

Barbara Montgomery Dossey and Susan Luck

May 26, 1873. The eclipse of the sun has begun. 7.36 A.M. The eclipse of the sun is at its full. 8.28 A.M. The eclipse of the sun has ended. 9.24 A.M. After this a dearth of great eclipses of the sun visible in this country succeeds for years. On August 1, 1999, at 12 minutes 20 seconds to 10 A.M., "local time," the next total solar eclipse in England is to occur, we are told... What will the world be on August 11, 1999? What we have made it.

Florence Nightingale, 1873

LOOKING AHEAD...

After reading this chapter, you will be able to:

- Define the Integrative Nurse Coach Leadership Model© (INCLM) five components.
- Identify your leadership qualities and capacities in each INCLM component.
- Use the INCLM to guide your Integrative Nurse Coach leadership endeavors.
- Examine polarities in your personal and professional endeavors.
- Explore nursing initiatives for addressing underserved populations.

DEFINITIONS

Authenticity: Consistency in a person's beliefs, values, and actions, which demonstrate what one believes to be her/his truth.

Complexity: A phenomenon that occurs at the boundary between order and chaos, or at the edge of chaos where an individual's health is influenced by the systems in which she/he lives and works.

Embodied awareness: A state of being mindful and consciously in the present moment, as change takes place in the present, not in the past or future.

Hardiness: Attitudes of change, commitment, and control that together provide the courage and motivation needed to turn stressful circumstances from potential calamities into opportunities for personal growth; more recently, the hardiness characteristics have been described as commitment, control, and challenge.

Integrative Nurse Coach leadership: A state of mindful awareness and beingness that embodies strengths, purpose, values, ethics, and vision that holds to present and future expectations that can be shared with others in interprofessional collaboration; it includes opening to intuitive insights and inner wisdom, which allows caring, compassion, purpose empathy, authenticity, humility, and integrity to manifest.

Integrative Nurse Coach Leadership Model (INCLM): The INCLM five components are: (1) Nurse Coach Self-Development (Self-Reflection, Self-Assessment, Self-Evaluation,

Self-Care); (2) Integral Perspectives and Change; (3) Integrative Lifestyle Health and Wellbeing (ILHWB); (4) Awareness and Choice; and (5) Listening with HEART (Healing, Energy, Awareness, Resilience, Transformation).

Polarities: Interdependent pairs of different, competing, or opposite values or points of view that engage "both/and" thinking, rather than "either/or" thinking; each polarity has an identified upside (values) and downside (fears), and must be explored together to find one's life balance (personal life and work life, staff satisfaction and patient satisfaction) (Wesorick, 2014).

Situational awareness: Recognizing the many attitudes, patterns, beliefs, rules (spoken or unspoken), and processes among individuals and throughout organizations and communities. (Perlman, Horrigan, Goldblatt, & Maizes, 2014).

Skillpower: Implies integration of new information and skills that lead to changes in one's thinking and in lifestyle and work patterns.

Soul's purpose: Arises from sourcing that is a felt sense of profound meaning, intention, and focus about one's life and work.

Transdisciplinary dialogue: An approach where interprofessional colleagues come together to share knowledge and are willing to explore deep meaning that engages the human spirit and spiritual concerns, connections, ideas, and visioning and evolving possibilities rather than competition between and among.

Transparency: An intentional way to be clear, direct, and with no hidden agendas.

Wisdom: Sourcing action from the deepest place within and generating appropriate action for meeting challenges (Sharma, 2007).

Work spirit: Involves selflessness, which is being unself-consciously engrossed in the outcome of coaching clients and others, and engaging in projects, protocols, and tasks, rather than worrying about what others think.

WHAT WILL OUR WORLD BE IN 2020?

Florence Nightingale (1820–1910) often thought about the future, as seen in the chapter opening quote. Beginning in the 1870s, while frustrated with the many slow reform efforts, Nightingale engaged in a flurry of writing that centered on her belief that, although history unfolded according to certain laws, humans could make a difference in the future of humankind. She wrote that it would take 150 years to have the kind of nursing she envisioned, which is illustrated in **Figures 21-1** and **21-2**. She is a model for Nurse Coach leaders to be visionary thinkers and change agents. Inspired by the global celebrations of the bicentennial of the birth of Florence Nightingale in 2020, Nurse Coaches can ask, "What will our world be in 2020?"

Nightingale referred to her work as her "must" (Dossey, 2010). Nurse Coaches are focused on identifying their individual and collective "must," which is an intentional, mindful, focused mission for nurse coaching practice, education, research, and healthcare policy. Nurse Coach leaders understand the necessity of healing relationships with clients/patients, families, communities, and colleagues. As we increase our awareness of the deepest needs of the world, this knowledge continues to help all of us collaborate with interprofessional colleagues and concerned citizens alike—to identify our own "musts" (Beck, Dossey, & Rushton, 2014). This keeps us focused and empowered. Nightingale saw 19th-century problems and created 20th-century solutions. Nurse Coaches have seen 20th-century problems and are creating 21st-century solutions using the INCLM to guide their leadership endeavors as discussed next. See Chapter 1, Roots of Professional Nurse Coaching, Florence Nightingale's legacy, and the Nightingale Declaration, Figure 1-1.

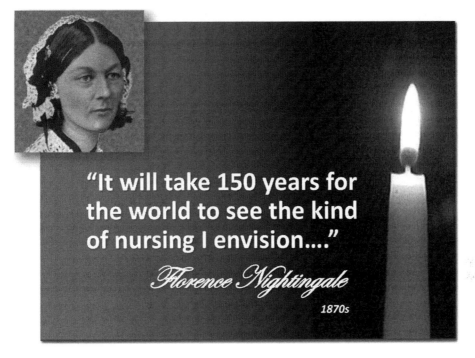

"It will take 150 years for the world to see the kind of nursing I envision...."

Florence Nightingale

1870s

Figure 21-1
Source: Copyright © NIGH World 2014. Used with permission by the Nightingale Initiative for Global Health. www.nightingaledeclaration.net

Nurse Coach leaders' mission is to cultivate and motivate others, instill confidence, and create cohesive teams and environments that lead to authentic integrative healthcare in institutions, clinics, and communities. They are masters of time management and emotional intelligence, communicating decisively, delegating effectively, and exhibiting a genuine love of others. Nurse Coach leaders are change agents and find their voice to engage in many interprofessional conversations about integrative healthcare. They thrive in environments that foster networking, change, collaboration, and an awareness of collective efforts to bring about integrative healthcare policy and healthcare transformation (Luck, 2010).

INTEGRATIVE NURSE COACH LEADERSHIP MODEL (INCLM)

Using the INCLM, this chapter explores how to be effective Nurse Coach leaders and live and work with authenticity and integrity. We are at a turning point in the history of the world where many Nurse Coaches, other interprofessional health and wellness coaches, clients/patients, and concerned citizens are ready to take the necessary steps leading to healthy people living on a healthy planet—local to global.

The INCLM expands Nurse Coaches' visibility in how to engage in the art and science of Nurse Coach leadership endeavors and create a culture of health for individuals and communities. The INCLM components shift the current focus from the medical model to a comprehensive understanding of the complexity of human nature and healing for healthcare and society (Dossey, 2013). Healing and integrative healthcare will never be

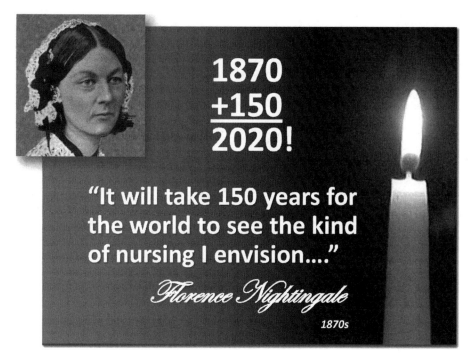

1870
+150
2020!

"It will take 150 years for
the world to see the kind
of nursing I envision...."

Florence Nightingale

1870s

Figure 21-2
Source: Copyright © NIGH World 2014. Used with permission by the Nightingale Initiative for Global Health. www.nightingaledeclaration.net

achieved with the current and outmoded management culture of "fix" and "cure" using the latest technologies at all costs while asking caregivers to work harder and not smarter.

The structure of the INCLM is seen in **Figure 21-3** and listed in **Table 21-1**. All content components are viewed as an overlay together. The Nurse Coach enters into a unique relationship with the client/patient and others of trust and mutual respect that reflects healing, the integration of the metaparadigm in a nursing theory (nurse, person, health, environment [society]), and patterns of knowing in nursing (personal, empirics, aesthetics, ethics, not knowing, sociopolitical). The INCLM five components are represented as a five-circle Venn diagram: (1) Nurse Coach Self-Development, (2) Integral Perspectives and Change, (3) Integrative Lifestyle Health and Wellbeing, (4) Awareness and Choice, and (5) Listening with HEART. The outside dotted circle denotes the constant exchanging movement of the energy field and internal and external healing environments that impact all aspects of health and wellbeing. [*Note*: The components of the Theory of Integrative Nurse Coaching (TINC) and the INCLM are the same. See Chapter 2 and the Theory of Integrative Nurse Coaching (TINC) for a description of healing, the metaparadigm in nursing, patterns of knowing in nursing, the five INCLM components, and specific book chapters for more details.] In the next section, each of the INCLM five components is discussed from a leadership perspective.

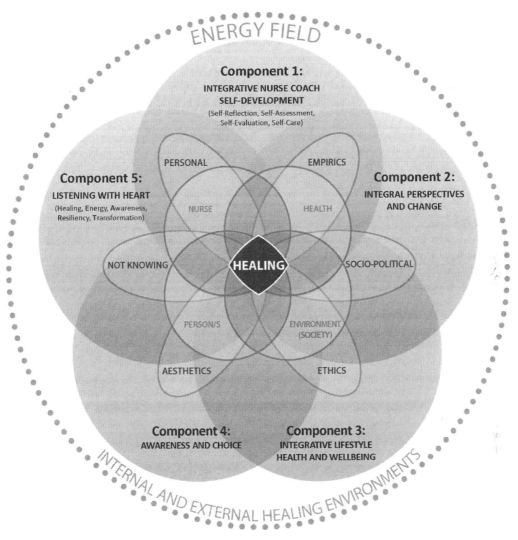

Figure 21-3 Integrative Nurse Coach Leadership Model (INCLM).
Legend: The INCLM is an overlay of Healing, Metaparadigm in a Nursing Theory, Patterns of Knowing in Nursing, TINC Five Components, and Energy Field and Internal and External Healing Environments).
Source: Copyright © 2014 by the International Nurse Coach Association. www.inursecoach.com

Table 21-1 Integrative Nurse Coach Leadership Model (INCLM) Five Components.

Component 1:	Integrative Nurse Coach Self-Development (Self-Reflection, Self-Assessment, Self-Evaluation, Self-Care)
Component 2:	Integral Perspectives and Change
Component 3:	Integrative Lifestyle Health and Wellbeing (ILHWB)
Component 4:	Awareness and Choice
Component 5:	Listening with HEART (Healing, Energy, Awareness, Resilience, Transformation)

Source: Copyright © 2014 by the International Nurse Coach Association. www.inursecoach.com

INCLM Component 1: Nurse Coach Self-Development

Integrative Nurse Coach leaders practice and embody aspects of self-development, which includes four areas: self-reflection, self-assessment, self-evaluation, and self-care. See Chapters 2 and 22 for details. These four components enhance Nurse Coaches' leadership capacities for mindfulness in the moment and their search for a deeper self-understanding and renewal of the human spirit, leading to personal and integrative leadership transformation in healthcare that can be sustained (Kreitzer, 2014; Perlman, Horrigan, Goldblatt, & Maizes, 2014). Through self-development, Nurse Coach leaders are inspired, reflective leaders who identify their strengths, purpose, values, ethics, and spiritual vision (Freshwater, Taylor, & Sherwood, 2008; Johns, 2013). They embody an integrated life of health and well-being, and hold a vision of future expectations. This vision includes having a plan or idea, being able to share it with others for interprofessional collaboration, and aiming towards desired integrative outcomes.

Nurse Coaches realize that self-development is crucial in leadership and one's ability to be in the present moment when coaching clients/patients, and in thinking creatively in all nurse coaching endeavors. This also helps them move through the dark nights of the soul and identify strategies that can guide one through life's challenging ordeals (Moore, 1994). As the self is renewed through these four self-development components, it is easier to give attention to what it means to be called to service in healing.

Self-development leads to body–mind–spirit hardiness—commitment, control, and challenge—also referred to as psychological hardiness (Kobasa, 1979; Kobasa, Maddi, & Kahn, 1982). The first is *change*, wherein individuals feel open to change and are willing to take risks. These individuals see life events as challenges and not problems, and they thrive on challenges. The second characteristic refers to *commitment*. Individuals feel committed to family, friends, work, and goals, and are deeply engaged in what they are doing. The third characteristic is *control*. Individuals have a sense of personal power and control over life and perceive their body–mind–spirit as an integrative unit. Hardiness characteristics not only apply to staying healthy, but they also have tremendous potential for adapting to more effective health promotion strategies if chronic illness is present.

More recently, Maddi (2004, 2006) has characterized hardiness as a combination of three attitudes (commitment, control, and challenge) that together provide the courage and motivation needed to turn stressful circumstances from potential calamities into opportunities for personal growth. Bartone (2006) considers hardiness as something more global than mere attitudes, and as a broad personality style or generalized mode of functioning (cognitive, emotional, and behavioral qualities). He also incorporates commitment, control, and challenge as affecting how one views one's self and interacts with the world. Inspired by the hardiness research, the INCLM "C" qualities and actions are listed in **Table 21-2**. Nurse Coach leaders strive to be mindful and embody the INCLM Component 1 leadership qualities and capacities listed in **Table 21-3**. In the next section, INCLM Component 2: Integral Perspectives and Change is discussed.

Table 21-2 Integrative Nurse Coach Leadership "C" Qualities and Actions.

Caring	Collective vision	Consciousness expanding
Challenges	Commitment	Contributor
Change	Communicator	Control
Change agent	Compassion	Cooperation
Charisma	Competent	Core values
Choices	Concentration	Courage
Clarity	Conceptualizer	Creativity
Co-creator	Confidence	Critical thinker
Collaborator	Connector	Curiosity

Source: Copyright © 2014 by the International Nurse Coach Association. www.inursecoach.com

Table 21-3 INCLM Component 1: Nurse Coach Self-Development Qualities and Capacities.

A Nurse Coach leader strives to:

- Cultivate the capacity of being in the present moment to open up to intuition, insights, and inner wisdom, which allows caring, empathy, authenticity, humility, and integrity to manifest.
- Acknowledge her/his own pain and suffering, remembering that it is the story told to self that encompasses the physical, mental, emotional, spiritual, cultural, or environmental.
- Explore her/his own shadow (a composite of personal characteristics and potentials that have been denied expression in life and of which a person is unaware) to move forward in life's journey.
- Be alert to personal judgments and prejudices, and practice gratitude, loving kindness, and self-forgiveness.
- Identify her/his soul's purpose and passion and reflect qualities of "being with" and "in collaboration with."
- Let go of attachments and daily disappointments about how things should be.

Source: Copyright © 2014 by the International Nurse Coach Association. www.inursecoach.com

INCLM Component 2: Integral Perspectives and Change

Nurse Coach leaders are aware of an integral perspective that is a comprehensive way to organize multiple phenomenon of human experience related to four perspectives of reality: (1) individual interior (personal/intentional); (2) individual exterior (physiology/behavioral); (3) collective interior (shared/cultural); and (4) collective exterior (systems/structures). See Chapter 14 for details.

With an integral framework, perspective, and consciousness, Nurse Coach leaders are curious about what matters most to each client and the chosen topic and desired goals in each coaching session, while skillfully asking relevant questions to explore each quadrant as appropriate. They find awareness of an integral perspective extremely useful in inter-professional collaboration as it assists with addressing the whole of any situations. Perlman et al. (2014) describe situational awareness as being aware of the many attitudes, patterns, beliefs, rules (spoken or unspoken), and processes among individuals and throughout the organizations and communities. When any of these quadrants is not addressed, the desired outcomes are usually not accomplished. Using an integral perspective, Nurse Coach leaders can clearly articulate, document, analyze statistical data, design protocols, and translate true integrative healthcare that can be sustained.

Nurse Coach leaders' purpose and mission reflects wholeness as a goal, and is interdependent, dynamic, open, fluid, and continuously interacting with changing variables that can lead to greater complexity and order (Dossey, 2013). From an integral perspective,

Nurse Coach leaders exhibit authenticity in their inner and outer individual and collective endeavors, that is, they are consistent with their beliefs and values, and act on what they believe to be their truth. This authenticity also leads to transparency, which is an intentional way to be clear, direct, and with no hidden agendas. It also invites opportunities from others and appreciates all contributors into creative collaborate so that change can be translated for sustained change towards the health of individuals or interprofessional teams and institutions, and in communities. This helps to build trusting relationships and leads to successful completion of endeavors.

An integral perspective assists the Nurse Coach leader to be flexible in the change process and to be with uncertainty, ambiguity, and complexity. Thus, the Nurse Coach leader is more likely to adapt to new situations while assisting others in the midst of constant chaos and change. Nurse Coach leaders practice shared leadership, recognizing that the power among group members is contagious and each individual has the potential to intellectually stimulate others. When leadership is shared, it empowers others to develop creative outlets and new ideas.

Change implies flexibility and shows that lifestyle patterns and habits are learned behaviors and do not need to be permanent. Nurse Coach leaders experiment and notice what occurs when clients/patients try new ways of relating with friends, family, and colleagues, as well as integrating new healthier behaviors. Changing detrimental or risky habits is essential for wellbeing. The more we choose effective lifestyle patterns, the better we learn the change process. Changing and taking risks are an important part of life. Often when people do not change, they conclude they do not have the willpower to change. Willpower is a myth that does not lead to insight that effects long-lasting lifestyle changes. Rather, we can think in terms of "skillpower". Skillpower implies integration of new information and skills that lead to changes in lifestyle patterns. The more we are challenged in changing lifestyle, the more consistently we select positive changes because with increased awareness, the fear of change is lessened.

Nurse Coach leaders strive to be mindful and embody the INCLM Component 2 leadership qualities and capacities listed in **Table 21-4**. In the next section, INCLM Component 3: Integrative Lifestyle Health and Wellbeing (ILHWB) is discussed.

Table 21-4 INCLM Component 2: Integral Perspectives and Change Qualities and Capacities.

A Nurse Coach leader strives to:

- Practice deep listening with another to be present and focused with intention to understand what another person is expressing or not expressing.
- Speak her/his heart-centered truth, which awakens the conscious awareness of connection from "me" to "we" to "all of us."
- Engage in conscious awareness of "entering into" a conversation or dialogue with others where stories, worldviews, beliefs, priorities, and values related to the present moment or collective endeavors can be better understood and appreciated.
- Be aware of relating with others where all integral perspectives are shared in an appropriate manner so that there are fewer hidden interpretations.
- Recognize aspects of change as hidden assumptions and values, and remember that unwritten rules are always present and not known until they are broken.
- Notice political and power (control) dynamics and create a win/win dialogue as the "we" of group takes ownership and responsibility for change and innovation.

Source: Copyright © 2014 by the International Nurse Coach Association. www.inursecoach.com

INCLM Component 3: Integrative Lifestyle Health and Wellbeing (ILHWB)

Nurse Coach leaders recognize that the ILHWB is a personalized approach in coaching clients/patients and working in communities. The ILHWB deals with primary prevention and underlying causality through a whole-person perspective rather than traditional labels and codes for symptoms and diagnoses of disease. See Chapters 7–10 for details.

Nurse Coach leaders address complexity, which is often referred to as a phenomenon that occurs at the boundary between order and chaos, or at the edge of chaos (Davidson, Ray, & Turkel, 2011). Human beings are complex, are living in complex systems, are evolving in nonlinear ways, and are influenced by the systems in which they live (Mitchell et al., 2013).

By exploring the implications of complexity science as it pertains to the ILHWB, Nurse Coach leaders recognize that a major reason that our healthcare system has failed is that it did not deal with complexity; it remained locked into an autocratic hierarchy where traditional practitioners and administrators believed that they knew the most appropriate information about treatment and protocols. The old hierarchal system did not consider the emerging new story of clients/patients acknowledging their cultural beliefs and perceptions that influence their health and healing process. In today's world, those who desire ILHWB information may form new beliefs and want to be partners and active participants in their own healthcare, as they have been informed by the Internet and friends about treatment protocols and much more. Integrative Nurse Coach Leaders recognize that many nontraditional practitioners and healers who wanted to collaborate and participate with allopathic (or Western-oriented) practitioners have also been excluded; they are an integral part of the integrative healthcare team.

Nurse Coach leaders see organizations as self-organizing fields of dynamic complexity and chaos. Through integrative leadership Nurse Coaches engage with clients/patients and their communities in the emergence from chaos to a natural order that incorporates desired healthy lifestyle and new behaviors. Nurse Coach leaders are always incorporating ILHWB coaching principles in their analyzing, communicating, exchanging, surveying, involving, synthesizing, investigating, interviewing, mentoring, developing, creating, researching, and teaching. They listen to others and co-create new scenarios for what is possible, leading to change for and with clients/patients, and with cultural and organizational transformation and strategies for sustained change. Nurse Coach leaders strive to be mindful and embody the INCLM Component 3 leadership qualities and capacities listed in **Table 21-5**. In the next section, INCLM Component 4: Awareness and Choice is discussed.

Table 21-5 INCLM Component 3: Integrative Lifestyle Health and Wellbeing (ILHWB) Qualities and Capacities.

The Nurse Coach leader strives to:

- Consider all factors that influence health, wellness, and disease, and that include the bio–psycho-social–spiritual–cultural–environmental aspects.
- Develop ILHWB behaviors and skills with a personal action plan and steps to achieve health that assist in "walking the talk" of health and wellbeing.
- Recognize her/his unique position to engage self and others in the process of meaningful and new health-promoting strategies.
- See organizations as self-organizing fields of complexity and chaos that have the capacity to be true integrative healthcare institutions, clinics, and community centers that have an ILHWB focus.

(continues on next page)

Table 21-5 (*Continued*).

- Integrate meaningful recognition and gratitude for all healthcare team members so that their hearts are open and they feel appreciated for their work of service.
- Create exterior healing environments that incorporate nature and the natural world when possible such as with outdoor and indoor healing gardens, use of green materials with soothing colors, and sounds of music and nature when possible.

Source: Copyright © 2014 by the International Nurse Coach Association. www.inursecoach.com

INCLM Component 4: Awareness and Choice

Nurse Coach leaders have an awareness of being mindful and consciously choosing to use skills to stay in the present moment as change takes place in the present, not in the past or future. See Chapters 11–13 for details. Through embodying awareness and choice in both personal and professional endeavors, Nurse Coach leaders have the ability to inspire others through a caring charisma that imparts deep humility, empathy, and compassion.

Nurse Coach leaders strive to be mindful and embody the INCLM Component 4 leadership qualities and capacities listed in **Table 21-6**. In the next section, INCLM Component 5: Listening with HEART is discussed.

Table 21-6 INCLM Component 4: Awareness and Choice Qualities and Capacities.

A Nurse Coach leader strives to:

- Use mindful, conscious awareness so that all endeavors will source from the soul's purpose.
- Maintain forward movement while promoting positive change and living and working from core values.
- Promote health and wellbeing to open the paths of creativity and innovation and decrease obstacles and barriers.
- Use personal strategies to find balance in the midst of complexity, chaos, change, and transition, knowing that a natural order will emerge.

Source: Copyright © 2014 by the International Nurse Coach Association. www.inursecoach.com

INCLM Component 5: Listening with HEART

Listening with HEART© (**H**ealing, **E**nergy, **A**wareness, **R**esiliency, **T**ransformation) captures the dynamic elements within all the INCLM components that are threaded throughout this book.

Nurse Coach leaders strive to embody healing, energy, awareness, resilience, and transformation in all their endeavors through a deep "work spirit" that arises from a sense of meaning and "soul's purpose" (Sharma, 2004, 2007). Work spirit is related to increased resilience, effectiveness, productivity, and individual satisfaction, which contribute to positive results (Maddi & Khoshara, 2005). It is also directly related to how much responsibility one is willing to take to change the course of one's life. Work spirit also involves selflessness, which is being unself-consciously engrossed in the outcome of coaching clients and others and engaging in projects, protocols, and tasks, rather than worrying about what others think.

Nurse Coach leaders have abundant energy and always appear to be "on a roll" or "in a flow state." They experience a different sense of time, and have a sense of higher order and oneness. Their state of mind is positive and open to new ideas, and a full sense of self is manifest. They work with self and others to produce greater results. Exhibiting hardiness characteristics, Nurse Coach leaders can make frequent shifts in thinking and

---

releasing old mindsets, knowing that patterns and processes in any project create the whole, rather than focusing on isolated parts. They value input from colleagues and seek meaningful relationships, remembering to praise co-workers' talents and resources. They focus on win/win situations.

Those organizations that offer praise, rewards, and encourage risk-taking and problem-solving while not punishing individuals for mistakes, also increase individual work spirit.

Nurse Coach leaders strive to be mindful and embody the INCLM Component 5 leadership qualities and capacities listed in **Table 21-7**. In the next section, Nurse Coach leadership in transformational dialogues and organization change is discussed.

Table 21-7 INCLM Component 5: Listening with HEART Qualities and Strategies.

A Nurse Coach leader strives to:

- Recognize healing as a lifelong journey of seeking harmony and balance in one's own life and in family, community, and global relations. It is an emergent process of the whole system, bringing together aspects of one's self and the body–mind–spirit–culture–environment at deeper levels of inner knowing, leading towards integration and balance, with each aspect having equal importance and value.
- Identify the energy exchange with self and others towards desired goal/s and steps forward with transformational change and how to sustain the change.
- Notice the resilience of self and clients and group members as a positive trait involving the capacity to cope with daily life challenges.
- Understand the way individuals come together for meaningful work, setting priorities, use of technologies, and any aspect of the technological environment.

Source: Copyright © 2014 by the International Nurse Coach Association. www.inursecoach.com

TRANSFORMATIONAL DIALOGUE AND ORGANIZATIONAL CHANGE

Nurse Coaches possess the capacities necessary as change agents to bring their skills and vision to transform their organizations in the spirit of collaboration and willingness to take risks and actions toward change. Through an integrative, integral, and holistic lens, Nurse Coaches understand the diversity of an organization and can facilitate fostering an authentic healing environment where all participants are valued, respected, and can collectively explore together their hopes and their challenges.

Vignette

Nurses at a large metropolitan hospital were leaving their jobs due to discontentment over work conditions, which included long hours. In their exit interview, they were asked why they were leaving. The majority of nurses reported that they still loved being a nurse. They were challenged by feeling undervalued and overworked, and felt the personal hardship on their own health at work that also impacted their personal relationships beyond the hospital. They voiced complaints about poor communication among nurse colleagues and essentially no communication with other interprofessional team members operating in their silos.

Alarmed at the number of older nurses opting for early retirement, the hospital administration valued their experience. These nurses recalled a time when they could spend time with patients and their families, listen to their stories, hold a hand, and comfort family members, and they longed for that time, when caring was valued over efficiency and technology.

Administration acknowledged that they were in a moral nursing crisis. Jane, a Nurse Coach on the staff, was a team manager in transition care. The nurses on this team were not exiting in droves. Thus, Jane was asked to meet with other nurse managers to explore the dynamics breeding discontent across the system.

Facilitating Awareness and Change

When facilitating change and transformation in a system or organization, Nurse Coaches approach their role as change agents by asking the following questions to nursing leadership and with other interprofessional team members. Working with nursing managers and administrators, Nurse Coaches may explore:

- What has been most successful with the nurses (and others) on your team?
- What works now? Or what has worked in the past?
- What are the strengths of your nurse team (individually and collectively)?
- What is the best experience (dream, imagine) for the nurses on your team?
- What are the elements needed to optimize the work environment for the nurses on your team?
- What do you envision is the best possible outcome in working as a team?
- What would your team (specialty) look like if you could maximize the qualities and core values?
- What are the possibilities?
- What are the next steps?
- What are you hoping for as an interprofessional team?

Nurses Coach leaders create opportunities for transdisciplinary dialogues and approaches to integrative healthcare where each individual's story is heard and valued as part of the energetic whole. In an integrative model with an integral perspective, a transdisciplinary approach means that professionals and all other members of the healthcare team (clerical, dietetic, medical, physical therapy, housekeeping, etc.) come together as a whole to share knowledge and authentic communication, and are willing to explore deep meaning that engages the human spirit and spiritual concerns. They emphasize connections with each other rather than silos of specialization; there is "visioning possibilities with," "evolving ideas with," "collaboration with," rather than "competition between and among."

Nurse Coaches have a commitment to new approaches and the courage and spirit to "walk the talk" with creativity and inspiration. All participants acknowledge and respect different approaches in collaborative and interprofessional dialogues, and welcome other possibilities in integrative healthcare with new elements in one's knowing, doing, and being (Integrative Nurse Coach Certificate Program, n.d.; Watson Caring Science Institute, n.d.).

Nurse Coach leaders exhibit synergy; that is, they are involved in discovering common threads when there appears to be nothing but opposites and problems and conflicts. However, Nurse Coach leaders see these opposites as polarities that are part of the fabric of history and found everywhere, and are indestructible and unavoidable; they are present in our personal preferences, group dynamics, and organizational issues. Wesorick (2014) describes "polarities" as interdependent pairs of different, competing, or opposite values or points of view. Polarities are about "both/and" thinking, rather than "either/or" thinking. Each polarity has an identified upside (values) and downside (fears). Nurse Coach leaders are challenged to recognize these polarities and work with others to see how to experience the upside and dynamic interdependence of each pole, and to achieve a higher purpose.

Common "life polarities" are home life and work life, activity and rest, self and others, candor and diplomacy, and gentle love and tough love. Some common "healthcare polarities" are doing and caring, recruitment and retention, tradition and innovation, framework-driven change and project-initiative-driven change, autonomous care and standardized care, integrated competency and individual competency, mission and margin, hospital interest and physician interest, staff satisfaction and patient satisfaction, and patient safety and staff freedom (Wesorick, 2014).

Polarity thinking is everywhere and can assist us with integrative healthcare transformation. Wesorick (2014) believes that many of the cultural shadows that haunt us today and prevent us from reaching a high ground of a healthy work culture and integrated care are the result of trying to fix problems that are already polarities. For example, we often hear that a hospital unit needs to get their patient satisfaction scores up. However, the staff satisfaction is often neglected and the staff is asked to do more with less. The challenge is to balance staff satisfaction and patient satisfaction, and this requires a different approach. One cannot neglect one over the other; both need to be given attention at the same time.

Synergy awareness allows Nurse Coach leaders to recognize those Individuals who exhibit dysergy, which is the opposite of synergy, as they focus on an isolated action that promotes one function that impedes the progress of another person or the group working together. These individuals tend to work alone or evoke unnecessary competition among colleagues. They exhibit poor communication skills, aggressiveness, and insecurity, and they emphasize win/lose outcomes and reject meaningful interaction from co-workers.

Nurse Coach leaders have an identified purpose that can be shared and clearly communicated with clients/patients, supervisors, managers, and all team members. They recognize individual strengths and talents and channel creative energy toward the organizational goals. See Chapter 5 on strengths. To further Nurse Coach leadership qualities and capacities, health disparity issues are discussed in the next section.

NURSE COACH LEADERSHIP AND HEALTH DISPARITY ISSUES

Nurse Coach leaders have as their goal to improve one's quality of life to maintain health, live well with chronic illness, or to move through the end-of-life with comfort care and ease. With a renewed focus on prevention and wellness promotion in healthcare reform, Integrative Nurse Coach leaders are uniquely positioned to coach and engage individuals in behavior change, promote healthier lifestyles, and sustain these new health behaviors—local to global. As seen in Chapter 1, Table 1-3, in the overview of the extant Nurse Coach and nurse coaching literature review, Nurse Coaches are engaged as leaders, in shifting from the nurse expert to the nurse coaching role of "being with" clients/patients in one-to-one coaching sessions, telephonic coaching, laser coaching for short sessions and in clinical settings, and group coach settings in hospitals, clinics, corporations, schools, and the community.

Nurse Coach leaders are aware of addressing the health disparity issues in the underserved populations and the importance of recognizing the social determinants and environmental determinants of health. The *social determinants of health* are the economic and social conditions under which individuals live that affect their health. The *environmental determinants of health* are any external agent (biological, chemical, physical, social, or cultural) that can be linked to a change in health status that is involuntary, i.e., breathing unwanted secondhand smoke, whereas active tobacco smoking is a behavioral determinant. Disease and illness are often a result of detrimental social, economic, and political forces. To further address these concerns, Nurse Coach leadership initiatives are discussed in the next section.

Nurse Coach Initiatives

A Nurse Coach exemplar led by Meg Jordan (2013), the Integrative Wellness Coaching (IWC) Model and Leadership Pilot Project, brought integrative wellness coaching to homeless and low-income individuals. This project was undertaken to assess the feasibility of the health coaching model and general responsiveness of individuals and families that received it. It also identified principles of communication that reflected core values in working with marginalized, under-represented, and underserved populations.

Rather than a focus on cultural competency, Jordan and her team realized that the focus should be on structural competency. This implies that practitioners and healthcare organizations apply the coaching skills to reduce the health inequalities by acting on the social policies, institutional structures, and environmental conditions that determine mental and physical health. Shifting the thinking from cultural competency to structural competency allowed this project team, using health coaching skills, to address the social and economic determinants where the health disparity was firmly rooted.

This project clearly showed how different coaching approaches were needed with the homeless on the streets at three to six months, and those who had at least some support from an agency with basic housing. The coaching outcomes were most successful with individuals in shelters and least successful with those living on the street. Coaching the very poorest (street dwellers and those in temporary shelters) required more attention to the upstream needs of safe housing, access to healthcare, education, job training, and freedom from violence.

This project clearly revealed the downstream consequences of upstream social and environmental policies. In order to close the gap of unmet needs of the marginalized and underserved individuals, this project team concluded that the social, clinical, and personal needs of individuals must be matched with programs and alliances. When this is done, it cuts across boundaries and can link physicians, health coaches, and social sector workers together as they already know how to connect these people with resources (Jordan, 2013).

Nurse Coach leaders are engaged in the Nurses Workgroup of Health Care Without Harm (HCWH, n.d.) and the Luminary Project (Luminary Project, n.d.), which features over 200 nurse stories that address environmental problems and health challenges, and illuminate the way towards safe hospitals; communities with clean air, land, and water; and children born without toxic chemicals in their bodies. These nurse leaders are addressing the "precautionary principle" described as follows: "When an activity raises threats of harm to human health or the environment, precautionary measures shall be taken, even if some cause-and-effect relationships are not fully established scientifically. This implies 'better safe than sorry' and is common sense to most and why experts call the precautionary principle the 'duh' principle. Its emphasis is on 'suspects'; if there is a suspicion about a harmful environment or substance, even though all of the evidence is not in, remove the person from the situation or stop the use of suspected harmful substances; emphasis is on *zero* contamination and pollution of our environments as acceptable, not minimal/moderate" (Raffensperger & Tickner, 1999). Nurse Coach leaders are applying the principles of ecological sustainable health that focuses on the protection of the quality of life on earth, the environment, and the earth's natural resources; this is synergistic with human health and planetary wellbeing and connected to the web of life. See Chapter 9 on Environmental Health.

Nurse Coach leaders are raising their voices and concerns through the wider public promotion of healthcare—to influence other groups and to dialogue and collaborate with other disciplines and the media. They are visibly advocating for a new healthcare paradigm in all sectors including community and public health, hospice and palliative care, disease management, mental health, oncology, and environmental health initiatives, to name a few areas where nurse leaders have been instrumental in implementing new innovative integrative initiatives.

The examples that follow are the Nurse Coach chapter coauthors and their initiatives and endeavors. In 2004, Susan Luck established the EarthRose Institute (ERI) (Earth-Rose Institute, n.d.), which was established in response to the growing need for disseminating information, providing education, and doing collaborative research on the environmental links to women's and children's health. The primary ERI goal is preventing exposures to toxic compounds in the home, workplace, food chain, and community. ERI works with women, communities, institutions, nurses and healthcare providers, and other organizations on advocacy and health policy issues related to environmental health on a local and global level. The ERI is committed to being a bridge that brings scientific research and information to diverse communities. Another ERI initiative, the Integrative Nursing Institute (INI), was established to respond to the crisis in healthcare and nursing and offers innovative solutions through education and ongoing professional development.

In 2004, Nurse Coach and Nightingale scholar, Barbara Dossey, with Deva-Marie Beck, a Nightingale scholar and global nurse activist, with several other global activists and concerned citizens, began the Nightingale Initiative for Global Health (NIGH) (NIGH, n.d.) and crafted the Nightingale Declaration for a Healthy World (Nightingale Declaration, n.d.). See Chapter 1, Figure 1-1. NIGH is a grassroots, nurse-inspired movement to increase global public awareness about the priority of human health. This inclusive, collaborative, and synergistic initiative gives nurses a voice and creates new opportunities for them to discover possibilities for their unique contributions towards health and wellbeing for all. They honor the legacy of Florence Nightingale and other nurses, midwives, and healthcare workers, past and present, who have shown by their example how personal actions can make a significant difference. They seek to engage the values and wisdom of millions of nurses and concerned citizens and to act as a catalyst for the transformation of individuals, communities, and society for the achievement of a healthy world. To raise the voices of Nurse Coach endeavors, emerging media capacities are discussed next.

EMERGING MEDIA CAPACITIES

Nurse Coach leaders are actively engaged in global discussion and networking, to share "Nurse Coach news stories" to wider audiences about the Nurse Coach role in health coaching through the emerging media capacities—first in community-based print journalism, radio and video broadcasts, and later through emerging Internet capacities such as blogs, Facebook, and face-to-face meetings (Beck et al., 2014). With new communication tools unparalleled in human history, now is the time for Nurse Coaches to find the courage and confidence to use these tools for the dynamic and innovative promotion of health at local, regional, national, and global levels. This will widen the scope of nurse coaching practice—to widely communicate the concerns we care about most with everyone else.

Two exemplars are the missions of Barbara Glickstein, a public health nurse consultant and broadcast journalist, and Diana Mason, Rudin Professor of Nursing. Together they are the co-directors, Center for Health, Media & Policy at Hunter College, City University of New York. For the past 25 years, Glickstein and Mason have produced and hosted *Healthstyles*, an award-winning, weekly program on New York City listener-sponsored public radio, that provides ongoing coverage of issues that make a difference in our everyday lives. Glickstein has consulted with Nurse Coaches to show how to effectively use media tools to demonstrate strategies for health and wellbeing, and to become trusted voices that can address many issues impacting health and nursing coaching practice.

Our challenge as Nurse Coaches is to develop further collaborative pathways to impact positive interprofessional relationships with healthcare colleagues—as well as with journalists, broadcasters, multimedia professionals, and other national and international networking groups. Our Nurse Coach practices can incorporate further development of networking and communications capacities and media-related interviewing, writing, and Internet skills.

Reflecting upon Nightingale's global legacy of activism, advocacy, and transformation—and the possibilities for what we can achieve in our time—we as Nurse Coaches can consider following these seven recommendations (Beck et al., 2014; NIGH, n.d.):

- Make health—and activating positive health determinants—a top priority in human affairs.
- Value and sustain nurses in their caring to achieve health goals everywhere.
- Collaborate across disciplines and cultures to promote health in community settings.
- Think global; act to create and sustain local health literacy for everyone, across the lifespan.
- Make media a catalyst for nursing and for health.
- Keep health holistic, integrative, and transdisciplinary.
- Answer your own "calling," your "must".

SUMMARY

- The Integrative Nurse Coach Leadership Model (INCLM) has five components that are as follows: (1) Nurse Coach Self-Development (Self-Reflection, Self-Assessment, Self-Evaluation, Self-Care); (2) Integral Perspectives and Change; (3) Integrative Lifestyle Health and Wellbeing; (4) Awareness and Choice; and (5) Listening with HEART (**H**ealing, **E**nergy, **A**wareness, **R**esiliency, **T**ransformation). All five components are *fully integrated* and have equal value.
- The INCLM guides nurse coaching practice, education, research, and healthcare policy.
- The INCLM five components have identified leadership qualities and strategies to guide all nurse coaching endeavors.
- The INCLM recognizes polarities as interdependent pairs of different, competing, or opposite values or points of view, which are about "both/and" thinking, rather than "either/or" thinking.
- Nurse Coach leaders are challenged to recognize polarities and work with others to see how to experience the upside and dynamic interdependence of each pole, and to achieve a higher purpose.
- Decent care is a comprehensive care continuum approach that is integral, integrative, and holistic, whereby individuals are afforded dignity and a destigmatized space to take control of their own destinies.
- To decrease the health disparities of the underserved population, the gap must be closed in the unmet social, clinical, and personal needs with programs and alliances that cut across boundaries and link physicians, Nurse Coaches, other professional and lay health coaches, and social sector workers who already know how to connect people with resources.

NURSE COACH REFLECTIONS

After reading this chapter, the Nurse Coach will be able to bring awareness and personal insight to the following questions:

- How does the Integrative Nurse Coach Leadership Model (INCLM) guide me in my personal and professional coaching endeavors?
- How do I model Nurse Coach leadership?
- What are my special ways to cultivate the capacity of being in the present moment to open up to intuitive insights and inner wisdom?
- What do I experience when I know that I am working from my soul's purpose?

REFERENCES

Bartone, P. T. (2006). Resilience under military operational stress: Can leaders influence hardiness? *Military Psychology 18*, S131–S148. doi:10.1207/s15327876mp1803s_10. Retrieved from http://en.wikipedia.org/wiki/Hardiness_(psychological)

Beck, D. M., Dossey, B. M., & Rushton, C. H. (2014). Global activism, advocacy, and transformation: Florence Nightingale's legacy for the twenty-first century. In M. J. Kreitzer & M. Koithan (Eds.), *Integrative nursing*. New York, NY: Oxford University Press.

Davidson, A. W., Ray, M. A., & Turkel, M. C. (2011). *Nursing, caring, and complexity science: For human-environment well-being*. New York, NY: Springer.

Dossey, B. M. (2010). *Florence Nightingale: Mystic, visionary, healer*. Philadelphia, PA: F. A. Davis.

Dossey, B. M. (2013). Nursing: Integral, integrative, and holistic—local to global. In B. M. Dossey & L. Keegan (Eds.), *Holistic nursing: A handbook for practice* (6th ed., pp. 1–57). Burlington, MA: Jones & Bartlett Learning.

EarthRose Institute (ERI) (n.d.). Retrieved from http://www.earthrose.org

Freshwater, D., Taylor, B. J., & Sherwood, G. C. (Eds.) (2008). *The international textbook of reflective practice in nursing*. Chichester, UK: Wiley-Blackwell.

Healthcare Without Harm (HCWH) (n.d.). Retrieved from http://hcwh.org

Integrative Nurse Coach Certificate Program (n.d.). Retrieved from http://inursecoach.com/programs

Integrative Nursing Institute (INI) (n.d.). Retrieved from http://www.integrativenursing-institute.org

Johns, C. (2013). *Becoming a reflective practitioner* (4th ed.). Hoboken, NJ: Wiley-Blackwell.

Jordan, M. (2013). Health coaching for the underserved. *Global Advances in Health and Medicine 2*(3), 75–82.

Kobasa, S. C. (1979). Stressful life events, personality, and health – Inquiry into hardiness. *Journal of Personality and Social Psychology 37*(1), 1–11. doi:10.1037/0022-3514.37.1.1. PMID 458548. Retrieved from http://en.wikipedia.org/wiki/Hardiness_(psychological)

Kobasa, S. C., Maddi, S. R., & Kahn, S. (1982). Hardiness and health: A prospective study. *Journal of Personality and Social Psychology, 42*, 168–177. Retrieved from http://en.wikipedia.org/wiki/Hardiness_(psychological)

Kreitzer, M. J. (2014). Whole-systems healing: A new leadership path. In M. J. Krietzer & M. Koithan (Eds.), *Integrative nursing* (pp. 47–55). New York, NY: Oxford University Press.

Luck, S. (2010). Changing the health of our nation: The role of nurse coaches. *Alternative Therapies in Health and Medicine, 16*(5), 78–80.

Luminary Project (n.d.). Retrieved from http://www.theluminaryproject.org

Maddi, S. R. (2004). Hardiness: An operationalization of existential courage. *Journal of Humanistic Psychology 44*(3), 279–298. doi:10.1177/0022167804266101. Retrieved from http://en.wikipedia.org/wiki/Hardiness_(psychological)

Maddi, S. R. (2006). Hardiness: The courage to grow from stresses. *Journal of Positive Psychology 1*(3), 160–168. doi:10.1080/17439760600619609. Retrieved from http://en.wikipedia.org/wiki/Hardiness_(psychological)

Maddi, S. R., & Khoshara, D. (2005). *Resilience and work: How to succeed, no matter what life throws at you.* New York, NY: AMACOM.

Mitchell. G. J., Cross, N., Wilson, M., Biernacki, W. W., Adib, B., & Rush, D. (2013). Complexity and health coaching: Synergies in nursing. *Nursing Research & Practice.* Article ID238620.

Moore, T. (1994). *Care of the soul: A guide for cultivating depth and sacredness in everyday life.* New York, NY: Harper Perennial.

Nightingale, F. (1873). What will our religion be on August 11, 1999? *Fraser's Magazine,* (July), 28–36.

Nightingale Declaration for a Healthy World (n.d.). Retrieved from http://www.nightingaledeclaration.net/the-declaration

Nightingale Initiative for Global Health (NIGH) (n.d.). Retrieved from http://www.nightingaledeclaration.net

Perlman, A., Horrigan, B., Goldblatt, E., & Maizes, V. (2014). The pebble in the pond: How integrative leadership can bring about transformation. *Explore 10*(5S), S1–S4.

Raffensperger, C., & Tickner, J. (1999). *Protecting public health and the environment: Implementing the precautionary principle.* Washington, DC: Island Press.

Sharma, M. (2004). Conscious leadership at the crossroads of change. *Shift 12,* 17–21.

Sharma, M. (2007). World wisdom in action: Personal to planetary transformation. *Kosmos,* Fall/Winter, 31–35.

Watson Caring Science Institute (WCSI, n.d). Retrieved from http://www.watsoncaringscience.org

Wesorick, B. (2014). Polarity thinking: An essential skill for those leading interprofessional integration. *Journal of Interprofessional Healthcare 1*(1), Article 12. Retrieved from http://www.jihonline.org/jih/vol1/iss1/12

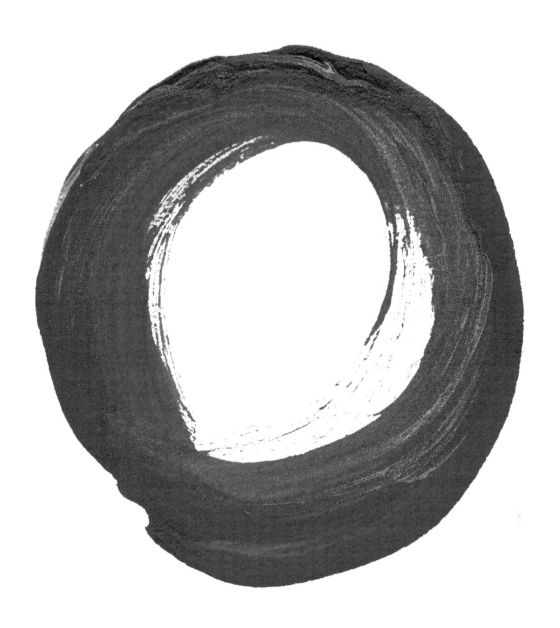

CORE VALUE 5
Nurse Coach Self-Development

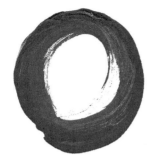

CHAPTER 22

Nurse Coach Self-Development

Deborah McElligott

Quiet in our own rooms—we have bustle every day—a few minutes of calm...—how indispensable it is, in this ever increasing hurry of life! When we live 'so fast' do we not require a breathing time, a moment or two daily, to think where we are going.

Florence Nightingale, 1873

LOOKING AHEAD...

After reading this chapter, you will be able to:

- Define the four components in Nurse Coach self-development (self-reflection, self-assessment, self-evaluation, self-care).
- Examine the concept of the wounded healer.
- Explore self-development principles and strategies.

DEFINITIONS

Healing: An emergent process of the whole system bringing together aspects of one's self and the body–mind–emotion–spirit–environment at deeper levels of inner knowing, leading toward integration and balance, with each aspect having equal importance and value. Healing involves those physical, mental, social, and spiritual processes of recovery, repair, renewal, and transformation that increase wholeness and often (though not invariably) order and coherence (Hess et al., 2013, p. 50).

Self-assessment: A centered, dynamic, and ongoing *informal* caring process where one uses her/his inherent wisdom to identify personal patterns, concerns, and opportunities (Hess et al., 2013, p. 4). Formal self-assessment may occur through the use of standardized wellness tools or in collaboration with a healthcare professional who provides additional data to the client, who then engages in self-assessment.

Self-care: The process of engaging in health related activities (including health promoting behaviors, feelings, and attitudes) in order to adopt a healthier lifestyle, and enhance balance and wellbeing (McElligott, 2013, p. 831). Self-care may occur throughout the lifespan as one uses compassion-focused awareness, reflective choices, and self-determined actions and behaviors in a meaningful way.

Self-development: A process where one takes personal responsibility for her or his learning and development, often involving self-reflection, self-assessment, self-evaluation, and self-care as an integral process.

Self-evaluation: Exploration of our understanding, experiences, and behaviors; may include the measurement of self-care actions through the use of a tool or a specific goal to determine if, how and why, desired, specific outcomes have been achieved.

Self-reflection: An inner awareness of our thoughts, feeling, judgments, beliefs, and perception that opens the process for "the intentional and conscious use of self" (Levin & Reich, 2013, p. 247).

THE INTEGRAL WHOLE AND SELF-DEVELOPMENT

Nurse Coach self-development is the first component in the Theory of Integrative Nurse Coaching (TINC) and involves four areas: self-reflection, self-assessment, self-evaluation, and self-care. These areas cannot be separated, just as the Nurse Coach cannot be divided into parts, but exists as an integral whole. This chapter will assist the Nurse Coach to deepen her/his own personal exploration of self-development in order to knowingly and effectively participate in the nurse coaching process. The willingness to model and commit to lifelong self-development and learning are described as two of the qualities of the Nurse Coach. See Chapter 2 and Chapter 21, Tables 21-3 to 21-7 for Nurse Coach qualities and capacities.

While discussing the self-development of the Nurse Coach as an individual, one must recognize the important relationship of the Nurse Coach's self-development to the nurse coaching process and nurse coaching competencies. The self-development of the Nurse Coach is both a necessity and the foundation for the needed competencies in the role. This role requires more than the acquisition of knowledge, it involves the integration of the whole person, using a range of skills to assist the client to move towards desired goals (Donner & Wheeler, 2013). See Chapter 4 for Nurse Coach competencies.

The Nurse Coach self-development, guided by nursing theory and practice, is paramount to the success and longevity of the Nurse Coach's career. This also mirrors one's own healing journey or transformation to wholeness in all phases of life and includes self-care through the dying or transition process.

While each of these four areas is vital in the development of the Nurse Coach, self-reflection is a uniting thread throughout. Reflection, part of self-care and nurse coaching, "integrates the critical thinking mind with the intelligent compassion of the heart" (Levin & Reich, 2013) and may be seen in each component of the self-development process. For example, reflection occurs with the self-assessment with or without an assessment tool. Once assessment is completed, reflection occurs again to derive meaning from developing a self-care plan and desired practice. Self-evaluation of one's goals and actions involves reflection and is another continuous process.

The Nurse Coach role recognizes the fluidity of the changing health promoting process and honors the individual's knowledge and expertise. The inner wisdom is brought forth to dance throughout the self-development process. Dossey (L. Dossey, 1982, pp. 72–81) describes this as the *biodance* as we are participating in an endless exchange with all living things, with planet Earth in which all living organisms participate, and at the energetic and cosmic level as well. This energetic dance exists not only as we live, but also as we die.

Nurse Coaches continuously explore self-development and the art of healing so that in coaching sessions they can move with ease between the expert nurse role of knowing, being a educator, and symptom management, to the Nurse Coach role of "not fixing" and assisting the client to access her or his own inner wisdom. In the next section, healing and the wounded healer are explored.

HEALING AND THE WOUNDED HEALER

Healing is a person's lifelong journey of seeking harmony and balance in one's own life; it involves those physical, mental, social, and spiritual processes of recovery, repair, renewal, and transformation that increase wholeness and often (though not invariably) order and coherence. Healing is an emergent process of the whole system bringing together aspects of one's self and the body–mind–spirit–culture–environment process at deeper levels of inner knowing, leading toward integration and balance, with each aspect having equal importance and value. Thus, healing can lead to more complex levels of personal understanding and meaning, and may be synchronous but not synonymous with curing (Dossey, 2013). See Chapter 14 for discussion on integral perspectives and change.

There is a part of us that always needs healing. No one has total freedom from stress or illness, although many try to hide from the fact. Yet, the more we hide from our woundedness, the more we set ourselves up for body–mind–spirit risks and symptoms, referred to as the wounded healer. This is the wounded healer that is a concept derived from Greek mythology, specifically, the myth of Chiron, the centaur, who could not be healed (Dossey, 2013). This myth is described in **Table 22-1** and suggests that even the greatest healers suffer and must confront their own suffering.

Table 22-1 The Myth of Chiron.

The Myth of Chiron
Chiron was a centaur, half man and half horse, who was skilled in healing. Along with other centaurs, Chiron was invited to the cave of Heracles. Pholos, also a centaur, had delivered a jar of wine to Heracles. The scent of the wine intrigued the other centaurs, and they began to drink. Because they were not accustomed to drinking, they became intoxicated and began to fight. During the battle, one of the arrows shot by Heracles hit Chiron in the knee. Heracles tended Chiron, the wounded healer. The point of the arrow had been dipped in the poison of the hydra, thus the wound was incurable. Chiron, an immortal, could not be cured but could not die. From his cave, Chiron taught many heroes his great knowledge of healing. One of the students was Aesclepius, who gained knowledge of the healing herbs and the power of acknowledging one's *woundedness*.

Source: From Dossey, B. M. (2013). Nursing: Integral, integrative, and holistic—local to global. In B.M. Dossey & L. Keegan (Eds.), *Holistic nursing: A handbook for practice* (6th ed.), (pp. 1–57). Burlington, MA: Jones & Bartlett Learning.

As Nurse Coaches increase their healing and self-awareness, they recognize their suffering and more consistently enter into a state of being authentic. Authenticity implies consistency between inner experiences/outer expression and congruence between beliefs, behaviors, and values. We must learn to embrace our limitations, as well as to recognize our strengths. All great healers acknowledge their inherent weaknesses and fallibilities. Likewise, the Nurse Coach must find time in a fast paced life to take that step of self-engagement in the healing process, and recognize one's woundedness.

As the Nurse Coach participates in the healing process, aspects of suffering may be transformed and he/she moves from fragmentation to a wholeness, experiencing serenity, interconnectedness, and a new sense of meaning (McElligott, 2010). In contrast, when a Nurse Coach and a client come together with both denying their woundedness, the outcome is mechanical at best. Neither the Nurse Coach nor the client is able to use her/his inner wisdom to activate self-healing. Both have devalued this innate potential. Inner healing does not flow from the Nurse Coach to the client; the Nurse Coach cannot give inner healing to the client, for it already exists within the client. Rather, the Nurse Coach acts as a facilitator to evoke the client's process of inner healing.

As Nurse Coaches recognize their personal attitudes, beliefs, and stressors, their self-development can be a source of creativity and spontaneity. Hence, acknowledging our own stressors opens us to creativity in coaching. Being a Nurse Coach requires work on the self, our imperfect, fallible self. We must affirm our weaknesses and strengths, and acknowledge our inadequacies. It is only then that we know a powerful part of our being and allow new strengths to be born. See Chapter 5 on Strengths. It is the use of self, in a loving and compassionate way, that provides us with our most powerful instrument in the nurse coaching process and in healing. This transformative healing occurs as a positive, subjective, unpredictable process, where one often has a new sense of wholeness as life is reinterpreted and new meanings developed (McElligott, 2010). We recognize that this healing process is different than curing and may even occur as one is transitioning from this life. To deepen this understanding of healing, the next section discusses of each of the four components of self-development.

SELF-DEVELOPMENT

Self-Reflection

Self-reflection is the inner awareness of our consciousness—our thoughts, feelings, judgments, beliefs, and perceptions, and our connections to something greater than ourselves (Dossey, 2013) as developed in the Theory of Integrative Nurse Coaching. See Chapter 2. As we deepen our capacity for personal healing, we enhance our healing presence in the Nurse Coach relationships.

Self-reflection has been described as an act of service, and as a preparation for the deeper relationships with self and others (Levin & Reich, 2013). The daily practice of self-reflection and reflective skills such as mindfulness, presence, deep listening, and skillful questioning enable the Nurse Coach to comfortably use these skills with clients in the face of ambiguity, providing access to many ways of knowing. It takes practice and skill to hold the space, as well as trust in the nurse coaching process to allow the client's wisdom to unfold. Practice is needed as self-reflection occurs best during the relaxation phase where the parasympathetic system supports more choices in awareness. As most nurses report numerous stressors in their lives, we need to develop self-reflection to change that neuronal wiring so often focused on combating various stressors. For an in-depth discussion of awareness and choice, see Chapters 11, 12, and 13.

Through reflection, the nursing practice in the Nurse Coach model changes—from "doing to" to "being with", from "responsible for" to "responsible to"—all statements of the new relationship that are nourished by reflective skills. Self-reflection allows one to move from specialized to integrated and interconnected, in relationship with the integral whole. This self-reflection in action, not unique, but yet essential to the nurse coaching process, has been termed reflective practice (Johns, 2013). The Nurse Coach is a reflective practitioner using mindfulness and awareness throughout each coaching encounter. As seen in **Figure 22-1**, self-reflection occurs throughout the cycle of self-development as an integral part of the process.

Self-Assessment

Nurse Coaches must first identify their own wellbeing through the centered, dynamic, and ongoing caring process of self-assessment, if they are to be effective coaches. They need to use their inherent wisdom, that inner knowing, to identify personal patterns, concerns,

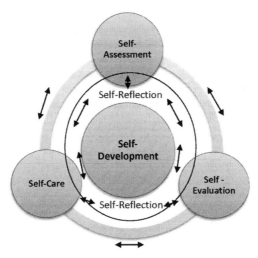

Figure 22-1 The Cycle of Self-Development.
Source: Copyright © 2014 by Deborah McElligott.

and opportunities that support meaning and wholeness in their life. Wellness is an evolving process that does not just happen but aligns with self-development, requiring ongoing self-reflection, self-assessment, self-evaluation, and self-care. Self-assessment may be done in a formal structured manner or informally as part of daily life.

Formal self-assessment involves valid and reliable tools, interactions with healthcare professionals, including health coaches, and structured time or sessions to accomplish the desired task. Before you read further, answer the questions in **Table 22-2**. Theories such as the Theory of Integrative Nurse Coaching (Chapter 2) and tools such as the Integrative Health and Wellness Assessment™ (IHWA) (Chapter 6) support an integrative, integral, and holistic self-assessment.

Table 22-2 Integrative Health and Wellness Assessment (IHWA). (See Chapter 6 and Appendix C-2, IHWA long form.)

Integrative Health and Wellness Assessment (IHWA)

Formal Self-Assessment:

Questions to answer after completion of IHWA (See Chapter 6)
- Was this easy or challenging?
- What did you learn about yourself and the eight areas of wellness—Life Balance and Satisfaction, Relationships, Spiritual, Mental, Emotional, Physical (exercise, nutrition, weight), Environmental, Health Responsibility?
- How ready are you to make changes?
- How important is your goal to you?
- How confident are you in your ability to reach your SMART goal (see Chapter 15)?

Before reading further, reflect on the questions seen in **Table 22-3**. Informal self-assessment often occurs throughout the day of the Nurse Coach as one engages in self-reflective practice and activities such as meditative practice, journaling, *tai chi*, yoga, imagery, prayer, poetry, and other forms of narrative. This assessment may also occur with the short form of the IHWA (Appendix C-1, short form). It is important to note that the short form is just a prompt for reflection and discussion, and not meant as a medical assessment. Throughout the assessment process we are focusing on our self as an integral whole and identifying the balance or lack of, in the various aspects of the cognitive, emotional, somatic, interpersonal, spiritual, and moral lines of development. See Chapter 14.

While assessment of the integral whole is familiar to holistic practitioners, it is often an "ah-ha" moment, for other healthcare professionals and the community at large. This moment may be described as a new sense of self-awareness. Self-awareness has been ascribed many meanings, from becoming the object of one's attention, understanding one's values and beliefs and their impact on our environment, to the simple recognition of self. As a process, self-awareness has been described as knowingly using insights and presence to guide authentic behavior in creating a "healing interpersonal environment" (Eckroth-Bucher, 2010). Thus, self-assessment can be seen as part of self-development and directly related to self-reflection and self-awareness.

Table 22-3 Reflections: Informal Wellness/Self-Assessment.

Reflections: Informal Wellness/Self-Assessment
Pause for a moment and reflect on these questions: • What are the key elements in my wellness program? • Do I have a positive self-image? • Do I have a positive attitude? • How is my self-discipline? • Do I use an integration of body–mind–spirit? • What mindful practices do I have? • Do I see wellness as a fluctuating state that I can continuously participate in creating? • Do I see my health as affected and determined by family, friends, job, and environment? • Do I think that I can learn new wellness behaviors? • Is the responsibility for staying well mine or someone else's?

Self-Evaluation

Self-evaluation invites us to reflect and explore many areas of our understanding, and experience of deep attention, intention, presence, and healing as seen in **Table 22-4**. Each of these areas of understanding is needed to care for ourselves and also applies to our clients. Through self-evaluation we learn to declare our attention of a somatic awareness of how to be centered, grounded, and balanced. Intention is a conscious awareness of being in the present moment to help facilitate the healing process; it is a volitional act of love that has a quality of resonance in our total beingness. Presence is the essential state or core in healing of approaching an individual in a way that respects and honors her/his essence. It is relating in a way that reflects a quality of "being with" and in collaboration with rather than "doing to."

Through the assessment, reflection, and self-evaluation, we develop our self-image that is the way we view ourselves; a positive self-image means that we view ourselves as worthy human beings. How often do we see ourselves with the same loving compassion that we extend to others? We must continue to develop keenly all of our senses and see ourselves as well in all respects—physical, mental, emotional, social, and spiritual. A positive attitude means that we like and respect ourselves in all that we do. To thrive in this life, we have to learn to respect our body–mind–spirit. We also have to teach ourselves self-discipline.

Table 22-4 Reflection: Self-Evaluation.

Self-Evaluation
Reflect and act on the following steps:

- Search for patterns and antecedents or precipitants of stress and anxiety.
- Identify positive feelings and emotions.
- Emphasize our human values.
- Assess any pain and disease as valuable signals of internal conflict, not as being totally negative.
- Place emphasis on achieving maximal body–mind–spirit wellness.
- View our own body–mind–spirit as equal factors, with one element never being more important than the others.
- Explore life's meaning more deeply.

Self-discipline embodies the idea of being calm and consistently following positive wellness patterns, such as relaxation, exercise, play, and good nutrition. Body–mind–spirit integration means that we see ourselves as a whole. We learn to "walk our talk" of integration in the personal and professional aspects of our lives. We must learn how to have compassion and loving kindness that is an open, gentle, and caring state of mindfulness. We are part of a whole universe, and we must see this relationship in terms of interacting wholes that are different from the sum of the parts. We must feel a keen sense of balance and relatedness between who we are, where we are, and how we interact with everyone. Evaluation and creation of a positive self-image enhances the life of the Nurse Coach as well as the coaching process. We enter into a shared experience (or field of consciousness) with the client and others that promotes healing potential and an experience of wellbeing. To further evaluate your state of health, consider ways that you might deeply explore life's meaning as discussed in Chapter 5.

As mentioned earlier, as the self-development process is not stagnant or linear, the self-evaluation may occur after self-assessment, or after the development of the self-care plan. It may be sparked by self-reflection, somatic responses, or interactions with others. Throughout our day, as we enter into a shared experience (or field of consciousness) with our environment, including others, we either increase or decrease our healing potential and experience of wellbeing. Application of the wellness model to our own lives can assist us in feeling whole and inspired about life.

Just as self-evaluation aids in the self-development of the Nurse Coach, self-evaluation during the coaching process assists the Nurse Coach in further role development and the deepening of coaching skills. Self-reflection has subtle differences depending on whether the Nurse Coach is evaluating her/his self in general, or her/his role during the Nurse Coach process. Both reflections for self and reflection on the coaching process will deepen our experience of understanding our present way of life, feelings, and personal habits. Take a moment to reflect on the questions in **Table 22-5**.

Table 22-5 Self-Evaluation for the Nurse Coach and the Nurse Coaching Process.

Self-Evaluation for the Nurse Coach	Self-Evaluation for the Nurse Coaching Process
• How do I let go of fixed ideas about myself and others? • How can I be more aware of ways to bear witness to my own joy as well as my own suffering and that of others? • How can I welcome everything that occurs? • What allows me to embrace all experiences directly? • How can I use all the ingredients of my life?	• Are my personal needs/issues/ desires impinging my client/work? • Am I cultivating a capacity for deep listening/mindful presence? • Am I aware of the client's vulnerability and how it is revealed? • Am I identifying and understanding the goal the client is expressing? • Am I opening the client to new perspectives and new ways of seeing?

Self-Care

Self-care assists us with having balance in our life as we initiate and perform activities on our own behalf to maintain wellbeing. It includes the ability to respond to choices and activities that lead to integration of body, mind, and spirit. Self-care is about valuing who we are and recognizing that we must care for ourselves in order to be able to serve others. It is our willingness to experience and face our fears, worries, and self-deceptions.

Caring for ourselves also means that we will be able to bring more of ourselves to all aspects of our lives. Self-care directly relates to health promotion and self-responsibility, and often involves deliberate actions. See Chapter 15. These actions are learned behaviors, therefore, naturally culturally specific (McElligott, 2013). Thus, a focus on self-care necessitates an individualized approach, or specific group coaching skills. Self-responsibility, a key component of self-care and wellness, resides within each of us. It is through these areas that we focus on maximizing wellness.

Self-care in nursing is rooted in Florence Nightingale's legacy and expands to the need for nurses to care and support each other and the environment (Dossey et al., 2005). Current nursing literature supports the need for self-care in nurses to improve patient-centered care, prevent burnout, and decrease turnover in institutions (McElligott et al., 2010). National and international agendas support the need for self-care and health-promoting behaviors in everyone. Thus, self-care for the Nurse Coach involves caring for one's self, others, and our environment as well as coaching others in the vital area of self-care, empowering them to reach their maximum health potential. See Chapters 7, 8, and 9.

A focus on self-care necessitates attention to the six lines of development mentioned in Chapter 14. Throughout the self-development process, how do we focus on our cognitive, emotional, somatic, interpersonal, spiritual, and moral lines of development? Combining the lines of development with the four areas of self development (self-reflection, self-assessment, self-evaluation, and self-care) offers many strategies for self-care.

Principles of Self-Care. In self-care planning we must develop and incorporate four basic and critical factors: (1) a positive self-image, (2) a positive attitude, (3) self-discipline, and (4) integration of body–mind–spirit. Each person will develop and incorporate these factors in her or his own unique way. The following elements of self-care are very useful. Reflect on the reminders in **Table 22-6**.

Table 22-6 Reminders for Relecting on Life's Journey.

Reflections for Life's Journey
• Cultivate compassion and equanimity.
• Give your best effort; don't be attached to outcomes.
• Practice radical optimism.
• Remember the truth of impermanence.
• Give no fear.
• Realize joy on the path of service.
• Discover a place of rest in the midst of things.

Self-Care Plan. Develop a plan for doing your work in a way that is restorative, mindful, and wholesome. See your limits with compassion and a schedule that is sane. Identify those practices and activities that can refresh you (Halifax, Dossey, & Rushton, 2007). As you focus on the development of a self-care plan, incorporate "islands of care and nourishment" to assist with lifelong healing. As a Nurse Coach, create and revise your own self-care strategies as seen in **Table 22-7**. Self-care assists us to stay alert to present moment events. What ways do you care for yourself? Design a care plan that includes strategies that allow a kind of internal rhythm and presence within, a dynamic flow state. Include SMART goals in your care plan as described in Chapter 15. Without a plan, self-care usually remains low on the list of priorities.

Table 22-7 Self-Care Plan Strategies.

Self-Care Plan Strategies
Your self-care plan may include some of the following ideas:
• Journaling behaviors (food, activity) and feelings
• Recognizing not-knowing and bearing witness as a basis for self-compassion
• Strengthening your tolerance for difference
• Remembering that there is no one right way to create your plan
• Using relaxation, imagery, massage, play, exercise, nutrition, arts and crafts
• Integrating contemplative perspectives and practices
• Cultivating a belief system that supports well-being
• Maintaining a commitment to well-being
• Working with a partner for support and feedback
• Creating a community for practice, support, and feedback
• Being aware of one's limits
• Contemplating and realizing the profound benefits of serving others
• Becoming unattached to outcomes

Strategies for Self-Development. As we discuss strategies for self-development, note the need to develop new strategies in the face of ambiguity—for ourselves and our clients (Mitchell et al., 2013). Health care is continuously changing, as are the needs of the communities, families, and clients we serve. The importance of healthy lifestyles cannot be overemphasized, as many chronic illnesses are related to poor lifestyle choices and behaviors (Vincent & Sanchez-Birkhead, 2013). As our personal wellness/healing journey is constantly unfolding, so must our self-development. Strategies for self-development are based on the four components and dance in the cycle of life. These components outline strategies for our self-development as individuals and as the Nurse Coach. This role differs from previous nursing roles as we are not focused on quickly stabilizing heart rhythms or lab results, but coaching a new awareness in clients and empowering them to adopt choices leading to balance, meaning, and wellness.

While self-development focuses on the "I" in the integral process, it does not negate the need to care for and involve the other three quadrants, the "We", "It", and "Its" (Dossey, 2013). See Chapter 14. It also provides the skills to lead clients/patients through reflective practices or imagery to assist them in developing their mindful practice. See Chapters 11 and 12 and Appendix F.

Developing a reflective practice enables the Nurse Coach to be mindful when working with clients, and to be comfortable holding the space and not focused on "fixing" every problem, but honoring the person's own wisdom. This mindfulness occurs knowing we are complex systems interacting with our families, society, and all parts of our environmental field, bringing our histories, including our past experiences and woundedness, into the coaching relationship, but not having them interfere.

SUMMARY

- Nurse Coach self-development is an integral, lifelong journey encompassing phases of woundedness, healing, and seeking and finding meaning.
- Nurse Coach self-development includes four areas—self-reflection, self-assessment, self-evaluation, and self-care.
- Nurse Coach self-development is supported by the Theory of Integrative Nurse Coaching and other nurse theorists.
- Nurse Coach self-development both mirrors and impacts one's own unfolding healing journey, ever increasing in complexity.
- Self-development directly relates to the Nurse Coach's ability to offer a healing presence, hold the sacred space, and reflect with the client and allow inner wisdom to unfold.

NURSE COACH REFLECTIONS

After reading this chapter, the Nurse Coach will be able to bring awareness and personal insight to the following questions:

- What new awareness do I have related to my self-development?
- Have I developed a self-reflective process?
- What new awareness do I have about my self-assessment?
- How do I evaluate my self-care?
- What practices and activities revitalize me?
- How does my self-care affect the coaching process?

REFERENCES

Donner, G., & Wheeler, M. (2013). Health coaching a natural fit. *The Canadian Nurse, 109*(6), 35.

Dossey, B. M. (2013). Nursing: Integral, integrative, and holistic—local to global. In B. M. Dossey & L. Keegan (Eds.), *Holistic nursing: A handbook for practice* (6th ed., pp. 1-57). Burlington, MA: Jones & Bartlett Learning.

Dossey, L. (1982). *Space, time and medicine* (pp. 72-81). Boston, MA: Shambhala.

Dossey, B. M., Selanders, L., Beck, D. M., & Attewell, A. (2005). *Florence Nightingale today: Healing leadership global action.* Silver Spring, MD: American Nurses Association.

Eckroth-Bucher, M. (2010). Self Awareness. A Review and analysis of a basic nursing concept. *Advances in Nursing Science, 33*(4), 297–309.

Halifax, J., Dossey, B. M., & Rushton, C. H. (2007). *Being with dying: Compassionate end-of life training guide.* Santa Fe, NM: Prajna Mountain Press.

Hess, D. R., Dossey, B. M., Southard, M. E., Luck, S., Schaub, B. G., & Bark, L. (2013). *The art and science of nurse coaching: The provider's guide to coaching scope and competencies.* Silver Spring, MD: Nursesbooks.org.

Johns, C. (2013). *Becoming a reflective practitioner* (4th ed.). Hoboken, NJ: Wiley-Blackwell.

Levin, J. D., & Reich, J. L. (2013). Self-reflection. In B. M. Dossey & L. Keegan (Eds.), *Holistic nursing: A handbook for practice* (6th ed., pp. 247–259). Burlington, MA: Jones & Bartlett Learning.

McElligott, D. (2010). Healing: From concept to practice. *Journal of Holistic Nursing, 28*(4), 251–259.

McElligott, D. (2013). The nurse as an instrument of healing. In B. M. Dossey & L. Keegan (Eds.), *Holistic nursing: A handbook for practice* (6th ed., pp. 827–842). Burlington, MA: Jones & Bartlett Learning.

McElligott, D., Capitulo, K., Morris, D., & Click, E. (2010). The effect of a holistic intervention on the health promoting behaviors of registered nurses. *Journal of Holistic Nursing, 28*(3), 175–183.

Mitchell, G., Cross, N., Wilson, M., Biernacki, S., Wong, W., Adib, B., & Rush, D. (2013). Complexity and health coaching: Synergies in nursing. *Nursing Research and Practice.* Article ID 238620. Retrieved from http://dx.doi.org/10.1155/2013/238620

Nightingale, F. (1873). *Address from Miss Nightingale to the probationer-nurses in the 'Nightingale Fund' at St. Thomas's Hospital, and the nurses who were formerly trained here* (p. 2). London, UK: Spottiswoode. (Privately printed).

Vincent, A., & Sanchez-Birkhead, A. (2013). Evaluation of the effectiveness of nurse coaching in improving health outcomes in chronic condition. *Holistic Nursing Practice, 27*(3), 148–161.

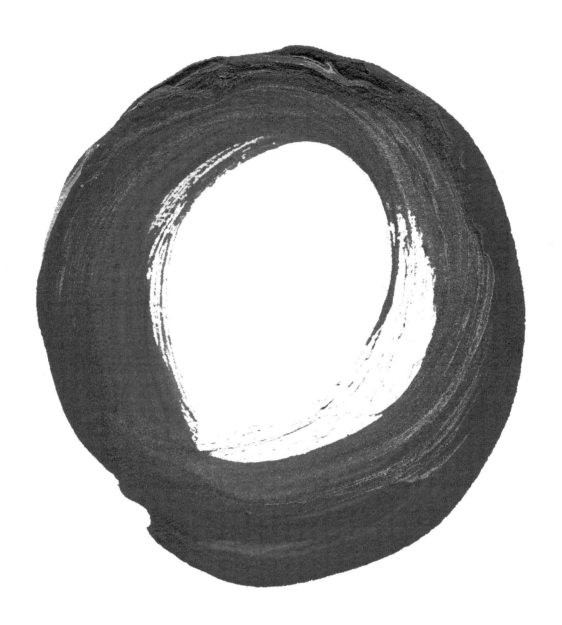

APPENDICES

*Nurse Coaching Resources
and Toolkit*

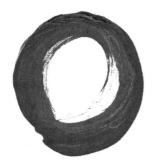

Nurse Coach and Client Guiding Principles and Agreement

Source: Copyright © 2014 by International Nurse Coach Association, 640 N.E. 124th Street, North Miami, FL 33161. For permission to use, contact www.inursecoach.com/contact/contact-us

APPENDIX A-1: NURSE COACH AND CLIENT GUIDING PRINCIPLES

Nurse Coaches join in a coaching and discovery process with clients to increase awareness of desired healthy lifestyle goals, life balance/satisfaction, behavioral change, and much more. These Nurse Coach and client guiding principles bring clarity to this dynamic coaching relationship/partnership.

Nurse Coach

- I will listen with full presence to the client's concerns and hopes in a safe, supportive environment (e.g, in person, at the office, or via Skype) to increase trust and self-exploration of health and wellness goals.
- I will respect the client as the authority for her/his own health and wellbeing.
- I will support the client's inner wisdom, intuition, and innate ability to determine the next steps in her/his process for best possible outcomes.
- I will involve the client in formulating SMART goals (Specific, Measurable, Achievable, Realistic, Time-lined) in her/his action plan.
- I will obtain the client's consent to coach in vulnerable areas and will maintain confidentiality.
- With permission, I will offer guidance and health education for specific health concerns and/or conditions (acute/chronic), nutrition, exercise, stress management, and other areas related to overall lifestyle health and wellbeing.
- I will recommend other healthcare professionals when I feel issues are outside my scope of practice and experience.
- I will be punctual and keep scheduled appointments.

Client

- I am aware that the key to my wellbeing is me.
- I am ready to make changes and to sustain change for increasing my health and wellbeing.
- I will commit to assessing my readiness for change and create an action plan towards my goals.
- I will explore new ideas, behaviors, and actions that may involve risk-taking and fear of failure and/or fear of success.
- I will take responsibility for learning new lifestyle behaviors.
- I will be open and honest so that I can access my deeper wisdom and become more self-aware.
- I will integrate self-reflection and self-care practices each day.
- I will explore obstacles towards my goals and notice my unique responses to these challenges.
- I will be punctual and keep scheduled appointments.

Nurse Coach: _____ Date: _____

Client: _____ Date: _____

APPENDIX A-2: NURSE COACH AND CLIENT AGREEMENT

Services

Coaching is a relationship of respect between the Nurse Coach and client/patient. As a Nurse Coach, I have a rich background and experience in lifestyle health and wellbeing. I will recognize your unique story, beliefs, values, history, and culture. Together, through the coaching and change process we will explore your various challenges, obstacles, and successes. (*Note*: Coaching is for individuals who are emotionally and psychologically healthy and is in no way considered or construed as any type of therapy. If needed, the Nurse Coach will refer the client to another qualified professional.)

Coaching Approach

Coaching is a collaborative partnership where trust is established. My coaching approach is integrative, integral, holistic, and skilled. This means that I see you as a whole person from many perspectives. Together, we will identify the topics and concerns that you want to work on towards change and those areas that arouse energy and excitement.

We will focus on your strengths and values to move you towards healthier lifestyle behaviors, and how you can sustain and integrate new patterns, strategies, goals, and action plans. Throughout our coaching sessions, I will share many strategies that may be new for you, such as awareness practices, relaxation, and imagery, to enhance your success.

Confidentiality

As the Nurse Coach, I will keep private any information that is shared in a coaching session. At no time, either directly or indirectly, will it be shared. As the client, you are free to share any part of the coaching sessions with others.

Conflict of Interest

If a conflict of interest arises, you and I will work together and discuss and take steps to resolve it respectfully and objectively. If this cannot be accomplished, the coaching agreement will be terminated and a referral to another professional will be made.

Session Day/Time

The coaching session will be conducted in person or on the phone at an agreed-upon day, time, and place. If the coaching session is by phone, you (client) will agree to call me (Nurse Coach) at the agreed-upon time and phone number.

We both agree to start and finish on time. If you are more than 10 minutes late for the coaching session, I will assume you have cancelled the session, and I will still need to bill you for the session.

In between coaching sessions, you are free to contact me at an agreed-upon time. We can communicate via e-mail, text, or phone.

Cancellation

If the coaching session needs to be cancelled or rescheduled, please allow at least 24 hours in advance of the scheduled session to notify me. If this is not done, you will be billed for the session. If I need to reschedule with you, I will give you a 24-hour notice.

Client Responsibilities

I see you as resourceful, accountable, and responsible for engaging in the agreed-upon action plans. Change requires an awareness, readiness, and commitment that is a call to action.

Coaching Fees and Terms of Agreement

Opening Discovery Session. The Nurse Coach may offer a free 30-minute consultation session to the potential client to introduce the coaching process and various strategies used in coaching. At the end of this time, a decision will be made about forming a coaching relationship.

Three-Month Commitment. A 3-month period is time to create a new vision for health and wellbeing, and to prioritize goals and action plans. It also allows opportunities to experience change and learn strateiges to sustain and integrate these changes into daily life.

The sessions can be two (2), 30- or 60-minute session in person, on the phone, or via Skype, or one (1) 90-minute session each month for three months. Between the sessions, the Nurse Coach can provide support to the client via exchanges of e-mails, text, or phone calls. The 3-month fee is $_____.

Monthly Agreement. Following the 3-month coaching commitment, the Nurse Coach and client can discuss monthly sessions. This may be done by either two (2) 30- to 60-minute coaching sessions or one (1) 90-minute session each month as agreed upon. If the client decides not to move forward with coaching, the agreement can be cancelled in writing or by phone within two weeks of the scheduled session with no charge. The monthly fee is $_____.

Hourly Sessions. The hourly rate is $_____. The Nurse Coach offers support between sessions.

Payment. You may pay by check or credit card (when available). (Nurse Coach will add information if she/he contracts with insurance companies or other agencies.)

The Nurse Coach and Client Agreement will be (**circle**: 3-month, monthly, or hourly) and begins:

Date: _____ Time: _____

Nurse Coach: _____ Date: _____

Client: _____ Date: _____

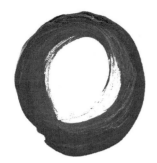

Coaching Sessions

Source: Copyright © 2014 by International Nurse Coach Association, 640 N.E. 124th Street, North Miami, FL 33161. For permission to use, contact www.inursecoach.com/contact/contact-us

APPENDIX B-1: NURSE COACH SESSION NOTES

Client/Age: _____

Session #: _____ Date: _____ Time: _____

Consent form (signed/verbal): _____ Referred by: _____

Client seeing other health professionals for: _____

Health summary (recent/pending surgery, tests, X-rays, chemotherapy, etc.): _____

Client's narrative: _____

_____

IHWA completed/Date: _____ IHWA parts complete, date, comments (see below):

Life balance and satisfaction/Date: _____

Relationships/Date: _____

Spiritual/Date: _____

Mental/Date: _____

Emotional/Date: _____

Physical (nutrition, weight, exercise)/Date: _____

Environmental (internal/external)/Date: _____

Health responsibility/Date: _____

Client's chosen topic/s for session: _____

Awareness practice/s and response/s: _____

_____

Other Nurse Coach interventions used (circle/add more: affirmations, appreciative inquiry, contracts, energy practices, imagery, motivational interviewing, somatic awareness): _____

_____

Nurse Coach Process (6 steps; not a linear process)

1. Establishing Relationship and Identifying Readiness for Change (Assessment):
Client strengths (What makes you feel good about yourself? What do you want me to know about you?): _____

_____

Internal motivation to change: _____

External motivation to change: _____

Desired areas for change: _____

Readiness for change (circle one): now—within 2 weeks—next month—in 6 months—in a year

Priority for making change: now—within 2 weeks—next month—in 6 months—in a year

Confidence/ability to make a positive change: now—within 2 weeks—next month—in 6 months—in a year

2. Identifying Opportunities, Issues, and Concerns (Diagnosis): _____

3. Establishing Client-Centered Goals (Outcomes Identification): (SMART: Specific, Measurable, Action-oriented, Realistic, Time-lined): _____

_____

_____

4. Creating the Structure of the Coaching Interaction (Planning): _____

_____

_____

5. Empowering and Motivating Client to Reach Goals (Implementation): (Strengths, Obstacles, Barriers) _____

_____

_____

6. Assisting Client to Determine the Extent to which Goals were Achieved (Evaluation):

_____

_____

Summary Plan: _____

_____

_____

Nurse Coach: _____ Date: _____ Next Session Date: _____

APPENDIX B-2: GROUP COACHING GUIDELINES

Integrative Nurse Coach Group Coaching Model

Group coaching is grounded in the Integrative Nurse Coaching core competencies. See Chapter 4. Nurse Coaches facilitate group coaching to bring clients/patients into the coaching conversation and discovery process. (*Note*: This is *not* the traditional nurse-led support groups that are focused on education around certain diseases, nutrition, exercise, stress management, etc.).

This coaching conversation is a supportive and dynamic group process that facilitates clients/patients in making lifestyle changes and/or while living with chronic health challenges (heart disease, cancer, diabetes, etc.). It is a strategy for increasing effective goal setting for positive health, human flourishing, and desired clinical outcomes. Within a group coaching setting, the Nurse Coach is alert to the clients'/patients' diverse personalities and style preferences.

The success for treating chronic conditions depends in large part on the ability of clients/patients to follow self-care recommendations that are often perceived as complex. It is not simply a lack of motivation that causes these failures, though lack of motivation may play a part. Major challenges for clients/patients living with both acute and chronic conditions are:

- following treatment plans that healthcare providers recommend
- insufficient knowledge of the condition or its treatment
- lack of the self-confidence or skills to manage the condition well
- lack of adequate support from family members or friends to initiate and sustain the structure for behavioral lifestyle changes
- physical impairments, such as poor vision, that may complicate necessary tasks (daily weighing, preparing daily medications, giving injections such as insulin, or monitoring blood sugar and blood pressure)

Group Coaching Benefits

- increased understanding of self-reflection, self-assessment, self-evaluation, self-care
- improved health behaviors (e.g., exercise, nutrition, awareness practices)
- improved positive mood
- increased confidence (self-efficacy)
- perceived social support
- improved health-related quality of life
- enhanced resilience
- identified strengths
- increased chronic disease symptoms management
- taking medications as prescribed
- developing an expanded holistic, integrative perspective of the impact of lifestyle and behaviors on symptoms and potential positive outcomes

Integrative Nurse Coach Group Process Overview

Begin each group session with an awareness practice (Appendix F) to assist with:

- focusing awareness and choice around key issues,
- using the Integrative Health and Wellness Assessment (IHWA) for beginning the group conversation (IHWA short form, Appendix C-1 and IHWA long form, Appendix C-2),
- exploring stages of change through a group imagery or awareness practice,

- creating both individual and group goals, and
- developing a personal action plan and next steps (Appendices C-1 and C-2). The group may choose the same goal such as meal planning and healthier food choices to bring to the next group session. Journaling or drawing in the session and following can deepen the self-awareness process

In the next section, the group coaching circle process details are discussed.

Group Coaching Circle Process

The group coaching circle process is a reflective practice and a time to experience a unique conversation of group trust and wisdom. The Nurse Coach, as facilitator, uses her/his presence and intuition to be aware of the collective group energy and serve as a bridge to deepen understanding. Individuals are encouraged to speak honestly and constructively about their health and wellness change process (challenges, obstacles, barriers, resistance, etc.) to focus with attention and intention.

Circle Size

The circle can be composed of 2 or more people. The ideal circle is composed of 8–12 people and can be as many as 15–20 people. Several Nurse Coaches may facilitate the larger session, open the circle, give the guidelines, and bear witness to the process. The small group circle is an excellent model for processing the content. Respect and permission is given to any person who does not want to share.

Circle Setting

The circle may occur in diverse settings such as a community center, meeting room, hospital/clinic room, or in nature. Before beginning, the Nurse Coach will create a quiet and safe environment for all to participate and to be heard.

A circle is arranged with chairs for the number of participants. A small table is placed in the center of the circle. A "talking object" is placed on the table. It can be a stone, a shell, a family heirloom, a musical instrument, or another selected object that may have special meaning for the group. The person speaking holds the talking object and the group's undivided attention.

A small tea-light candle (battery-operated) may also be placed on the table. It will be turned on as the circle process begins.

Circle Guidelines for Participants

Circle guidelines are simple:

1. Speak truthfully and constructively.
2. Stay focused on the topic or theme.
3. Listen openly.
4. Be concise (go to essence).

There are also *three* requests: *confidentiality* is maintained, there are *no interrupt*ions, and there is no need to *"fix"* any person or any situation.

Beginning the Circle Process

- **Silence.** The circle begins in silence. Participants are invited to center and focus on the breath, and are invited to close or soften their eyes to deepen the experience. A short breathing practice may follow. The group is then asked to open their eyes and notice their inner state. The Nurse Coach will offer an intention for the circle while turning on the candle.

- **Weather report and/or opening question.** A technique for checking in and beginning the circle is to ask each participant for a "weather report" as a metaphor to represent where one is in the moment. Then each participant is asked to share just one word or a brief description to answer the question.

  If a participant has had a challenging day, her/his internal weather report may be described as "raining and storming with a small glimmer of blue sky." Another way to begin the circle is to ask a simple question such as, "What energizes you in the *present*?", "What is most alive for you right now?", or "What are you hoping for being here today?"

- **Choosing a topic and setting the time.** The Nurse Coach will invite the group members to explore a theme for the session that may take five minutes or so. Examples of topics might be how to deal with resistance and/or obstacles to change or various health-related issues. After the topic is chosen, the Nurse Coach will focus on anchoring the theme and invite all participants to recall or connect with their strengths around well-being throughout the session and to go to essence with a comment/s, remembering that all participants need time to share. Initially, effective circles last at least one hour.

- **Talking object.** Participants are instructed to speak only when holding the talking object. This practice removes the option to interrupt a speaker. In this way, each person can speak without being concerned about being cut off. Those who listen also have a chance to relax into a spacious quality of listening, hopefully without judgment or prejudice, listening not only to what is said, but also to what is not said.

- **Being in the moment.** Participants are encouraged to consider the following questions before speaking: "What is the truth of what is happening at this moment? Can I articulate what I see or feel? Is what I am saying truthful and constructive? Can I look into the moment and find what is true and clear? Am I able to bring this forward at this time? Can I trust and let go of my fear as I go deeper than what I know?"

- **"I" statements.** Participants are called to speak from personal experience, using "I" statements. Silence may also be an option for a participant. As one listens, many responses can arise such as memories, associations, insights, criticism, judgment, agreement, and so on. The Nurse Coach is aware of this back conversation.

- **Rising tension.** Tension may arise in a group, particularly when a participant moves past "I" statements and talks at length. When this occurs, the Nurse Coach will ask the speaker to pause, and invite the group to be in silence, and ask the group a reflective question, and ask if anyone else would like to speak to what has just been shared. It is important to review the circle guidelines throughout the session.

- **Closing the circle.** Allow time for all to speak at the end. Do a "pearl dive" or an "ah-ha" and invite anyone to share at least one take-away from the session. End with a brief reflective breath awareness or imagery practice. This can be followed by any information for future group coaching sessions. At the end of the group process, each person creates an individual action plan for her/his next steps.

Group Coaching Case Study

Mary is a 47-year-old single parent, recently diagnosed with type 2 diabetes, hyperlipidemia, and steady weight gain over the past three years. While balancing her demanding job and her two school-age children, the PA at her doctor's office told her she needed to change her lifestyle and begin to prepare healthy meals, begin simple physical activity, lose weight, and cope better with her fatigue and depression. She was offered medication that she refused. The other option was to attend a group coaching program led by an Integra-tive Nurse Coach at the local community center with a group of patients with diabetes.

Individual and Group Goal and Process

In Mary's first session, the group chose to discuss the topic of preparing healthy meals each day. They focused on how to develop SMART (**S**mart, **M**easurable, **A**chievable, **R**ealistic, **T**ime-lined) goals and shared how to create small, sustainable, and attainable action goals for healthy meals. They were asked to keep a diary and bring their successes and challenges to the next session the following week. They also discussed how to discover resilience and inner strengths around living with diabetes.

Group Coaching Process and the Nurse Coach Leadership Model (INCLM)

The above circle process steps can successfully be used in healthcare and interprofessional collaboration. For additional information, the reader is referred to Thompson, P. A., & Baldwin, C. (2005). *Peer-spirit circling for nursing leadership: A model for conversation and shared leadership in the workplace.* Washington, DC: American Organization of Nurse Executives and PeerSpirit, Inc.

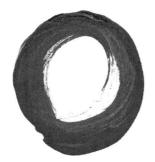

Integrative Health and Wellness Assessment

INTEGRATIVE HEALTH AND WELLNESS ASSESSMENT

Source: Copyright © 2014 by International Nurse Coach Association, 640 N.E. 124th Street, North Miami, FL 33161. For permission to use, contact www.inursecoach.com/contact/contact-us

INTEGRATIVE HEALTH AND WELLNESS ASSESSMENT™

This **INTEGRATIVE HEALTH and WELLNESS ASSESSMENT** (short form) is intended for informational purposes only. It is not a substitute for professional medical advice, diagnosis or treatment.

DIRECTIONS: This questionnaire contains statements about your present way of life, feelings, and personal habits. Please respond to each item as accurately as possible, and try not to skip any item. Indicate the frequency with which you engage in each item by shading (●) one of the following:

1 = Never   2 = Rarely   3 = Occasionally   4 = Frequently   5 = Always

Life Balance/Satisfaction   / 20   ① ② ③ ④ ⑤

1. I have balance between my work, family, friends, and self.   ○ ○ ○ ○ ○

2. I can release anxiety, worry, and fear in a healthy way.   ○ ○ ○ ○ ○

3. I use strategies (breathing, stretching, relaxation, meditation and imagery) to manage stress daily.   ○ ○ ○ ○ ○

4. I recognize negative thoughts and reframe them.   ○ ○ ○ ○ ○

Relationships   / 15

5. I create and participate in satisfying relationships.   ○ ○ ○ ○ ○

6. I feel comfortable sharing my feelings/opinion without feeling guilty.   ○ ○ ○ ○ ○

7. I easily express love and concern to those I care about.   ○ ○ ○ ○ ○

Spiritual   / 15

8. I feel that my life has meaning, value, and purpose.   ○ ○ ○ ○ ○

9. I feel connected to a force greater than myself.   ○ ○ ○ ○ ○

10. I make time for reflective practice (affirmation, prayer, meditation).   ○ ○ ○ ○ ○

Mental   / 15

11. I prioritize my work and set realistic goals.   ○ ○ ○ ○ ○

12. I ask for help/assistance when needed.   ○ ○ ○ ○ ○

13. I can accept circumstances and events that are beyond my control.   ○ ○ ○ ○ ○

©2014. International Nurse Coach Association. www.inursecoach.com
Contact the International Nurse Coach Association at programs@inursecoach.com
for permission to use the Integrative Health and Wellness Assessment™ (IHWA)
(short or long form) or about the format designed for software.

Nurse Coaching: Integrative Approaches for Health and Wellbeing

Emotional   / 20

❶ ❷ ❸ ❹ ❺

14. I recognize my own feelings and emotions. ○ ○ ○ ○ ○

15. I express my feelings in appropriate ways. ○ ○ ○ ○ ○

16. I practice forgiveness. ○ ○ ○ ○ ○

17. I listen to and respect the feelings of others. ○ ○ ○ ○ ○

Physical/Nutrition   / 20

18. I eat at least 5 servings of fruits and vegetables, and recommended whole foods (beans, nuts, etc.) daily. ○ ○ ○ ○ ○

19. I drink 6-8 glasses of water daily. ○ ○ ○ ○ ○

20. I eat real food. ○ ○ ○ ○ ○

21. I eat mindfully (concentrate on eating and not multi-tasking or eating in front of the TV). ○ ○ ○ ○ ○

Physical/Exercise   / 15

22. I do stretching or flexibility activities 2 or more days a week. ○ ○ ○ ○ ○

23. I do muscle-strengthening activities (i.e., free-weights, machines, resistance bands, body weight exercises, or carrying heavy loads) for all major muscle groups (legs, back, core, chest, arms) 2 or more days a week. ○ ○ ○ ○ ○

24. I do moderate-intensity aerobic activity (i.e., brisk walking, or any activity that makes you breathe harder with an increased heart rate) for at least 150 minutes (2 hours and 30 minutes) a week. ○ ○ ○ ○ ○

Physical/Weight   / 10

25. I maintain an ideal weight. ○ ○ ○ ○ ○

26. I have gained no more than 11 pounds in adulthood. ○ ○ ○ ○ ○

Environmental   / 15

27. I have a healthy non-toxic home environment. ○ ○ ○ ○ ○

28. I have a healthy non-toxic work environment. ○ ○ ○ ○ ○

29. I am aware of how my external environment affects my health and wellbeing. ○ ○ ○ ○ ○

©2014. International Nurse Coach Association. www.inursecoach.com

Health Responsibility   / 35   ❶ ❷ ❸ ❹ ❺

30. I believe I am key to my wellbeing and overall health, and   O O O O O
    address symptoms as they arise.

31. I know my blood pressure, triglycerides, cholesterol and glucose   O O O O O
    levels.

32. I am aware of my risk factors for disease.   O O O O O

33. I am not addicted to a substance or behavior (alcohol, drugs, sex, O O O O O
    food, gambling, shopping, exercise, internet).

34. I can work and do regular activities of daily life.   O O O O O

35. I avoid smoking or using smokeless tobacco.   O O O O O

36. I discuss/formulate a wellness plan with my primary healthcare   O O O O O
    provider, and if needed, take and know prescribed medications
    and possible side effects.

Total Score   / 180

©2014. International Nurse Coach Association. www.inursecoach.com

AREAS TO ADDRESS	SCORE	MY READINESS TO CHANGE 1= In one year 2= Within 6 months 3= Next month 4= In two weeks 5= Now	PRIORITY FOR MAKING CHANGE (1-5) 1= Never a priority 2= Very low priority 3= Medium priority 4= Priority 5= Highest priority	CONFIDENCE IN MY ABILITY TO DO IT (1-5) 1= Not at all confident 2= Not very confident 3= Somewhat confident 4= Confident 5= Very confident
Life Balance/Satisfaction	/ 20			
Relationship	/ 15			
Spiritual	/ 15			
Mental	/ 15			
Emotional	/ 20			
Physical/Nutrition	/ 20			
Physical/Exercise	/ 15			
Physical/Weight	/ 10			
Environment	/ 15			
Health Responsibility	/ 35			

©2014. International Nurse Coach Association. www.inursecoach.com

4

ACTION PLAN

Please list 3 changes that you can implement into your current lifestyle over the next 3 months:

1. _____
_____
_____
_____
_____
_____
_____

2. _____
_____
_____
_____
_____
_____
_____

3. _____
_____
_____
_____
_____
_____
_____

Additional changes, comments, thoughts:
_____
_____
_____
_____
_____
_____
_____
_____
_____
_____

©2014. International Nurse Coach Association. www.inursecoach.com

INTEGRATIVE HEALTH AND WELLNESS ASSESSMENT™

This **INTEGRATIVE HEALTH and WELLNESS ASSESSMENT** (long form) is intended for informational purposes only. It is not a substitute for professional medical advice, diagnosis or treatment.

DIRECTIONS: This questionnaire contains statements about your present way of life, feelings, and personal habits. Please respond to each item as accurately as possible, and try not to skip any item. Indicate the frequency with which you engage in each item by shading (●) one of the following:

1 = Never   2 = Rarely   3 = Occasionally   4 = Frequently   5 = Always

Life Balance/Satisfaction

	①	②	③	④	⑤
1. I have a balance between my work, family, friends, and self.	○	○	○	○	○
2. I appreciate who I am.	○	○	○	○	○
3. I am satisfied with my work and/or profession.	○	○	○	○	○
4. I feel joy and gratitude.	○	○	○	○	○
5. I am hopeful about the future.	○	○	○	○	○
6. I look forward to going to work each day.	○	○	○	○	○
7. I give time and resources to people and causes I admire.	○	○	○	○	○
8. I am comfortable with my financial situation.	○	○	○	○	○
9. I am coping well with life.	○	○	○	○	○
10. I focus on my strengths.	○	○	○	○	○
11. I get 6-8 hours of uninterrupted sleep each night.	○	○	○	○	○
12. I wake up feeling rested and alert.	○	○	○	○	○
13. I use strategies (breathing, stretching, relaxation, imagery, meditation) to manage stress daily.	○	○	○	○	○
14. I use daily positive self-talk and affirmations.	○	○	○	○	○
15. I set realistic goals.	○	○	○	○	○
16. I can release anxiety, worry, and fear in a healthy way.	○	○	○	○	○
17. I manage my time to meet my personal goals.	○	○	○	○	○
18. I take time for leisure activities (gardening, hobbies, etc.).	○	○	○	○	○
19. I take short breaks for play, laughter, and humor each day.	○	○	○	○	○
20. I recognize negative thoughts and reframe them.	○	○	○	○	○
21. I take on no more than I can manage.	○	○	●	○	○

©2014. International Nurse Coach Association. www.inursecoach.com
Contact the International Nurse Coach Association at programs@inursecoach.com
for permission to use the Integrative Health and Wellness Assessment™ (IHWA)
(short or long form) or about the format designed for software.

Relationships

	①	②	③	④	⑤
1. I create and participate in satisfying relationships.	○	○	○	○	○
2. I have people in my life that I trust and can go to for support and guidance.	○	○	○	○	○
3. I feel comfortable sharing my feelings/opinions without needing approval from others.	○	○	○	○	○
4. I am able to set boundaries and say no to others without feeling guilty.	○	○	○	○	○
5. I clearly express my needs and desires.	○	○	○	○	○
6. I am happy with the quality and quantity of nurturing physical contact (hugs, bodywork, partner yoga) I have with others.	○	○	○	○	○
7. I easily express love and concern to those I care about.	○	○	○	○	○
8. I do my part in establishing and maintaining relationships.	○	○	○	○	○
9. I feel comfortable with my sexuality.	○	○	○	○	○
10. I am happy with the quality and quantity of sexual intimacy in my life right now.	○	○	○	○	○
11. I can talk about feelings related to death and other losses with friends and/or family.	○	○	○	○	○
12. I have taken actions to ensure that my end of life care is as I would want it to be (Health Care Proxy, Living Will, Power of Attorney).	○	○	○	○	○

Spiritual

	①	②	③	④	⑤
1. I feel that my life has meaning, value, and purpose.	○	○	○	○	○
2. I feel connected to something greater than myself.	○	○	○	○	○
3. I feel in touch with my inner wisdom.	○	○	○	○	○
4. I have experiences of feeling awe and wonder.	○	○	○	○	○
5. I feel joyfulness and gratitude.	○	○	○	○	○
6. I follow a spiritual and/or religious practice.	○	○	○	○	○
7. I make time for reflective practice (affirmation, prayer, meditation).	○	○	○	○	○
8. I feel that I am growing and changing in positive ways.	○	○	○	○	○
9. I have a community that will be there for me in times of need (illness, crisis, death).	○	○	○	○	○

©2014. International Nurse Coach Association. www.inursecoach.com

Mental _____

                                  ① ② ③ ④ ⑤

1. I am open and receptive to new ideas and experiences.   ○ ○ ○ ○ ○

2. I use my imagination in considering new choices or possibilities. ○ ○ ○ ○ ○

3. I am interested in and knowledgeable about many topics. ○ ○ ○ ○ ○

4. I prioritize my work and set realistic goals. ○ ○ ○ ○ ○

5. I enjoy developing new skills and talents. ○ ○ ○ ○ ○

6. I can let go of unwanted thoughts. ○ ○ ○ ○ ○

7. I am aware of the connection between my thoughts, emotions, and health. ○ ○ ○ ○ ○

8. I ask for help/assistance as needed. ○ ○ ○ ○ ○

9. I am committed and disciplined when I take on new projects. ○ ○ ○ ○ ○

10. I follow through and work on decisions with clarity and actions steps. ○ ○ ○ ○ ○

11. I take important challenges as needed. ○ ○ ○ ○ ○

12. I can accept circumstances and events that are beyond my control. ○ ○ ○ ○ ○

Emotional _____

1. I recognize my own feelings and emotions. ○ ○ ○ ○ ○

2. I laugh freely and openly. ○ ○ ○ ○ ○

3. I include my feelings when making decisions. ○ ○ ○ ○ ○

4. I express my feelings in appropriate ways. ○ ○ ○ ○ ○

5. I recognize my intuition. ○ ○ ○ ○ ○

6. I can learn from my mistakes. ○ ○ ○ ○ ○

7. I am compassionate with myself. ○ ○ ○ ○ ○

8. I practice forgiveness. ○ ○ ○ ○ ○

9. I am authentic in my communication(s). ○ ○ ○ ○ ○

10. I listen to and respect the feelings of others. ○ ○ ○ ○ ○

11. I enjoy new challenges or experiences. ○ ○ ○ ○ ○

12. I seek guidance if necessary. ○ ○ ○ ○ ○

©2014. International Nurse Coach Association. www.inursecoach.com

Physical/Nutrition

	1	2	3	4	5
1. I eat a nutritious breakfast daily.	O	O	O	O	O
2. I eat at least 5 servings of vegetables and fruits daily.	O	O	O	O	O
3. I eat whole foods (grains, beans, seeds, nuts).	O	O	O	O	O
4. I am aware that high fat foods (i.e., trans fats, fried foods) are not healthy.	O	O	O	O	O
5. I drink 6 to 8 glasses of water daily.	O	O	O	O	O
6. I read labels for ingredients.	O	O	O	O	O
7. I eat "real" food.	O	O	O	O	O
8. I eat organic and/or local produce.	O	O	O	O	O
9. I eat my meals at home.	O	O	O	O	O
10. I have access to healthy food choices.	O	O	O	O	O
11. I am aware of foods that affect my digestion.	O	O	O	O	O
12. I am aware of any food sensitivities or food allergies.	O	O	O	O	O
13. I have a daily bowel movement.	O	O	O	O	O
14. I chew my food thoroughly.	O	O	O	O	O
15. I eat mindfully (concentrate on my eating, not multi-tasking or eating in front of the television).	O	O	O	O	O
16. I refrain from eating late at night.	O	O	O	O	O
17. I am aware of portion size and how much food I need.	O	O	O	O	O
18. I feel energy after eating.	O	O	O	O	O

Physical/Exercise

	1	2	3	4	5
1. I include exercise and/or movement as part of my daily routine.	O	O	O	O	O
2. I recognize when my body is in need of exercise and movement.	O	O	O	O	O
3. I do stretching or flexibility activities 2 or more days a week.	O	O	O	O	O
4. I do muscle-strengthening activities (i.e., free-weights, machines, resistance bands, body weight exercises, or carrying heavy loads) for all major muscle groups (legs, back, core, chest, arms) 2 or more days a week.	O	O	O	O	O
5. I do moderate-intensity aerobic activity (i.e., brisk walking, or any activity that makes you breathe harder with an increased heart rate) for at least 150 minutes (2 hours and 30 minutes) a week.	O	O	O	O	O
6. I am aware of the connection between exercise and health.	O	O	O	O	O
7. I recognize my resistance to a regular exercise plan.	O	O	O	O	O
8. I feel comfortable exercising in public places (gym, park, class).	O	O	O	O	O

©2014. International Nurse Coach Association. www.inursecoach.com

④

Physical/Weight

	①	②	③	④	⑤
1. I maintain my ideal weight.	○	○	○	○	○
2. I have gained no more than 11 pounds in adulthood.	○	○	○	○	○

Environmental

	①	②	③	④	⑤
1. I have a healthy, non-toxic home environment.	○	○	○	○	○
2. I have a healthy, non-toxic work environment.	○	○	○	○	○
3. I am aware of how my external environment affects my health and wellbeing.	○	○	○	○	○
4. I share environmental awareness with others in my workplace and community.	○	○	○	○	○
5. I make healthy environmental choices when I can.	○	○	○	○	○
6. I check my home for mold.	○	○	○	○	○
7. I use a water filter in my home.	○	○	○	○	○
8. I use natural pesticides whenever possible in my home, garden, or lawn.	○	○	○	○	○
9. I take precautions with my hobbies or work that involves chemicals (painting, stained glass, woodwork).	○	○	○	○	○
10. I refrain from using a flea collar or other topical chemical treatment on my pets.	○	○	○	○	○
11. I live in a smoke-free environment.	○	○	○	○	○
12. I am aware that what I apply to my skin absorbs into my body.	○	○	○	○	○
13. I read labels and check ingredients for my personal care products.	○	○	○	○	○
14. I use environmentally-friendly cleaning products in my home and/or workplace.	○	○	○	○	○
15. I dry clean clothes and remove the plastic before hanging them in my closet.	○	○	○	○	○
16. I microwave my food in glass and avoid plastics.	○	○	○	○	○
17. I use my cell phone and hold it away from my ear or use an earpiece or headset.	○	○	○	○	○
18. I purchase new products (shower curtain, carpeting, furniture) and ventilate the area or leave the product outside until the "off-gas" smell disappears.	○	○	○	○	○

©2014. International Nurse Coach Association. www.inursecoach.com

Health Responsibility

	①	②	③	④	⑤
1. I believe I am key to my wellbeing and overall health.	○	○	○	○	○
2. My overall health is excellent.	○	○	○	○	○
3. I receive yearly physical exams.	○	○	○	○	○
4. I know my risk factors for disease.	○	○	○	○	○
5. I pay attention to my physical wellbeing and address symptoms as they arise.	○	○	○	○	○
6. I am aware of any unusual weight loss, fever, etc., and seek the advice of my primary healthcare provider.	○	○	○	○	○
7. I have had a baseline eye examination and get regular eye examinations as recommended for my age.	○	○	○	○	○
8. I practice good oral hygiene (flossing, toothpicks, dental cleaning).	○	○	○	○	○
9. I receive regular dental preventive care (teeth cleaning every 6 months).	○	○	○	○	○
10. I check my skin for changes or suspicious moles.	○	○	○	○	○
11. I recognize changes in bowel patterns and seek professional consultation if not corrected by lifestyle change.	○	○	○	○	○
12. I know my blood pressure, cholesterol, triglycerides, and glucose levels.	○	○	○	○	○
13. I avoid smoking or the use of smokeless tobacco.	○	○	○	○	○
14. I can work and do regular activities of daily life.	○	○	○	○	○
15. I buckle my seatbelt when driving or when riding as a passenger.	○	○	○	○	○
16. I avoid talking on my cell phone when driving or doing critical tasks.	○	○	○	○	○
17. I have been free of pain or injury for the last 6 months.	○	○	○	○	○
18. I am not addicted to a substance or behavior (alcohol, drugs, sex, food, gambling, shopping, exercise, internet).	○	○	○	○	○
19. I have completed a personal health record and know where to access it.	○	○	○	○	○
20. I discuss/formulate a wellness plan with my primary healthcare provider, and if needed, take and know prescribed medications and possible side effects.	○	○	○	○	○

©2014. International Nurse Coach Association. www.inursecoach.com

6

AREAS TO ADDRESS	MY READINESS TO CHANGE 1= In one year 2= Within 6 months 3= Next month 4= In two weeks 5= Now	PRIORITY FOR MAKING CHANGE (1-5) 1= Never a priority 2= Very low priority 3= Medium priority 4= Priority 5= Highest priority	CONFIDENCE IN MY ABILITY TO DO IT (1-5) 1= Not at all confident 2= Not very confident 3= Somewhat confident 4= Confident 5= Very confident
Life Balance/Satisfaction			
Relationship			
Spiritual			
Mental			
Emotional			
Physical/Nutrition			
Physical/Exercise			
Physical/Weight			
Environment			
Health Responsibility			

©2014. International Nurse Coach Association. www.inursecoach.com

LIFE BALANCE and SATISFACTION ACTION PLAN

Please list 3 changes that you can implement into your current lifestyle over the next 3 months:

1.

2.

3.

Additional changes, comments, thoughts:

RELATIONSHIPS ACTION PLAN

Please list 3 changes that you can implement into your current lifestyle over the next 3 months:

1.

2.

3.

Additional changes, comments, thoughts:

SPIRITUAL ACTION PLAN

Please list 3 changes that you can implement into your current lifestyle over the next 3 months:

1.

©2014. International Nurse Coach Association. www.inursecoach.com

8

2. _____
_____
_____
3. _____
_____
_____
_____

Additional changes, comments, thoughts:
_____
_____

MENTAL ACTION PLAN

Please list 3 changes that you can implement into your current lifestyle over the next 3 months:
1. _____
_____
_____
2. _____
_____
_____
3. _____
_____
_____

Additional changes, comments, thoughts:
_____
_____

EMOTIONAL ACTION PLAN

Please list 3 changes that you can implement into your current lifestyle over the next 3 months:
1. _____
_____
_____
2. _____
_____
_____
3. _____
_____
_____

©2014. International Nurse Coach Association. www.inursecoach.com

Additional changes, comments, thoughts:

_____
_____

NUTRITION ACTION PLAN

Please list 3 changes that you can implement into your current lifestyle over the next 3 months:

1. _____
_____
_____

2. _____
_____
_____

3. _____
_____
_____

Additional changes, comments, thoughts:

_____
_____

EXERCISE ACTION PLAN

Please list 3 changes that you can implement into your current lifestyle over the next 3 months:

1. _____
_____
_____

2. _____
_____
_____

3. _____
_____
_____

Additional changes, comments, thoughts:

_____
_____

©2014. International Nurse Coach Association. www.inursecoach.com

10

WEIGHT MANAGEMENT ACTION PLAN

Please list 3 changes that you can implement into your current lifestyle over the next 3 months:

1. _____

   _____

   _____

2. _____

   _____

   _____

3. _____

   _____

   _____

Additional changes, comments, thoughts:

_____

_____

ENVIRONMENTAL ACTION PLAN

Please list 3 changes that you can implement into your current lifestyle over the next 3 months:

1. _____

   _____

   _____

2. _____

   _____

   _____

3. _____

   _____

   _____

Additional changes, comments, thoughts:

_____

_____

HEALTH RESPONSIBILITY ACTION PLAN

Please list 3 changes that you can implement into your current lifestyle over the next 3 months:

1. _____

   _____

   _____

©2014. International Nurse Coach Association. www.inursecoach.com

11

2. _____
_____
_____
3. _____
_____
_____

Additional changes, comments, thoughts:
_____
_____

©2014. International Nurse Coach Association. www.inursecoach.com

APPENDIX C-3: PERSONAL HEALTH RECORD

PERSONAL HEALTH RECORD (Age_____)

THIS PERSONAL HEALTH RECORD DOES NOT PROVIDE MEDICAL ADVICE. It is intended for informational purposes only. It is not a substitute for professional medical advice, diagnosis or treatment. Never ignore professional medical advice in seeking treatment. If you think you may have a medical emergency, immediately call your doctor or dial 911.

BLOOD PRESSURE

_____ Systolic (high number) (<120 desirable)

_____ Diastolic (low number) (<80 desirable)

BLOOD GLUCOSE (Fasting)

_____ Glucose (<100 desirable)

_____ If elevated, Hemoglobin A1c

BLOOD LIPIDS (Fasting)

_____ Total cholesterol (<200 desirable)

_____ HDL, good cholesterol (>50 women, >40 men desirable)

_____ LDL, bad cholesterol (<130 desirable)

_____ C-Reactive Protein (CRP)

_____ Homocysteine

HEIGHT in inches (without shoes)

Height at age 35 _____

Height at age 55 _____

WEIGHT in pounds (without shoes)

Current _____

1 year ago _____

3 years ago _____

5 years ago _____

10 years ago _____

BODY MASS INDEX (BMI)

Underweight = <18.5

Normal weight = 18.5–24.9

Overweight = 25.0–29.9 Obesity = >30

(Please see Body Mass Index tables on pp. 455–456.)

WAIST MEASUREMENT (in inches)

_____ (>35 for women or >40 for men indicates increased disease risk.)

WOMEN—Check all that apply:

❑ I discuss when to have a PAP smear with my primary healthcare provider.

❑ I discuss when to have a mammogram or thermogram with my primary healthcare provider.

❑ I discuss when to have a colonoscopy with my primary healthcare provider.

MEN—Check all that apply:

❑ I discuss when to have a prostate exam with my primary healthcare provider.

❑ I discuss when to do self-testicular exams with my primary healthcare provider.

❑ I discuss when to have a colonoscopy with my primary healthcare provider.

I take the following daily supplements:

_____   _____

_____   _____

I take the following medications (including prescription, non-prescription medications for anxiety, mood, sleep or depression):

_____   _____

_____   _____

_____   _____

FAMILY HISTORY (in immediate family, alive or deceased)

Select one for each of the following:

Y = Yes and is not under control

C = Yes and is under control via treatment/medication

N = No or not applicable

Cancer	❑ Y	❑ C	❑ N

Please specify type(s) _____

Cardiovascular Disease (heart attack, coronary heart disease, heart surgery, congestive heart failure, stroke before age 65 in women and age 55 in men)	❑ Y	❑ C	❑ N
Diabetes	❑ Y	❑ C	❑ N
High Blood Pressure	❑ Y	❑ C	❑ N
High Cholesterol	❑ Y	❑ C	❑ N
Obesity	❑ Y	❑ C	❑ N
Mental Illness	❑ Y	❑ C	❑ N

Please specify type(s) _____

Alzheimer's Disease	❑ Y	❑ C	❑ N
Suicide	❑ Y	❑ C	❑ N
Other	❑ Y	❑ C	❑ N

Please specify _____

PERSONAL HISTORY

I have been informed by my primary healthcare provider on the following health problems:

Arthritis	❏ Y	❏ C	❏ N
Asthma	❏ Y	❏ C	❏ N
Bowel Polyps	❏ Y	❏ C	❏ N
Back Problems (sciatica, musculoskeletal)	❏ Y	❏ C	❏ N
Cancer (including skin cancer melanoma)	❏ Y	❏ C	❏ N

Please specify type(s) _____

Chronic Bronchitis or Emphysema (COPD)	❏ Y	❏ C	❏ N
Cardiovascular Disease (angina, heart attack, heart surgery, congestive heart failure, stroke before age 65 in women and age 55 in men)	❏ Y	❏ C	❏ N
Diabetes	❏ Y	❏ C	❏ N
Chronic Bronchitis or Emphysema (COPD)	❏ Y	❏ C	❏ N
High Blood Pressure (140/90 or higher)	❏ Y	❏ C	❏ N
High Cholesterol (200 or higher)	❏ Y	❏ C	❏ N
Mental Illness	❏ Y	❏ C	❏ N

Please specify type(s) _____

CURRENT SYMPTOMS (within last month)

Heart flutters or frequent palpitations	❏ Y	❏ C	❏ N
Chest pain	❏ Y	❏ C	❏ N
Unusual shortness of breath	❏ Y	❏ C	❏ N
Dizziness or fainting	❏ Y	❏ C	❏ N
Temporal sensations of tingling, numbness, light-headedness	❏ Y	❏ C	❏ N
Restricted blood flow (to head, neck, legs)	❏ Y	❏ C	❏ N
Lower leg symptoms (calf muscle pain, tenderness, redness, swelling)	❏ Y	❏ C	❏ N
Trouble sleeping	❏ Y	❏ C	❏ N
Back pain or sciatica in last month	❏ Y	❏ C	❏ N

Frequent urination or unusual thirst	❏ Y	❏ C	❏ N
Vision problems	❏ Y	❏ C	❏ N
Memory loss	❏ Y	❏ C	❏ N
Increased fatigue	❏ Y	❏ C	❏ N
Digestive problems	❏ Y	❏ C	❏ N
Bowel changes	❏ Y	❏ C	❏ N
Hot flashes (hot flushes or night sweats)	❏ Y	❏ C	❏ N

Source: Used with permission. Dossey, B. M., Luck, S., & Schaub, B. G. (2012). *Nurse Coaching: Integrative Approaches for Health and Wellbeing*. North Miami, Florida: International Nurse Coach Association. www.inursecoach.com

APPENDIX C-4: BODY MASS INDEX (BMI) TABLES

Find the appropriate height in the left hand column. Label **Height**. Move across to a given weight (in pounds). The number at the top of the column is the **BMI** at that *height* and *weight*. Pounds have been rounded off.

http://www.nhlbi.nih.gov/guidelines/obesity/bmi_tbl.htm

BMI Table 1

BMI	19	20	21	22	23	24	25	26	27	28	29	30	31	32	33	34	35
Height (inches)	Body Weight (pounds)																
58	91	96	100	105	110	115	119	124	129	134	138	143	148	153	158	162	167
59	94	99	104	109	114	119	124	128	133	138	143	148	153	158	163	168	173
60	97	102	107	112	118	123	128	133	138	143	148	153	158	163	168	174	179
61	100	106	111	116	122	127	132	137	143	148	153	158	164	169	174	180	185
62	104	109	115	120	126	131	136	142	147	153	158	164	169	175	180	186	191
63	107	113	118	124	130	135	141	146	152	158	163	169	175	180	186	191	197
64	110	116	122	128	134	140	145	151	157	163	169	174	180	186	192	197	204
65	114	120	126	132	138	144	150	156	162	168	174	180	186	192	198	204	210
66	118	124	130	136	142	148	155	161	167	173	179	186	192	198	204	210	216
67	121	127	134	140	146	153	159	166	172	178	185	191	198	204	211	217	223
68	125	131	138	144	151	158	164	171	177	184	190	197	203	210	216	223	230
69	128	135	142	149	155	162	169	176	182	189	196	203	209	216	223	230	236
70	132	139	146	153	160	167	174	181	188	195	202	209	216	222	229	236	243
71	136	143	150	157	165	172	179	186	193	200	208	215	222	229	236	243	250
72	140	147	154	162	169	177	184	191	199	206	213	221	228	235	242	250	258
73	144	151	159	166	174	182	189	197	204	212	219	227	235	242	250	257	265
74	148	155	163	171	179	186	194	202	210	218	225	233	241	249	256	264	272
75	152	160	168	176	184	192	200	208	216	224	232	240	248	256	264	272	279
76	156	164	172	180	189	197	205	213	221	230	238	246	254	263	271	279	287

BMI Table 2

BMI	36	37	38	39	40	41	42	43	44	45	46	47	48	49	50	51	52	53	54
Height (inches)	Body Weight (pounds)																		
58	172	177	181	186	191	196	201	205	210	215	220	224	229	234	239	244	248	253	258
59	178	183	188	193	198	203	208	212	217	222	227	232	237	242	247	252	257	262	267
60	184	189	194	199	204	209	215	220	225	230	235	240	245	250	255	261	266	271	276
61	190	195	201	206	211	217	222	227	232	238	243	248	254	259	264	269	275	280	285
62	196	202	207	213	218	224	229	235	240	246	251	256	262	267	273	278	284	289	295
63	203	208	214	220	225	231	237	242	248	254	259	265	270	278	282	287	293	299	304
64	209	215	221	227	232	238	244	250	256	262	267	273	279	285	291	296	302	308	314
65	216	222	228	234	240	246	252	258	264	270	276	282	288	294	300	306	312	318	324
66	223	229	235	241	247	253	260	266	272	278	284	291	297	303	309	315	322	328	334
67	230	236	242	249	255	261	268	274	280	287	293	299	306	312	319	325	331	338	344
68	236	243	249	256	262	269	276	282	289	295	302	308	315	322	328	335	341	348	354
69	243	250	257	263	270	277	284	291	297	304	311	318	324	331	338	345	351	358	365
70	250	257	264	271	278	285	292	299	306	313	320	327	334	341	348	355	362	369	376
71	257	265	272	279	286	293	301	308	315	322	329	338	343	351	358	365	372	379	386
72	265	272	279	287	294	302	309	316	324	331	338	346	353	361	368	375	383	390	397
73	272	280	288	295	302	310	318	325	333	340	348	355	363	371	378	386	393	401	408
74	280	287	295	303	311	319	326	334	342	350	358	365	373	381	389	396	404	412	420
75	287	295	303	311	319	327	335	343	351	359	367	375	383	391	399	407	415	423	431
76	295	304	312	320	328	336	334	353	361	369	377	385	394	402	410	418	426	435	443

Source: Retrieved from http://www.nhlbi.nih.gov/guidelines/obesity/bmi_tbl.htm

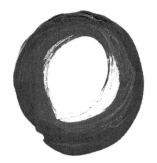

APPENDIX **D**

Integral Perspectives

Source: Copyright © 2014 by International Nurse Coach Association, 640 N.E. 124th Street, North Miami, FL 33161. For permission to use, contact www.inursecoach.com/contact/contact-us

APPENDIX D-1: SIX LINES OF DEVELOPMENT

Directions: Reflect on the six lines of development that we can consciously touch in relation to self, others, and the natural world. Explore behaviors, capacities, and strengths you wish to develop and integrate.

Line of Development	Low	Medium	High	Reflections
Cognitive: *Awareness of what is*				
Emotional: *Awareness of spectrum of emotions*				
Somatic: *Awareness of body/mind*				
Interpersonal: *Awareness of how I relate to others*				
Spiritual: *Awareness of ultimate issues and meaning*				
Moral: *Awareness of what to do*				

APPENDIX D-2: INTEGRAL SELF-DEVELOPMENT CIRCLE

Directions: Reflecting on the integral process is a way to connect all areas of our life and how to name behaviors and actions that lead to health and wellbeing. Place statements about you and your relationship to self and others that are working in each quadrant. Identify areas you want to change. Each quadrant represents one-fourth of reality. Leaving any quadrant out is incomplete. A change in one quadrant creates a change in all the other quadrants. "I"—my meaning; "IT"—my body and actions; "WE"—our shared meaning and relationships; "ITS"—group process, systems, structure.

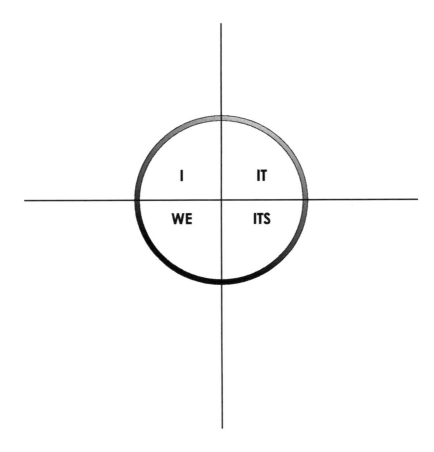

APPENDIX D-3: LOVINGKINDNESS REFLECTION

Directions: Focus your attention on your solar plexus, your chest area, and your "heart center". Breathe in and out at your own pace, and focus your awareness on your heart center. Let go of any areas of self-judgment, self-hatred, mental blockage, or numbness. Choose the phrases below that are personally meaningful to assist you with being present for suffering, transforming suffering, forgiveness, and coming home. At the end of this reflective practice period, rest in openness, inviting the feeling of gratitude to be present within and for others.

Being Present for Suffering

- May the power of lovingkindness sustain me.
- May I be happy, healthy, and strong.
- May I be free of mental suffering or distress.
- May I be free of physical pain and suffering.
- May I be able to live in this world, peacefully, joyfully, and with ease.
- May I find the inner resources to be present for suffering.
- May I fully face life (or death), loss, and sorrow.
- May I accept things as they are.
- May I be open to the pain of grief.
- May I accept my pain, knowing that it does not make me bad or wrong.
- May I accept my suffering, knowing that I am not my suffering.
- May I accept my anger, fear, and sadness, knowing that they do not limit the openness of my heart.
- May I be open with others and myself about my experience of suffering.
- May all living things everywhere, known and unknown, be happy, peaceful, and free of suffering.

Transforming Suffering

- May sorrow show me the way to compassion.
- May I realize grace in the midst of suffering.
- May this experience in some way be a blessing for me.
- May love fill and heal my body and mind.
- May I be peaceful and let go of expectations.
- May I find peace and strength that I may use my resources to help others.
- May I receive the love and compassion of others.
- May all those who are grieving be released from their suffering.
- May I offer love, knowing that I cannot control the course of life, suffering, or death.

Forgiveness

- May I let go of guilt and resentment.
- May I forgive myself for mistakes made and things left undone.
- May I forgive and be forgiven.
- May I forgive myself for not meeting my loved one's needs.
- May I accept my human limitations with compassion.

Coming Home

- May I be open to the true nature of life.
- May I open to the unknown as I let go of the known.
- May I offer gratitude to those around me.
- May I and all beings live and die peacefully.

Adapted by Barbara M. Dossey. Source: Halifax, J., Dossey, B. M., & Rushton, C. H. (2007). *Being with dying: Compassionate end-of-life-care* (pp. 78–79). Santa Fe, NM: Prajna Mountain Publishers.

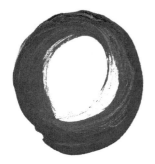

Lifestyle Health and Wellbeing Tools

Source: Copyright © 2014 by Susan Luck. Integrative Nursing Institute. Miami, Florida. For permission to use, contact www.inursecoach.com/contact/contact-us

APPENDIX E-1: INTEGRATIVE LIFESTYLE HEALTH AND WELLBEING NURSE COACH INTAKE

Reflect on your current health and what motivated you to seek a Nurse Coach at this time.

- What does being healthy mean to you?
- Describe your vitality and energy recently (over the past 3–6 months).
- Do you believe you hold the key to your wellbeing?

Sleep/Rest

Describe your sleeping patterns/habits.

- Do you have challenges falling asleep?
- Do you feel rested upon awakening?

Stress

- Are you aware of where you hold on to stress in your body?
- How do you handle life's stressors?
- Do you have supportive loving relationships?

Food Patterns

Ask yourself the following questions:

- Am I aware of how what I eat affects how I feel?
- Do my food choices support my health and wellbeing?
- What is the meaning of food in my life?
- Am I aware of emotional factors that influence my food choices, eating patterns, and behaviors?
- Do I follow any specific food plan?
- Are there foods that I avoid?
- Reflecting on my eating patterns and choices, what works and what do I want to change?
- What are my activity levels, and how do I plan to meet my needs?
- What factors, unique to me, influence my food planning and choices?
- What does my body need to be nourished?
- What are the psychological factors that influence my eating behaviors?
- What are the positive and negative associations with food that are unique to me?
- Do I choose foods that nurture my body/mind?
- Do I eat when I am hungry?
- Are there foods that I crave?
- Do I have known food allergies?
- What does my body need to enhance my energy and vitality?

Environmental

- Do I live in a healthy environment?
- Do I work in a healthy environment?
- Do I experience environmental sensitivities?
- Do I pay attention to the impact of the environment on my health?
- Am I aware of how the products I choose to use might be affecting my health?

APPENDIX E-2: SYMPTOMS CHECKLIST

This tool can assist the client and Nurse Coach to increase awareness of lifestyle factors that may act as triggers for common symptoms and to explore lifestyle changes that might be helpful to integrate into the client's personal wellness plan.

Have you experienced any of the following symptoms within the recent past (2–4 weeks)? If yes, please describe:

- prolonged fatigue
- chronic pain
- mental fogginess or trouble concentrating or poor memory and recall
- digestive problems
- increased anxiety or mood changes
- exercise intolerance (feeling exhausted following activity)
- less than 6–8 hours of sleep a night and often wake up tired
- irritable, weak, or tired if a meal is missed

APPENDIX E-3: READINESS FOR LIFESTYLE CHANGE SCALE

On a scale of 1–5 (5 = very willing)
To improve my health and wellbeing:

- I am willing to examine my lifestyle choices   1 2 3 4 5

- I am willing to learn a relaxation technique and practice daily.   1 2 3 4 5

- I am willing to engage in regular physical activity.   1 2 3 4 5

- I am willing to explore new ways of eating.   1 2 3 4 5

- I am willing to partner with a Nurse Coach for a minimum of 3 sessions.   1 2 3 4 5

APPENDIX E-4: EATING PATTERNS SURVEY

Name: _____

Date: _____

Current weight: ___ height: ___

Do you have an ideal body weight (IBW)? _____

Do you follow a special food plan? (i.e., vegan, guten or dairy free, high protein, high carbohydrates etc.). Describe:

Do you avoid certain foods? Describe:

Check all of the factors that apply to your current lifestyle and eating patterns.

☐   fast eater

☐   love to eat

☐   erratic eating patterns

☐   eat too much

☐   dislike "healthy" food

☐   eat more that 50% of meals away from home

☐   travel frequently

☐   non-availability of healthy foods

☐   do not plan meals

☐   do not like to cook

☐   reliance on convenient foods

☐   poor snack choices

☐   have a negative relationship with food

☐   struggle with eating issues

☐   emotional eater

☐   eat too much under stress

☐   eat too little under stress

☐   confused about what to eat

APPENDIX E-5: FOOD AWARENESS JOURNAL

Name: _____   Date: _____

Record the time you start and finish a meal/snack each day for 3 days (minimum). Record everything you eat and drink for all meals and snacks.

Be specific about preparation and as accurate as possible about amounts. Record any symptoms that occur after consumption (note time of onset). Symptoms may include any changes in skin, breathing, sinus congestion, digestive function, mood changes, drowsiness, fluid retention, etc. This information will help identify which (if any) foods you may be sensitive to.

Record EVERY encounter with food (meals/snacks). **Time** = start and finish; **Place** = specific room (LR, Kit, etc.), restaurant, car; **Activity** = during meal (TV, music, etc.); **With Whom** = specific person(s) present while eating; **Position** = sit, stand, lying; **Mood** = before you began eating; **Hunger** = before meal (0–3); **Food** = e.g., 1 cup steamed spinach, 2 medium dried apricots, sandwich: 4 oz roast beef, ½ cup shredded romaine, 2 slices onion, 1 thick slice tomato, 1 Tbsp real mayo.

It will also help to identify eating patterns and behaviors around food and food choices.

Date/Time	Food/Amount/Preparation	Symptoms/Observations

What did you notice about your eating pattern and choices?

APPENDIX E-6: CREATING HEALTHY EATING PATTERNS AND BEHAVIORS

Along with keeping a food journal (E-5), reflect on your eating experiences. The next step in this process is to ask yourself,

- What does healthy eating mean to me?
- What do I need to nourish myself—mind, body, and spirit?
- Do certain foods, or in combination, affect how I feel? (my digestion?, energy?, pain...?)
- How much time did I spend eating my last meal?
- How hungry was I when I ate my last meal?
- How do my emotions affect my eating choices and patterns?
- Do I take time at work to sit down when I eat?
- Do I chew, digest, and assimilate my food?
- How large are my portion sizes?
- What time is my evening meal? How long before I go to bed?
- How often do I focus on eating without doing other activities at the same time? Sometimes ___ Always ___ Rarely ___ Never ___
- What other activities do I engage in simultaneously with a meal or snack?
- What are my biggest challenges to changing the way that I eat? Describe:

Plan: I am willing to increase my awareness of my eating behaviors and patterns.

Food for thought:
- I will put my fork down between bites.
- I will chew my food more slowly.
- I will sit down when eating.
- I will purchase foods to have available at home and at work to support my health goals.
- I will savor the taste, aroma, and texture of my food and know it is nourishing every cell in my body.
- I will change an eating behavior unique to me.

List 1 to 3 new eating behaviors to begin the change process.

1. _____

2. _____

3. _____

Creating a Healing Eating Environment

Reflection: How many different specific locations do I eat in? Consider each room in the house or each place in the office as a separate location. _____

Tip: Eat in a single place in a single room at home and, if it applies, at work.

Reasoning: People tend to make subconscious associations. If you have routinely enjoyed a big bowl of ice cream in the living room, just entering that room may trigger the thought even if you are not hungry.

Select a Designated Eating Space in which ALL meals and snacks will be consumed. If you must eat at your desk, clear it off to create a peaceful eating atmosphere that separates the meal from work (i.e., keep a placemat and real utensils in a drawer).

Designated Eating Space at home: _____

_____

Designated Eating Space at work: _____

_____

Tip: When I am eating, I will only eat!

Reasoning: Just as an association between food and a particular room may be made, so can eating and engaging in a particular activity. If have you eaten in front of the TV, when the program ends do you feel full or recall eating? If the brain has been distracted and satiety does not get "registered," it is more likely to consume more food or snacks. The goal is to be more mindful and aware and includes the appearance, aroma, flavor, and portions of food during a meal. This helps you form a new relationship with food and keeps you focused on your goal of consuming healthful foods in appropriate portions.

Plan: Set a goal for the number of meals per week you will eat without any associated activity. Each week, try to increase this number.

Additional Tip: Avoid heated conversation, quick-tempo music, or talk radio; avoid reading the paper, talking on your phone, watching TV, etc.

Consider creating a healing environment while eating (i.e., soft background music, soft or natural light, quiet conversation).

Exploring Emotions, Feelings, and Eating Behaviors

Reflection: What are my emotional triggers that influence my eating behaviors? Review the different emotions you may experience and how they influence your food choices.

Tip: Try to eat only when you are relatively relaxed. Upon the first thought of food, think about how you are feeling and whether the hunger you think you have is really hunger? What else might be triggering the desire to eat? Are you seeking comfort? A moment to celebrate? What other feelings are unique for you?

Reasoning: We may eat when we feel happy or when we are sad; we eat to relax, and we eat to feel more awake and alert; we eat when we are angry, and we eat when we are joyful; we celebrate with food, and we mourn with food. This seems to be the human experience although it is also culturally based and learned behavior. The biological reason for food is, of course, is to provide nutrients to nourish and sustain health.

Plan: List the most common emotions that you associate with your specific eating behaviors or food choices. Consider new possibilities and healthier choices when experiencing emotional stressors.

Evaluate a meal when you were feeling frustrated or angry. Did it affect your food preference and eating behaviors at the time? Are there foods you choose and that you can identify that accompany specific feelings?

Mood/Emotion: _____

Reflection: _____

Establishing Healthy Eating Patterns

Reflection: Who do you spend mealtime with at work and home and socially? Consider more time with individuals who are supportive and have a positive influence upon you and your food choices and may assist you in meeting your goals.

Reflection: Am I eating because I am hungry? Review your journal over the past 3 days. Compare the amounts of food consumed in the comparison to the ratings for hunger.

Tip: Often our schedules dictate when we have to eat. Ideally, strive to eat when you are actually hungry if you have control of mealtimes. If you do not, be sure to choose portions according to your degree of hunger.

Reasoning: Many times people eat because others are eating in social settings, because they are in the habit of eating at a certain time or in a certain place, or for any number of other reasons having little if anything to do with their body sending signals that it needs fuel and nutrients.

Plan: Learn the signals your body sends when it needs nourishment. One way to do this is to delay a meal by 30–60 minutes or even skip one meal entirely. (DO NOT DO THIS if you are hypoglycemic, diabetic, or on medications.) During this time, become very aware of how you are feeling. Do you get sleepy, weak, or jittery? Do have anxiety, lose concentration, get a headache, or feel irritable? What signals does your body use to let you know it needs food? What do you crave?

Slight hunger signs: _____

Moderate hunger signs: _____

Strong hunger signs: _____

Once you learn how to rate your hunger, determine the amount of food it takes to satisfy your needs. Choose accordingly, and every now and then stop, put down your knife and fork, sit back for 2–5 minutes, and determine how much more you really need. Taking 20 minutes for a meal as discussed above is crucial to avoid overeating. If you eat slowly you will also get the signals your body sends to tell you have had enough food for the time being. If you chew your food well it will assist in all of your digestive processes.

Choose foods that are less likely to trigger blood sugar response and cravings.

These behavioral tips can be challenging to master. Tackle the behaviors you have identified that need to be changed—one at a time. Take a week or two, or even a month to work on one behavior and then move on to another. Whether you are 18 or 80 years old, there is always the possibility for changing behaviors! If you have difficulties with any modifications, your integrative Nurse Coach will guide you to enhance your success.

APPENDIX E-7: EATING WITH AWARENESS REVIEW

In assessing eating patterns and behaviors, the following guidelines are reviewed. These guidelines support optimizing digestion, absorption, assimilation, and elimination and promote optimal health and wellbeing.

Taking time for the eating experience can help to reduce cravings, control portion sizes, and enhance one's eating experience. This approach optimizes cellular and physical energy and can lower inflammation and associated symptoms triggered by an inflammatory response.

- **Eat in a setting where you feel relaxed.** These practices will all help with the digestive process, including absorption to assimilation of nutrients.
- **Chew thoroughly.** The process of digestion begins in the mouth where enzymes are secreted in saliva to break down food. Explore the texture in your mouth. If we do not properly chew and make our food morsels smaller, indigestion and other digestive problems can occur. The act of eating allows us to be mindful, and in the moment, of our exchange of energy within our foods.
- **Eat mindfully.** Become increasingly aware of how what you eat nurtures your body/mind. At the end of each meal, leave a small amount of food on your plate. Take time to feel your satiety. Breathe. Digest. Step away from the table. Observe your physical sensations. With gratitude and a sense of abundance, know you have nurtured and cared for yourself.
- **Choose foods to support your health and wellbeing.** Avoid processed, packaged, fast, and prepared foods. Broil, steam, or bake to avoid fried foods. Fresh is always best. Choose organic or local produce whenever possible.
- **Sample a variety of flavors.** By consuming small amounts of diverse herbs and flavors, you enhance taste and pleasure while benefiting from nature's chemical properties that can support your health.
- **Choose a palette of colors.** Ensure that you get enough of the important phytonutrients that assist in healthy cellular communication, intracellular energy exchange, detoxification, and nutritional balance.
  - Orange: apricots, butternut squash, cantaloupe, carrots, mangoes, nectarines, oranges, papayas, peaches, persimmons, pumpkin, tangerines
  - Yellow/green: green apples, artichokes , asparagus, avocados, green beans, broccoli, Brussels sprouts, green cabbage, cucumbers, green grapes, honeydew melon, kiwi, lettuce, lemons, limes, green onions, peas, green pepper, spinach, zucchini
  - Blue/purple: purple kale, purple cabbage, purple potatoes, eggplant, purple grapes, blueberries, blackberries, boysenberries, raspberries, raisins, figs, plums
  - Red: beets, red cabbage, cherries, cranberries, pink grapefruit, red grapes, red peppers, pomegranates, red potatoes, radishes, raspberries, rhubarb, strawberries, tomatoes, watermelon

APPENDIX E-8: GLUTEN-FREE FOOD PLAN

A gluten-free plan is completely free of all foods derived from the protein gluten found in many grains. Gluten shows up unexpectedly in many processed foods that contain additives, flavorings, stabilizers, or thickening agents. Read labels.

It is recommended to follow an elimination plan for 3 weeks to observe changes.

Type of Food	Foods Allowed	Foods to Avoid
Beverages	• vegetable juice • carbonated or mineral water • coffee, tea • almond, rice, hemp, or coconut milk	• coffee substitutes • Postum, Ovaltine • ale, beer • instant coffee if wheat flour added
Breads	• breads made from rice, gluten-free oats, sorghum, garbanzo bean, arrowroot, tapioca, soybean, corn, pure buckwheat, or potato flours • gluten-free baking mixes • rice crackers and cakes	• wheat, rye, kamut, spelt, and barley (flours, bread, rolls, crackers) • pancakes, breads, muffins, biscuits, and waffles from commercial mixes, unless stated "gluten-free" • all crackers, pretzels, bread crumbs, breaded foods made from above grains
Cereals	• amaranth, millet, or corn cereal • quinoa, rice/cream of rice, cream of buckwheat, oatmeal • puffed corn or rice	• all products made with wheat, rye, barley, kamut, spelt, farro, and wheat germ
Desserts	• desserts made with allowed flours • meringues • rice pudding • apple sauce • plain yogurt with fresh fruit	• commercial ice creams • ice cream cones • prepared puddings • mixes • homemade puddings thickened with flour • pies, pastries • cakes, cookies, doughnuts
Fruits	• all	• none
Meats, fish, eggs, cheese (if not lactose- or casein-intolerant)	• all meats, poultry, and fish prepared without breading • eggs	• breaded meat, poultry, fish, patties, croquettes and loaves with bread crumbs • canned meats, dishes with coldcuts and frankfurters (unless guaranteed pure meat) • creamed sauces, gravies, cheese spreads, spreads with wheat flour

(*continues on next page*)

(*Continued*).

Type of Food	Foods Allowed	Foods to Avoid
Potatoes/pasta/grains	• white and sweet potatoes • rice and bean thread noodles and pasta • quinoa/corn pasta	• spaghetti, noodles, macaroni, dumplings made from wheat, spelt, kamut • barley soup or pilaf
Vegetables	• unlimited—raw, steamed, baked	• any prepared with bread crumbs or cream sauces

As you eliminate gluten, become aware of any changes in symptoms, including digestion, cognitive function, and aches and pains. Refer back to symptoms checklist (Appendix E-2) after 1 week and note any changes.

APPENDIX E-9: MEDITERRANEAN FOOD PLAN: AN ANTI-INFLAMMATORY APPROACH

Inflammation is typically part of the body's natural response to infection, injury, food sensitivities, allergens, and other foreign substances in the body, including chemicals in our environment. Removing inflammatory triggers is an important intervention to calm down the inflammatory response.

As a Nurse Coach and nurse educator, the following evidence-based guidelines can be helpful to share with clients and families.

Anti-inflammatory choices: fish (wild salmon, halibut, mackerel), nuts, and pure unprocessed oils. Emphasis on reducing saturated/trans fats (animal fats, processed oils) and replacing with quality monounsaturated/polyunsaturated fats (avocado, olive oil, seeds, nuts, omega-3-rich eggs). Avoid foods high in saturated animal fats in fatty meats, whole milk dairy products, and trans fats (in hydrogenated oils, processed foods).

Proper fatty acid composition: Foods rich in unsaturated fats include legumes, seeds, and nuts as part of the daily diet. Lower consumption of commercially produced animal products. Maintain a high level of healthy omega-3 essential fatty acids, including walnuts, flax seeds, and fish oils.

Healthy fish: Choose low-mercury, low-toxin seafood, including wild salmon, scallops, and flounder. Avoid farm-raised fish.

Predominantly plant-based diet: Increase plant-based foods including vegetables and fruits. Emphasize cruciferous vegetables, flavonoid-rich fruits (especially red/purple/blue/black fruits including all berries) with high levels of phytonutrients and antioxidants, vitamins, and minerals.

Healthy protein: Plant-based proteins including beans and whole grains (alkaline preferred): quinoa, millet, buckwheat. Choose pasture-raised, chemical-free animal products.

Elimination food plan: Gluten- and casein-free plan for minimum of 3 weeks if suspected of sensitivity or symptoms including altered digestion, low energy, or any other symptoms. Observe changes. See symptoms checklist, Appendix G-8.

Low toxic burden: Minimizes toxic burden of food: avoid added hormones, pesticides, antibiotics, and all artificial additives and preservatives.

Choose organic: Fruits and vegetables and animal products whenever possible (local produce is the next best choice).

High fiber content: Fiber helps slow the insulin response and optimize digestive health, elimination, and detoxification pathways (minimum 35 g/day).

Optimize all elimination pathways: skin, kidneys, respiration, bowels.

Lower glycemic load: Avoid large meals. Eat smaller, more frequent meals and snacks to keep blood sugar/insulin levels in desirable ranges.

Additional Lifestyle Factors to Lower Inflammation

Exercise moderately: 3–5 times a week, including brisk walking (along with weight loss plan as needed).

Manage stress: Relaxation and mindfulness practices.

Get adequate (restful) sleep: Elevated cortisol can trigger inflammation.

Elimination Plans

These plans can be explored with clients along with awareness practices to self-assess effectiveness of this personalized approach.

Comprehensive elimination diet: Eliminate alcohol, caffeine, sugar, citrus, corn, dairy, soy, egg, gluten-containing grains, and red meats/processed meats for a specified time period (3 weeks minimum) followed by intentional re-introduction of foods slowly to determine food triggers.

Modified elimination diet: A modified diet to eliminate specific trigger foods per individual need, based on known triggers and/or laboratory assessment or a gluten-free plan with self-awareness practices to identify possible food triggers are very useful. See Appendix G-9.

Gastrointestinal support: Probiotic replacement. Increase fiber, exercise, and elimination of refined foods for healthy digestion and elimination. Increase intake of clean fluids.

Source: Used with permission. Luck, S. (2013). Nutrition. In Dossey, B. M., & Keegan L. *Holistic nursing: A handbook for practice* (6th ed., pp. 261–293). Burlington, MA: Jones & Bartlett Learning.

APPENDIX E-10: HYPOGLYCEMIC FOOD PLAN

Hypoglycemia or low blood sugar occurs when the level of sugar in the blood drops to below 70 milligrams per deciliter. Symptoms can include weakness, sweating, dizziness, confusion and shakiness. Symptoms can be avoided by following a food plan that keeps blood sugar levels stable throughout the day and by planning healthy meals in advance.

If you have any of these symptoms or any from the symptoms checklist (Appendix E-2), you may want to consider the following approach:

- Eliminate caffeine, soda, fruit juices, white flour, white sugar, white rice, and white bread.
- Increase fluids—filtered water, herbal teas, and green juices.
- Limit fruits—2/day in 4 portions. Avoid grapes and bananas (highest in sugar).
- Consume unlimited vegetables—raw, steamed, or baked depending on your preference (*Note*: carrots, peas, and beets are highest in sugar).
- Consume several smaller meals throughout the day (3 small meals + 3 snacks). Each serving should consist of protein (fish, chicken, beans, whole grains, nuts, eggs, or dairy).

Sample healthy snacks and/or small meals to integrate into your food plan:

- hummus with vegetables or crackers (gluten-free if needed)
- 2 tablespoons almonds, sunflower seeds, or walnuts
- avocado slices with tomatoes (guacamole) and "handful" of chips
- 2 tablespoons almond or peanut butter on celery or crackers
- boiled egg with 1 slice whole-grain or gluten-free bread
- salmon salad or sardines on bed of lettuce with olive oil and lemon juice
- 3 oz grilled chicken breast with steamed or grilled asparagus or green beans
- 3 oz grilled fish with ½ sweet potato
- 1 cup lentil soup with ½ cup brown rice or quinoa
- 3 oz tofu with mixed vegetables
- low-fat plain Greek yogurt with 1/3 cup berries (blueberry, raspberry, strawberry)
- Mediterranean salad with garbanzo beans, olives, tomatoes, feta cheese

APPENDIX E-11: EXERCISE AND MOVEMENT SURVEY

Rate your motivation for including exercise into your life   ☐ Low ☐ Medium ☐ High

Do you participate in any of the following activities?

Activity Type	Frequency per Week	Duration
Stretching		
Walking		
Cardio/aerobics		
Running		
Yoga (Pilates)		
Swimming		
Sports (tennis, spinning, volleyball, etc.)		
Others		

APPENDIX E-12: EXERCISE AND MOVEMENT CALENDAR

Name _____ Date _____ Age _____

Circle the benefits you are hoping for. *My goal is to:*

- Improve my sleep.
- Lose weight.
- Improve my mood.
- Improve my endurance.
- Unload daily stress.
- Slow down my aging process.
- Decrease pain.
- Improve mental function and decrease risk of dementia.
- Improve my immune system.
- Improve strength and build muscle.
- Reduce my risk for injuries.
- Improve my cholesterol.
- Decrease my blood pressure.
- Reduce my risk of stroke and heart attack.
- Improve my performance in a sport.
- Improve my tone and look better.
- OTHER

Record in each box the activity you engaged in and the amount of time. If you did nothing that day, write a note to describe why you did not exercise.

Monday	Tuesday	Wednesday	Thursday	Friday	Saturday	Sunday

Summarize weekly observations on your strengthening, flexibility, and accomplishments on the back of this sheet.

APPENDIX E-13: EXERCISE AND MOVEMENT GUIDELINES

Goal-setting: Set up goals for what you want to accomplish and how you will do it. Find time every day for movement and/or exercise. Writing down your plan, your program, and your goals ahead of time helps you achieve them. Set up a weekly routine, and log your workouts.

Regular routine: Developing consistent habits is the key to excellent fitness.

Many small steps go a long way: Make a habit of taking advantage of the many small things in your everyday life that give you more strength and endurance. Park your car further away from work or if possible, walk or bike to and from work. Take the stairs. Stretch and do isometrics at your desk, at meetings, while waiting in line, etc. Small bouts of mini workouts throughout the day can be effective and add up to a workout at the end of your day.

Variety: Overall fitness is best achieved by a variety of exercise routines that contribute to strength, endurance, flexibility, balance, and coordination. Mix it up with different activities and training modes that challenge you and work your whole body. Try new forms of movement, dance, and exercise routines. Long walks can be mixed with a yoga session, a dance night, and a zumba or gym workout.

Get your heart beating: Make at least half of your workouts "huff and puff" workouts, where you really get your heart beating. Intervals are great at building speed, endurance, strength, cardio health, and raising your metabolic rate to burn more calories throughout the day.

Exercise with others: Find a walking buddy or join a gym, yoga studio, tennis club, swim club, bike club, etc. Working out regularly and together is more fun and more effective. You make new friends, get more motivation, get some valuable tips, and keep it fun and consistent by exercising with others.

Eat a whole-foods clean diet: Optimize your training goals by eating an antioxidant-rich and anti-inflammatory plant-based diet for more stamina, flexibility, and capacity. With vigorous strength training, more protein is needed. With vigorous, long-distance cardio exercise, more complex carbs are needed. For best results, follow a Mediterranean, vegetarian, or paleolithic diet.

Drink enough liquids: Drink at least half your liquid intake as water. A recovery drink with some protein (whey) or a protein-rich meal are helpful in muscle recovery directly after a workout.

Use the right equipment, shoes, and clothing: Find out what is needed for the best comfort and performance for the exercise you are pursuing. The wrong equipment, gear, shoes, or clothes can make your efforts less comfortable, effective, or safe.

Learn about your activity, and get help, coaching, and advice: A personal trainer, coach, magazines, websites, apps, DVDs, CDs, and books can all give you more knowledge, motivation, and inspiration to keep moving, keep improving, and stay on track.

APPENDIX E-14: ENVIRONMENTAL HEALTH PREVENTION STRATEGIES

- **Choose your food wisely.** Eat as organically as possible. Limit animal fats as chemicals get stored in fat, including endocrine disruptors and heavy metals that accumulate in the food chain. The higher your animal protein source, the greater the potential toxic load. Choose seasonal and local foods. Fish consumption: Avoid fish like tuna and swordfish that may contain high levels of synthetic chemicals. Wild-caught salmon and cod are better choices.

- **Avoid pesticides.** If you cannot buy all organic food, try to pick and choose. Certain crops are more heavily sprayed than others. The Environmental Working Group database (www.ewg.org) offers guidelines on the fruits and vegetables containing both the highest pesticide residues and the lowest. Produce containing the highest pesticide levels include: peaches, apples, bell peppers, celery, nectarines, strawberries, cherries, lettuce, grapes, pears, spinach, and potatoes. Wash all fruits and vegetables thoroughly before consuming, or peel them if they are not organically grown.

- **Support your body's natural ability to detoxify.** Use a sauna or steam bath to sweat out toxins. Use a dry loofa skin brush. Drink filtered water. Increase fiber found in whole grains, beans, vegetables, fruits, seeds (flax), and nuts. Eat cruciferous vegetables high in glucosinolates and sulforaphane, including watercress and broccoli. Include green tea, curcumin, alpha lipoic acid, and resveratrol to support detoxification pathways.

- **Take precautions with cell phones and electromagnetic fields (EMFs).** Use the speaker function or an earpiece to decrease your exposure. Avoid sleeping with your phone under your pillow or in your pocket or bra.

- **Preparing for pregnancy and breastfeeding.** Be vigilant about chemicals. Become aware of what you can eliminate to be the healthiest you can be in preparation for pregnancy. Follow guidelines on fish for pregnant women listed at: www.american-pregnancy.org/pregnancyhealth/fishmercury.htm. Be aware of chemicals in your foods and in your personal care products when breastfeeding.

- **Know your water supply.** Find out whether your local community's water testing program checks for hormone-disrupting chemicals and heavy metals. Not all household filters work effectively on chemicals, and, unfortunately, not all bottled water is checked either. Read your water quality reports. If you drink purified water out of plastic bottles, do not leave the bottles in your car or the hot sun for any length of time; heat activates the molecules in the plastic, which increases the rate at which the polycarbons leach into the water. Filter your tap water—both for drinking and bathing/showering as your skin absorbs contaminants.

- **Avoid using plastics.** According to ongoing research, avoid bisphenol A in plastics. The "safest" plastics are marked with the recycling codes 2, 4, and 5. Never let infants chew on soft plastic toys and avoid microwaving food in a plastic bowl or covered in plastic wrap. A good rule of thumb is that the softer the plastic, the more chemicals. Buy in bulk and store foods in glass jars. Reuse hard plastic tubs. Limit use of plastic bags and cling wrap products. Assess the amount of plastic in your life and try to reduce it by five. For example: Bring a reusable mug to your local coffee stop. Buy a refillable glass or earthenware water jug. Invest in glass food storage containers that can be washed and reused for a lifetime. Use reusable cloth totes for groceries. Replace your vinyl shower curtain with one made of fabric.

- **Evaluate kitchen ware.** Replace your non-stick pots and pans with ceramic or glass cookware. Avoid aluminum pots and pans.

- **Avoid artificial fragrances.** Look for products that are fragrance-free. One artificial fragrance can contain hundreds of potentially toxic chemicals. Avoid synthetic fragrances in perfumes, air fresheners, and scented candles.
- **Evaluate your personal product use.** Become aware of what you put on your skin. Women are using an average of 12 products daily with over 60 total ingredients. Men use 6 products with over 80 ingredients. Check out your products at www.safecosmetics.org
- **Exercise your rights as a consumer.** Never doubt the power of consumer demand. Ask for green products when you do not see them in your neighborhood stores. If you have a talent for organizing and recruiting people, use it to develop community ordinances regarding the use of chemicals in public places. Encourage young people to learn more about environmental issues and to pursue research into redesigning the future.
- **Become an environmental detective.** Investigate the chemicals in your home, work, and community. Take action steps to create healthier environments.
- **Become an environmental advocate.** Support local and federal clean air and water initiatives. Support elected officials who make a clean environment their priority.

Together, we can create a healthier future for us all.

For more information, see:
Environmental Working Group: www.ewg.org
Earthrose Institute: www.earthrose.org

Source: Used with permission. Luck, S. (2013). Environmental health. In Dossey, B. M., & Keegan, L. *Holistic nursing: A handbook for practice* (6th ed., pp. 633–677). Burlington, MA: Jones & Bartlett Learning.

APPENDIX E-15: COMMON ENDOCRINE DISRUPTORS, HEALTH RISKS, AND PREVENTION TIPS

Living in today's world presents many environmental challenges. The following is a list of common hormonal and endocrine disruptor chemicals (EDCs) that we encounter in our daily lives. After reviewing this list, reflect on your personal and workplace environment and how you can begin to lower your toxic exposures and your "body burden" by making new choices.

Bisphenol A (BPA)

Health Risks

Bisphenol A (BPA) is a synthetic hormone and one of the most studied for its links to breast and other cancers, reproductive problems, obesity, early puberty, and heart disease. BPA is a polycarbonate plastic used primarily to manufacture durable epoxy resins and strong, clear polycarbonate plastic. It is used in a multitude of products ranging from protective food can linings, to bullet-resistant security shields used by police officers, to medical supplies including IV tubing.

References

1. Rochester, J. R. (2013). Bisphenol A and human health: A review of the literature. *Reproductive Toxicology, 42*(12), 132–155. doi:10.1016/j.reprotox.2013.08.008

2. Rochefort, H. (2013). Bisphenol A and hormone-dependent cancers: Potential risk and mechanism. *Médecine Sciences (Paris), 29*(5), 539–544. doi:10.1051/medsci/2013295019

3. Lee, H. A., Kim, Y. J., Lee, H., Gwak, H. S., Park, E. A., Cho, S. J., Kim, H. S., Ha, E. H., & Park, H. (2013). Effect of urinary bisphenol A on adrogenic hormones and insulin resistance in preadolescent girls: A pilot study from the EWHA birth & growth cohort. *International Journal of Environmental Research and Public Health,* 10(11), 5737–5749. doi:10.3390/ijerph10115737

Prevention Tips

- Choose fresh (or frozen) instead of canned products since most food cans are lined with BPA.
- Avoid plastics marked with a "PC" for polycarbonate, or label #7.
- Avoid plastic water bottles.
- Avoid microwaving in plastic (including covering with plastic wrap; use glass or paper).
- Avoid thermal paper (supermarket receipts) as it is often coated with BPA. Wash hands after handling.

◇ Find more tips at:

http://www.ewg.org/bpa/.
http://www.factsaboutbpa.org/bpa-safety/bpa-basics#sthash.ZwNKr5WM.dpuf

The Environmental Working Group (EWG) has become a leader in environmental advocacy that empowers people to live healthier lives in a healthier environment. They combine consumer choice and civic action with breakthrough research for an informed public. www.ewg.org

Dioxin

Health Risks

Dioxins form during many industrial processes when chlorine or bromine is burned in the presence of carbon and oxygen. Dioxins can disrupt the delicate ways that both male and female sex hormone signaling occurs in the body. Recent research has shown that exposure to low levels of dioxin in the womb and early in life can both permanently affect sperm quality and lower the sperm count in men during their prime reproductive years. Dioxins are very long-lived, build up both in the body and in the food chain, are potent carcinogens, and can also affect the immune and reproductive systems.

References

1.   Manuwald, U., Velasco, M., Berger, J., Manz, A., & Baur, X. (2012). Mortality study of chemical workers exposed to dioxins: Follow-up 23 years after chemical plant closure. *Occupational and Environmental Medicine, 69*(9), 636–642. doi:10.1136/oemed-2012-100682

2.   Marques, M., Laflamme, L., & Gaudreau, L. (2013). Estrogen receptor α can selectively repress dioxin receptor-mediated gene expression by targeting DNA methylation. *Nucleic Acids Research, 41*(17), 8094–8106. doi:10.1093/nar/gkt595

3.   Papoutsis, A. J., Selmin, O. I., Borg, J. L., & Romagnolo, D. F. (2013, October). Gestational exposure to the AhR agonist 2,3,7,8-tetrachlorodibenzo-*p*-dioxin induces BRCA-1 promoter hypermethylation and reduces BRCA-1 expression in mammary tissue of rat offspring: Preventive effects of resveratrol. *Molecular Carcinogenesis,* advance online publication. doi:10.1002/mc.22095

Prevention Tips

The ongoing industrial release of dioxin has meant that the American food supply is widely contaminated. Products including meat, fish, milk, eggs, and butter are most likely to be contaminated.

*   Lower your exposure by eating fewer animal products.
*   Choose grass-fed and naturally raised animal products.

Atrazine

Health Risks

Atrazine is the common name for an herbicide that is widely used to kill weeds. Atrazine is used on crops such as sugarcane, corn, pineapples, sorghum, macadamia nuts, and on evergreen tree farms and for evergreen forest regrowth. Atrazine is a potent endocrine disruptor. Researchers have found that exposure to even low levels of the herbicide can turn male frogs into females that can produce completely viable eggs. Atrazine is widely used on the majority of corn crops in the United States, and due to runoff, is a pervasive drinking water contaminant.

References

1.   Tyrone, B. H., Case, P., Chui, S., Chung, D., Haeffele, C., Haston, K., Lee, M., Mai, V. P., Marjuoa, Y., Parker, J., & Tsui, M. (2006). Pesticide mixtures, endocrine disruption, and amphibian declines: Are we underestimating the impact? *Environmental Health Perspectives, 114* (Suppl. 1), 40–50.

2.   Hayes, T. B., Anderson, L. L., Beasley, V. R., de Solla, S. R., Iguchi, T., Ingraham, H., Kestemont, P., & Willingham, E. (2011). Demasculinization and feminization of male gonads by atrazine: Consistent effects across vertebrate classes. *Journal of Steroid Biochemistry and Molecular Biology, 127*(1–2), 64–73. doi:10.1016/j.jsbmb.2011.03.015

3.   Omran, N. E., & Salama, W. M. (2013, November). The endocrine disrupter effect of atrazine and glyphosate on *Biomphalaria alexandrina* snails. *Toxicology and Industrial Health.* Advance online publication. doi:10.1177/0748233713506959

Prevention Tips

- Buy organic produce including corn and corn-based products.
- Purchase a drinking water filter certified to remove atrazine.
- Read herbicide labels when purchasing for use in gardens and small farms.

◇   Find more tips at:

   http://www.ewg.org/report/ewgs-water-filter-buying-guide/
   http://www.atsdr.cdc.gov/PHS/PHS.asp?id=336&tid=59

Phthalates

Health Risks

Phthalate esters of phthalic acid are mainly used as plasticizers and are added to plastics to increase their flexibility. They are found in a wide variety of common products including plastics, cosmetics, pharmaceuticals, baby care products, building materials, modeling clay, automobiles, cleaning materials, and insecticides. Phthalates are readily absorbed through the skin. Phthalates are considered to be endocrine disruptors because of their complex effects on several hormonal systems including the estrogen and androgen hormone systems. Research has linked phthalates to hormone changes, lower sperm count, less mobile sperm, birth defects in the male reproductive system, obesity, diabetes, and thyroid irregularities. Studies have shown that nail salon workers, exposed to phthalates and other chemicals, have high rates of infertility and birth defects in offspring.

References

1.   Albert, O., & Jégou, B. (2014). A critical assessment of the endocrine susceptibility of the human testis to phthalates from fetal life to adulthood. *Human Reproduction Update, 20*(2), 231–249.

2.   Lambrot, R., Muczynski, V., Lécureuil, C., Angenard, G., Coffigny, H., Pairault, C., Moison, D., ... & Rouiller-Fabre, V. (2009). Phthalates impair germ cell development in the human fetal testis in vitro without change in testosterone production. *Environmental Health Perspectives, 117*(1), 32–37. doi:10.1289/ehp.11146

3.   Mankidy, R., Wiseman, S., Ma, H. & Giesy, J. P. (2013). Biological impact of phtha-
        lates. *Toxicology Letters, 217*(1), 50–58. doi:10.1016/j.toxlet.2012.11.025

4.   Schecter, A., Lorber, M., Guo, Y., Wu, Q., Yun, S. H., Kannan, K., Hommel, M., ... &
        Birnbaum, L. S. (2013). Phthalate concentrations and dietary exposure from food
        purchased in New York State. *Environmental Health Perspectives, 121*(4), 473–479.
        doi:10.1289/ehp.1206367

Prevention Tips

*   Avoid plastic food containers, children's toys (some phthalates are already banned in
    children's products), and plastic wrap made from PVC, which has the recycling label
    #3.
*   Read the labels and avoid products that simply list added "fragrance," since this catch-
    all term sometimes means hidden phthalates.
*   Personal care products may also contain phthalates.

◇   Find phthalate-free personal care products with EWG's Skin Deep Database:

    http://www.ewg.org/skindeep/

Perchlorates

Health Risks

Perchlorates are very reactive chemicals that are used mainly in explosives, fireworks, and
rocket motors and as a component in rocket fuel. They contaminate much of our produce
today. They are soluble in water and generally have high mobility in soil as they are released
into the air and eventually settle primarily via rainfall and enter the body through food or
water. The main target organ for perchlorate toxicity in humans is the thyroid gland. Perchlorate has been shown to partially inhibit the thyroid's uptake of iodine. Metabolism and
endocrine function can be altered in adults and is critical for proper brain and organ development in infants and young children.

References

1.   EPA (U.S. Environmental Protection Agency) (2014, March). *Emerging Contami-
        nants Fact Sheet – Perfluorooctane Sulfonate (PFOS) and Perfluorooctanoic Acid
        (PFOA)*. http://www2.epa.gov/sites/production/files/2014-04/documents/fact-
        sheet_contaminant_pfos_pfoa_march2014.pdf

2.   Blount, B. C., Pirkle, J. L., Oserloh, J. D., Valentin-Blasini, L., & Caldwell, K. L. (2006).
        Urinary perchlorate and thyroid hormone levels in adolescent and adult men and
        women living in the Unites States. *Environmental Health Perspectives,* 114(12),
        1865–1871. doi:10.1289/ehp.9466

3.   Leung, A. M., Braverman, L. E., He, X., Schuller, K. E., Roussilhes, A., Jahreis, K., &
        Pearce, E. (2012). Environmental perchlorate and thiocyanate exposures and infant
        serum thyroid function. *Thyroid,22*(9), 938–943. doi:10.1089/thy.2012.0058

4.   Schreinemachers, D. M. (2011). Association between perchlorate and indirect indi-
        cators of thyroid dysfunction in NHANES 2001-2002, a cross-sectional, hypothe-
        sis-generating study. *Biomarker Insights, 6*, 135–146. doi:10.4137/BMI.S7985

Prevention Tips

- Clean produce well.
- Reduce potential effects by making sure you are getting enough iodine in your diet and use iodized salt.
- Reduce perchlorate exposure in your drinking water by using a water filter.

◇ Find more tips at:

http://www.ewg.org/report/ewgs-water-filter-buying-guide

Flame (Fire) Retardants

Health Risks

Brominated flame retardants (BFRs) are a group of compounds that have received much attention in recent years. Also known as polybrominated diphenyl ethers (PBDEs), they have been found in people and wildlife around the globe. These chemicals can imitate thyroid hormones in our bodies and disrupt normal function and metabolic activity.

References

1. Eskenazi, B., Chevrier, J., Rauch, S. A., Kogut, K., Harley, K. G., Johnson, C., Trujillo, C., Sjodin, A., & Bradman, A. (2013). In utero and childhood polybrominated diphenyl ether (PBDE) exposures and neurodevelopment in the CHAMACOS study. *Environmental Health Perspectives, 121*(2), 257–262. doi:10.1289/ehp.1205597

2. Johnson, P. I., Stapleton, H. M., Mukherjee, B., Hauser, R., & Meeker, J. D. (2013). Associations between brominated flame retardants in house dust and hormone levels in men. *Science of the Total Environment, 445–446*, 177–184. doi:10.1016/j.scitotenv.2012.12.017

3. Du, G., Hu, J., Huang, H., Qin, Y., Han, X., Wu, D., Song, L., Xia, Y., & Wang, X. (2013). Perfluorooctane sulfonate (PFOS) affects hormone receptor activity, steroidogenesis, and expression of endocrine-related genes in vitro and in vivo. *Environmental Toxicology and Chemistry, 32*(2), 353–360. doi:10.1002/etc.2034

Prevention Tips

- Better toxic chemical laws that require chemicals to be tested before they go on the market would help reduce our exposure.
- Use a vacuum cleaner with a HEPA filter, which can cut down on toxic-laden house dust.
- Avoid reupholstering foam furniture and removing old carpet as the padding underneath may contain PBDEs.

◇ Find more tips at:

http//www.ewg.org/pbdefree/

Lead

Health Risks

Lead has been linked to multiple health effects, including brain damage, lowered IQ, hearing loss, miscarriage, premature birth, increased blood pressure, kidney damage, and nervous system problems. Lead may affect the body by disrupting hormones. Children are the most vulnerable. Research has also shown that lead can disrupt hormone signaling and the stress response implicated in high blood pressure, diabetes, anxiety, and depression.

References

1.   Chen, A., Kim, S. S., Chung, E., & Dietrich, K. N. (2013). Thyroid hormones in relation to lead, mercury, and cadmium exposure in the National Health and Nutrition Examination Survey, 2007–2008. *Environmental Health Perspectives, 121*(2), 181–186. doi:10.1289/ehp.1205239

2.   Turker, G., Ozsoy, G., Ozdemir, S., Barutçu, B., & Gökalp, A. S. (2013). Effect of heavy metals in the meconium on preterm mortality: Preliminary study. *Pediatrics International, 55*(1), 30–34. doi:10.1111/j.1442-200X.2012.03744.x

3.   Woimant, F., & Trocello, J. M. (2014). Disorders of heavy metals. *Handbook of Clinical Neurology. 120*, 851–864. doi:10.1016/B978-0-7020-4087-0.00057-7

Prevention Tips

•   Take caution when removing old paint, which is a major source of lead exposure.
•   When doing home renovations, purchase home kits to test for lead on surfaces and in dust and use a mask as dust may contains lead in older homes.
•   Using a good water filter can reduce your exposure to lead in drinking water, especially from older pipes.

◇   Find more tips at:

       http://www.ewg.org/report/ewgs-water-filter-buying-guide/

Arsenic

Health Risks

Arsenic is omnipresent in our natural environment. In small amounts, arsenic can cause skin, bladder, and lung problems. Arsenic can interfere with normal hormone functioning in the glucocorticoid system, which regulates how our bodies process sugars and carbohydrates and has been linked to weight gain/loss, protein wasting, immunosuppression, insulin resistance (which can lead to diabetes), osteoporosis, growth retardation, and high blood pressure.

       Many outdoor wood structures such as playgrounds and decks have been treated with copper-chromated arsenate as a wood preservative.

References

1.   Apostoli, P., & Catalani, S. (2011). Metal ions affecting reproduction and development. *Metal Ions in Life Sciences, 8*, 263–303.

2.   Farzan, S. F., Karagas, M. R., & Chen, Y. (2013). In utero and early life arsenic expo-sure in relation to long-term health and disease. *Toxicology and Applied Pharma-cology, 272*(2), 384–90. doi:10.1016/j.taap.2013.06.030

3.   Gardner, R. M., Kippler, M., Tofail, F., Bottai, M., Hamadani, J., Grander, M., ... & Vahter, M. (2013). Environmental exposure to metals and children's growth to age 5 years: A prospective cohort study. *American Journal of Epidemiology, 177*(12), 1356–1367. doi:10.1093/aje/kws437

4.   Liu, J., Yu, L., Coppin, J. F., Tokar, E. J., Diwan, B. A., & Waalkes, M. P. (2009). Fetal arsenic exposure appears to facilitate endocrine disruption by postnatal diethyl-stilbestrol in neonatal mouse adrenal. *Chemico-Biological Interactions, 182*(2–3), 253–258. doi:10.1016/j.cbi.2009.07.023

Prevention Tips

•   Have your water tested and check your local water assays with your local municipality.
•   Reduce your exposure by using a water filter that lowers arsenic levels.
•   Avoid arsenic-treated wood including children's playgrounds.

◇   Find more tips at:

        http:// www.ewg.org/report/ewgs-water-filter-buying-guide/

Mercury

Health Risks

Mercury, a naturally occurring metal in the environment, has increased primarily though burning of coal and is found in the oceans and then enters the food chain, absorbed in contaminated seafood. The Food and Drug Administration (FDA) estimates that most peo-ple are exposed, on average, to about 50 ng of mercury per kilogram of body weight per day (50 ng/kg/day) in the food they eat. Pregnant women are the most at risk from the toxic effects of mercury as research shows that it concentrates in the fetal brain and can interfere with brain development. Mercury is also used in dental amalgams and in health-care. According to WHO, mercury is being phased out of healthcare by 2020 globally. According to the CDC, 75% of one's total daily mercury exposure depends on the number of amalgam fillings one has and the amount of fish consumed, mostly as methylmercury. Exposure from other less common sources includes mercury spills. Mercury is also known to bind directly to hormones that regulate the menstrual cycle and ovulation, interfering with normal signaling pathways. The metal may also play a role in diabetes and has been shown to damage cells in the pancreas that produce insulin, which is critical for the body's ability to metabolize sugar. Research also implicates elevated mercury with high blood pressure.

References

1.   Chen, A., Kim, S. S., Chung, E., & Dietrich, K. N. (2013). Thyroid hormones in relation to lead, mercury, and cadmium exposure in the National Health and Nutrition Examination Survey, 2007–2008. *Environmental Health Perspectives, 121*(2), 181–186. doi:10.1289/ehp.1205239

2. Knazicka, Z., Lukac, N., Forgacs, Z., Tvrda, E., Lukacova, J., Slivkova, J., Binkowski, L., & Massanyi, P. (2013). Effects of mercury on the steroidogenesis of human adrenocarcinoma (NCI-H295R) cell line. *Journal of Environmental Science and Health. Part A, Toxic/Hazardous Substances & Environmental Engineering, 48*(3), 348–353. doi:10.1080/10934529.2013.726908

3. Woimant, F., & Trocello, J. M. (2014). Disorders of heavy metals. *Handbook of Clinical Neurology, 120*, 851–864. doi:10.1016/B978-0-7020-4087-0.00057-7

Prevention Tips

- Limit amount of seafood known to have mercury, including tuna and swordfish.
- Check old mercury (amalgam) fillings and consider replacing with safer materials.
- Check mercury levels in blood or other testing with a functional medicine practitioner.
- Follow EPA guidelines for pregnant women (and women preparing for pregnancy).
- Avoid fish containing high levels of mercury, including swordfish, king mackerel, tuna, tilefish.

◇ Find more tips at:

http://www.atsdr.cdc.gov/phs/phs.asp?id=112&tid=24
http://www.epa.gov/hg/exposure.htm
http://www.mayoclinic.com/health/pregnancy-and-fish/PR00158
http://water.epa.gov/scitech/swguidance/fishshellfish/outreach/advice_index.cfm

Perfluorinated chemicals (PFCs)

Health Risks

Perfluorinated chemicals (PFCs) are water-resistant and have unique properties to make materials resistant to stains and oils, as well. They are widely used in diverse applications including as refrigerants, pharmaceuticals, and agrichemicals. PFCs persist in the environment as persistent organic pollutants (POPs). Ninety-nine percent of Americans tested have this group of chemicals in their bodies as they are resistant to biodegradation in the environment. One particularly notorious compound called PFOA has been linked to decreased sperm quality, low birth weight, kidney disease, thyroid disease, and high cholesterol, among other health issues. Scientists continue to research how PFOA affects the human body as animal studies have found that PFCs most affect thyroid and sex hormone levels.

References

1. Du, G., Hu, J., Huang, H., Qin, Y., Han, X., Wu, D., Song, L., Xia, Y., & Wang, X. (2013). Perfluorooctane sulfonate (PFOS) affects hormone receptor activity, steroidogenesis, and expression of endocrine-related genes in vitro and in vivo. *Environmental Toxicology and Chemistry, 32*(2), 353–360. doi:10.1002/etc.2034

2. Ji, K., Kim, S., Kho, Y., Paek, D., Sakong, J., Ha, J., Kim, S., & Choi, K. (2012). Serum concentrations of major perfluorinated compounds among the general population in Korea: Dietary sources and potential impact on thyroid hormones. *Environment International, 45*, 78–85. doi:10.1016/j.envint.2012.03.007

3.   Wen, L. L., Lin, L. Y., Su, T. C., Chen, P. C., & Lin, C. Y. (2013). Association between serum perfluorinated chemicals and thyroid function in U.S. adults: The National Health and Nutrition Examination Survey 2007–2010. *Journal of Clinical Endocrinology and Metabolism, 98*(9), E1456–1464. doi:10.1210/jc.2013-1282

Prevention Tips

- Avoid non-stick pans as well as stain- and water-resistant coatings on clothing, furniture, and carpets.
- Read labels on commercial stain removal and cleaning products.

◇   Find more tips at:

   http://www.saferchemicals.org/resources/chemicals/pfc.html

Organophosphate pesticides

Health Risks

Organophosphates are a large group of chemicals that have many domestic and industrial uses, most commonly used as insecticides and pesticides that target the nervous systems (neurotoxic) of insects. The United States Environmental Protection Agency lists organophosphates as very highly acutely toxic to bees, wildlife, and humans. Despite multiple studies linking organophosphate exposure to effects on brain development, behavior, and fertility, they are still among the more common pesticides in use today. Many in this group can lower testosterone and alter thyroid hormone levels.

References

1.   Jayachandra, S., & D'Souza, U. J. (2013). Pre- and postnatal toxicity of diazinon induces disruption of spermatogenetic cell line evidenced by increased testicular marker enzymes activities in rat offspring. *Journal of Environmental Pathology, Toxicology and Oncology, 32*(1), 73–90.

2.   Verma, R., & Mohanty, B. (2009). Early-life exposure to dimethoate-induced reproductive toxicity: Evaluation of effects on pituitary-testicular axis of mice. *Toxicological Sciences, 112*(2), 450–458. doi:10.1093/toxsci/kfp204

Prevention Tips

- Buy organic produce whenever possible.
- Avoid topical use of organophosphates as repellent. Use essential oils.
- Read labels in commercial household insecticides and choose natural options (lemon juice and white vinegar).

◇   Find more tips at:

   EWG's Shopper's Guide to Pesticides in Produce, which can help you find the fruits and vegetables that have the fewest pesticide residues.
   http://www.experience-essential-oils.com/homemade-insecticides.html
   http://www.ewg.org/foodnews/

Glycol Esters

Health Risks

Glycol esters are common solvents in paints, cleaning products, brake fluid, and cosmetics. The European Union says that some of these chemicals "may damage fertility or the unborn child" and lower sperm counts. Children who were exposed to glycol ethers from paint in their bedrooms had substantially more asthma and allergies.

Prevention Tips

- Avoid products with ingredients such as 2-butoxyethanol (EGBE) and methoxydiglycol (DEGME).
- Purchase "green paint" and other supplies that have lower levels of toxic solvents.

◇ Find more tips at:

Guide to Healthy Cleaning: http://www.ewg.org/guides/cleaners/
http://www.ewg.org
http://www.ncbi.nlm.nih.gov/pubmed/22398195

Triclosan

Health Risks

Triclosan is an antimicrobial that is used in a range of consumer products including tooth-pastes, soaps, household cleaning supplies, and used in hospitals as a hand washing dis-infectant. Triclosan has the potential to both alter gut microbiota and disrupt thyroid and endocrine function. It has been shown to disrupt reproductive hormone activity and brain cell signaling, hinder muscle function, and bring on allergies. Triclosan can affect body weight according to recent research using National Health and Nutrition Examination Sur-veys (NHANES) from 2003 to 2008. The study used urinary testing and concluded that triclosan exposure is associated with increased BMI and weight gain. According to another recent study in the *Journal of Allergy Research*, levels of the antimicrobial EDCs, triclosan, and parabens were significantly associated with allergic sensitization and the potential role of antimicrobial EDCs in allergic disease and suppressed immune function. Triclosan's effectiveness as an antibacterial agent is also questionable. An FDA panel recently con-ceded that soap with triclosan is no better against bacteria than hand-washing with plain soap and water. The FDA is currently reviewing the safety of triclosan.

References

1. Lankester, J., Patel, C., Cullen, M. R., Ley, C., & Parsonnet, J. (2013). Urinary triclosan is associated with elevated body mass index in NHANES. *PLoS One, 8*(11), e80057. doi:10.1371/journal.pone.0080057

2. Savage, J. H., Matsui, E. C., Wood, R. A., & Keet, C. A. (2012). Urinary levels of tri-closan and parabens are associated with aeroallergen and food sensitization. *Journal of Allergy and Clinical Immunology, 130*(2), 453–60. doi:10.1016/j.jaci.2012.05.006

Prevention Tips

- Advocate for safer cleaning and hand washing products in the workplace environment.
- Use safe antimicrobial alternative soaps whenever possible.

◇ Find more tips at:

http://www.sfgate.com/health/article/Triclosan-fears-lead-to-alternative-soaps-4160267.php
http://www.fda.gov/forconsumers/consumerupdates/ucm205999.htm
http://www.mayoclinic.com/health/triclosan/AN02141

Adapted from Environmental Working Group 2014. www.ewg.org
Adapted by Susan Luck from Environmental Working Group. www.ewg.org
Copyright © 2014 by the International Nurse Coach Association. www.inursecoach.com

APPENDIX E-16: TIPS FOR SLEEPING WELL

Sleep is one of the great mysteries of life, and research is discovering how essential "good sleep" is for our overall health and wellbeing.

As you become more aware of your sleeping habits and patterns and how sleep affects you, the following may provide some helpful tips for improving the quality of your sleep, falling asleep more easily, sleeping through the night, and feeling rested and alert when you awake in the morning.

Research Review:

- Restorative sleep is essential for optimizing health and wellbeing.
- Six to eight hours per night seems to be the optimal amount of sleep for most adults.
- Sleep deprivation has become epidemic in our modern lives. Sleep deficit can have serious, far-reaching effects on our mental and physical wellbeing.

Create Your Bedtime Ritual: Establish a Bedtime Routine

In preparation for winding down at the end of your day and easing into transition from wakefulness to drowsiness, *what is your ritual for promoting restful sleep*? Observe your current patterns and possible new behaviors.

The key is to find healthful tools that assist you in feeling more relaxed, then repeat them each night to help you release the tensions of the day.

What can assist you in your transition at the end of your day?

You may want to explore the benefits of evening meditation, deep breathing techniques, soothing sounds and music, relaxation tapes, and using aromatherapy or essential oils.

Creating a Healing Sleep Environment

As you become aware of what your unique patterns and behaviors are, ask yourself, *what can I change that will promote restorative sleep?* Become aware of sound, light, and the energy field of electronic equipment that is near your bed (or head). Dim the lights in preparation for sleep.

- **Sleep in complete darkness, or as close to it as possible.** Even the tiniest bit of light in the room can disrupt your internal circadian clock and your pineal gland's production of melatonin and serotonin. (Avoid turning on any light at all during the night, even when getting up to go to the bathroom.)
- **Wear an eye mask to block out light.**
- **Become aware that TV—the light and the images—could interfere with sleep.**
- **Cover windows with blackout shades or drapes.** Light signals your brain that it is time to wake up and starts preparing your body to be awake and alert.
- **Temperature of your room:** When you sleep, your body's internal temperature drops to its lowest level, generally about four hours after you fall asleep. Research shows that a cooler bedroom may be most conducive to sleep, since it mimics your body's natural temperature drop.
- **Remove electrical devices next to your bed** (or keep them preferably at least 3 feet from your bed; remove the digital clock from view). Replace jarring alarm clock sounds with chimes, birds singing, etc. to not awake and begin your day startled.

Lifestyle Tips for Improved Sleep

- **Reduce or eliminate caffeine, alcohol, sugar, and medications in the evening hours.** Alcohol has been shown to interfere with entering the deeper stages of sleep where your body does most of its healing. Adjust your medication, if possible, to an earlier time in your day.
- **Exercise earlier in the day** to avoid being overstimulated at night. Yoga and evening stretches can be helpful for releasing the tensions of your day. Studies show morning exercise is best for weight loss and overall health.
- **Enjoy a hot bath, shower, or sauna before bed.** When your body temperature is raised in the late evening, it will fall at bedtime, facilitating slumber. The temperature drop from getting out of the bath signals your body it is time for bed.
- **Wear socks to bed.** Feet often feel cold before the rest of the body. A study has shown that wearing socks to bed reduces night waking (or place a hot water bottle near your feet at night).
- **Eat lighter meals in the early evening.** Avoid the need to digest food at night as the body's natural cycle is to detoxify and prepare to eliminate waste products in the early morning hours.
- **Lower your intake of fluids within 2 hours of going to bed.** This will reduce the likelihood of needing to get up and go to the bathroom, or at least minimize the frequency.
- **Become aware of food sensitivities** that can cause inflammation and reactions, including congestion and GI distress in the night.
- **Avoid before-bed snacks, particularly grains and sugars.** These can raise your blood sugar and delay sleep. Later, when blood sugar drops too low (hypoglycemia), you may wake up and be unable to fall back asleep.
- **Journal your thoughts.** If you find yourself in bed with your mind racing, it might be helpful to keep a journal next to you and write down your thoughts before bed so you can release them to ease your mind and return in the morning to reflect on them.

APPENDIX E-17: PERSONALIZED LIFESTYLE PLAN

LIFE BALANCE & SATISFACTION

- Goals

- Activity

- Agreement/Commitment

STRESS MANAGEMENT

- Goals

- Activity

- Agreement/Commitment

RELATIONSHIPS

- Goals

- Activity

- Agreement/Commitment

SPIRITUAL

- Goals

- Activity

- Agreement/Commitment

MENTAL
- Goals

- Activity

- Agreement/Commitment

EMOTIONAL
- Goals

- Activity

- Agreement/Commitment

NUTRITION
- Goals

- Activity

- Agreement/Commitment

EXERCISE
- Goals

- Activity

- Agreement/Commitment

ENVIRONMENTAL

*   Goals

*   Activity

*   Agreement/Commitment

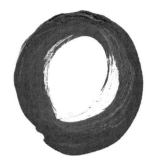

Awareness Practices

BREATH AWARENESS

MEANING, PURPOSE, INNER WISDOM

IMAGERY REHEARSAL

Source: Copyright © 2014 by Bonney Schaub. Adapted from Schaub, B. G., & Schaub, R. (1997). *Healing addictions: The vulnerability model of recovery*. Albany, NY: Delmar Publishers.
For permission to use, contact www.huntingtonmeditation.com/contact-us

APPENDIX F-1: BREATH AWARENESS AND AUTO-SUGGESTION

1. Close your eyes and bring your attention to the sensation of breath passing through your nostrils.
2. Don't do anything to your breathing...just notice it...
3. Now silently, in your imagination, say "My right hand feels warm and heavy...my right hand feels warm and heavy"
4. Continue repeating this for several minutes.
5. Slowly, at your own pace, begin to turn your attention toward noticing what you are experiencing...
6. Now, slowly, bring your awareness back to the room and when you're ready, open your eyes.

Dates and times of practice	Notes

APPENDIX F-2: HANDS ON BELLY WITH ENERGY BALL

1. Get yourself comfortable in your chair, uncross your legs, and place your feet flat on the floor...
2. Allow your shoulders to drop and rest your hands on your belly, just below your navel...
3. Now, bring your awareness to the sensation of hands in contact with your belly...
4. Notice the sensation of your hands in touch with the fabric of your clothing...
5. Notice any other tactile sensations...skin touching skin...skin in contact with the air in the room...
6. Now notice the sensation of the weight of your hands resting on your belly...
7. Notice the temperature of your hands...are certain places warmer or cooler?
8. Now that you've noticed so many sensations of your hands, notice that you can become aware of even subtler sensations...inside the skin sensations such as tingling... or pulsing...just allow yourself to be absorbed in noticing...
9. Now lift your hands, and hold them with palms facing, at about waist height, as if you were holding an inflated balloon and bring all your awareness to noticing that space between your palms...
10. Just notice the space between your palms...being curious...if you notice any sensations as you do this play with this a bit, slowly moving your hands a little closer or farther apart...
11. Whenever you feel ready, gently place your hands back on your belly, reconnect with your breath and notice the rise and fall of your belly...
12. At your own pace, slowly bring your awareness back to the room and when you are ready, open your eyes.

Dates and times of practice	Notes

APPENDIX F-3: LET GO

1. Begin by noticing your breath...noticing the sensation of breath passing through your nostrils...
2. Notice the in breath...and then the out breath...the inhalation...and now the exhalation...
3. Every time you become aware of a distracting thought, or noise or sensation, just notice it and return to noticing your breath...
4. Every time you exhale, let go of any tightness or tension you notice and allow yourself to be more deeply held by the chair...notice all the places your body is in contact with your chair....and really allow the chair to hold you...
5. Now repeat, silently to yourself, a simple three-word phrase over and over again in your mind...as you inhale say your name...as you exhale say let go...
6. Continue to slowly repeat this for several minutes...as you become distracted, just bring your awareness back to this phrase.
7. Okay, now let go of the words and keeping your eyes closed, just notice how you are... take your time and when you are ready, open your eyes.

Dates and times of practice	Notes

APPENDIX F-4: HANDS ON BELLY WITH MEMORY OF FEELING CALM

1. Close your eyes and rest your hands on your belly just below your navel...
2. Bring your awareness to noticing the sensation of the rise and fall of your belly with each breath...as soon as you are aware of being distracted, just come back to your hands...
3. Bring your awareness back to your hands noticing the tactile sensations of your hands touching each other...becoming aware of any distractions and choosing to bringing your awareness back to your hands...
4. Now, reflect back on the last few days and reconnect with an experience, it can be any time at all, when you felt a sense of inner calm or contentment...even if it was just for a moment or two...take your time and when you feel ready, open your eyes...

Dates and times of practice	Notes

APPENDIX F-5: CONNECTING WITH BREATH—EXHALING FOR TWICE AS LONG AS INHALING

1. Place your hands on your belly...
2. Close your eyes and bring your awareness to your breath...
3. Breathing in and out through your nose, notice the length of your inhalations and exhalations...
4. Allow yourself to exhale for twice as long as you inhale...the length of the breath doesn't matter, it's the long exhalation that is important...you can inhale for a count of 3 and exhale for 6 or inhale for 4 and exhale for 8, whatever feels comfortable to you...
5. Be patient with yourself...it may take a few tries to do this...
6. Allow that long exhalation to be a sigh, releasing...a letting go...
7. Let go and allow the chair to hold you...take your time...
8. Stay with counting the inhalation and exhalation...and then let go of counting and just stay with focusing on the long exhale...on letting go

Dates and times of practice	Notes

APPENDIX F-6: BREATH AWARENESS WITH INNER DIALOGUE

1. Take a moment to notice your breath...inhaling and exhaling through your nose...allow yourself to put all your attention here...
2. Notice the sensation of breath passing through your nostrils...if you notice any distractions, just acknowledge them and then return to noticing your breath...
3. Distractions are normal...you can notice and choose to come back to breath...notice that there is a slight cool sensation as the inhaled air passes through your nose...take a moment to explore that sensation...
4. Now become aware of the sensation of your exhaled air...it's warmer...sometimes it's actually difficult to feel because your breath has traveled into your lungs and become warmed by your body...
5. Now allow yourself to just focus on your breath in any way that you like...
6. Notice what you are experiencing right now...
7. Now from this quiet place, allow yourself to reconnect with (person X)...
8. Notice what are you feeling right now...
9. Now take a moment and if there is anything you need to communicate to X, allow yourself to do so in your imagination...
10. When you feel ready, open your eyes and take some notes on what you have experienced...

Dates and times of practice	Notes

APPENDIX F-7: CENTERING FOR STRESS REDUCTION

One simple technique to practice for yourself is counting breaths. Counting breaths is a first step in many forms of meditation.

1. Begin by just noticing your breath...stay with this for a few moments...
2. Now begin to count each exhaled breath starting with one and counting up to 10...
3. When you are distracted before you reach 10, go back to starting at 1...

This is a very challenging practice. It will be difficult to reach 10. The practice is not a test; rather, it is about becoming aware of all the distractions we are challenged by and learning that we can return to focus.

It is helpful to set a designated length of time that you want to practice, e.g., 5 minutes, and set a timer. This will free you from the inner chatter of wondering how long you have been doing it. As you continue to practice you will be able to extend the length of time for practice.

Dates and times of practice	Notes

APPENDIX F-8: WILLINGNESS

1. Take a few moments to reflect on a goal you have for yourself...it can be any kind of goal as long as it is a real possibility and not just a fantasy...
2. Close your eyes and bring attention to your breathing...
3. In your imagination, experience a path extending from where you are to the top of a tall hill...now, imagine your goal and place it on the top of the hill...
4. Now, starting from where you are, experience yourself willing to travel along the path...As you move along, become aware of the obstacles that try to pull you off the path...Notice these obstacles...Now, reconnect with your sense of purpose and your willingness to reach your goal...
5. Experience yourself on the top of the hill and fully identify with achieving the goal...allow yourself to feel what this would be like...
6. Identify with this success and imagine seeing the world from this place...

Dates and times of practice	Notes

APPENDIX F-9: CONNECTING WITH MEANING AND PURPOSE

1. Close your eyes or just lower them if you prefer and begin by bringing your awareness to your breath...follow your breathing...just noticing it...the sensation of the inhalation and the exhalation...
2. As you do this, allow your chair to hold you, allow your shoulders to drop, letting your arms feel heavy...just letting go and staying connected to your breath...
3. Now, let your awareness go into your imagination...into your memory and reconnect with a time when you experienced a sense of meaning and purpose in your life, a sense of wholeness...take your time and let the details come to you...
4. And now begin to realize what the essence of that time was...What was at the heart of it for you?...take your time...
5. Allow yourself to deeply connect with what you were experiencing...What allowed it to happen?...What supported it?...take your time...
6. Now, let go of the practice and turn your attention to noticing how you are right now... take as much time as you need...and when you feel ready, at your own pace, begin to come back to the room...

Dates and times of practice	Notes

APPENDIX F-10: CONNECTING WITH INNER GUIDE

1. Lower or close your eyes...relax your shoulders and begin to follow your breath...
2. Begin to reflect on something you are wondering about at this point in your life...perhaps something about a decision you are trying to make...or something about yourself you are trying to understand better...or something about which you need guidance...
3. Identify the question you are asking yourself. What's the question that gets to the heart of the matter? It's okay if you don't get it exactly.
4. And now for a moment return to your breath...
5. Now, begin to move from your breath to your imagination...and begin to imagine a road or path stretching out in front of you...one you know or one you create...
6. Get a sense of walking on this road or path...What's around you?...
7. And now begin to imagine, in the distance, a wise being or a wisdom figure of any kind...any kind at all...coming toward you...
8. Ask your question...and be open to whatever happens...take as much time as you want...

Dates and times of practice	Notes

APPENDIX F-11: IMAGERY FOR STRESS REDUCTION—CONNECTING WITH A SAFE PLACE

1. Begin by noticing your breath...stay with this a few moments...
2. Now, use the power of your imagination to experience yourself in a safe place...it can be an actual place or a place you have created.
3. Really experience what it feels like to be there.
4. Notice what it is about this place that allows this experience of safety and peacefulness.
5. Know that this place of sanctuary is available to you in your imagination whenever you need it.

Dates and times of practice	Notes

APPENDIX F-12: IMAGERY REHEARSAL FOR RELEASING WORRY AND FEAR

1. Begin by centering with your breath...noticing the inhalation and the exhalation...
2. Imagine the situation you are worrying about...noticing what you imagine will happen from beginning to end...
3. Now, pause and return to centering yourself.
4. Now, imagine the situation again, this time experiencing it in slow motion...very slowly and notice the point at which it starts to go wrong...
5. Now, pause and return to centering yourself...
6. Re-play the situation again in your imagination but now this process, imagine a successful outcome...
7. Rehearse this new answer again, feeling the success and noticing what this is like in as much detail as possible...

Dates and times of practice	Notes

Index

professional nurse coaching
  defined, 3
  See nurse coaching
professional practice evaluation
  competencies, 82
Professional Testing Corporation of New York
  (PTC), xxii, 11
psychosynthesis
  defined, 211
purpose. *See* meaning

Q
qualitative research
  basic statistical approaches, 377–378t
  defined, 368
  methodologies and selected research
    designs, 374t
quality of life
  defined, 123
quality of practice
  competencies, 80
quantitative research
  defined, 368
  methodologies and selected designs, 374t
  results, 376–380

R
reflective listening, 317–318
  four types of, 318t
reflective practice, 86
  defined, 86
Reich, Jennifer L., 97–98
relational knowing, 56–59
  defined, 52
  vignette, 57–59
  See also embodied knowing
relationships, 112–113
relaxation response
  defined, 239
reliability
  defined, 368
  of research tool, 380
religion, 101
research, 367–384
  competencies and, 80
  contributing to, 382–383
    PICOT question template, 383
    data collection and measurement,
      375–376
    evidence-based practice and,
      368–369
  future directions, 383–384
  key sections of a research article, 371–373t
  measurement and data collection, 375–376
  methods, 373–375

Nurse Coach as consumer of, 370t
  qualitative and quantitative, 368, 374t
    results of studies using, 376–380
  problems and questions, 369
  reading and understanding report,
    370–373
  relevant, finding, 369, 371t
research tools
  choosing, 380
  See also Integrative Health and Wellness
    Assessment (IHWA)
resiliency
  as element of HEART, 41, 42t, 396–397
resistance
  as motivational interviewing principle, 318
  defined, 314
resource utilization
  competencies, 82
respect in nurse coaching ethics, 56
rituals, 341–343
  characteristics, 342
  defined, 336
  examples of, 354t
  in education, 354
  structure, 341
  three phases of, 343
  traditional and self-generated, 341
rituals of healing, 341–343, 341t
  guide to getting well, 342–343t
  See also rituals
Rogers, Martha, 303
RULE, 321
  definition of acronym, 321t
rulers, 320
  readiness ruler, 321f
  sample conversation using, 320t
Rushton, Cynda, 59

S
Schaub, Bonney Gulino, 8, 30, 358
scope of practice. *See* nurse coaching
secondary source
  defined, 368
self-assessment
  as part of self-development, 38–39,
    410–412
  defined, 407
  in IHWA, 411t
  reflections, 412t
self-care
  as part of self-development, 39, 414–416
  defined, 407
  plan strategies, 415t
  reflection, 415t
self-care techniques, 250–252

VERMONT STATE COLLEGES

0 0003 0899927 5

Hartness Library
Vermont Technical College
One Main St.
Randolph Center, VT 05061

Hartness Library
Vermont Technical College
One Main St.
Randolph Center, VT 05061

29444152R00308

Made in the USA
Middletown, DE
19 February 2016